Endoscopic Surgery
for Gynaecologists

Endoscopic Surgery for Gynaecologists

Edited by

Chris Sutton
The Royal Surrey County Hospital, Guildford, UK
and

Michael P. Diamond
Vanderbilt University Medical Center, Nashville, USA

W.B. SAUNDERS COMPANY LTD

London   Philadelphia   Toronto   Sydney   Tokyo

This book is printed on acid free paper

W.B. Saunders Company Ltd 24–28 Oval Road
London NW1 7DX

The Curtis Center
Independence Square West
Philadelphia, PA 19106–3399

55 Horner Avenue
Toronto, Ontario M8Z 4X6, Canada

Harcourt Brace & Company (Australia) Pty Ltd,
30–52 Smidmore St
Marrickville, NSW 2204, Australia

Harcourt Brace Japan Inc.
Ichibancho Central Building, 22–1 Ichibancho
Chiyoda-ku, Tokyo 102, Japan

A catalogue record for this book is available from the British Library.

ISBN 0-7020-1578-4

Typeset by Photo graphics, Honiton, Devon
Printed and bound in Hong Kong by Dah Hua

Contents

Contributors   ix
Preface   xii

INTRODUCTION

1   The History and Development of Endoscopic Surgery   3
A. GORDON

LAPAROSCOPIC SURGERY

Techniques and Equipment

2   Setting up a Service: Instrumentation and Administration   11
G.W. PATTON Jr

3   A Practical Approach to Diagnostic Laparoscopy   21
C.J.G. SUTTON

4   New Laparoscopic Techniques   28
H. REICH

5   Delivery Systems for Laser Laparoscopy   40
Y. TADIR, J. NEEV AND M.W. BERNS

6   Electrosurgery   51
R.C. ODELL

7   Tissue Effects of Different Lasers and Electrodiathermy   60
J. KECKSTEIN

8   Laparoscopic Use of the Argon Beam Coagulator   71
J.F. DANIELL

9   New Developments in Equipment for Insufflation and Smoke
         Evacuation   77
         A. GALLINAT

10   Clinical Results of Laser and Electrosurgery   84
         T. TULANDI

Laparoscopic Tubal Surgery

11   Laser Neosalpingostomy and Fimbrioplasty   90
         J.B. DUBUISSON, J. BOUQUET DE JOLINIÈRE AND L. MANDELBROT

12   Non-laser Fertility-promoting Procedures   96
         V. GOMEL AND M.G. MUNRO

13   Ectopic Pregnancy   105
         J.L. POULY, C. CHAPRON AND A. WATTIEZ

14   Techniques of Mass Sterilization   113
         S.S. SHETH

Laparoscopic Ovarian Surgery

15   Laparoscopic Ovarian Surgery: Preoperative Diagnosis and
         Imaging   123
         L. DE CRESPIGNY

16   Laparoscopic Ovarian Surgery and Ovarian Torsion   134
         A.J.M. AUDEBERT

17   Endo-ovarian Surgery for Ovarian Endometriomas   142
         I. BROSENS

18   Endoscopic Surgical Approach to the Treatment of
         Anovulation due to Polycystic Ovary Syndrome—Ovarian
         Drilling   147
         G.T. KOVACS

19   Laparoscopic Treatment of Tubo-ovarian Abscess   154
         D.A. JOHNS

Laparoscopic Uterine and Pelvic Surgery

20   Laparoscopic Uterine Nerve Ablation for Intractable
         Dysmenorrhoea   159
         C.J.G. SUTTON AND N. WHITELAW

21   Laparoscopic Myomectomy   169
         J.B. DUBUISSON, F. LECURU AND H. FOULOT

22   Laparoscopic Pelvic Lymphadenectomy   172
         D. QUERLEU AND E. LEBLANC

23 Laparoscopic Assisted Vaginal Hysterectomy (LAVH) 179
D.A. JOHNS

24 Laparoscopic Appendicectomy and Colposuspension 187
R. MACDONALD

Laparoscopic Surgery for Endometriosis and Adhesions

25 Pathology and Pathogenesis of Endometriosis 192
R.P.S. JANSEN

26 Diagnosis of Endometriosis: Laparoscopic Appearances 200
A.S. COOK AND J.A. ROCK

27 Peritoneal Endometriosis: New Aspects in Two-dimensional
and Three-dimensional Evaluation 207
M. NISOLLE, F. CASANAS-ROUX AND J. DONNEZ

28 Laser Vaporization of Endometriosis 215
J.R. FESTE

29 Non-laser Resection of Endometriosis 220
D.B. REDWINE

30 Laparoscopic Treatment of Advanced Endometriosis 229
D.C. MARTIN

31 Laparoscopic Treatment of Bowel Adhesions (Enterolysis) 238
J.F. DANIELL

32 Prevention of Adhesion Reformation 245
L.B. SCHWARTZ AND M.P. DIAMOND

HYSTEROSCOPIC SURGERY

33 Initiating a Hysteroscopic Programme and Hysteroscopic
Instrumentation 253
M.S. BAGGISH

34 Diagnostic Hysteroscopy: Technique and Documentation 263
K. WAMSTEKER AND S. DE BLOK

35 Rigid and Flexible Optical Systems for Hysteroscopy 277
E. CORNIER

36 Distension Media and Fluid Systems 282
R. GARRY

37 Hysteroscopic Metroplasty 291
N. WHITELAW

38 Trans-cervical Resection of the Endometrium (TCRE)   294
J.A.M. BROADBENT AND A.L. MAGOS

39 Endometrial Electroablation   307
T.G. VANCAILLIE

40 Nd:YAG Laser Ablation of the Endometrium   317
M.H. GOLDRATH AND R. GARRY

41 Electroresection of Fibroids   327
J. HAMOU

42 Nd:YAG Laser Hysteroscopic Myomectomy   331
J. DONNEZ

43 Lysis of Intrauterine Adhesions (Asherman's Syndrome)   338
R.F. VALLE

44 Hysteroscopic Tubal Occlusion   345
F.D. LOFFER

45 Hazards and Dangers of Operative Hysteroscopy   355
B. VAN HERENDAEL

THE FUTURE

46 Radiofrequency Endometrial Ablation (RaFEA)   365
J.H. PHIPPS AND B.V. LEWIS

47 Circumferential Nd:YAG Endometrial Destruction   372
M.D. JUDD AND S.G. BOWN

48 Laser Microsurgery and Manipulations of Single Cells   379
Y. TADIR, J. NEEV AND M.W. BERNS

49 Photodynamic Therapy   387
W.R. KEYE

Directory of Manufacturers   393

Index   397

Contributors

Alain J.M. Audebert MD, Institut Robert B. Greenblatt, 4 rue Vauban, 33000 Bordeaux, France

Michael S. Baggish MD, Department of Obstetrics and Gynecology, Ravenswood Hospital Medical Center, Chicago, IL 60640-5205, USA

M.W. Berns PhD, Beckman Laser Institute, Department of Surgery, University of California, Irvine, CA 92715, USA

Sjoerd de Blok MD PhD, Onze Lieve Vrouwe Gasthuis, Le Oosterparkstraat 179, 1091 HA Amsterdam, The Netherlands

J. Bouquet de Jolinière MD, Clinique Universitaire Port Royal, 123 Boulevard Port Royal, 75014 Paris, France

Steve G. Bown MD, FRCP, National Medical Laser Centre, The Rayne Institute, 5 University Street, London WC1E 6JJ, UK

J.A. Mark Broadbent MRCOG, Minimally Invasive Therapy Unit, University Department of Obstetrics and Gynaecology, The Royal Free Hospital, Pond Street, London NW3 2QG, UK

Ivo Brosens MD, PhD, Department of Obstetrics and Gynaecology, University Hospital Gasthuisberg, B 3000 Leuven, Belgium

F. Casanas-Roux BS, Clinique Trocadero, 74 Avenue Paul Doumer, 75116 Paris, France

Charles Chapron MD, Polyclinique Gynécologie Obstétrique, Médecine de la Reproduction, CHU de Clermont Ferrand, Université de Clermont Ferrand, 13 Bd Charles de Gaulle, 63003 Clermont-Ferrand Cedex, France

Andrew S. Cook MD, Fertility Physicians of Northern California and Fertility and Reproductive Health Institute of Northern California, 2191 Mowry Avenue, Suite 600A, Freemont, CA 94538, USA

E. Cornier MD, Clinique Trocadero, 74 Avenue Paul Doumer, 75116 Paris, France

James F. Daniell MD, 2222 State Street, Suite A, Nashville, TN 37203, USA

Lachlan de Crespigny MD, BS, FRCOG, FRACOG, Royal Women's Hospital, Melbourne, Australia

Michael P. Diamond MD, Division of Reproductive Endocrinology and Infertility, Department of Obstetrics and Gynecology and Surgery, C-1100 Medical Center North, Vanderbilt University Medical Center, Nashville, TN 37232-2515, USA

J. Donnez MD, PhD, Department of Gynaecology, Catholic University of Louvain, Clinique Universitaires St Luc, Avenue Hippocrate 10, B-1200 Brussels, Belgium

Jean B. Dubuisson MD, Clinique Universitaire Port Royal, 123 Bd de Port Royal, 75014 Paris, France

Joseph R. Feste MD, Ob/Gyn Associates, 7550 Fannin Street, Houston, TX 77054, USA

H. Foulot MD, Clinique Universitaire Port Royal, 123 Bd de Port Royal, 75014 Paris, France

Adolf Gallinat MD, Altonaer Strasse 59, 2000 Hamburg 36, Germany

Ray Garry MD FRCOG, Women's Endoscopic Laser Foundation, South Cleveland Hospital, Marton Road, Middlesbrough, Cleveland TS4 3BW, UK

Milton H. Goldrath MD, Sinai Hospital of Detroit, Department of Obstetrics and Gynecology, 6767 West Outer Drive, Detroit, MI 48235, USA

Victor Gomel MD, Department of Obstetrics and Gynaecology, Faculty of Medicine, University of British Columbia and University Hospital, Vancouver BC, Canada V6H 3V5

Alan G. Gordon FRCS, FRCOG, Department of Obstetrics and Gynaecology, BUPA Hospital Hull and East Riding, Lowfield Road, Anlaby, Hull HU10 7AZ; Honorary Consultant Gynaecologist, Princess Royal Hospital, Hull, UK

Jacques Hamou, Université Paris XI, Hôpital Antoine Béclère, Chausée de la Muette 2, 75016 Paris, France

Robert P.S. Jansen MD FRACP FRACOG FRCOG CREI, Department of Reproductive Endocrinology and Infertility, Royal Prince Alfred Hospital, Sydney 2050, Australia

D. Alan Johns MD, Richland Medical Center, 3700 Rufe Snow Drive, Fort Worth, TX 76180, USA

Michelle D. Judd MRCOG, National Medical Laser Centre, The Rayne Institute, 5 University Street, London WC1E 6JJ, UK

Jörg Keckstein MD, Department of Obstetrics and Gynaecology, University of Ulm, Prittwotzstrasse 43, D-7900 Ulm, Germany

William R. Keye MD, Division of Reproductive Endocrinology, William Beaumont Hospital, Suite 344, 3535 West 13 Mile Road, Royal Oak, MI 48073, USA

Gabor T. Kovacs FRCOG FRACOG, Department of Obstetrics and Gynaecology, Monash University, Box Hill Hospital, Nelson Road, Box Hill, Victoria, Australia

Eric Leblanc MD, Centre Oscar Lambret, Lille, France

F. Lecuru MD, Clinique Universitaire Port Royal, 123 Bd de Port Royal, 75014 Paris, France

B. Victor Lewis MD FRCS FRCOG, Watford General Hospital, Vicarage Road, Watford, Hertfordshire, UK

Franklin D. Loffer MD, Gynecologic Endoscopy, Maricopa Medical Center, Phoenix, AZ 85013, USA

Russell Macdonald FRCS, MRCOG, The Hillingdon Hospital, Pield Heath Road, Uxbridge, Middlesex UB3 3NN, UK

Adam Magos MD MRCOG, Minimally Invasive Therapy Unit, University Department of Obstetrics and Gynaecology, The Royal Free Hospital, Pond Street, London NW3 2QG, UK

L. Mandelbrot MD, Clinique Universitaire Port Royal, 123 Bd de Port Royal, 75014 Paris, France

Dan C. Martin MD, Reproductive Surgery PC, 910 Madison Avenue, Suite 805, Memphis, TN 38103, USA

Malcolm G. Munro MD, Department of Obstetrics and Gynecology, University of California Los Angeles, Los Angeles, CA, USA

J. Neev PhD, Beckman Laser Institute, Department of Surgery, University of California, Irvine, CA 92715, USA

M. Nisolle MD, Infertility Research Unit, Department of Gynaecology, Catholic University of Louvain, Clinique Universitaires St Luc, Avenue Hippocrate 10, B 1200 Brussels, Belgium

Roger C. Odell, Electroscope Inc., 4890 Sterling Drive, Boulder, CO 80301, USA

Grant W. Patton Jr MD, South Eastern Fertility Center, PA, 900 Bowman Road, Suite 108, Mount Pleasant, SC 29464, USA

Jeffrey H. Phipps MD MRCOG, Department of Obstetrics and Gynaecology, George Eliot Hospital, College Street, Nuneaton, Warwickshire, UK

Jean-Luc Pouly MD, Polyclinique Gynécologie Obstétrique, Médecine de la Reproduction, CHU de Clermont-Ferrand, Université de Clermont Ferrand, 13 Bd Charles de Gaulle, 63003 Clermont-Ferrand Cedex, France

Denis Querleu MD, Centre Hospitalier de Roubaix, Cliniques Universitaire de Chirurgie Gynécologique et Mammaire Cancérologie, Pavillon Paul Gellé, 91 Avenue Julien Lagache, 59100 Roubaix, France

David B. Redwine MD, 2190 NE Professional Court, Bend, OR 97701, USA

Harry Reich MD, Wyoming Valley Obstetrics and Gynecology Association, 480 Pierce Street, Suite 205, Kingston, PA 18704, USA

John A. Rock MD, Department of Obstetrics and Gynecology, The Union Memorial Hospital, 201 E University Parkway, Baltimore, MD 21218, USA

Lisa Barrie Schwartz MD, Yale University School of Medicine, Division of Reproductive Endocrinology and Infertility, Department of Obstetrics and Gynecology, 333 Cedar Street, New Haven, CT 06510, USA

Shirish S. Sheth MD FACS FICS FCPS FICOG FAMS, Sheth Maternity and Gynaecological Nursing Home, 2/2 Navjeevan Society, Lamington Road, Bombay 400 008, India

Chris J.G. Sutton MA FRCOG, Department of Obstetrics and Gynaecology, The Royal Surrey County Hospital, Egerton Road, Guildford, Surrey GU2 5XX, UK

Yona Tadir MD, Beckman Laser Institute, Department of Surgery, 1002 Health Science Road, University of California, Irvine, CA 92715, USA

Togas Tulandi MD FRCS(C) FACOG, Division of Reproductive Endocrinology and Infertility, Professor of Obstetrics and Gynaecology, Royal Victoria Hospital, Women's Pavillion, 687 Pine Avenue, West, Montreal, Quebec, Canada H3A 1A1

Rafael F. Valle MD. Department of Obstetrics and Gynecology, Prentice Women's Hospital and Maternity Center, 333 East Superior Street, Chicago, IL 60611-3095, USA

Thierry G. Vancaillie MD, Center for Gynecologic Endosurgery, University of Texas HSC, Medical Center Tower II, 7940 Floyd Curl Drive, Suite 260, San Antonio, TX 78229, USA

Bruno van Herendael MD, Algemeen Ziekenhuis Jan Palfijn, Lange Bremstraat 70, 2170 Merksem-Antwerpen, Rekening 001-0665027-71, Belgium

Kees Wamsteker MD PhD, Verloskunde-Gynaecologic, Spaarne Ziekenhuis, Van Heythuizenweg 1, PO Box 1644, 2003 BR Haarlem, The Netherlands

Arnaud Wattiez MD, Polyclinique Gynécologie Obstétrique, Médecine de la Reproduction, CHU de Clermont Ferrand, Université de Clermont Ferrand, 13 Bd Charles de Gaulle, 63003 Clermont-Ferrand Cedex, France

Naomi Whitelaw MRCOG, Department of Obstetrics and Gynaecology, Royal Surrey County Hospital, Egerton Road, Guildford, Surrey GU2 5XX, UK

Preface

During the past few years, enormous progress has been made in the field of endoscopic surgery, not only in gynaecology but also in many other surgical disciplines. We have passed the days when we were able to perform destructive procedures with the use of electro-surgery, haemostatic clips and various lasers and are entering a phase when most gynaecological procedures traditionally performed by laparotomy can now be performed by a minimally invasive technique. Many of these advances have been due to the skill and enthusiasm of a small group of pioneering surgeons who have also been responsible for a revolution in surgical instrumentation and technology in order to adapt to the very different requirements for operating under endoscopic vision.

We therefore believe that the time is right to gather from all over the world the leading experts in this new type of surgery. We have been very careful in our choice of contributors, and are grateful to each and every one of them for sharing their experience with us. This is a truly international collaborative work; when reading the various chapters it must be borne in mind that many of the authors write and speak in a language other than English and inevitably some of the syntax is lost in the translation. Nevertheless, the book underlines the fact that progress in minimally invasive surgery is a result of pioneering surgery in many countries throughout the world. We are sure that readers will be stimulated by these developments and innovations.

The pace of change has been so great over the last few years that inevitably new developments occurred whilst this book was in preparation. Already it is becoming obvious that we are entering a reparative and reconstructive phase in this type of work and we eagerly await the development of new suturing and sealing techniques, whether by staples or laser activated tissue glues. Developments in photo-dynamic therapy and energy sources such as ultrasonic scalpels may well replace many of the procedures, techniques and modalities that we are using now. It is particularly encouraging that many of the innovations and developments are no longer commercially driven, and that endoscopic surgery is beginning to feel the need to prove its effectiveness to the scientific community by a number of well designed prospective comparative trials that are becoming available.

It is always difficult to predict the future, but this much seems certain: the trend to minimally invasive surgery is bound to continue because the chief benefits are felt by the patients whom we serve in ridding them of unsightly scars, prolonged hospital stays and long periods of convalescence. Those gynaecologists who are unfamiliar with these techniques will almost certainly have to realign their thoughts because this revolution is almost certain to be consumer driven.

CHRIS SUTTON
MICHAEL P DIAMOND

Introduction

1

The History and Development of Endoscopic Surgery

ALAN GORDON

BUPA Hospital Hull and East Riding, Hull; Princess Royal Hospital, Hull, UK

Early Endoscopy

For centuries physicians have been attempting to investigate human body cavities and their contents in order to advance their knowledge of disease. The earliest descriptions of endoscopic examinations were from the Kos school led by Hippocrates (460–375 BC) who described a rectal speculum which was remarkably similar to the instruments in use today. Similar speculae were discovered in the ruins of Pompei and the Babylonian Talmud written in 500 AD described a siphopherot, a tube made of lead, which acted as a vaginal speculum. In these early years, ambient light was used, later to be augmented by the sun's rays reflected through a mirror. In the middle ages more efficient light sources were used with gradually increasing complexity of the viewing 'endoscope'. Most physicians used endoscopic techniques to explore the nasal and aural cavities but occasional attempts were recorded of visualization of the rectum and vagina.

The father of modern endoscopy was Bozzini (1806) who attempted to observe the interior of the female urethra using a tube and candle light and, incidentally, was censured by the Medical Faculty of Vienna for 'undue curiosity'. Half a century later Desormeaux (1865) presented to the Academy of Medicine in Paris the first satisfactory description of a cystoscope. He used it to examine the bladder and urethra and incorporated a lamp burning alcohol and turpentine with a chimney to enhance the flame. Pantaleoni (1869) adapted the telescope for hysteroscopy and was able to

identify an intrauterine polyp in a 60-year-old woman with postmenopausal bleeding and cauterize it with silver nitrate. Interestingly, he had treated the same woman 3 years earlier for a nasal polyp which she had had for 30 years. The technique did not gain the acceptance he had hoped for because most of his students left claiming that they had not been able to see anything at all with the hysteroscope!

The development of telescopes with lens systems began in the late nineteenth century when Nitze (1879) produced a telescope in association with Reinicke, a Berlin optician. Later the electric light which had been invented by Edison in 1879, was added and when a separate operating channel was incorporated into the telescope, the potential for modern endoscopy and endoscopic surgery was realized and the complexity of the viewing 'endoscope' gradually increased.

Hysteroscopy

Diagnostic Hysteroscopy 1900–1950

The early years of the twentieth century saw an increasing interest in endoscopy resulting from the development of improved light sources and optical lenses. Progress in hysteroscopy and the development and acceptance of the technique were slow because of the greater difficulty of distending the uterus as compared with producing distension of the bladder for cystoscopy or with the introduction of the pneumoperitoneum for laparoscopy. The thickness of the uterine walls, the small size of the cavity and the tendency of the endometrium to bleed on contact provided further obstacles which were difficult to overcome. The available light sources combined with the early lens systems produced poor image quality and, even with the use of hysteroscopes with a diameter of 12 mm, limited their value. In addition, the light bulbs were on the distal end of the telescope which produced excessive heat and were prone to failure.

In 1907 David described the use of a cystoscope with an internal light and lens system to examine the uterine cavity. His hysteroscope had a distal bulb but he improved the design by sealing the end of the telescope to prevent blockage with blood. Rubin (1925) used CO_2 as a distension medium but also introduced fluid distension with water to try to wash away blood which obscured vision. He also suggested that visually directed biopsy was possible and introduced scissors and fulguration loops to amputate pedunculated fibroids and polyps. Others developed hysteroscopes with multiple channels to allow suction as well as insufflation and channels for the introduction of operating instruments. Transparent rubber balloons were placed over the objective lens to inflate the uterus and were intended to allow uninterrupted vision although they were not always successful.

Diagnostic Hysteroscopy 1950–1970

The first fibreoptic hysteroscopes were developed by Mohri (1971) and, at about the same time, he made the first attempts at transuterine salpingoscopy. The lens quality and light sources of the time prevented clear images being obtained and it was many years before flexible endoscopy became popular and produced satisfactory results. The superior images obtained with the rod lens designed by Hopkins of Reading in 1953 and the use of cold light illumination invented by Fourestiere et al. in Paris (1952) have revolutionized endoscopy and allowed the great advances of the past three decades.

Improved distension media were introduced in the 1970s by Edstrom and Fernstrom (1970) who used 32% dextran 70 (Hyskon), Levine and Neuwirth (1972) who used 30% dextran and Lindemann (1972) who demonstrated the safety of CO_2 provided the flow rate and intrauterine pressure were kept within limits.

Operative Hysteroscopy

By 1970 diagnostic hysteroscopy had become an accepted technique even though it was not widely practised. The reluctance of many gynaecologists to learn the technique may be attributed to the difficulty the inexperienced physician experiences in obtaining a good view every time. However, the realization that hysteroscopy may be used as a means of access to the uterine cavity to perform therapeutic procedures has altered opinion and now hysteroscopy is increasing in popularity.

Initially forceps and scissors were passed alongside the hysteroscope to excise polyps and pedunculated fibroids, to remove misplaced intrauterine devices and to divide synechiae. Scissors and forceps of varying strength were incorporated in the hysteroscope, strong rigid ones for thick adhesions and to excise uterine septa, semi-rigid or flexible ones for visually directed biopsies. These techniques were not easy and have now been supplanted by electro- and laser surgery.

The other major advance in recent years has been the introduction of lightweight, high-resolution cameras which allow surgery to be performed using a video screen instead of through the lens viewing. This not only makes training easier and safer but also allows the surgeon to work in comfort and to be assisted by his theatre staff. They have the same view of the operation as he has instead of only being able to see the back of his head and having little idea of the nature of his technique.

Robert Neuwirth (Neuwirth and Amin, 1976), working in New York, has been one of the foremost endoscopists in introducing electrosurgery. He described the use of the urological resectoscope to remove pedunculated submucous fibroids, either dividing its pedicle or shaving it off the uterine wall. As experience in this field has grown, so the indications and operability of fibroids with a greater intramural component have increased. It is now acceptable to operate on fibroids which have as little as 10% of their volume in the uterine cavity. If necessary the operation is performed in stages and the fibroid is treated with gonadotrophin releasing hormone (GnRH) agonists to reduce its size and vascularity.

The possibility of electrosurgery being used to remove the endometrium in patients with menorrhagia and thus avoid hysterectomy was realized by DeCherney and Polan (1983) who described the first endometrial resection. This has become the hysteroscopic operation which has excited both lay and medical opinion in that it can be used in some 65% of cases of menorrhagia with a cure rate of up to 85% and takes only 20 minutes to perform. In addition, the patient can go home in a few hours and be back at work in a few days. Electrosurgery has also replaced scissor dissection in the treatment of uterine septa and, in the simple septate uterus, has rendered laparotomy obsolete.

Hysteroscopic surgery is also one of the procedures which is suited to the use of laser. Milton Goldrath of Detroit (Goldrath *et al.*, 1981) reported on the use of neodymium:YAG laser to photovaporize the endometrium with the same advantages to the patient and surgeon as electrosurgery and, possibly, greater safety. Laser may also be used for myomectomy and resection of septa which will be discussed in detail later in this book.

Laparoscopy

Diagnostic Laparoscopy 1900–1940

Although the earliest attempts at gynaecological endoscopy involved the vagina and uterus because of their seemingly easy access, laparoscopy was initially the more popular and, potentially, the more useful technique. In 1901 Dr Georg Kelling, Professor in Dresden, described to the German Biological and Medical Society in Hamburg the examination of the stomach and oesophagus in the human and also the use of a cystoscope to visualize the viscera of a dog using air filtered through cotton wool to produce a pneumoperitoneum. In the same year, von Ott (1901) from Petersburg described the inspection of the abdominal cavity of a pregnant woman through a culdoscopic opening using a head mirror to reflect light. It was Jacobaeus (1910) who first referred to the word 'laparoscopy' when he published his description of the inspection of the human peritoneal, thoracic and pericardial cavities. Only one month later Kelling reported 45 laparoscopies and described the appearance of the liver, tumours and tuberculosis. The technique became popular mainly with general physicians for the diagnosis and treatment of tuberculosis and liver disease and to them must go much of the credit for the development of laparoscopy during the following 40 years. The first American description of laparoscopy was by Bernheim (1911) who used a 1.0 cm proctoscope with ambient light to inspect the abdominal cavity.

Further developments in the early years of the century include the adoption of the Trendelenburg position by Nordentoft in Copenhagen (1912), the use of carbon dioxide for insufflation by Zollikoffer in Switzerland (1924) and the introduction by Veress in Budapest (1938) of the modern spring-loaded needle which he devised to introduce the pneumothorax in the treatment of pulmonary tuberculosis.

Operative Laparoscopy 1930–1960

The earliest attempts at therapeutic laparoscopy were by general surgeons who performed adhesiolysis. These included Fervers (1933) who used oxygen as the distension medium and experienced 'great concern' at the audible explosion and flashes of light produced by the combination of oxygen and a high frequency electric current within the abdominal cavity. At the same time, John Ruddock (1934) described an optical system with biopsy forceps and coagulation. The first reported use of the laparoscope for the diagnosis of ectopic pregnancy was by Hope (1937) although gynaecologists had been using the laparoscope before that time. The first suggestion that female tubal sterilization could be performed by fulguration was by Bosch (1936) in Switzerland and Anderson (1937) in the United States although the first actual sterilization was probably performed by Power and Barnes (1941).

Techniques were developing in parallel in several countries at that time but, because of political constraints, language difficulties and the problems in communication produced by distance, it is sometimes difficult to be certain of the exact sequence of events. In the USA laparoscopy was virtually abandoned from the early 1940s until the late 1960s and culdoscopy was performed in most centres. In Europe laparoscopy continued to be practised under the influence of Raoul Palmer (1948) in Paris and, later Hans Frangenheim in Konstanz. Palmer popularized the use of monopolar electricity to carry out tubal sterilization which was highly effective but resulted in a number of complications from burns to adjacent organs. The technique was first described in the English language by Steptoe (1967) who recommended a double-puncture technique with coagulation and division of the tube. Frangenheim (1972) introduced bipolar electrocoagulation both for sterilization and for control of bleeding at about the same time as Kurt Semm of Kiel (1972) introduced endotherm coagulation in which no electric current passes through the body. Thermal tubal sterilization was largely replaced in the middle 1970s by mechanical methods using spring loaded clips (Hulka *et al.*, 1975) or silastic rings (Yoon and King, 1975).

Operative Laparoscopy 1970–

The major development in instrumentation since bipolar electrocoagulation and endocoagulation has been the introduction of a variety of forms of laser and their application to laparoscopic surgery. Carbon dioxide laser which is transmitted along a solid lens system was the first to be used extensively and was introduced to Europe by Maurice Bruhat of Clermont Ferrand (Bruhat *et al.*, 1979) and to the USA by James Daniell of Nashville (Daniell and Brown, 1982). Since then lasers transmitted along flexible fibreoptic cables have increased in popularity and include Nd:YAG, KTP and Argon lasers. All of these physical modalities form the basis of modern laparoscopic surgery.

It is now common practice to perform both conservative and radical surgery for ectopic pregnancy, reconstructive tubal surgery, excision of ovarian cysts, adhesiolysis for the sequelae of pelvic inflammatory disease and endometriosis and to remove even deep-seated endometriomata by laparoscopic surgery. Intraovarian surgery using a double-optic laparoscopic technique has been developed by Ivo Brosens of Leuven and the laparoscope is being used as a mode of access to perform advanced intra-abdominal surgery. The pelvic side walls can be explored in detail to perform lymphadenectomy, the laparoscope can be used to assist vaginal hysterectomy where the ovarian pedicles are difficult to reach and the general surgeons, who were the early exponents of laparoscopic surgery, have rediscovered the possibilities presented by the technique to perform cholecystectomy, repair of hernias and selective vagotomy. New developments at present under evaluation include the use of laparoscopic surgery for tubal and bowel anastomosis which, if their initial promise is upheld, will render laparotomy obsolete for many, if not most, conditions.

The Future

Endoscopic surgery must be the surgery of the future. The advantages to the patient and to the health services are immense in the saving of time in hospital, in postoperative recovery and in the early return to work. Initially the techniques may be difficult to learn but the advent of video monitoring has made training much easier and increased the safety of the operations.

Hysteroscopic surgery which is undergoing a dramatic upsurge in popularity will replace most hysterectomies and laparotomies for non-malignant intrauterine disease. It is highly likely, however, that newer techniques will eventually replace endometrial ablation and resection. Destruction of the endometrium by less invasive techniques such as radio frequency thermal ablation pioneered by Jeffrey Phipps and Victor Lewis at Watford (Phipps *et al.*, 1990), photodynamic therapy (Keye and Dixon, 1983) or by intrauterine hormone therapy are currently undergoing evaluation and preliminary results are encouraging.

Laparoscopic surgery with all the advantages which will be discussed in the following chapters of this book, must become a basic gynaecological technique replacing laparotomy for most non-malignant conditions. The advantages of this form of surgery are such that patients will demand it and it is imperative that gynaecologists are prepared to meet that demand.

The guidelines for safety and training have been laid down and must be adhered to. The advantages of endoscopic surgery are such that we owe it to our patients to exploit the full potential of these new forms of management.

References

Anderson ET (1937) Peritoneoscopy. *American Journal of Surgery* **35**: 136–139.

Bernkeim BM (1911) Organoscopy: cystoscopy of the abdominal cavity. *Annals of Surgery* **53**: 764–767.

Bosch PF (1936) Laparoskopische sterilization. *Schweizerische Zeitschrift für Krankenhaus und Anstaltswesen*.

Bozzini P (1806) Lichtleiter. Eine Erfindung zur Anschauung innerer Teile und Krankheiten. *Journal für Praktische Heilkunde* **24**: 107.

Bruhat MA, Mage G & Manhes H (1979) Use of CO_2 laser by laparoscopy. In Kaplan I (ed.) *Laser Surgery III. Proceedings of the Third International Congress on Laser Surgery*, p. 225. Tel Aviv: Jerusalem Press.

Daniell JF & Brown DH (1982) Carbon dioxide laser laparoscopy: critical experience in animals and humans. *Obstetrics and Gynecology* **59**: 761–764.

David C (1907) De l'endoscopie de l'utérus après avortement et dans les suites de couches à l'état pathologique. *Bulletin of Society of Obstetrics, Paris, December*.

DeCherney AH & Polan ML (1983) Hysteroscopic management of intrauterine lesions and intractable uterine bleeding. *Obstetrics and Gynecology* **61**: 392–397.

Desormeaux AJ (1865) *De l'Endoscopie et de ses Applications au Diagnostic et au Traitement des Affections de l'Uretre et de la Vessie*. Paris: Baillière.

Edstrom K & Fernstrom I (1970) The diagnostic possibilities of a modified hysteroscopic technique. *Acta Obstetrica et Gynecologica Scandinavica* 49: 327.

Fervers C (1933) Die laparoskopie mit dem Cystoskope. Ein Beitrag zur Vereinfachung der Technik und zur endoskopischen Strangdurchtrennung in der Bauchole. *Medizinische Klinik* 29: 1042–1045.

Fourestiere M, Gladu A & Vulmiere J (1943) La péritoneoscopie. *Presse Medicale* 5: 46–47.

Frangenheim H (1972) *Laparoscopy and Culdoscopy in Gynaecology*. London: Butterworth.

Goldrath MH, Fuller TA & Segal S (1981) Laser photovaporization of endometrium for the treatment of menorrhagia. *American Journal of Obstetrics and Gynecology* 140(1): 14–19.

Hope R (1937) The differential diagnosis of ectopic pregnancy by peritoneoscopy. *Surgery, Gynecology and Obstetrics* 64: 229–234.

Hopkins HH (1953) On the diffraction theory of optical images. *Proceedings of the Royal Society* A217: 408.

Hulka JF, Omran K, Phillips JM et al. (1975) Sterilization by spring clip. *Fertility and Sterility* 26: 1122–1131.

Jacobaeus HC (1910) Uber due Moglichkeit die Zystoskopie bei Untersuchlung seroser Hohlungen anzerwerden. *Munchen Medizinische Wochenschrift* 57: 2090–2092.

Kalk H (1929) Erfahrungen mit der Laparoskopie. *Zeitschrift für Klinische Medizin* 111: 303–348.

Kelling G (1902) Uber Oesophagoskopie, Gastroskopie und Koelioskopie. *Munchner Medizinische Wochenschrift* 49(1): 22–24.

Keye WR Jr & Dixon J (1983) Photocoagulation of endometriosis by the argon laser through the laparoscope. *Obstetrics and Gynecology* 62: 383–386.

Levine RU & Neuwirth RS (1972) Evaluation of a method of hysteroscopy with the use of 30% dextran. *American Journal of Obstetrics and Gynecology* 113: 696.

Lindemann H-J (1972) The use of CO_2 in the uterine cavity for hysteroscopy. *International Journal of Fertility* 17: 221.

Mohri T (1971) Demonstration of the Machida hysteroscope. In *Proceedings of the Seventh World Congress on Fertility and Sterility*, Tokyo and Kyoto, October 1971.

Neuwirth RS & Amin JH (1976) Excision of submucous fibroids with hysteroscopic control. *American Journal of Obstetrics and Gynecology* 126: 95–99.

Nitze M (1879) Beobachtung- und Untersuchungsmethode für Harnohre, Harnblase und Rectum. *Wiener Medizinische Wochenschrift* 29: 649–652.

Nordentoeft S (1912) Uber Endoskopie geschlossener Kavitaten mittels meines Trokar-Endoskopes. *Verhandlungen der Deutschen Gesellschaft für Gynäkologie* 41: 78–81.

von Ott DO (1901) Ventroscopic illumination of the abdominal cavity in pregnancy. *Zhurnal Akrestierstova I Zhenskikh Boloznei* 15: 7–8.

Palmer R (1948) La coelioscopie. *Bruxelles-medical* 28: 305–312.

Pantaleoni DC (1869) On endoscopic examination of the cavity of the womb. *Medical Press Circular* 8: 26–27.

Phipps JH, Lewis BV, Roberts T et al. (1990) Treatment of functional menorrhagia with radio frequency endometrial ablation. *Lancet* 335: 374–376.

Power FH & Barnes AC (1941) Sterilization by means of peritoneoscopic fulguration: a preliminary report. *American Journal of Obstetrics and Gynecology* 41: 1038–1043.

Rubin IC (1925) Uterine endoscopy, endometroscopy with the aid of uterine insufflation. *American Journal of Obstetrics and Gynecology* 10(3): 313–327.

Ruddock JC (1934) Peritoneoscopy. *Western Journal of Surgery* 42: 392–405.

Semm K (1977) *Atlas of Laparoscopy and Hysteroscopy*. Philadelphia: Saunders.

Steptoe PC (1967) *Laparoscopy in Gynaecology*. London: Livingstone.

Veress J (1938) Neues Instrument sur Ausfuhrung von Brust-oder Bachpunktionen und Pneumothoraxbehandlung. *Deutsche Medizinische Wochenschrift* 64: 1480–1481.

Yoon IB & King TM (1975) A preliminary and intermediate report of a new laparoscopic ring procedure. *Journal of Reproductive Medicine* 15: 54–56.

Zollikoffer R (1924) Zur Laparoskopie. *Schweizerische Medizinische Wochenschrift* 5: 264–265.

Laparoscopic Surgery

Techniques and Equipment
Laparoscopic Tubal Surgery
Laparoscopic Ovarian Surgery
Laparoscopic Uterine and Pelvic Surgery
Laparoscopic Surgery for Endometriosis and Adhesions

2

Setting up a Service: Instrumentation and Administration

GRANT W. PATTON JR

Southeastern Fertility Center, Mount Pleasant, South Carolina, USA

Introduction

Gynaecological endoscopic surgery has changed and continues to evolve rapidly. This text discusses operative laparoscopic and hysteroscopic techniques that are generations away from laparoscopic tubal ligation. The magnitude of change is reflected in the rapidity with which general surgeons have embraced laparoscopic cholecystectomy and prepare to test each abdominal surgical procedure through the laparoscope. Certainly laparoscopic hysterectomy is becoming common, as are the extensive conservative procedures discussed in later chapters. The sense of change is critical when evaluating operating room design since this area has also changed dramatically and will continue to do so in the years ahead.

Operating room arrangement may include a number of luxuries, but must include certain basic equipment, since the setup will have significant impact on surgical technique. Nowhere is this more apparent than the standard that operative laparoscopy should be performed by viewing the monitor rather than peering down the telescope. In many respects a well designed and equipped operating room leads the surgeon to a higher level of surgical expertise.

It is our goal in this chapter to describe a fundamental approach to operating room (OR) layout and equipment that permits the endoscopic surgeon to function comfortably at various levels of surgical expertise. The design for the surgeon who performs occasional operative laparoscopic surgery will not differ from that used in the most

complicated endoscopic procedures. Obviously the number of instruments will vary but the OR layout will not, thus permitting the surgeon to move with ease from the simple vaporization of endometriosis to excision of a large endometrioma and lysis of adhesions with minimal changes in layout or staffing. Combined operative hysteroscopic, laparoscopic procedures would be easily performed in this setting, as would laparoscopic hysterectomy and cholecystectomy.

Overall Concept

Successful operative laparoscopy requires three essential ingredients:

1. surgical skill
2. a well designed and equipped OR
3. a surgical team

The discussion that follows will assume that the surgeon is aware of his level of surgical expertise and operates comfortably at that level. That different levels of skill exist among various gynaecological surgeons is obvious to the operating room staff, as well as to fellow surgeons. Operative gynaecological endoscopy permits the surgeon to get in quickly over his or her head and requires discipline on the part of the surgeon to know when to stop.

This chapter will discuss a concept of operating room design for operative laparoscopy that integrates the surgical team into this design much as an architect must consider function when designing a building. It is the author's opinion that operative laparoscopy hinges on the ability of the surgeon to use the team members successfully.

Technique and Team

The right-handed surgeon stands on the patient's left side, while the left-handed surgeon usually stands on the opposite side of the patient. The need for a high degree of hand–eye coordination during these procedures means that moving from one side of the table to the other during operative laparoscopy is difficult. A second surgeon, therefore, often makes a poor assistant because of this orientation. In most cases, a well trained nursing assistant familiar with the surgeon's technique and comfortable working across the table will complement the surgeon's approach, as experience teaches this individual to anticipate surgical moves and equipment changes.

The author would counsel residents and fellows against operating on the opposite side of the table while working with an attending physician, a point that also applies to physicians attending a surgical preceptorship.

Scrub Nurse

This individual should be utilized efficiently. In the author's OR, the scrub nurse stands at the foot of the table between the patient's legs. She hands equipment to the surgeon from either the surgeon's side table or the back instrument table, holds the uterine manipulator and manipulates second puncture instruments when necessary. Naturally he/she checks to see that various instruments, suction, cautery, etc. are properly attached. Most importantly, the scrub nurse cleans and cares for the equipment, which in this day of delicate instrumentation is a major role. This individual is also responsible for sending instruments to be repaired and for recommending that new instruments be ordered when necessary.

Biomedical Technician

This new position is critical to the success of a high-technology operating room. This individual may not be assigned to a specific operating room, but rather functions to oversee the equipment in a number of ORs, yet be able to step into an operating procedure and adjust the video, light source, laser, or correct other potential trouble spots. This individual should be trained in electronic, digital and analogue equipment, with specific training in the video and laser instrumentation specifically utilized. He/she must also develop OR expertise and assume a clinical role to some degree, thereby developing a sensitivity to equipment needs of specific surgeons and procedures. The primary goal of this individual is to avoid crisis management by keeping all equipment in good working order and by teaching team members to use all instruments comfortably. The biomedical technician should also function as the laser nurse and assume responsibility for in-service instruction for those individuals who will be running the specific lasers in the operating room. In a large operating room suite, it is essential to train a number of nurses and OR technicians to act in the role of the biomedical technician. This training should include laser operation and is designed to provide personnel available to assume this role when necessary during operative laparoscopic procedures in a number of ORs.

Circulating Nurse

This is the 'captain of the team', knowledgeable in the roles of other team members, able to help each when necessary, and able to relate to the surgeon. Communication with the surgeon is most critical to successful operative laparoscopy, particularly when a procedure goes poorly. There is an element of tension present during operative laparoscopic surgery that does not exist during a microsurgical procedure. Perhaps it is the threat of bleeding, the possibility of a bowel or bladder injury, the fear of fatigue during prolonged procedures. Whatever the problem, the circulator should help everyone deal with the situation and provide support when and where it is needed. She may check the light source, call the biomedical technician, find a lost instrument, adjust the suction, turn up the stereo, and in general maintain the rhythm. The circulating nurse is specifically responsible for operation of the bipolar and monopolar electrosurgical generators. She also adjusts the wall suction, adjusts laser and electrosurgical pedals for appropriate use during an operative procedure. It is expected that this individual will be familiar with all laser units and able to operate them when necessary; however, during an operative procedure the biomedical technician (laser nurse) in attendance should be primarily responsible for this equipment.

In many ways the circulating nurse orchestrates the procedure as much as the surgeon. During endoscopic procedures by a young or inexperienced surgeon, she must hold the procedure together. This is obviously an important role beyond the scope of the traditional circulating nurse.

Summary

These four individuals must be able to function comfortably within the operating room designed for operative laparoscopy (Figure 2.1). It is clear that all hospital operating room services will not be able to maintain identical team members for all surgeons. The principle that these four roles are essential to successful operative laparoscopy is critical, however.

Instrumentation for Endoscopic Surgery

Video

Perhaps the most difficult area to maintain at a high level is the quality of the video picture. A high quality camera with both focus and zoom adjustments is essential. This camera is attached to the telescope lens before placing the telescope into the abdominal cavity. The camera is white balanced when necessary and the camera–telescope unit inserted through the trocar sleeve. A beam splitter is not used since it reduces light to the video picture, and secondly, after adequate surgical experience produces no improvement in surgical technique. The surgeon must learn to work from the monitor and break the old habit of looking through the telescope. This has been easier for general surgeons who learned laparoscopic surgery by working from the monitor, and most difficult for those gynaecological surgeons accustomed to keeping the field of view to themselves.

Two monitors are the gold standard, providing ease of viewing for both surgeon and assistant. A single video screen placed at the foot of the table will work, but limits the role of the scrub nurse and is inconvenient for the assistant and occasionally for the surgeon. One video screen works, but two improve the quality and ease of surgery.

The author uses two Storz cameras and two 20-inch high resolution Sony monitors placed on floor stands that move easily. The monitors are wired above through the ceiling with flexible cables that permit adequate mobility. Ceiling-mounted monitors are very convenient for specific procedures but have the limitation of movement so critical during newer laparoscopic procedures (Figure 2.2).

Figure 2.1 Photograph of operating team essential for operative laparoscopy. Team includes circulating nurse, surgeon, scrub nurse, surgical assistant and biomedical technician.

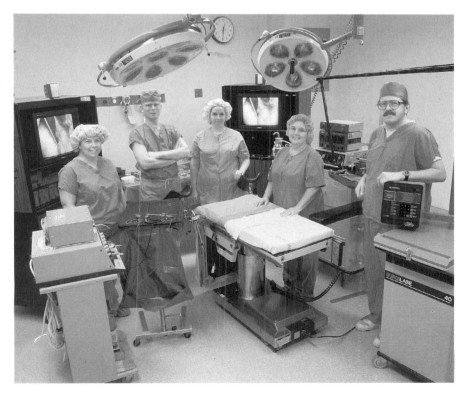

Figure 2.2 Photograph of operating room equipped for operative laparoscopy. Anaesthesia equipment has been removed.

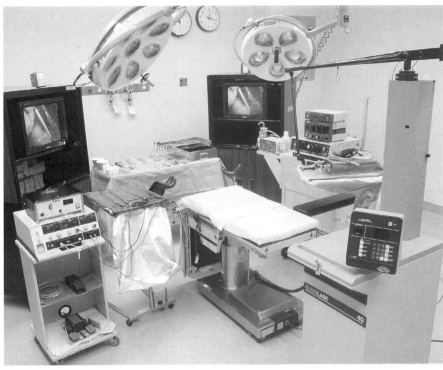

Light Source

The old 150 W light source has been superseded; at least it is not useful during operative laparoscopy. The xenon light is extremely useful; however, the automatic adjustment used on early models that permitted the light source to adjust the light requirement is no longer of value since the new video cameras perform this function more successfully. The xenon units are reliable, the bulb lasts many hours (warranty covers 400–500 hours of operating time) and, in general, are a major advance over earlier light sources. A 150 W halogen light sold by Stryker is promising, but requires a complete surgical setup including camera, cable, light source and video monitor. This three-chip camera and accessories were not found superior to the older Storz camera.

Electrosurgical Generator

A surgical technique that combines sharp incision with scissors and coagulation of specific vessels with bipolar current has become a standard approach of laparoscopic surgeons dealing with extensive pelvic adhesions and fimbrial occlusion. A fine tip monopolar electrode has also been employed when necessary in an effort to mimic microsurgical technique.

The standard Wolfe bipolar coagulating instrument is of value when used with the Kleppinger bipolar forceps to coagulate significant bleeding vessels. The tip of the instrument remains hot for short intervals following coagulation and should be used as a probe or grasping forceps with care. Storz Instrument Co. recently introduced a series of bipolar forceps that vary in size from micro to a macro size equivalent to the Kleppinger. An advantage of this new design is the ability of the forcep blades to close smoothly on an object rather than retract during closure, as occurs with the Kleppinger forceps. The new bipolar forcep has been a pleasure to use. Extensive bipolar coagulation during laparoscopic hysterectomy procedures may require the Kleppinger forceps, however. A fine tip monopolar electrode is incorporated into the Corson instrument, permitting suction and irrigation as needed during the cutting procedure. The Bard, Valley Lab or Bircher electrosurgical generators provide monopolar and bipolar current and are useful with macro and micro bipolar forceps as well as a microelectrode when necessary. Recently the argon beam coagulator has been utilized for haemostasis with good results. Reintroduction of the technique by Bircher includes a long 10 mm tip useful as a second-puncture instrument during operative laparoscopy. A smaller 5 mm tip will soon be available. This instrument provides both coagulation and monopolar current. The ability to provide both bipolar and argon beam coagulation, as well as monopolar cutting is essential during operative laparoscopy. Again, this is an area in which availability is essential, since coagulation may be required at short notice if bleeding occurs. Monopolar cutting and coagulation may be used by individual surgeons and should be discussed prior to a surgical procedure, as should the use of the argon beam coagulator. In the author's operating room, these instruments are assembled and placed on the surgeon's small instrument table for easy access.

Laser

A carbon dioxide laser technique utilizing a third generation sealed tube CO_2 laser is also used for lysis of adhesions, excision of endometriosis and other operative laparoscopic procedures. The KTP and Nd:YAG fibre lasers can serve this purpose but have been found most effective when significant coagulation is required, i.e. during a myomectomy procedure. The surgeon must discuss his surgical technique with the operating room staff prior to the actual procedure in order to permit adequate preparation of instruments and placement of individual lasers. As discussed earlier, the operating endoscopic OR staff must be well trained in both electrosurgical and laser techniques and comfortable moving from one to the other. When the carbon dioxide laser is utilized during operative laparoscopy, the articulating arm of the laser is attached to the operating laparoscope (12 mm, 6° operating telescope with a 6 mm operating channel), and the telescope placed in the warming unit for later use. The arm is usually covered with a sterile drape. A word should be said concerning the articulation of the CO_2 laser with the endoscope. In early model lasers, a joystick attachment was used to permit laser beam alignment. This is no longer used and the articulating arm should attach directly to the laparoscope. This articulation will contain only a fixed focus lens which differs from a variable focus lens used to produce variable degrees of a defocused beam. Misalignment of the laser beam in this situation is caused by either a loose attachment of the coupler or misalignment of the beam through the articulating arm due to improper mirror adjustment that might have occurred by bumping the arm or hitting it against a stationary object. This is easily detected by the biomedical technician and should be corrected. In this regard, the biomedical technician or a substitute should be able to monitor beam alignment during the procedure and advise the surgeon and staff regarding problems with alignment, suggesting simple solutions such as condensation inside the telescope channel and other causes discussed earlier. After a period of time the circulating nurse will also be able to fill this role.

Smoke Evacuation

Most laser companies market a free-standing smoke exhaust unit which prevents smoke and plume from contaminating the operating room environment and hospital suction systems. These units are satisfactory but usually noisy. A second option involves use of an in-line filter attached to the hospital OR suction line. These disposable in-line filters have been found to be completely satisfactory and do not appear to permit contamination of the main hospital system. Recently, Northcutt has marketed a CO_2 insufflation device that recirculates the gas and removes smoke and plume from the system.

Telescope and Instruments

The author performs an operative laparoscopic procedure utilizing a zero degree 10 mm panoview diagnostic telescope which produces an excellent picture and permits careful exploration of the pelvic area. Once the operative approach has begun, he changes to a 12 mm, 6° operating laparoscope, although one could use the operating telescope throughout. An angled 30° lens on a diagnostic telescope will assist in evaluating the anterior abdominal wall and is used by general surgeons in inguinal hernia repair. The smaller lens and lower number of fibre bundles contained in the 12 mm operating telescope reduce light and the quality of the video picture. Successful use of this telescope requires high intensity light and a high quality camera. A good quality video picture will often deteriorate during a difficult operative procedure when the early contrast of tissues is blunted by the colour red (blood) and dark blue (methylene blue), yet the quality of the video image must be maintained throughout.

Telescope Warmer

Numerous techniques are helpful in an attempt to prevent fogging of the telescope lens during operative laparoscopy. One of these is the use of a solution termed 'ultrastop' placed on the lens, and the author has found that warming the telescope preoperatively is also helpful. An electrical unit that is thermostatically controlled permits warming of a maximum of four telescopes. In practice, the diagnostic and operating telescopes are placed in the warming unit during OR setup. The temperature is maintained at 40–50°C and the telescopes reach this stable temperature within 5–10 minutes.

A further refinement to maintain clear vision at all times is the lens irrigation system recently introduced by ACMI.

Individual Operating Instruments

A selection of operating instruments should be available and, if possible, the surgeon should discuss these with the scrub nurse prior to the surgical procedure. At least two 5 mm or two 5.5 mm puncture trocars and sleeves are of value, one containing a stopcock and vent for smoke exhaust. The need for both 5 mm and 5.5 mm sleeves has been eliminated since the new Nezhat suction irrigation cannula has been reduced to 5.0 mm. The pyramidal trocar tip is safer to use. The author prefers re-usable metal trocars and sleeves, but has found that a combination of metal and disposable trocars is a great convenience. Disposable trocars have gained popularity in general surgery, and permit flexibility when the number of second punctures varies. A metal trocar and sleeve pass through the fascia and peritoneum with little resistance under better control than the older model Teflon sleeve. The disposable trocars are also easy to use and permit removal of tissue with little hang up on the flap valve which is not as easy with the permanent metal units. In an effort to reduce cost the metal trocar and sleeves are used primarily by the author with disposable units employed when necessary.

Each surgeon will express his preference for second-puncture accessory instruments. A selection of these instruments is important, however, in order to deal with the unusual surgical occurrence.

Basic Instruments

1. Grasping forceps:
   3 mm alligator, flat pancake forceps,
   3, 5 mm needle drivers
2. Scissors—5 mm
   Semm micro-dissecting scissors
   Semm Hook scissors
   Sharp cutting scissors
   'Scissors must cut, not cauterize or tear'
3. Suction, irrigation:
   Single instrument with dual function control, permitting easy digital control of both suction and irrigation
   Nezhat (Cooper): Updated Nezhat–Dorsey (Storz)

The Nezhat–Dorsey Suction Irrigation System has replaced the older stage aqua purator. The basic components of this system are: adjustable pressure unit, re-usable variable-tip cannulas, and disposable trumpet valve and tubing. The hospital wall suction is attached to this unit as well.

4. Bipolar cautery:
   Kleppinger, bipolar microforceps, Storz bipolar instruments (Manhes instrument style)
5. Monopolar current:
   2 mm micro tip, Corson suction irrigation unit
   5 mm suction cannula, scissors, forceps
6. Other:
   Angled backstop (deflecting)
   Oviduct forceps
   Grasping forceps for suturing
   Deflecting mechanism for laser fibre

CO_2 Insufflation

The original 1 litre per minute CO_2 insufflator used for diagnostic laparoscopy was modified by Wolfe to deliver 3 litres of CO_2 per minute and termed 'high flow', yet this unit has passed the way of the 150 W light source. This early model appears archaic today in light of the need for higher flow insufflation and rapid smoke exhaust.

Second generation insufflators delivered three rates of flow which included 1, 3, 5–6 litres of CO_2 per minute. Third generation insufflators, popularized during laparoscopic cholecystectomy techniques, and in general use today, deliver 9–10 litres per minute and are pressure controlled. A microprocessor monitors intra-abdominal pressure and adjusts gas flow accordingly. Of interest, the Storz insufflators also contain an air pump that may be used to assist during suction procedures when necessary. Recently a small company, Northgate Inc., has marketed an insufflator that delivers 14 litres of CO_2 per minute, and removes smoke and plume during a recycling process. A second generation high-flow insufflator is mandatory, and a third generation model of great help, particularly during extensive operative procedures utilizing a laser technique.

Equipment Summary

Obviously, laparoscopic equipment used for diagnostic procedures as well as tubal ligation will not suffice for modern operative laparoscopic procedures. Neither will the early CO_2 insufflator, telescope, nor early model beam-splitting cameras be adequate. The hospital must, therefore, purchase new equipment suitable for individual procedures. Successful operative gynaecological laparoscopy requires those instruments mentioned earlier. These instruments, team and the OR layout to be noted later will suffice for virtually all laparoscopic procedures, including those now being performed by many general surgeons.

Operating Room Design

The basic OR design permits easy adaptation to various gynaecological endoscopic surgical procedures. Figure 2.3 is a diagram of the author's operating room arrangement, arranged for a typical laparoscopic procedure. Photographs of this arrangement are shown in Figures 2.1 and 2.2. It is apparent that the staff has also anticipated the possibility that the surgeon may wish to utilize an operative laparoscopic technique. This typical arrangement, permitting transition from a diagnostic to an operative approach, is accomplished with minimal confusion. Disposal equipment such as the suction irrigation handle, tubing and trocars can be opened once the surgeon decides to proceed with operative laparoscopy.

The primary (back) instrument table (Figure 2.4), utilized primarily by the scrub nurse, contains all laparoscopic instruments for diagnostic laparoscopy as well as those instruments the surgeon prefers during an operative approach. The selection of operative instruments should be made prior to surgery since individual surgeons will have different preference. Extra instruments such as needle holders should be kept in sterile packages in a drawer of the laparoscopy cart (Figure 2.5).

The surgeon's instrument table is usually a draped jumbo Mayo stand containing electrosurgical instrumentation, including the macro and micro bipolar forceps, a monopolar needle instrument and the argon beam coagulator. These instruments should be available at all times in the event that unexpected bleeding occurs. Additional selected instruments such as a favourite forceps or grasping instrument can also be placed here for easy access. This table can also act as an interchange between surgeon and scrub nurse with placement of instruments on this table either for anticipated use by the surgeon or anticipated removal by the scrub nurse.

The laparoscopy cart, is a compact unit. The light source, high flow insufflator and camera power box are stacked on top with a suction irrigation unit on the side platform. An electric panel on the back of the cart permits all of these instruments to be plugged into a single source and use of a single electrical cord from the cart to an electrical outlet. Additional instruments that may be required during laparoscopy are kept in the drawers.

The biomedical cart, shown in the diagram (Figure 2.6), permits storage of instruments and equipment used by the biomedical technician. These tools, cords, instruments, bulbs, etc. are available for immediate use as needed during an operative procedure. On top of the cart are the character generator used with the video system and a video mixer that permits two camera images to appear on a single video monitor screen.

Figure 2.3 Diagram of operating room layout. 1, KTP/YAG laser; 2, video display monitors; 3, operating instruments table; 4, video supply cart; 5, patient table with stirrups; 6a, surgeon; 6b, scrub nurse; 6c, operating room technician; 6d, bio-medical technologist; 6e, circulating nurse; 7, endoscopic supply cart with CO_2 insufflator and suction machine; 8, surgeon's instrument table; 9, electro-surgical cart; 10, CO_2 laser; 11, warming tray for endoscopes; 12, VCR power source and cassette storage; 13, stereo.

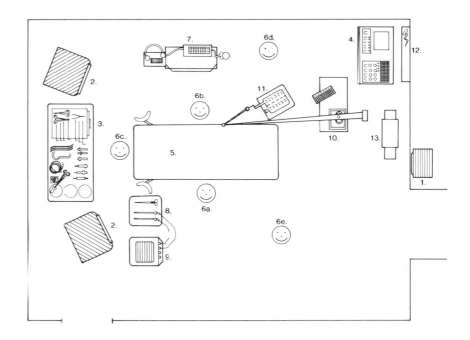

Figure 2.4 Back instrument table.

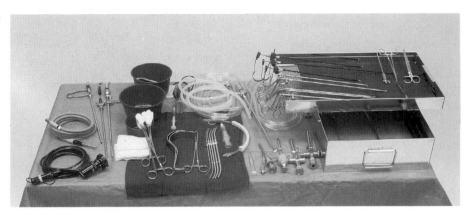

Figure 2.5 Photograph of laparoscope cart consisting of mobile cart with drawers, endoscopic light source, CO_2 insufflator, camera power source and irrigation system.

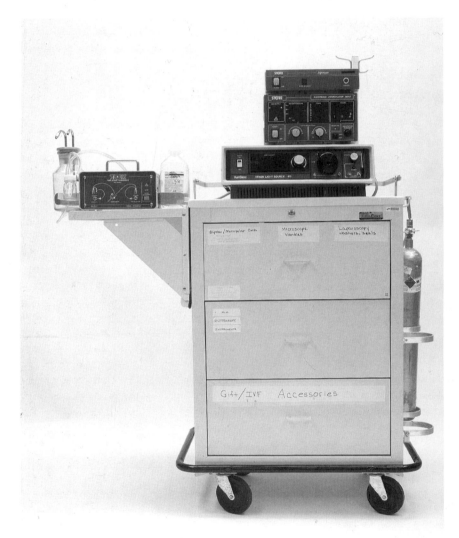

Behind this cart one can see the wall cabinet that contains the camera power source for both the laparoscope and operating microscope camera, as well as a one-half-inch VCR. A three-quarter-inch VCR could also be placed in this cabinet.

Video monitors mounted on large mobile carts are easily moved to accommodate comfortable viewing by surgeon and assistant. This system permits adaptation to operative hysteroscopy as well as both laparoscopic hysterectomy and laparoscopic cholecystectomy.

Electrosurgical generators are placed on the patient's left side just behind the surgeon's instrument table. This will include the argon beam coagulator when it is used.

The CO_2 laser is placed to the right of the patient's shoulder, somewhat behind the anaesthesia machine and is moved into the surgical

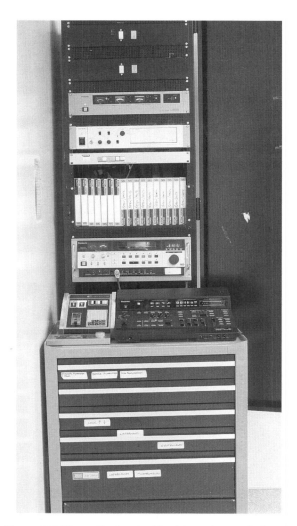

Figure 2.6 Biomedical cart with video mixer and character generator. Wall-mounted power source is shown in background.

field when needed. The operating laparoscope is usually attached to the CO_2 articulating arm and placed in a warmer during initial setup. In this design, a single weakness is the need to move the telescope warmer table and tray out of the field when using the CO_2 laser.

The KTP and YAG lasers used during operative laparoscopy and hysteroscopy are stored in the hall and placed to the left of the patient at shoulder level when needed. The fibre may be positioned on either side of the surgeon for his comfort.

Operative Hysteroscopy

Hysteroscopy is frequently used during evaluation of patients who may also require diagnostic laparoscopy as well as an operative endoscopic procedure. The ability to incorporate hysteroscopy

easily into the OR setup is essential. This is accomplished by using a small Mayo size stand for hysteroscopic instruments placed next to the main instrument table, and a second stand on which is placed a high-intensity light source and video camera power source. Both are easily incorporated into the OR design as discussed below.

OR Team

The OR team used for operative laparoscopy remains the same during operative hysteroscopy. These individuals must be trained in basic hysteroscopic technique, become familiar with types of operative hysteroscopy and, of course, safety procedures involving the use of equipment, particularly the YAG and KTP lasers.

Equipment

The telescope used during operative hysteroscopy is a 4 mm, 30° telescope usually inserted through a double operating channel. Recently Baggish has designed a hysteroscope sleeve that includes three channels permitting insertion of a flexible instrument or laser fibre through one, and fluid or suction exhaust through a second accessory channel. Urological instrumentation, including the Olympus Ignasius resectoscope, typically employed during transurethral prostatectomy, has been of great value during operative hysteroscopy, permitting resection of submucus myomas and a uterine septum, as has the use of the KTP and YAG laser fibres. Distension of the uterine cavity with dextron 70 (Hyskon) during a diagnostic procedure has been a standard, and recently glycine and 3% sorbitol have been used under pressure to increase distension of the uterine cavity and improve the ability to use the resectoscope for a prolonged interval without fear of overloading the patient with excessive fluid. These subjects are discussed in Chapter 34 on operative hysteroscopy.

Light Source

Adequate light is necessary during operative hysteroscopy now performed in a fashion similar to operative laparoscopy, in which the video camera is attached to the telescope, and the surgeon views the procedure by observing the video monitor. A xenon light source similar to that used during operative laparoscopy is used for hysteroscopy and the same video camera used during laparoscopy can be used interchangeably.

Dual Image Video Hysteroscopy/Laparoscopy

Many operative hysteroscopic procedures are facilitated by the ability to visualize the laparoscopic view of the uterus and tubes during the procedure. This is particularly useful during tubal cannulation in which, while inserting the cannula through the tubal ostia, the surgeon is able to view the fallopian tube and passage of the catheter through this structure. Additional uses include concurrent laparoscopy and falloposcopy and exploration of the common bile duct during laparoscopic cholecystectomy. In order to view images from two cameras on the monitor at the same time, a video mixer is used. Two high-quality cameras are, therefore, necessary and two xenon light sources also used in order to carry out concurrent laparoscopy and hysteroscopy.

Two monitors are not absolutely necessary during operative hysteroscopy since both assistant and surgeon may view a single monitor. However, concurrent laparoscopy may make a second monitor necessary and clearly two monitors are an obvious convenience.

Two cameras are used, one with the hysteroscope and the second is attached to a diagnostic laparoscope. The images from both cameras can be displayed on a single video monitor by using a video mixer. The video mixer permits display of images from both cameras on a single video monitor.

The Future

The use of endoscopic procedures will continue to grow in the years ahead. Once the province of the reproductive surgeon, operative laparoscopy will soon be a must for the practising gynaecologist who performs hysterectomy and routine procedures such as salpingo-oophorectomy. Reproductive surgeons will take the lead, however, in advanced techniques often involving two cameras. Falloposcopy will become commonplace and essential in grading tubal mucosa, assisting in the choice of surgical repair or *in vitro* fertilization. Transvaginal ultrasound will be combined with laparoscopy to identify intramural fibroids and ovarian cysts.

The general surgeons will attempt all abdominal procedures through the laparoscope, and with technological advances in automatic staplers, may be able to do bowel resection in addition to cholecystectomy and herniorrhaphy. Here, too, the use of two cameras will assist in common bile duct exploration as well as internal location of a bowel polyp or intestinal mass, permitting exact resection.

3

A Practical Approach to Diagnostic Laparoscopy

CHRIS SUTTON

The Royal Surrey County Hospital, Guildford, Surrey, UK

During the past few years laparoscopy has become one of the most frequently performed operations in gynaecological departments. Initially it was used for occlusion of the fallopian tube as a simple method of female sterilization as well as for the diagnosis of pelvic pain and infertility but increasingly it is used for operative procedures which are described in detail in this section of the book. Before embarking on such procedures it is essential that each surgeon develops a safe technique for the insufflation of the abdomen, insertion of the laparoscope and the various ancillary probes and instruments.

Complications and Consenting the Patient

Modern laparoscopy is essentially a safe procedure and serious complications are rare. One of the pioneering examples of detailed surgical audit was the Confidential Enquiry into Gynaecological Laparoscopy conducted on behalf of the Royal College of Obstetricians and Gynaecologists by Professor GVP Chamberlain which revealed an overall complication rate of 34/1000 and a mortality rate of 0.08/1000 (Chamberlain and Brown, 1978). A much larger survey from West Germany, reporting operative laparoscopies as well, drew attention to the relative safety of laparoscopic surgery in the hands of experienced operators. Major complications, requiring laparotomy or re-laparoscopy, were four times greater with operative compared to diagnostic procedures but

the rate was only 3.8/1000 with an overall mortality for all procedures of only 0.05/1000 (Riedel et al., 1986).

The most dangerous time for direct trauma is when the Veress needle and the first trocar and cannula are being introduced blindly especially in a patient who has had previous surgery. Injuries to the bowel, urinary tract and pelvic organs contributed 1.8, 0.2 and 3.4/1000 complications in the RCOG series. Once the laparoscope has been introduced the other trocars are inserted under direct vision but in spite of all precautions to avoid injury to blood vessels in the abdominal wall they are still a significant factor in the morbidity of laparoscopic surgery with a rate of 2.5/1000 (Chamberlain and Brown, 1978). Certain patients such as the grossly obese or the very thin are particularly at risk of problems during the initial insertion of the Veress needle and laparoscope. Major direct trauma injuries and diathermy accidents, which if involving the bowel may lead to faecal peritonitis with an associated mortality of 50% (Thompson and Wheeless, 1973), may require laparotomy and patients should be consented for this should the need arise during laparoscopic surgery.

Contraindications

The subject has been well reviewed by Gordon and Magos (1989) and the absolute and relative contraindications are listed in Table 3.1.

Table 3.1 Contraindications to laparoscopy

Absolute
    Mechanical and paralytic ileus
    Large abdominal mass
    Generalized peritonitis
    Irreducible external hernia
    Cardiac failure
    Recent myocardial infarction
    Cardiac conduction defects
    Respiratory failure
    Severe obstructive airways disease
    Shock

Relative
    Multiple abdominal incisions
    Abdominal wall sepsis
    Gross obesity
    Hiatus hernia
    Ischaemic heart disease
    Blood dyscrasias and coagulopathies

Abdominal distension secondary to bowel obstruction is an absolute contraindication because of the dangers of bowel trauma and perforation. An irreducible hernia is only likely to be exacerbated, and possibly made ischaemic, by the added pressure of a pneumoperitoneum. Similarly intraperitoneal gases under pressure are also likely to aggravate the anaesthetic risks associated with severe respiratory and cardiac disease due to the effects on acid–base balance, myocardial contractility, venous return and blood pressure.

Patients should be haemodynamically stable and clinical shock is therefore a contraindication and, if due to a ruptured ectopic pregnancy, is a reason for immediate laparotomy to stem the haemorrhage rather than subjecting the patient to the further delay implicit in setting up for a laparoscopy.

Relative contraindications depend rather on the experience of the laparoscopic surgeon and the anaesthetist. Previous abdominal scars require special skill in the direction of introducing instruments and employing special techniques such as the Z- introduction of Semm described below. Alternatively the insufflation of CO_2 can be achieved through the posterior fornix or even through the uterine fundus.

Patients with hiatus hernia pose a special problem and the Trendelenburg position should be limited to 15° of downward tilt and the intra-abdominal pressure should not exceed 10 mmHg. Some authorities have advocated direct insertion of the laparoscopic trocar without prior pneumoperitoneum as a safer approach in patients with this condition (Dingfelder, 1978).

Laparoscopic surgery should be kept to the minimal possible time in patients with ischaemic heart disease and bleeding disorders should be corrected before laparoscopic surgery in the same way as they would be before conventional surgery.

Anaesthetic Considerations (contributed by Dr Gareth Jenkins, Consultant Anaesthetist, Royal Surrey County Hospital, Guildford)

In our unit patients are usually admitted on the day of operation and are not usually given a premedication although, if particularly anxious, they are given oral benzodiazepine. Intravenous induction of anaesthesia is achieved with propofol (Diprivan) and muscle relaxation with atracurium (Tracrium). Endotracheal intubation is used for all patients since we feel that a laryngeal mask is inherently unsafe, particularly for prolonged procedures. We do not use a gastric tube to empty stomach contents since all our patients are starved for at least 6 hours before operation. The operation is conducted under intermittent positive pressure ventilation with oxygen, nitrous oxide and enflurane or isoflurane. Analgesia is achieved with fentanyl and metoclopramide is employed as an antiemetic.

At the end of the procedure residual paralysis is rapidly reversed with neostigmine 2.5 mg and glycopyrrolate 0.5 mg and diclofenac 100 mg is inserted rectally as a suppository for postoperative analgesia. After that most patients only need oral analgesics and can go home with a responsible adult accompanying them 4 hours later but, it must be admitted that after lengthy procedures, most patients benefit from an overnight stay in hospital and can then be safely discharged the following day. The nursing staff and many of the patients seem to prefer this and they are much more likely to retain information concerning their operation when it is imparted to them the following day.

Preparation and Positioning the Patient

Our patients are routinely catheterized prior to laparoscopy unless we can be absolutely sure that they have voided just before their arrival in the operating suite. If extensive surgery is likely in the vicinity of the large bowel as occurs with complete obliteration of the cul-de-sac with endometriosis, it is advisable to administer a mechanical bowel preparation such as the polyethylene glycol-based isosmotic solution GoLytely or Colyte. Prophylactic antibiotics are not used routinely but can be administered in prolonged cases and whenever an increased risk of infection seems likely.

The patient is placed in a modified lithotomy position once they are anaesthetized and care is taken to abduct the thighs slowly and symmetrically. Pads are placed between the poles and the calf muscles and diathermy pads are carefully attached to ensure wide and uniform application to the skin. Lower abdominal, pubic and perineal hair is not shaved and if this is deemed necessary by overzealous operating room staff any shaving should be performed in the anaesthetic room immediately prior to surgery. Shaving of patients on the wards several hours beforehand with the inevitable serosanguinous discharge from cut hair follicles produces a perfect culture medium for *Staphylococcus aureus*. This is an ideal way to ensure wound infections and introduces a totally avoidable risk factor into laparoscopic surgery.

The patient is supine until after the initial insertion of the Veress needle and then is placed in a steep Trendelenburg position of about 30°. It is therefore essential to have a non-slip mattress or shoulder braces, otherwise the assistant who is attempting to antevert the uterus is prevented from so doing. Some laparoscopic surgeons employ Trendelenburg positions as steep as 40° and have reported no adverse effects (Reich, 1989) although there is likely to be some protestations from the anaesthetists until they become familiar with the ventilation pressure changes induced by this degree of tilt.

Insufflation of the Abdominal Cavity with CO_2

A vertical incision is usually made deep inside the inferior aspect of the umbilicus which is, after all, the scar resulting from the sloughing of the umbilical cord and therefore overlies the area where skin, deep fascia and parietal peritoneum meet. The Veress needle is inserted, initially almost at right angles, and advanced through the layers of the abdominal wall, feeling each layer as it is penetrated, for about 1 cm before angling it forwards towards the hollow of the sacrum. Although a vertical incision is the most popular, other incisions, such as an elliptical one beneath the rim, can be made depending on the actual configuration of the navel, to produce a better

cosmetic result. Nevertheless the incision should still be within the umbilicus since this minimizes the chance of the peritoneum tenting away from the end of the needle and producing surgical emphysema of the anterior abdominal wall.

After insertion the needle is connected to a CO_2 insufflator flowing at 1 litre per minute with a pressure only slightly above that registered when the needle was tested prior to insertion. The abdomen is percussed for the characteristic uniform tympanitic sound that signifies that the gas is flowing into the abdominal cavity. Once liver dullness is lost the patient is tilted head down at an angle of 30–40° and as long as there is no appreciable rise in insufflation pressure the controls are switched to deliver a fast flow of gas until about 3 litres of CO_2 have been introduced to distend the peritoneal cavity.

A muffled sound on percussion or asymmetric swelling of the abdomen is suggestive of failure to perforate the peritoneum, which can be very thick and elastic, especially in obese patients, resulting in surgical emphysema. If the surgeon is uncertain that insufflation is intraperitoneal the Veress needle should be removed and re-inserted before too much surgical emphysema has developed. If a second attempt at insertion is unsuccessful insufflation should be attempted elsewhere—either through a suprapubic incision into the uterovesical pouch or even transfundally. This latter approach is used almost exclusively by some gynaecologists and requires strict aseptic preparation of the lower genital tract and careful uterine sounding to measure the distance from the cervix to the internal surface of the fundus. The Veress needle is pushed through the myometrium with the patient in a steep Trendelenburg position until a loss of resistance signifies fundal perforation.

The induction of a pneumoperitoneum can be particularly difficult in very obese patients, often due to the thickness and elasticity of a peritoneum densely infiltrated with adipose tissue. In some patients who weigh in at 120 kg or more we use longer trocars and needles but these instruments must never be used for women of a normal habitus since they would pose a very real risk of penetrating pelvic organs, particularly the fundus of the uterus or, more seriously, the great vessels. The correct siting of the Veress needle can also be very difficult, paradoxically, in the very thin when the tactile recognition of the separate layers is often absent.

Insertion of the Umbilical Trocar and Laparoscope

If the abdominal cavity is well distended it is not necessary to lift up the anterior abdominal wall during insertion of the trocar because this can give rise to unpleasant bruising. The gas can be forced into the lower abdomen by simply pressing on the upper abdomen with the left hand whilst the trocar is inserted in the palm of the right hand with the index finger acting as a guard to allow only a few centimetres of the sharp end to penetrate the peritoneum. Once inserted the trocar is angled almost horizontally and pushed forwards towards the anterior pelvis, taking care to avoid the major vessels as they course over the sacral promontory. This is particularly important on the rare occasion when laparoscopy is performed on an achondroplastic dwarf since the true conjugate of the pelvis is considerably reduced, thus exposing the aorta and inferior vena cava to serious risk of laceration and the inevitable catastrophic haemorrhage which ensues.

Other organs at risk of damage by the trocar are the full bladder and rarely, the transverse colon, a low slung stomach or pelvic kidney, either naturally occurring or following renal transplantation. Previous abdominal surgery used to be considered a contraindication to laparoscopy and certainly loops of bowel adherent to a midline scar are at risk of perforation and such patients should have had a bowel preparation such as GoLytely. The Veress needle and the trocar should be angled at 45° away from the scar but great care must be taken to introduce only the sharp tip of the trocar just inside the peritoneum before checking the site visually with the laparoscope. An alternative technique in these patients is the Z-puncture technique of Semm (1989) where a 5 mm trocar is inserted proximal to the peritoneum and penetration of a thin translucent sheet of peritoneum is selected visually, thus avoiding adherent bowel or omentum.

Initial Inspection

Following insertion of the laparoscope the surgeon should consciously perform an anatomical tour of the pelvis to identify any structures that could be harmed if inadvertently hit with the laser beam or electrodiathermy. This first step is vital to ensure the safety of operative laparoscopy and should never be omitted since no two pelvises are identical and anatomical variations, particularly concerning the course of the ureter, are not unusual.

The pelvic side wall is inspected to determine the position of the ureters which can occasionally lie close to the uterosacral ligaments but usually run 1–2 cm laterally. They can be 'palpated' with a blunt probe and often the characteristic peristaltic movements can be recognized beneath the peritoneal surface. In extreme cases they can be dissected out with the CO_2 laser, scissors and aquadissection (Reich, 1990) or illuminated by special ureteric catheters (Rocket, London, UK) but although such measures may be justified during laparoscopic hysterectomy or a difficult dissection of an ovary plastered onto the pelvic side wall by endometriosis they should not be necessary for most operative laparoscopic procedures. Once the anatomical landmarks have been established the surgeon should carefully inspect the pelvis for evidence of any pathology, particularly endometriosis, which can be responsible for dysmenorrhoea. The laparoscope when held close to the peritoneal surface can provide 8× magnifications and close inspection may reveal subtle or atypical appearances (Jansen and Russel, 1987) described in detail in Chapters 25 and 26. Figure 3.1 shows some of these changes with vesicles (sago grains) and white scarring (powder puff burns) with abnormal vessels radiating out of an endometriotic lesion lying perilously close to the ureter. The ovarian fossa and posterior surface of the ovary must also be inspected for evidence of endometriosis and subovarian adhesions and, in the absence of ovarian ultrasound or nuclear magnetic resonance (NMR)

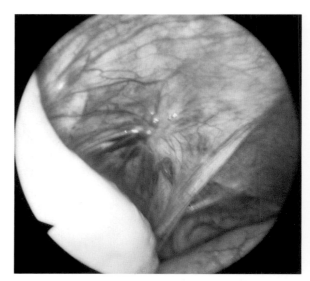

Figure 3.1 Atypical endometriosis on back of broad ligament close to ureter.

imaging techniques, the ovaries may have to be 'needled' for the presence of haemosiderin to avoid missing ovarian endometriomas.

It is impossible to perform an adequate diagnostic laparoscopy with a single puncture technique and nearly all operative procedures require additional punctures in the suprapubic area or in one or other iliac fossa.

Insertion of the Suprapubic Probe

This probe is inserted through a 5 mm trocar introduced via a small incision placed centrally just above the pubic bone or at the left end of an imaginary Pfannenstiel incision in the hair-bearing area of the mons veneris so that no visible scar remains following the procedure. Since a full bladder would be punctured by a stab at this site it is imperative that the bladder is emptied before the start of the operation by catheterization using a sterile technique. An alternative to a rigid metal probe is to use a suction–irrigation instrument to wash off residual carbon deposits and cool the tissues if laser or electrosurgery is being used. Some of these devices are not as strong as the rigid stainless steel probes and since they are expensive great care must be taken not to distort them whilst applying pressure to the posterior aspect of the cervix to delineate the uterosacral ligaments prior to a laparoscopic uterine neurectomy. Some surgeons prefer to use flexible fibre lasers in which case the suction–irrigation probe is inserted in the right iliac fossa as described below and the central channel of the probe is used to conduct the silicone quartz fibre which transmits the laser energy.

Insertion of the Second Operative Trocar

An incision is made either at the right-hand end of an imaginary Pfannenstiel incision just above the pubic hairline or higher in the right iliac fossa just lateral to the deep inferior epigastric vessels. These vessels—an artery flanked by two veins (venae comitantes)—can bleed profusely if accidentally punctured and this is an accepted and unfortunate hazard of operative laparoscopy. Transillumination of the abdominal wall will often pick out the superficial vessels but cannot be relied upon to locate the deeper vessels, especially

in a well covered woman. These must routinely be located by direct vision of the peritoneal surface of the anterior abdominal wall where they run just lateral to the umbilical ligaments—the obliterated umbilical artery (Figure 3.2). A finger tapping the skin lightly from above can be identified and it is moved to an avascular area lateral to these vessels and the incision made at this site. The 5 mm trocar is inserted there, preferably with a self-retaining thread to prevent it sliding during instrument movements, and a 3 mm sleeve reducer should be available to introduce endocoagulators, biopsy forceps and scissors without losing the pneumoperitoneum. Please note that the trocar, when introduced lateral to the rectus sheath, is very close to the external iliac vessels and the forefinger should always act as a guard to prevent deep insertion and the penetration of the peritoneum by the sharp trocar should always be conducted under direct vision so that perforation of these vessels can be avoided (Figure 3.3).

Most operative laparoscopy can be performed through these three trocars but it is occasionally necessary to employ a fourth 12 mm port which is usually placed just beneath the umbilicus in the midclavicular line. This is needed to introduce larger instruments such as the Semm morcellator and tissue extractor or the Endo-GIA stapling gun. In practice they are used for only a relatively short time during complicated procedures such as hysterectomy and oophorectomy or for removing ectopic pregnancies or myomas. The development of reducing sleeves to enable smaller diameter instruments to be introduced through the large

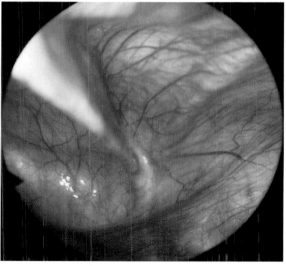

Figure 3.2 Obliterated umbilical artery and inferior epigastric vessels running parallel and to the right.

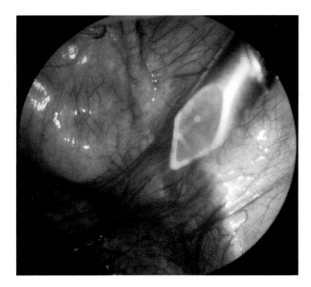

Figure 3.3 Second portal trocar inserted under direct vision to avoid damage to external iliac vessels.

trocars without loss of pneumoperitoneum represents a very real advance and is a classic example of how complex problems can be solved by very simple solutions. Care must be taken to keep the incisions well apart to avoid interference with other instruments: the, so-called 'clashing swords' effect, which can be annoying and frustrating for both the surgeon and the assistant. The laparoscopic surgeon should try to adopt a situation where the positioning of the trocars is constant for specific procedures to allow the surgeon and assistants to gain a certain familiarity with the technique. Incisions should be kept to the minimum necessary because multiple scars, albeit small, are unsightly and can be the site of implantation endometriosis (Figure 3.4).

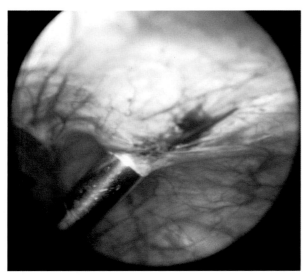

Figure 3.4 Endometriosis in previous laparoscopy scar.

Management of Profuse Bleeding during Trocar Introduction

The procedure outlined above to avoid puncturing the inferior epigastric vessels should always be followed but sometimes, regardless of the preventive measures taken, a large vessel is pierced and deep suture equipment should be immediately available. The bleeding can sometimes be very dramatic and if this occurs DO NOT REMOVE THE TROCAR because it is marking the track of insertion along which the bleeding vessel must be located. A strong suture on a straight needle should be passed directly beside the trocar and retrieved inside the abdomen with a needle holder and passed up on the other side of the trocar and extracted through the skin using a conventional needle holder. The procedure is then repeated to embrace the tissue occupied by the trocar in a Z-fashion then the trocar is removed and a knot carefully tied to achieve haemostasis. Unfortunately this often results in an untidy scar but if the trocar is removed and the excision extended it can be almost impossible to locate the bleeding point.

Closure

The umbilical incision is closed with a 4-0 Vicryl suture opposing deep fascia and skin dermis. The other incisions can be closed with plain catgut for day cases or Michel clips which are removed the following morning before the patient goes home. If large incisions are made for the removal of ovarian tumours or myomas it is important to close the rectus sheath with nylon, otherwise there is a risk of incisional hernia.

Postoperative Care

If the laparoscopic surgery is on a morning list the patient is usually able to go home, accompanied by a responsible adult, the same evening. Although the incisions are only small many of them have had a lot of surgery performed inside and should be warned to expect some soreness over the following week. Temperature elevation is unusual beyond the first day and they should be told to report any temperature rise beyond this. They should also be warned to expect some vaginal bleeding due to the intrauterine manipulator.

One of the problems of day-case surgery is that most patients suffer a degree of postanaesthetic amnesia and do not take in all that the surgeon tells them before discharge from the hospital. It is worthwhile preparing a 'fact sheet' telling them of the problems they might expect during the first week and some surgeons have the patients return 5 days later for a nurse to remove nylon sutures and answer any questions regarding problems that may have arisen since the operation.

References

Chamberlain GVP & Brown JC (1978) *Gynaecological Laparoscopy—The Report of the Working Party of the Confidential Enquiry into Gynaecological Laparoscopy.* London: Royal College of Obstetricians and Gynaecologists.

Dingfelder JR (1978) Direct laparoscopic trocar insertion without prior pneumo-peritoneum. *Journal of Reproductive Medicine* 21: 45–47.

Gordon AG & Magos AL (1989) The development of laparoscopic surgery. In Sutton CJG (ed.) *Laparoscopic Surgery. Baillière's Clinical Obstetrics and Gynaecology* 3, No. 3: 429–449.

Jansen R & Russel P (1986) Non-pigmented endometriosis: Clinical, laparoscopic and pathological definition. *American Journal of Obstetrics and Gynecology* 155: 1154–1159.

Reich H (1989) New techniques in advanced laparoscopic surgery. In Sutton CJG (ed) *Laparoscopic Surgery. Baillière's Clinical Obstetrics and Gynaecology* 3, No. 3: 655–681.

Reich H (1990) Aquadissection. In Baggish M (ed.) *Laser Endoscopy.* The Clinical Practice of Gynecology series, pp. 159–185. New York: Elsevier.

Reidel H-H, Lehmann-Willenbrock E, Conrad P & Semm K (1986) German pelviscopic statistics for the years 1978–1982. *Endoscopy* 18: 219–222.

Semm K & O'Neill-Freys I (1989) Conventional operative laparoscopy (pelviscopy). In Sutton CJG (ed.) *Laparoscopic Surgery. Baillière's Clinical Obstetrics and Gynaecology* 3, No. 3: 451–485.

Thompson BH & Wheeless CR Jr (1973) Gastrointestinal complications of laparoscopic sterilisation. *Obstetrics and Gynecology* 41: 669.

4

New Laparoscopic Techniques

HARRY REICH

Wyoming Valley GYN Associates, Kingston, Pennsylvania, USA

Operative laparoscopy requires another level of skill, facilities, and equipment far beyond the standard diagnostic and sterilization procedures of the 1970s and 1980s. Advanced laparoscopic surgery uses new techniques, similar to traditional techniques, to perform the same old procedure with better visualization. Laparoscopic procedures are not new procedures.

In the last 2 years, the general surgeon has incorporated laparoscopic surgery into accepted practice in their specialty. Over the past 20 years, the laparoscopic gynaecological surgeon has failed in this endeavour. The recent realization that the consumer will often elect a relatively non-invasive procedure over traditional surgery and the rapid expansion of the laparoscopic instrument and advertising (media) market will force the expert gynaecological surgeon to reconsider laparoscopy. Intraperitoneal laparoscopists should work together and laparoscopic surgery should become a specialty within itself: a fraternity of gynaecologists, general surgeons, urologists, and perhaps gastroenterologists.

This chapter will concentrate on laparoscopic techniques that are new to many surgeons, though some of these techniques have been known for over 20 years. Ideas and techniques are not listed in any particular order of importance and only reflect this author's preferences.

Preoperative Evaluation

Endovaginal ultrasound is done to evaluate the pelvis in cases involving a pelvic mass, retrocervical nodules, or fibroids. A CA-125 assay, which uses a monoclonal antibody that reacts to an antigen found in most non-mucinous ovarian cancers, is obtained when a mass is present. Intravenous pyelograms are rarely done preoperatively but should be obtained when abdominal pain persists after surgery on or near the ureter. Prior to laparoscopic surgery, there are no indications for CT scan or MRI that justify their expense; this author has no experience with these procedures and believes that laparoscopy is better for diagnosis.

Preoperative Preparation

Leuprolide acetate depot suspension (Lupron Depot), 3.75 mg i.m., is often administered after ovulation in the cycle preceding surgery to avoid operating on ovaries containing a corpus luteum. Patients are encouraged to hydrate and eat lightly for 24 hours before admission. When extensive cul-de-sac involvement with endometriosis is suspected, either clinically or from another doctor's operative record, a mechanical bowel preparation is advised (polyethylene glycol-based isosmotic solution: GOLYTELY or Colyte). Lower abdominal, pubic, and perineal hair is *not* shaved. Patients are encouraged to void on call to the OR, and a Foley catheter is inserted only if the bladder is distended or a long operation anticipated. Antibiotics (usually cefoxitin) are administered in all cases lasting more than 2 hours, at the 2-hour mark.

Equipment

High Flow CO₂ Insufflators

High flow CO_2 insufflation up to 10–15 l/min is necessary to compensate for the rapid loss of CO_2 during suctioning. Models to filter smoke produced by electrosurgery or laser from the CO_2 gas still work poorly. The ability to maintain a relatively constant intra-abdominal pressure between 10 and 15 mmHg during long laparoscopic procedures is essential. Higher pressure settings may be used during initial insertion of the trocar, with the setting lowered thereafter in order to diminish the development of subcutaneous emphysema. High pressure settings may be used to control venous bleeding, but only for short periods to avoid the possibility of CO_2 embolism and delayed bleeding.

30° Tiltable OR Table

Operating room tables capable of 30° Trendelenburg's position are extremely valuable for advanced laparoscopic surgical procedures, especially when the deep pelvis is involved. Unfortunately these tables are rare, and this author has much difficulty when operating in other institutions with the limited degree of body tilt that can be obtained.

For the past 16 years this author has used steep Trendelenburg's position (20–40°), with shoulder braces and the arms at the patient's sides. Presently, the hand-controlled Champagne model 600 (Affiliated Table Company, Rochester NY) is used; this author knows of no electronically controlled tables capable of this degree of body tilt. This author's patients have experienced no adverse effects from steep Trendelenburg's position.

Uterine Manipulators

A Valtchev uterine mobilizer (Conkin Surgical Instruments, Toronto, ON, Canada) is the best available single instrument to antevert the uterus and delineate the posterior vagina throughout complicated cases. The uterus can be anteverted to about 120° and moved in an arc about 45° to the left or right by turning the mobilizer around its longitudinal axis. Four interchangeable detachable uterine obturators of various length and diameter ranging from 3 mm thickness and 4.5 cm length to 10 mm thickness and 10 cm length are available. Two cannulas for injection of dye, measuring 3 mm thick by 3.5 or 5 cm in length, are also available.

With this device in the anteflexed position, the cervix sits on a wide acorn which is readily visible between the uterosacral ligaments when the cul-de-sac is inspected laparoscopically. The 100 mm length, 10 mm thick obturator is used for uterine manipulation during hysterectomy. The 50 mm length, 3 mm thick acorn cannula is used for most other procedures, including cul-de-sac dissections and as a backstop during laser culdotomies.

Rectal and Vaginal Probes

If a Valtchev uterine mobilizer is not available, a sponge on a ring forceps is inserted into the posterior vaginal fornix and a no. 81 French rectal probe (Reznik Instruments, Skokie, IL, USA) is placed in the rectum to define the rectum and posterior vagina in endometriosis and adhesion cases with some degree of cul-de-sac obliteration and to open the posterior vagina (culdotomy). In addition, a no. 3 or 4 Sims curette or Hulka uterine elevator is placed in the endometrial cavity to antevert the uterus markedly and stretch out the cul-de-sac. The rectal probe and intraoperative rectovaginal examinations remain important techniques even when the Valtchev is available. Whenever rectal location is in doubt, it is identified by placing a probe.

Trocar Sleeves

Trocar sleeves are available in many sizes and shapes. For most cases, 5.5 mm cannulas are adequate. Newer electrosurgical electrodes which eliminate capacitance and insulation failures (Electroshield from Electroscope, Boulder, CO, USA) will require 7/8 mm sleeves. Laparoscopic stapling is performed through 12/13 mm ports.

Short trapless 5 mm trocar sleeves with a retention screw grid around its external surface are used (Richard Wolf, Vernon Hills, IL, USA; Apple Medical, Bolton, MA, USA). These trocar sleeves facilitate efficient instrument exchanges and evacuation of tissue while allowing unlimited freedom during extracorporeal suture tying. With practice, a good laparoscopic surgical team makes instrument exchanges so fast that little pneumo-peritoneum is lost. Once placed, their portal of exit stays fixed at the level of the anterior abdominal wall parietal peritoneum, permitting more room for instrument manipulation (Reich and McGlynn, 1990).

US Surgical disposable trocar sleeves with adjustable locking retention collars (Reich screw grid design) hold their position well for stapling, but their trap makes extracorporeal suturing cumbersome. Their retention collars are used to prevent any company's 10 mm trocar sleeve from sliding out of the umbilicus and to stabilize their 12.5 mm sleeve during stapling.

Positioning of Patient

All laparoscopic surgical procedures are done under general anaesthesia with endotracheal intubation and an *orogastric* tube. The routine use of an orogastric tube is recommended to diminish the possibility of a trocar injury to the stomach and to reduce small bowel distension. The patient is flat (0°) until after the umbilical trocar sleeve has been inserted and then placed in steep Trendelenburg's position (20–30°). Lith-otomy position with the hip extended (thigh parallel to abdomen) is obtained with Allen stirrups (Edgewater Medical Systems, Mayfield Heights, OH, USA) or knee braces, which are adjusted to each individual patient before she is anaesthetized. Anaesthesia examination is always performed prior to preparing the patient.

Positioning of Video Equipment

The video monitor is placed opposite the surgeon if only one is available. The monitor is on the patient's right, the surgeon on her left, and a specially trained assistant between the patient's legs. The circulating nurse tends the video recorder (two tapes: one for the patient and the other for the surgeon), irrigation supply, laser, etc. This arrangement requires some hand–eye adjustment for the surgeon, since the monitor is rotated 90° from the plane of surgery. However, it avoids neck and back strain from twisting to see a monitor placed between the patient's legs, especially if the surgeon operates with instruments in the left hand and laparoscope in the right. Hand–eye coordination (almost mirror-

image) is extremely difficult for the assistant, who often assumes a passive role of maintaining retraction or grasper positions achieved by the surgeon. Mirror-image operating skills are attain-able after extensive training and will greatly increase the efficiency of the surgical team.

Scrubbing

Laparoscopy was never thought to be a sterile procedure before the incorporation of video with the laparoscope, as the surgeon operated with his head in the surgical field, attached to the laparoscopic optic. Since 1983, this author has maintained a policy of not scrubbing for laparos-copy and not sterilizing or draping the camera or laser arm. Infection has been rare: less than one per 200 cases. This author attributes this to his policy of absolute haemostasis *per* underwater examination, copious irrigation and clot evacu-ation, and leaving 2–4 litres of Ringer's lactate in the peritoneal cavity at the end of each operation. Bacteria grow poorly in Ringer's lactate solution especially if all blood clot is evacuated from the peritoneal cavity. The umbilical incision is closed with a single 4–0 Vicryl suture opposing deep fascia and skin dermis, with the knot buried beneath the fascia to prevent the suture from acting like a wick to transmit bacteria into the soft tissue or peritoneal cavity.

Hysteroscopy

CO_2 hysteroscopy is done on all laparoscopic surgical patients with a uterus while pneumoperi-toneum is being developed to 20–25 mmHg for safe trocar insertion. All indicated hysteroscopic surgery is done after the laparoscopic portion of the case using the resectoscope attached to a continuous flow controlled distension irrigation system (CDIS, Zimmer, Warsaw, IN, USA), which pumps sorbitol into the uterus for distension at a constant intrauterine pressure of 80 mmHg. Two new techniques were recently introduced to increase safety during high-voltage resectoscope surgery.

Bulldog Clamps

Prior to resectoscope myomectomy procedures, tubal lavage with indigo carmine dye is done.

Visualization of blue dye in the infundibulopelvic ligament vessels during tubal lavage signifies direct communication to the venous system, making fluid overload likely. When this dye is seen coursing through the infundibulopelvic ligament vessels, bulldog clamps inserted through the 10 mm umbilical cannula are applied to the infundibulopelvic ligaments to decrease the risk of fluid overload in these high-risk women.

Underwater Resectoscope Surgery

The uterus is submerged in an isotonic electrolyte solution instilled laparoscopically to prevent thermal burn of intraperitoneal organs by dispersing current near the uterine serosa. For endometrial ablation, high voltage electrosurgery is used: 80 W of spray coagulation current from an Aspen laboratory electrosurgical generator (5000 V peak) through a resectoscope roller cylinder (Wolf). For fibroids, 100–140 W cutting current is used through a wire loop electrode for cutting and 60–80 W coagulation current for fulguration of bleeding vessels.

Incisions

For most pelvic procedures, the operative incisions are limited to three: 10 mm umbilical, 5 mm right, and 5 mm left lower quadrant. Three puncture sites in the anterior abdominal wall are sufficient for 90% of laparoscopic procedures. Large puncture sites or incisions bordering on minilaparotomy for tissue extraction should be replaced by an umbilical extension or a laparoscopic culdotomy approach.

Lower Quadrant Lateral to the Deep Epigastric Vessels

Placement of the lower quadrant trocar sleeves lateral to the deep epigastric vessels and just above the pubic hairline is preferred, as it avoids the rectus muscle, while making a tract through the external oblique, internal oblique, and transversalis fascia, which is easily identifiable for replacement of the trocar sleeve during suturing and specimen excision. These vessels, an artery flanked by two veins (venae comitantes), are located by direct inner laparoscopic inspection of the anterior abdominal wall. They are found lateral to the lateral umbilical ligament (obliterated umbilical artery), and cannot be consistently found by traditional transillumination. The left lower quadrant puncture is the major portal for operative manipulation. The right trocar sleeve is used for atraumatic grasping forceps to retract tissues as needed.

Ninth Intercostal Space

Special entry techniques are necessary in patients who have undergone multiple laparotomies, or who may have extensive adhesions either clinically or from another doctor's operative record. If CO_2 insufflation is not obtainable through the umbilicus, Veress needle puncture is done in the left ninth intercostal space, anterior axillary line. The trocar is then inserted at the left costal margin in the midclavicular line, giving a panoramic view of the entire peritoneal cavity. Likewise when extensive adhesions are encountered initially surrounding the umbilical puncture, the surgeon should immediately seek a higher site. Thereafter, the adhesions can be freed down to and just beneath the umbilicus, at which time it becomes possible to establish the umbilical portal for further work.

Operative Techniques

Advanced laparoscopic surgical techniques used include aquadissection, scissors dissection, electrosurgery, laser, and suturing. Aquadissection and scissors dissection are used in preference to thermal energy sources.

Aquadissection

Aquadissection is broadly defined as the use of hydraulic energy from pressurized fluid to aid in the performance of surgical procedures. It differs from mechanical energy applied with a blunt probe, which is a unidirectional force, the direct prolongation of the surgeon's hand. The force vector with hydraulic energy is multidirectional within the volume of expansion of the noncompressible fluid. Installation of fluid under pressure displaces tissue, often resulting in the fluid creating cleavage planes in the least resistant spaces. In addition, the instillation of fluid under pressure into closed spaces or behind enclosed areas of adhesions produces oedematous, distended tissue on tension and with loss of elasticity, making further division easy and safe using blunt dissection, scissors dissection, laser, or electrosurgery.

Aquadissectors (suction-irrigators with the ability to dissect using pressurized fluid) should have a single channel to maximize suctioning and irrigating capacity. Separate suction and irrigation channels, either side by side or one inside the other, result in diminished suction capacity and reduced hydraulic effect. An aquadissector with a solid (not perforated) distal tip is necessary to perform atraumatic suction–traction–retraction, irrigate directly, and develop surgical planes (aquadissection). Small holes at the tip impede these actions and serve no purpose.

The Aqua-Purator (WISAP, Tomball, Texas, USA) was the first of the aquadissection devices. It delivers fluid under 200 mmHg pressure at a rate of 250 ml/10 s. One litre can be instilled in 35 seconds. The handle of the Aqua-Purator uses large staples to occlude separate suction and irrigation tubing, each of which funnels into a single-channelled tube. Aquadissection has not changed since this author's previous review (Reich, 1990); the market is crowded with other aquadissection devices, none of which comes near the suction and irrigating speed of the original.

Scissors that Cut

Scissors that actually cut most of the time are truly a new laparoscopic technique. Sharp dissection is the primary technique used for adhesiolysis to diminish the potential for adhesion formation; electrosurgery and laser are usually reserved for haemostasis. Straight scissors, 5 mm, with blunt, rounded, or sharp tips, are used to lyse thin and thick bowel adhesions sharply. Since scissors notoriously become dull after processing between cases, a large number and variety should be available to assure that some will cut. Blunt tipped, sawtooth scissors (Wolf), Manhes scissors (Storz, Culver City, CA, USA), and US Surgical disposable scissors all cut. Hook scissors are used when the surgeon can get completely around the structure being divided, but rarely maintain their sharpness.

Electrosurgery (Odell, 1987)

Electrosurgical knowledge and skill are essential. The terms 'cautery' and 'diathermy', when referring to electrosurgery, should be abandoned. Unipolar *cutting* current has been used by this author for 15 years without any complications from this energy source. More effective surgery can be done with electrosurgery than with a fibre laser. Electrosurgery at laparoscopy is safer than at laparotomy as it takes 30% more power to spark or arc in CO_2 than in room air; at the same electrosurgical power setting, less arcing occurs at laparoscopy.

Cutting current is used to both cut and coagulate, depending on the configuration of the electrode in contact with the tissue. The tip cuts, while the wide body coagulates. Unipolar *coagulation current* is used in close proximity to tissue, but not in contact, to fulgurate. This waveform uses voltages over 10 times that of cutting current and should not be used in contact with tissue. Coagulation current is modulated so that it is on only 6% of the time. The high voltage allows it to arc or spark for 1–2 mm, producing very good haemostasis with venous and arteriolar bleeding.

Bipolar desiccation for large vessel haemostasis of uterine and ovarian vessels has been done since 1983 (Reich and McGlynn, 1986; Reich, 1987). A more uniform bipolar desiccation process is obtained using a cutting current. Coagulating current is not used as it quickly desiccates the outer layers of the tissue, producing superficial resistance which may prevent deeper penetration. Large blood vessels are compressed and bipolar *cutting* current passed until complete desiccation is achieved, i.e. the current depletes tissue fluid and electrolytes until it ceases to flow between the forceps as determined by an ammeter or current flow meter (end-point monitor: Electroscope EPM-1, Boulder, CO, USA). In most cases, three contiguous areas are desiccated. Complete end-point desiccation results in full thickness coagulation (Soderstrom and Levy, 1987; Soderstrom *et al.*, 1989) fusion of collagen and elastic fibres (Sigel and Dunn, 1965), and vessel weld strength (Harrison and Morris, 1991). The ammeter provides a scientific measurement of complete coaptive desiccation, allowing the surgeon to make an objective decision of how much current is enough and when it is safest to divide. This author uses his right foot to activate the CO_2 laser, his left foot for the bipolar electrosurgical pedal, and hand controls for unipolar electrodes.

Argon Beam Coagulation

Beacon Labs (Boulder, CO, USA) made the first argon beam coagulator for laparoscopic use at this author's request in April, 1990. It uses argon gas at 2 l/min and high-voltage coagulation current to increase the spark or arc possible with conventional fulguration while penetrating the tissue very superficially.

Advantages of the argon beam coagulator include the ability to clear the operative site of surface blood and fluids, making the bleeding vessel or rent in that vessel visible by the gentle flow of argon gas as it moves towards the tissue, but before it is close enough to activate current. Conventional spray coagulation current at 80 W will arc approximately 1 cm through the argon gas with resultant superficial charring and haemostasis. As argon is cooler than CO_2, there is less smoke generated than with a conventional electrode. Uses include intraovarian bleeding after cystectomy, uterine haemostasis after myomectomy, and pelvic haemostasis after hysterectomy and endometriosis surgery.

Laser

Laser to this author means CO_2 laser. The physics are wrong with the fibre lasers as they coagulate before they cut and lack the precision and the ability that CO_2 laser possesses to operate across space. Some laser companies marketed their fibre laser line by not addressing surgeons' concerns with poor CO_2 laser beam alignment. Many surgeons put them in the corner and went to fibres. Others put an ice-pack between the laserscope coupler and their hand to prevent skin burns when using lasers with large raw beams and beam–coupler mismatches. The newer CO_2 lasers from Coherent (Palo Alto, CA, USA), Heraeus Lasersonics (Milpitas, CA, USA), and Sharplan (Tel Aviv, Israel) are fantastic instruments that do very fine work in an uncluttered field with a collimated (parallel) beam travelling through the operating channel of the laparoscope.

The passage of CO_2 gas through the laparoscope lumen, presently a necessity to purge this channel of debris, results in a decrease in both power delivered to tissue and power density at tissue because the 10.6 μm wavelength of the laser beam is the same as that of the purge gas. Power to tissue is reduced by 30–50% with a 7.2 mm laparoscopic operating channel (12 mm scope) and by 60% with a 5 mm operating channel (10 mm scope) (Reich et al., 1991b). While it is desirable to operate at high power density for a short time to minimize damage to surrounding tissue, the passage of CO_2 gas through the laparoscope lumen results in an increase in spot size and thus a reduction in power density (the concentration of laser energy on the tissue) at higher power settings. At high power settings with the CO_2 laser (80–100 W), a very large spot

size, 3–4 mm, is obtained which is extremely coagulative and provides very good haemostatic cutting. Considering these limitations with a Sharplan 1100 laser (Tel Aviv, Israel) through a 10 mm laparoscope with 5 mm operating channel, a setting of 20–35 W in superpulse mode is used for most procedures (<1000 W/cm² at the tissue) at between 80 and 100 W continuous mode to obtain a diffuse haemostatic effect for myomectomy and culdotomy.

Coherent has recently advanced CO_2 laser technology by modifying the 10.6 μm wavelength to 11.1 μm, resulting in little interference in power transmission from the purge gas (Ultrapulse 5000L). With this modification, settings of 10–20 W ultrapulse are used for precise cutting and 50–80 W for extirpative procedures. Also little power is lost in the Coherent coupler from the 6 mm raw beam.

Superpulse mode implies very high power (500 W), low-energy pulse released for brief surges (<50 mJ), theoretically allowing tissue to cool between spikes to reduce surrounding thermal effect. Ultrapulse delivers short duration high-energy pulses (>200 mJ) at the same high power (500 W), allowing longer cooling intervals between pulses with resultant reduced heat conduction and char-free vaporization. At the same average power, the superpulsed laser must produce five pulses to deliver as much energy as one ultrapulse.

Heraeus LaserSonics (Milpitas, CA) and Sharplan Laser (Tel Aviv, Israel) have recently introduced defocusing couplers for laparoscopy. With the Sharplan CVD (Continuously Variable Defocus) system, spot size can be controlled to obtain a 1 mm spot size for cutting and a much larger defocused spot size for coagulation (0.6–4.0 mm). Heraeus LaserSonics maintains a small spot size by performing rapid exchanges of gas through the operating channel of the operating laparoscope. This gas is exchanged faster than it can be heated up, a technique which also minimizes smoke in the peritoneal cavity while actively using the laser.

Suturing

Suturing is not as new as some like to think it is. A knot-pusher (Marlow Surgical, Willoughby, OH, USA) is used to tie in a manner very similar to the way one would hand tie suture at open laparotomy. This technique was developed in 1970 by H. Courtenay Clarke (Clarke, 1972). This device is just like an extension of the surgeon's fingers.

To suture with a straight needle (Figure 4.1),

Figure 4.1 (A) Clarke Knot-Pusher. (B) Application to a single tie. (C) The first throw of the knot is passed through the trapless trocar sleeve. (D) The second throw is passed through the trocar sleeve to secure the first. Reprinted with permission from The American College of Obstetricians and Gynecologists (*Obstetrics and Gynecology*, 1992, **79**: 143–147).

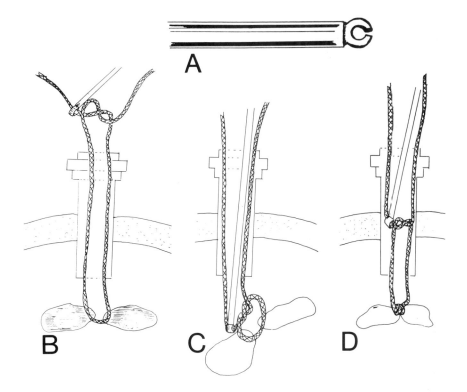

the surgeon applies the suture to the tissue, pulls the needle outside, and then, while holding both strands, makes a simple half-hitch, but not a surgeon's knot, which will not slip as well. The Clarke Knot-Pusher (Marlow Surgical) is put on the suture held firmly across the index finger and the throw is pushed down to the tissue. A square knot is made by pushing another half-hitch down to the knot to secure it, while exerting tension from above. Suture tying outside the peritoneal cavity is made easy by using trocar sleeves without traps, as traps make it very hard to slip knots down from outside the peritoneal cavity.

The Endoloop (Ethicon, Somerville, NJ, USA) and Surgitie ligating loop (US Surgical) are preformed knotted loops designed to fit over vascular pedicles and then be tightened. Over the last 15 years, this author has used it for appendectomies and omentectomies, but never for oophorectomy. Bipolar desiccation works better and eliminates any chance of slippage. Postoperative pelvic pain is less in desiccated pedicles; an endolooped pedicle leaves living cells distal to the loop to necrose, releasing lysozymes.

Recently, a technique to put any size curved needle into the peritoneal cavity through a 5 mm lower quadrant incision has been developed (Reich *et al.*, 1992). To do it, the lower abdominal incisions are placed lateral to the deep epigastric vessels, and, thus, lateral to the rectus muscle, as previously described. Upon removing the trocar sleeve, a tract is obvious and is very easy to get back into. To suture with a CT-1 needle, the

trocar sleeve taken out of the abdomen and loaded by grasping the end of the suture with a needle holder, pulling it through the trocar sleeve, reinserting the instrument into the sleeve, and grasping the suture about 2–3 cm from the needle (Figure 4.2). The needle driver is inserted into the peritoneal cavity through the original tract, as visualized on the monitor and the needle follows. Even large needles can be pulled into the peritoneal cavity in this manner. At this stage, the Semm straight needle holder is replaced with a Cook curved needle driver (Cook OB/GYN, Cook Urological, Spencer, IN, USA), and the needle driven through the tissue (Figure 4.3). Afterward, the needle is stored in the anterior abdominal wall parietal peritoneum (like a pincushion) for later removal after the suture is tied (Figure 4.4). The needle is cut, the cut end of the suture pulled out of the peritoneal cavity, and the knot tied with the Clarke Knot-Pusher. To retrieve the needle, the trocar sleeve is unscrewed after which the needle holder inside it pulls the needle through the soft tissue (Figure 4.5). The trocar sleeve is replaced with or without another suture.

Staples

The latest advance in laparoscopy surgery is the development of stapling devices. Disposable stapling instrumentation is used for large vessel haemostasis during laparoscopic cholecystectomy, oophorectomy, and hysterectomy.

Figure 4.2 (A) Short trocar sleeve in place. (B) Distal suture is loaded into the sleeve removed from the peritoneal cavity. (C) The suture is grasped 3 cm from the curved needle. Reprinted with permission from The American College of Obstetricians and Gynecologists (*Obstetrics and Gynecology*, 1992, **79**: 143–147).

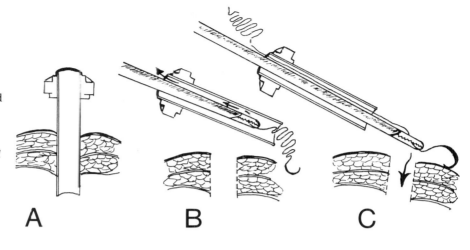

A   B   C

Figure 4.3 (A) Needle-holder is directed back through the original incision. (B) The sleeve is replaced over the needle-holder. (C) Suture is applied with the curved needle-holder. Reprinted with permission from The American College of Obstetricians and Gynecologists (*Obstetrics and Gynecology*, 1992, **79**: 143–147).

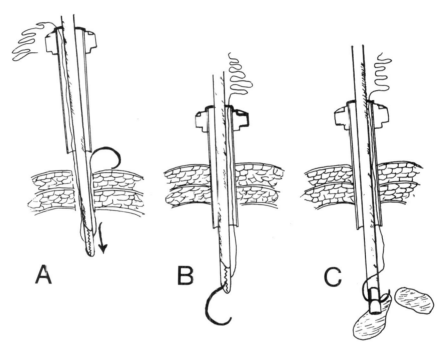

A   B   C

An automatic clip applier (Auto Suture ENDO CLIP Applier) stacks 20 clips of medium to large size (9 mm long when closed), which are made of titanium, an inert, non-reactive metal. The disposable loaded unit is designed for introduction through a 12 mm trocar sleeve. Skeletonization of vessels is necessary prior to application of this staple. When applied to vessels with overlying peritoneum, the staple will frequently slip off during further manipulation of the tissue.

A laparoscopic stapler (MULTI-FIRE ENDO GIA 30) places six rows of titanium staples, 3 cm in length, and simultaneously divides the clamped tissue. It consists of a disposable handle and shaft, the end of which contains a replaceable single-use stapling cartridge. The standard staple compresses on firing to 1.5 mm, while the vascular cartridge compresses to 1 mm. The disposable

handle is designed to fire up to four staple cartridges through a 12 mm cannula before being discarded. This instrument functions similarly to the gastrointestinal anastomosis stapler (GIA) that thoracic and general surgeons have used for the past 25 years.

This author worked with US Surgical in 1988, developing clips and staples for laparoscopic gynaecological work. Unfortunately, these products were never used in protocol studies, because the general surgeons entered the laparoscopic cholecystectomy market. US Surgical had clips available when laparoscopic cholecystectomy was first performed because they were developing them for gynaecology. The MULTI-FIRE ENDO GIA 30 stapler has just become available, though both devices were to be released at the same time. They had difficulty keeping up with the

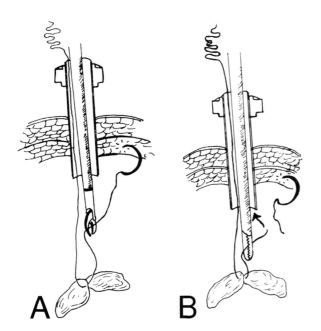

Figure 4.4 (A) Suture is cut 3 cm from the needle. (B) The cut end is pulled through the trocar sleeve and the needle is placed in the parietal peritoneum. Reprinted with permission from The American College of Obstetricians and Gynecologists (*Obstetrics and Gynecology,* 1992, **79**: 143–147).

demand for the Endoclip. The Endo-GIA is a very welcome addition in gynaecology, especially for hysterectomy with ovarian preservation, as it will divide the pedicle next to the uterus, the utero-ovarian ligament, very precisely; it was first used in laparoscopy by this author for appendectomy on 9 August, 1990 and two hysterectomies on 29 August, 1990.

During laparoscopic hysterectomy, the Endo-GIA is applied to the utero-ovarian ligament, round ligament, and fallopian tube pedicle. The Endoclip may be used to ligate the uterine artery after both it and the ureter have been skeletonized. Ureteral dissection should be an integral part of laparoscopic hysterectomy to prevent ureteral injury during uterine artery ligation.

Culdotomy (Reich, 1989)

A posterior *culdotomy* incision using CO_2 laser or electrosurgery through the cul-de-sac of Douglas into the vagina is preferable to a *colpotomy* incision using scissors through the vagina and overlying peritoneum because complete haemostasis is obtained while making the culdotomy incision. Vaginal bleeding greater than 100 ml is usual before all cuff bleeding is stopped after scissors colpotomy.

Despite frequent culdotomy incisions and a

relatively non-sterile technique, infection is rare. The culdotomy incision is closed from below or laparoscopically with interrupted, figure-of-eight, or running 0–Vicryl suture. Vaginal suturing is aided by the use of a lateral vaginal retractor used to spread the lateral vagina adjacent to the culdotomy incision (Euro-Med, Redmond, WA, USA; Simpson/Basye, Wilmington, DE, USA). This device is self-retaining with a thumb-ratchet release that keeps it open and in place. Vaginal suturing can be difficult if the vaginal incision becomes oedematous during the procedure, making exposure inadequate. In these cases, the surgeon may elect to close the culdotomy incision from above using 1–3 curved needle sutures (Vicryl on a CT-2) tied extracorporeally with the Clarke Knot-Pusher.

Tissue Removal

Specimens slightly larger than the 5 mm trocar channel are often removed by slipping the trocar sleeve upward on the biopsy forceps shaft out of the peritoneal cavity and then pulling the biopsy forceps with specimen out in one motion through the soft tissue of the anterior abdominal wall. The biopsy forceps are then reinserted through their exit tract and the trocar sleeve pushed back into the peritoneal cavity over the forceps.

Larger masses are removed through a cul-de-sac culdotomy. A new technique for unruptured ovaries or cysts is to insert an impermeable sac (LapSac: Cook OB/GYN) intraperitoneally through the culdotomy incision. This 5 × 8 inch nylon bag has a polyurethane inner coating and a nylon drawstring. It is impermeable to water and dye. The ovary with intact cyst is placed in the bag which is closed by pulling its drawstring. The sac is delivered by the drawstring through the posterior vagina, the bag opened and the intact specimen visually identified, decompressed, and removed.

For fibroids (or a large fibroid uterus), an 11 mm corkscrew device is screwed into the myoma vaginally through the culdotomy incision, the myoma put on traction, and further morcellated vaginally with scissors or scalpel if necessary until removal is completed. This can be a particularly time-consuming portion of the procedure. It is wise to change from laparoscopic stirrups (Allan stirrups or knee supports) to candy cane stirrups to obtain better hip flexion to permit assistance with vaginal sidewall retractors during long procedures. Self-retaining lateral vaginal wall retractors or Vienna retractors (Breisky-Navatril vaginal specula: Baxter Health Care Corp, McGaw

Figure 4.5 (A) Knot placement. (B) The needle end is retrieved. (C) The needle is removed from the peritoneal cavity after withdrawing the trocar sleeve, which is then replaced. Reprinted with permission from The American College of Obstetricians and Gynecologists (*Obstetrics and Gynecology*, 1992, **79**: 143–147).

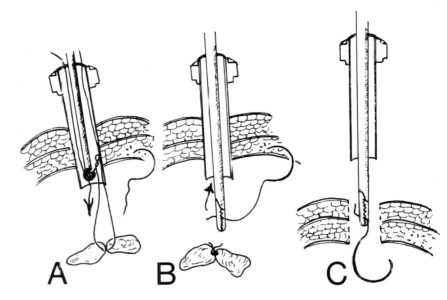

Park IL, USA) are considered for shorter procedures.

While morcellation of fibroids through anterior abdominal wall puncture sites is not practical with presently available instruments, future developments should solve this problem for the gynaecologist. Professor Semm and WISAP have recently developed a manual circular saw to core out 2 mm cylinders of fibromyomatous tissue while the fibroid is still in or attached to the uterus. This device is inserted through a 2 cm lower abdominal trocar sleeve and depends on a corkscrew inside it to fixate the fibroid prior to twisting the circular saw into it. Loss of resistance during the twisting indicates the base of the fibroid after which the cylindrical specimen is pulled free by traction, the specimen removed, and the instrument reinserted. After the bulk of the lesion is removed in this fashion, a claw forceps is substituted for the corkscrew in the device for traction and the compressible, fenestrated, remaining tissue is removed from the uterus through the 2 cm cannula. Professor Semm accomplishes supracervical hysterectomy using this same device after coring out the endocervical canal with a 1 cm circular saw. These 2 cm puncture sites require direct peritoneal and/or fascial closure with skin hooks to prevent hernias.

Cook Urological has developed a 1 cm motorized circular saw with suction for laparoscopic nephrectomy. After placement of the kidney into the LapSac, it is morcellated into small soft pieces which are sucked into the device until the LapSac is small enough to be pulled out of the umbilicus. This author has used this instrument for myoma morcellation during laparoscopic hysterectomy and myomectomy, and for fibroma oophorectomy. We are currently working on 2 and 3 cm versions for culdotomy morcellation.

Underwater Surgery at the End of Each Procedure (Reich, 1989)

At the close of each operation, an underwater examination is used to document complete intraperitoneal haemostasis in stages; this detects bleeding from vessels and viscera tamponaded during the procedure by the increased intraperitoneal pressure of the CO_2 pneumoperitoneum. The CO_2 pneumoperitoneum is displaced with 2–5 litres of Ringer's lactate solution, and the peritoneal cavity is vigorously irrigated and suctioned with this solution until the effluent is clear of blood products, usually after 10–20 litres. Underwater inspection of the pelvis is performed to detect any further bleeding which is controlled using the Vancaillie microbipolar forceps (Storz) to coagulate through the electrolyte solution.

First, complete haemostasis is established with the patient in Trendelenburg's position. Next, complete haemostasis is secured *per* underwater examination with the patient supine and in reverse Trendelenburg using underwater microbipolar coagulation. Finally, complete haemostasis is documented with all instruments removed, including the uterine manipulator.

To visualize the pelvis with the patient supine, the 10 mm straight laparoscope and the aquadissector are manipulated together into the deep cul-de-sac beneath floating bowel and omentum, and this area is alternately irrigated and suctioned until the effluent is clear both in the pelvis and the upper abdomen. During this copious irrigation procedure, clear fluid is deposited into the pelvis and circulates into the upper abdomen, displacing upper abdominal bloody fluid which is suctioned after flowing back into the pelvis. An 'underwater' examination is then performed to observe the completely separated tubes and ovaries and to confirm complete haemostasis.

The 'chopstick' manoeuvre refers to the synchronized moving of the actively irrigating aquadissector tip just in front of the distal end of the laparoscope to maintain a clear underwater view in a bloody field deep in the pelvis. Bloody fluid is diluted, circulated and aspirated. Individual blood clots are isolated, usually in the pararectosigmoid gutters, and aspirated.

A final copious lavage with Ringer's lactate solution is undertaken and all clot directly aspirated; at least 2 litres of lactated Ringer's solution are left in the peritoneal cavity to displace CO_2 and to prevent fibrin adherences from forming by separating raw operated-upon surfaces during the initial stages of reperitonealization. No other anti-adhesive agents are employed. No drains, antibiotic solutions, or heparin are used.

Adhesion Prevention

Dr Jaroslav Hulka said in 1988 that 'Reich's solution to pollution is dilution', and that opinion has not changed. This author currently believes that the following will reduce adhesions: a reduction of thermal damage to tissue, absolute haemostasis, clot evacuation, copious irrigation to dilute fibrin and prostaglandins arising from operated surfaces and bacteria, and leaving 2–4 litres of Ringer's lactate in the peritoneal cavity at the end of each operation to physically separate normal and compromised structures. Currently, lactated Ringer's solution (1–2 litres) postoperatively is widely used but has rarely been prospectively studied. Rose determined by weighing patients that lactated Ringer's solution is absorbed over 2–3 days (Rose et al., 1991).

The GORE-TEX Surgical Membrane is probably the best of the presently available surgical barriers. It is a non-absorbable inert membrane with pore size less than 1 μm. It is used after division of severe adhesions, e.g. retroperitoneal ovary, and is sutured in place. It is this author's belief that *Interceed* is impossible to use successfully laparoscopically as it requires absolute haemostasis at the applied site and no fluid. Bleeding from vessels and viscera tamponaded during the procedure by the increased intraperitoneal pressure of the CO_2 pneumoperitoneum cannot be detected without an underwater examination. This author suspects that bleeding from a raw site after the pneumoperitoneum is expelled results in the filling of the Interceed with blood, making it adhesiogenic.

Bowel Injury

Gastrointestinal injuries may occur during laparoscopic surgery, and the surgeon should be familiar with their management, in many cases laparotomy can be avoided, regardless of specialty training. Treatment of gynaecological conditions like rectal endometriosis requires special understanding. This author did the first laparoscopic repair of a small bowel trocar perforation in July 1988 and a planned full thickness resection of deep fibrotic rectal endometriosis in August 1989 (Reich et al., 1991a).

Small bowel perforation occurs at laparoscopic surgery while inserting umbilical or lower quadrant trocars in cases involving extensive small bowel adhesions. Small bowel perforation during small bowel adhesiolysis surgery for pain secondary to adhesions from multiple previous laparotomies is common, occurring in over 25% of these procedures. Despite the application of traction and countertraction to each adhesion, bowel punctures are inevitable as these adhesions are carefully cut.

Following recognition of a small bowel perforation, it can be repaired transversely with interrupted 3–0 Vicryl, silk, or PDS on a taper SH needle tied either externally or with intracorporeal instruments. Sterile milk is instilled into the bowel lumen prior to the closing of the last suture to detect leakage from the laceration and occult perforations near the small bowel mesentery.

In the bowel-prepared patient, injury to the anterior rectum can usually be repaired laparoscopically. Full-thickness penetration of the rectum may occur during the excision of rectal nodules of endometriosis. After excision of the nodule and identification of the rent in the rectum, a single or double-layered repair is done using 3–0 silk, Vicryl, PDS, or the MULTI-FIRE ENDO GIA 30. Stay sutures are placed at the transverse angles of the defect and brought out through the lower quadrant trocar sleeves which are then replaced in the peritoneal cavity over the stay suture. After closure, povidone-iodine (Betadine) solution is injected into the rectum through a no. 26 F Foley catheter with a 30 ml balloon, and an underwater examination is done to check for any leaks, which, if seen, are then reinforced. This author has had no late sequelae following five such procedures.

Concerning the unprepared bowel, the decision whether to repair laparoscopically depends on the amount of faecal spillage present. Should a large amount of faecal contamination occur, laparotomy followed by repair should be considered. Laparoscopic suture closure followed by copious irrigation until the effluent clears, may be satisfactory. We have found little indication for colostomy during the repair of bowel injuries noted during the course of a laparoscopic procedure.

The practice of performing a colostomy during treatment of bowel injury began following the report of Ogilvie who reported significant reductions in mortality following treatment of colon injuries during World War II (Ogilvie, 1944). In fact in 1943, the Surgeon General of the United States issued an order that all colon injuries sustained in battle should be treated by performing a colostomy (Office of the Surgeon General, 1943). In 1951, Woodhall and Ochsner reported their experience with primary repair without colostomy: their mortality rate fell from 23% to 9% with primary repair (Woodhall and Ochsner, 1951). In 1979, Stone and Fabian reported the first well controlled prospective randomized study on primary closure of traumatic colon perforations. Morbidity for the randomized colostomy group was 10-fold higher and average hospital stay 6 days longer (Stone and Fabian, 1979). Similar results were obtained by George *et al.* and Burch *et al.* (Burch *et al.*, 1986; George *et al.*, 1989). Thus, this author finds little indication for colostomy during the repair of bowel injuries noted during the course of a laparoscopic procedure.

References

Burch JM, Brock JC, Gevirtzman L et al. (1986) The injured colon. *Annals of Surgery* **203(6)** 701.

Clarke HC (1972) Laparoscopy—new instruments for suturing and ligation. *Fertility and Sterility* **23**: 274–277.

George SM Jr, Fabian TC, Voeller GR et al. (1989) Primary repair of colon wounds. *Annals of Surgery* **209(6)**: 728.

Harrison JD & Morris DL (1991) Does bipolar electrocoagulation time affect vessel weld strength? *Gut* **32(2)**: 188–190.

Odell R (1987) Principles of electrosurgery. In Sivak

M (ed.) *Gastroenterologic Endoscopy*, pp. 128–142. Philadelphia W.B. Saunders Company.

Office of the Surgeon General (1943) Circulation Letter, no. 178: October 23, 1943.

Ogilvie WH (1944) Abdominal wounds in the Western Desert. *Surgery, Gynecology and Obstetrics* **78**: 225.

Reich H (1987) Laparoscopic oophorectomy and salpingo-oophorectomy in the treatment of benign tubo-ovarian disease. *International Journal of Fertility* **32**: 233–236.

Reich H (1989) New techniques in advanced laparoscopic surgery. In Sutton C (ed.) Baillière's *Clinical Obstetrics and Gynaecology* 3, **No. 3**: 655–681.

Reich H (1990) Aquadissection. In Baggish M (ed.) *Laser Endoscopy*, The Clinical Practice of Gynecology series, pp. 159–185. New York: Elsevier.

Reich H & McGlynn F (1986) Laparoscopic oophorectomy and salpingo-oophorectomy in the treatment of benign tuboovarian disease. *Journal of Reproductive Medicine* **31**: 609.

Reich H & McGlynn F (1990) Short self-retaining trocar sleeves for laparoscopic surgery. *American Journal of Obstetrics and Gynecology* **162(2)**: 453.

Reich H, McGlynn F & Budin R (1991a) Laparoscopic repair of full-thickness bowel injury. *Journal of Laparoendoscopic Surgery* **1**: 119.

Reich H, MacGregor TS & Vancaillie TG (1991b) CO_2 laser used through the operating channel of laser laparoscopes: *in vitro* study of power and power density losses. *Obstetrics and Gynecology* **77**: 40–47.

Reich H, Clarke HC & Sekel L (1992) A simple method for ligating in operative laparoscopy with straight and curved needles. *Obstetrics and Gynecology* **79**: 143–147.

Rose BI, MacNeill C, Larrain R & Kopreski MM (1991) Abdominal instillation of high-molecular-weight dextran or lactated Ringer's solution after laparoscopic surgery: a randomized comparison of the effect on weight change. *Journal of Reproductive Medicine* **36**: 537–539.

Sigel B & Dunn MR (1965) The mechanism of blood vessel closure by high frequency electrocoagulation. *Surgery, Gynecology and Obstetrics* **10**: 823–831.

Soderstrom RM & Levy BS (1987) Bipolar systems—do they perform? *Obstetrics and Gynecology* **69**: 425–426.

Soderstrom RM, Levy BS & Engel T (1989) Reducing bipolar sterilization failures. *Obstetrics and Gynecology* **74**: 60–63.

Stone HH & Fabian TC (1979) Management of perforating colon trauma. *Annals of Surgery* **190(4)**: 430.

Woodhall JP & Ochsner A (1951) The management of perforating injuries of the colon and rectum in civilian practice. *Surgery* **29**: 305.

5

Delivery Systems for Laser Laparoscopy

Y. TADIR, J. NEEV AND M.W. BERNS

Beckman Laser Institute and Medical Clinic, University of California, Irvine, California, USA

Lasers are now frequently used in gynaecological endoscopic surgery. However, since the first introduction of carbon dioxide (CO_2) laser-operative laparoscopes (Bruhat *et al.*, 1979) and the design of special laser delivery cannula inserted at a separate suprapubic puncture (Tadir *et al.*, 1981), there have been many modifications in this surgical modality. Other laser wavelengths, as well as various rigid and flexible delivery systems, were designed to offer maximum safety and manoeuvrability.

The CO_2 laser, an ideal cutting beam, operates at the far infrared range (10 600 nm), is reflected by mirrors and is principally delivered through a rigid set of tubes. This beam is also transmitted through silver halide crystal fibres (Katzir and Arieli, 1982). However, technical difficulties such as power attenuation, the relatively large fibre diameter, and low flexibility, limit its cutting capabilities. Rigid (Baggish and ElBakrey, 1986; Tadir *et al.*, 1989) and flexible (Baggish *et al.*, 1988; Gannot *et al.*, 1992) hollow wave guides for the CO_2 laser, and contact Nd:YAG laser fibres offer several advantages and are thus more commonly used. It is the aim of this chapter to elucidate various technical and physical aspects that influence the design and the handling of delivery systems for laser laparoscopy.

CO_2 Laser

'Back Focal Length' and its Practical Relevance

A laser beam is unique in its directionality, brightness, coherence and monochromaticity. These properties set it apart from other light sources such as incandescent light (light bulbs) or even the sun. Directionality means that all the light energy (or photons, the energetic, massless particles of which light is composed) are emitted in one direction. Brightness relates to the very high concentration of photons per unit area. Coherence means that the energy emitted by the many atoms or molecules in the lasing medium are all emitted in phase or synchronously, and monochromaticity means that this energy is emitted at a single wavelength.

In order to increase laser effectiveness as a cutting/coagulating tool, special lenses with different refractive indexes are used. The distance between the lens and the focal point (the point where idealized light rays will converge after passing through the lens) is termed the 'back focal length' (BFL) (Figure 5.1). The shorter the BFL of a given lens (or lens system) the smaller the spot size (or 'waist') of a laser beam which passes through the lens, and the smaller the *depth of focus*. Depth of focus is defined as length along the beam direction of propagation where the laser's beam possesses its smallest waist (for a given lens system), and the beam is most

Figure 5.1 Depth of focus, spot size, and beam divergence are different in various delivery systems. (A) Long rigid laser laparoscope with 200–300 mm back focal length (BFL) lenses. Depth of focus is relatively large and defocusing of the laser beam is minimal. (B) Minimal free hand movements are causing significant defocusing effects due to the 100–150 mm BFL lenses. (C) Wave guides with short (6–15 mm) BFL lenses cause notable beam defocus which means safe 'optical backstop' (D) Wave guide without a lens. Beam divergence is minimal, and metal back stops are needed if vital organs might be hidden behind the 'lased' area.

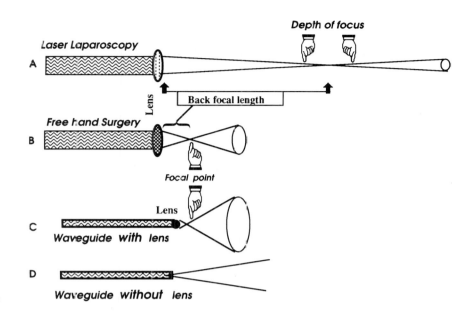

collimated (i.e. the beam of light in this region is neither diverging nor converging).

Laparoscopic application of the CO_2 laser through long and rigid cannula requires lenses with 200–300 mm BFL, which means long focal depth. For example, if the beam's minimum spot size (at the focal point) after passing through the lens is about 1 mm in diameter, the beam will remain relatively collimated 2 cm before and 2 cm behind the focal point with a diameter of approximately 1.1 mm. This means that power densities within the long range of the focal plane (which, in turn, determine the effects of the laser beam on tissue), remain similar to those at the focal point. Indeed, one of the main advantages of the CO_2 laser is that varying the power densities yields different effects on tissue. This is especially relevant in reproductive surgery where minimizing heating and heat conductance will prevent unwanted damage to adjacent tissues. Long focal length lenses limit the achievable minimum spot size of the beam at the waist, and thus results in lower power densities (energy per unit time per unit area). In turn, using very low power densities can superficially ablate endometrial implants or cause serosal shrinkage needed for fimbrial eversion during salpingostomy.

The Connection between Long Back Focal Length and Beam Misalignment

The CO_2 laser beam is reflected from the laser cavity to the target organ with mirrors. The movable articulated arm and the long BFL frequently cause misalignment, meaning that the beam is not centred at the distal port. In order to correct such misalignments, an endoscopic coupler was designed (Tadir et al., 1984). (A joystick, which controls a movable mirror, is placed before the laparoscope. The misalignment in beam position can be compensated for and restored to the desired location.) Several types of couplers are currently available. Some couplers contain a sliding lens known as 'continuous variable defocus' (CVD). A direct coupler that enables the interchangeable use of any operating laparoscope and laser arm is also available (Sharplan, Israel).

How can the Power Density be changed during Surgery?

As mentioned previously, changes of power density (PD = W/cm²) can offer more versatile tissue effects to this surgical modality. Minimal power density changes can be obtained by sliding the lens in the CVD coupler. However, in view of the long BFL and the wide focal plane, these changes are minimal. A simple way to reduce power density is by reducing the power output of the laser source. This process may be time consuming and the small spot size may still cause a cutting effect when superficial ablation is wanted. Significant reduction of the power density may be reached by moving the joystick and reflecting the beam on the inner cannula surface. The emerging beam profile will be crescent shaped instead of round, but effects on tissue may be superficial as needed (Figure 5.2). Another innovative modality for superficial tissue ablation on large areas, with minimal thermal damage to the underlying layers was recently introduced (Sharplan, Israel). The CO_2 laser beam is directed through the laparoscopic coupler (with its limited ability of defocusing the beam). An electronic rotating mechanism causes fast scanning of the exposed area next to the laparoscope. By reducing the power density, superficial effects in an area of 8–10 mm can safely be performed. This might be useful for procedures such as salpingostomy ('Bruhat manoeuvre'), endometriosis, and peritoneal ablation over vital organs.

Mechanical and Optical Backstops

The 'light scalpel', unlike any other cutting tool, acts in the non-contact mode. The lack of tactile feeling is unfamiliar to most surgeons and it takes some time to get used to it. The collimated beam of light may cause damage to organs located behind the 'lased' area. Several instruments and manoeuvres protect against such damage. In general, these can be divided into mechanical and optical methods. The various types of rigid cannulas, inserted in the suprapubic region (called 'second-puncture laser channel'), usually contain a metal tongue at the distal end (Tadir *et al.*, 1981). This part is located behind the cutting area and prevents further delivery of the beam. Adding such a tongue to the single-puncture operative laparoscope is impossible since it may obstruct visibility.

Donnez (Figure 5.3) has designed several types of metal probes that can be used as backstops when the beam is delivered through the operative laparoscope. Different configurations serve as an aid during tissue handling, and a channel for smoke evacuation is built into the device. It is important to note that the laser port and the viewing lens are parallel to each other. When the target area is too close to the tip of the laser laparoscope the He–Ne aiming beam is invisible and activating the laser might cause damage to other organs (Figure 5.4).

Short BFL laser probes (Tadir *et al.*, 1989) offer the advantage of a cutting effect at the focal plane

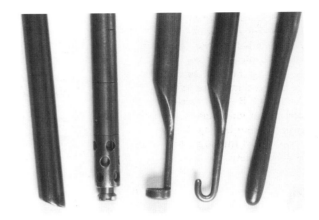

Figure 5.3 Donnez backstop set. Useful for laser laparoscopy when the beam is delivered through the operative laparoscope. Channels for smoke evaluation are built in the probes. (Courtesy of Prof. J. Donnez, Catholic University of Louvain, Brussels, Belgium.)

and lack of laser effect at a short distance behind the focal point. Beam divergence causes an 'optical backstop' and there is no need for any protecting devices. The main disadvantage of these probes is the short distance between the lens and the organ. Contamination of the lens with debris or blood might prevent further lasing. However, this device may be ideal for fimbriolysis and fimbrioplasty.

Another way to protect deep pelvic organs from unwanted damage of the CO_2 laser beam is by using fluid that absorbs the light and acts as a backstop. This can be achieved as part of the ongoing process of tissue irrigation or simply by applying the fluid at the lower pelvis, in the event that this is the area behind the dissected region.

Smoke Evacuation

One of the problems encountered during laser endoscopy is how to evacuate the smoke produced during tissue evaporation without compromising visibility and peritoneal cavity distension. Unlike laser thoracoscopy, where the ribs prevent chest collapse, and continuous suction is performed without any difficulty, the peritoneal cavity

Figure 5.2 Large 'crescent shape' spot of a CO_2 laser beam on tissue. The beam is reflected on the inner surface of the laser laparoscope if low power density is needed for superficial effects.

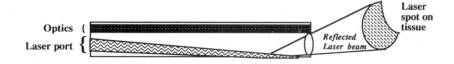

Figure 5.4 Location of CO_2 laser beam at various distances behind the laparoscopic objective. Activating the laser beam when the targets are at zones A through B might cause damage to vital organs. At zone C there is a sufficient area around the target to provide safety.

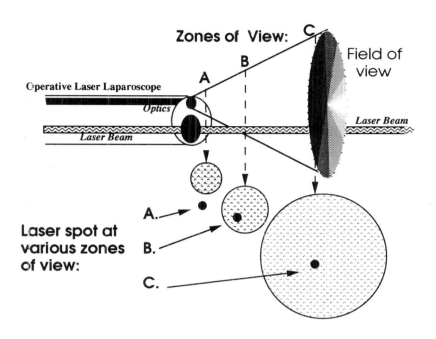

collapses if positive pressure is not maintained. Several methods allow smoke evacuation during laser laparoscopy:

1. High flow CO_2 gas insufflation.
2. Synchronized laser-suction unit activated by the laser apparatus with preset suction delay.
3. Ports for smoke evacuation:
   (a) double channel in the second puncture probe;
   (b) Veress needle placed suprapubically close to the 'lased' area and connected to smoke evacuator;
   (c) suction–irrigation probe (described later in this chapter) that can be used as a backstop as well as smoke evacuator;
   (d) Donnez backstop hooks (see above) that contain port for smoke evacuation (Figure 5.3).
4. Pressure valves designed to prevent the occurrence of overpressure during high gas inflow.
5. Closed system: plastic tubes and filters with in/outflow connected to the trocars.

Possible Power Attenuation during Laparoscopic Laser Surgery

Experience showed that there is a drop in the laser power at the laparoscope distal end, as compared to the power at the proximal end. To elucidate the cause of this power reduction and to define the actual effective power on tissue of beams delivered through different endoscopes, an experimental model was designed and tested (Tadir *et al.*, 1986). No significant power loss was noted when passing a CO_2 laser beam through a

CO_2 gas pressurized chamber in this model. However, a correlation between the internal diameter of an endoscope and the power output became evident. Effective power drops of 92%, 85%, and 48% were measured when a beam was delivered through three different types of laparoscopes. It was noticed that the reason for some power loss with long and narrow metal ports is caused by the thermal dissipation of laser energy while passing through the metal tube. If during surgery a power loss is noticed (or, if the rigid metal laparoscope is getting hot), the accuracy of beam alignment and proper coupling of the laparoscope to the laser arm should be checked. In other studies it was noticed that heated CO_2 gas (low or no flow) reduces beam transmission and effective power density in the pelvic cavity.

CO_2 Laser Fibres, Flexible Hollow Wave Guides and Rigid Probes

Optical fibres made of silver halide crystals are capable of transmitting CO_2 laser energy (Katzir and Arieli, 1982). Although the transmission losses are on the order of 1 dB/m, some limitations like flexibility, low cutting effects and high cost have prevented its clinical use in gynaecological endoscopy. Recent developments of CO_2 laser flexible hollow wave guides for laparoscopic use have been reported (Figures 5.5, 5.6) (Gannot *et al.*, 1992). They are made of a flexible plastic tube with two inner layers of metal ribbon and dielectric coating, with an inside diameter (i.d.) of 2.4, 1.9 and 1.0 mm. A 120 cm long wave guide

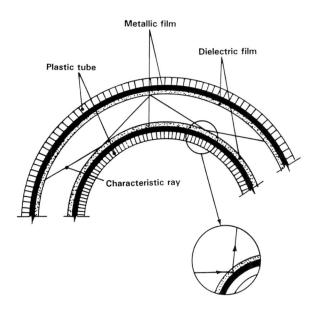

Figure 5.5 Reflection of CO_2 laser beam through flexible hollow wave guides for laparoscopic use. It is made of a plastic tube with two inner layers of metal ribbon and dielectric coating. (Courtesy of Prof. N. Croitoru, Tel Aviv University, Israel.)

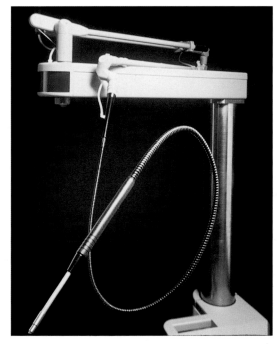

Figure 5.6 Flexible hollow wave guide connected to a CO_2 laser. (Courtesy of Sharplan Laser, Tel Aviv, Israel).

(1.9 mm i.d. at 50 W continuous wave (CW)) transmitted 90% of input power. Bending the tube at a radius of 220 mm reduced the transmission to 60%. These plastic CO_2 laser hollow wave guides enable surgeons to easily access areas that are

normally difficult to reach. Pelvic anatomy and satisfactory organ visibility allows workable laser transmission through rigid wave guides (Tadir *et al.*, 1989). These probes allow the passage of the CO_2 laser beam via standard laparoscopes. They are made of a rigid stainless steel tube with an inner hollow dielectric coating. The probe is attached to an articulated arm of a CO_2 laser system, thus enabling the degree of freedom needed to manipulate the probe. The outer diameters and lengths fit most of the standard operative channels of single-puncture laparoscopes and of the second-puncture suprapubic trocar sleeves. Spot size is dependent on the i.d. of the wave guide, usually in the range of ± 0.8 mm. Recently, probes with a conical tip (i.d. 0.4 mm) for non-contact surgery were presented (Levi, 1992) (Luxar, Bothell, WA, USA). Beam divergence beyond the tip of the straight probe is ± 7° and beyond the 0.4 mm conical tip is ± 14°. This means that changes of spot diameter, and power density, within a few millimetres are minimal. In order to get significant defocusing effects, miniature zinc selenide lenses (6.5 mm BFL and 17 mm BFL) were attached at the distal end (Tadir *et al.*, 1989). The efficacy of these probes was examined at 5 and 15 W and compared to the standard CO_2 laser laparoscope with the 340 mm BFL lens. These probes enable power density modulation and easy switching between precise cutting and superficial ablation by simply shifting the lens–target distance and time of exposure.

The particular location of a focusing lens with short BFL produces focus/defocus (cutting/ablating) effects in close distance. The lack of tissue damage at a few millimetres beyond the focal plane offers another safety feature known as 'optical' backstop (see above). The probe's optical transmission is less sensitive to misalignment than the 'first-generation' laser laparoscope. The miniature lens containing probes did not gain popularity because of the close proximity of the distal lens to the operation field (especially with the 6.5 mm BFL lens). This required reasonable care to avoid lens contamination which could result in degradation of transmission. However, with enhanced resolution of video images and a protective pointer next to the lens it might become useful, especially for new applications in general surgery and laser thoracoscopy. Other wave guides with built-in reflectors at the tip (Luxar, Bothell, WA, USA) can be used whenever poor accessibility dictates a different approach. Exposure to high temperatures generated by the laser beam may result in damage to the inner coating of the wave guide. In order to prevent such damage it is recommended that gas flow inside the inner channel will be applied. CO_2 gas is usually used for this purpose; however, it is important to note that CO_2 gas at high temperatures may significantly reduce beam transmission and thus, a constant flow is required. Nitrogen gas for cooling can also be used, but is not recommended because nitrogen is relatively insoluble and cases of nitrogen surgical emphysema have been reported which take about 10 days to resolve (Sutton and Macdonald, 1990).

Suction–Irrigation Probes

The principles of reconstructive pelvic microsurgery (careful tissue handling and continuous irrigation) are also relevant to laparoscopic surgery. Suction–irrigation probes were available prior to the era of laser laparoscopy. However, the increased need for fluid and smoke evacuation during laser surgery, and the specific requirements of some laser wavelengths, call for instrument modifications such as surface abrasion (to prevent laser reflection), variety of probe diameters, easy valve manipulation and a dedicated port for fibre insertion. The correct handling of these multipurpose devices is very important during laser laparoscopy, particularly since it may also serve as a backstop (see above).

Nd:YAG, KTP, and Argon Laser

Delivery of these laser beams (and others such as: Ho:YAG, argon pumped dye, flash lamp pumped dye, and Alexandrite lasers) via optical fibres makes them ideal energy sources for flexible endoscopy. Next to the CO_2, the other main lasers which are clinically used are the Nd:YAG, KTP, and argon.

The following practical aspects of their performance will be discussed.

1. thermal and non-thermal effects on tissue;
2. contact and non-contact laser surgery;
3. fibre guides.

Thermal and Non-thermal Effects on Tissue

One of the key questions concerning lasers operating in the near infrared and visible region of the spectrum is related to selective, site-specific thermal effects which are wavelength dependent.

Ophthalmic lasers serve as an ideal example of the unique advantages of wavelength selectivity and pulse duration specificity for specific applications. Procedures such as retinal photocoagulation with argon lasers, or applications of short Nd:YAG pulses for secondary cataract removal, rely principally on the strong variations in absorption characteristics between adjacent tissues (the argon emission lines in the green and blue are easily transmitted through the cornea and the lens but are strongly absorbed by the pigmented retina), or on ablation power threshold effects which can be accomplished by concentrating the photon flux in time (short pulses) and in space (highly focused beam). Other examples of lasers operating on the principle of selective absorption are the Ruby laser (694.3 nm, with pulse duration ranging between 15 and 70 ns) for tattoo removal and the flash lamp excited dye laser (e.g. the Candela SPTL-1 at 585 nm and 450 µs pulse duration) for removal of coloured skin lesions (congenital port wine stains).

The unique advantage of lasers over other surgical modalities is due to the potential penetration ability of the selected beam through superficial structures, without causing any damage on its way to the target area. The interaction between dyes such as porphyrin derivatives with laser light (known as photodynamic therapy, PDT) in order to initiate photochemical reactions is another approach for site-specific beam targeting. The current technology in laser laparoscopy, however, is in most instances based on direct thermal excitation of the target area. Some differences between such thermal systems still exist: Nd:YAG laser which is in the near infrared range is poorly absorbed by water, and thus results in deep coagulating effects. However, by using conical sculpted tips in a contact mode (as will be described later) cutting effects can become predominant. KTP lasers (which are frequency doubled Nd:YAG, emitting at 532 nm) as well as argon lasers (wavelengths 488–514 nm) fall in the visible part of the spectrum. Their absorption in water is poor and tissue penetration is relatively high. However, because of their strong interaction with absorption centres embedded in the tissue (such as small pigmented endometrial implants), the CW argon laser is useful in applications where selective ablation is required. KTP lasers, operating at a similar wavelength but with higher power and in pulse mode cuts more efficiently. These two examples show that even if similar wavelength and similar mechanisms (thermal) are dominating the interaction, different effects can result if power densities and modes of operation (pulsed versus CW) are used.

Contact and Non-contact Laser Surgery

Most surgical laser applications are in the non-contact mode. The lack of tactile feeling is probably the most unusual experience for beginners in that field. In clinical practice it is difficult to compare or predict effects on tissue just by referring to power or energy density. The distance between fibre tip and tissue, different tissue types, beam divergence caused by irregular fibre tips and other variations, may produce different effects. However, these variations are usually not critical, and the surgeon with considerable laser experience can achieve the desired effects, or switch from superficial cutting to deep coagulation by setting the proper laser parameters and correctly manipulating the delivery systems. Unlike the CO_2 laser, non-contact application of the visible/near infrared lasers through fluids is possible (and sometimes even recommended) (Tadir *et al.*, 1988). With the advent of sapphire tips (Daikyzono and Joffe, 1985) (SLT, Oaks, PA, USA), Nd:YAG laser surgery could be performed in the contact mode. Adding a sapphire contact tip to the laser fibre changes the energy deposition in the tissue. Within the tip, laser energy is focused and converted into heat, thus enabling the operator to heat and cut the tissue very rapidly. Using low powers (W), or by changing beam geometries at the contact surface, contact laser probes will cut, coagulate, vaporize or administer low levels of interstitial irradiation. These tips are made of synthetic crystal, have great mechanical strength and high melting temperature ($\sim$2000° C). The tips are designed in various shapes to bring about different tissue effect. Direct contact with tissue allows precise and controlled manipulation, and restores some of the tactile feeling that was lost with other non-contact laser techniques. Due to the geometric design and the optical properties, it is possible to determine the spot size, power density, and thus the effect on tissue. A general purpose scalpel (outside diameter (o.d.) = 0.2, 0.4, 0.6 and 0.8 mm), offers precise cutting while using the proximal side of the tip. The same tip will cause coagulation when the lateral portion is in contact with the tissue. A shorter conical probe permits more precise cutting and minimal lateral coagulation. Other probes (Figure 5.7) are the chisel, round and flat shape tips (o.d. = 1.8 mm), which produce more coagulation than cutting. By focusing the laser energy at the conical tip, power of

25 W (or even less) can cut and coagulate. This means that low cost Nd:YAG laser sources are capable of supplying the energies needed for most of the laparoscopic surgical applications. The main practical difference between various fibre delivery systems (i.e. with and without the probes) is related to its cooling mechanism. The fibre coupled with the contact tip requires a coaxial channel for the transmission of cooling medium.

Potential advantages of the Nd:YAG surgery over the CO_2 laser include improved haemostasis, decreased plume formation and the ability to incise adhesions without the need for a mechanical backstop. Effective transmission through fluids may be an advantage or a disadvantage depending on the type of procedure performed. The main disadvantages of the Nd:YAG systems (as compared to the CO_2 laser) are:

1. extent of tissue damage (similar to electrocautery), which may be critical in some areas (such as damage to the fallopian tube during reconstructive surgery); and
2. the need for disposable fibres.

More recently, contact fibres with conical and hemispherical sculpted tips (o.d. = 0.6, 0.8, 1.0 mm), have been introduced (Sharplan, Tel Aviv, Israel). Cutting, vaporization and coagulation effects may be obtained under similar conditions with different tip profiles. These fibres are delivered through an irrigation/aspiration probe, and the need for cooling is eliminated. Both types of contact tips were designed to perform similar tissue effects, and both have advantages and disadvantages.

Fibre Guides

Flexible fibres are introduced into the pelvis through rigid probes at various diameters. In order to allow for more complex manoeuvres it is possible (and suggested) to use combined irrigation/aspiration fibre guides, of which some even hold a steerable tip. Various probes with different design of the suction and irrigation control buttons are available. This tool, though simple, is of great use, and the better design may ease performance of lengthy and complicated laparoscopic procedures.

Other Lasers and Delivery Systems

The fields of laser physics and fibre technology have progressed rapidly in the last decade. New

Figure 5.7 Sapphire contact tips. From left to right: chisel probe (for cutting and coagulation), short cone (precise cutting), long cone (cutting), round (ablation), and flat probe (for deep coagulation). (Courtesy of SLT, Oaks, PA, USA.)

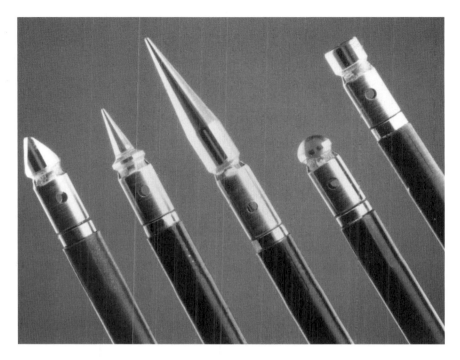

lasers in the visible range like the flash lamp dye (504/590 nm), and others in the infrared range such as Holmium:YAG (2.12 μm), Erbium:YAG (2.94 μm), and CO (5.4 μm) are becoming available for clinical evaluation. Each of these lasers has different effects on tissue, and may offer special advantages or disadvantages. It is beyond the scope of this chapter to compare or evaluate all these new devices; however, it is expected that some of them will be used in future endoscopic surgery. The same applies to optical fibre and wave guide developments. Recently, a flexible chalcogenide glass fibre (0.5 mm i.d.) for the Er:YAG laser was presented (Kubo *et al.*, 1992). This type of laser which has special cutting capabilities might be another potential candidate for endoscopic surgery, when coupled with flexible delivery systems.

The basic elements of flexible laser fibres include coating materials which are polymeric (silicone, nylon, Teflon, and acrylate), metallic (aluminium and gold) and inorganic components (oxides, carbides and nitrides). An example of a 'smart fibre' was recently introduced (Fibertome™, Dornier Medical Systems, Kennesaw, GA, USA). This fibre contains an optoelectronic control system which allows temperature controlled cutting of tissue with a bare fibre. A sensor in the fibretome measures the temperature at the fibre tip during cutting (in the contact or non-contact mode), and automatically reduces the power to a safe level, a fraction of a second before the fibre tip melts. The manufacturer claims that optimal laser power varies from 10 to 40 W, while the cutting temperature at the fibre tip can be set

to three different levels for variable cutting effects, speed, depth and necrotic zone. It is well known that hyperthermic effects in tissue cause irreversible tissue damage. An advanced, disposable, plastic introducer has been developed for interstitial tumour therapy. This device is designed for volume coagulation by the insertion of a frosted bare fibre. When the desired size of coagulation is reached, an alert signal, to stop the treatment, is derived from on-line monitoring of NADH concentration by laser-induced fluorescence measurements (Bethuan *et al.*, 1991). Other 'smart fibres' with tiny rotating mirrors (to allow beam orientation at different angles) are being tested for urological procedures (Johnson and Cromeens, 1992) and might be applicable to laparoscopy (Figure 5.8). It is too early to predict the potential use of these devices in endoscopic surgery; however, it undoubtedly does represent a new approach in combined technologies for delivery systems. Applying advanced endoscopic surgery safely (with or without the laser) requires knowledge of other assisting tools such as special grasping forceps, tools for removing specimens or dissected organs, and accessories for clamping or tying vessels and sealing open surfaces with tissue glue.

Imaging and Camera Guided Laser Surgery

During the past 5 years there has been an increasing tendency to use video cameras and

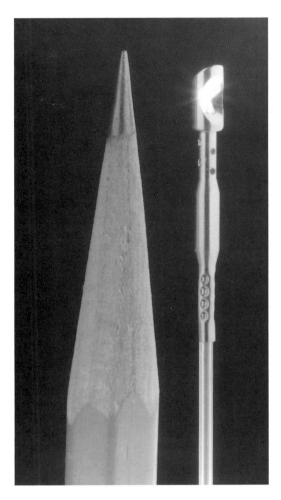

Figure 5.8 Flexible fibre with tiny rotating mirror (to allow beam orientation at different angles). Pencil tip serves as size reference. (Courtesy of Trimedyne, Irvine, CA, USA.)

computerized image processors in research as well as clinical facilities. When video cameras were first introduced for laparoscopic procedures, surgeons viewed the operative field through the eyepiece and the images were video recorded through the beam splitter. Poor image quality, minimal depth perception and above all conservatism and scepticism of the personnel has limited its acceptance. More recently, however, operations are performed in combination with video monitors for guidance (Figure 5.9). This approach offers several advantages:

1. magnification of the target organ and the pathological lesions;
2. more stable images and less fatigue to the surgeon;
3. improved team work and better assistance;
4. permanent documentation via recorded video files.

The increased market demand has stimulated

the industry to further develop high-resolution, lightweight endo-cameras and bright light sources. Miniaturization and steerable fibres enable further penetration and video imaging of narrow cavities like the fallopian tubes or the bile ducts. At present, depth perception is reasonable; however, there is no doubt that future developments will result in higher resolution and even three-dimensional images. Undoubtedly, within a few years most endoscopic procedures will be performed with endo-cameras. The incorporation of video monitors and bright light to the armamentarium of the endoscopic operating room (EOR) calls for some changes in the laser equipment, mainly the CO_2 and the Nd:YAG, both operating at the invisible (infrared) wavelength spectrum. The helium neon (He–Ne) beam, used as an aiming beam, was not sufficiently visible in the bright light field and required upgrading. A different dimension of precise depth and direction control of laser coagulation inside the body may be obtained with imaging devices like ultrasound or magnetic resonance imaging (MRI) (Jolez *et al.*, 1988). Potential benefits of these new approaches are being assessed in some medical centres.

Conclusions

Reproductive surgeons have encountered significant changes during the past 15 years. Reconstructive pelvic surgery has progressed from conventional to microsurgery. *In vitro* fertilization has made a significant impact on indications to surgery, and endoscopy offers in some cases an alternative approach. DeCherney (1985) has stated that the new laser technology has 'effected a major renaissance in endoscopic surgery. In this instance, the laser has a distinct advantage over unipolar electrocautery, because the area of damage may be greatly diminished'. It also has an advantage over sharp dissection in that it is haemostatic. He suggested that regarding the relationship with *in vitro* fertilization (IVF), 'the dictum that will surely emerge is that if reconstructive surgery cannot be done through the endoscope, it should not be done at all . . .'. It is neither expected nor required that the average surgeon will perceive and recognize the content of the 'black box' behind the laser beam. However, in order to gain maximum benefit of special effects that lasers might offer, and to overcome certain difficulties encountered during laparoscopic procedures, basic understanding of factors

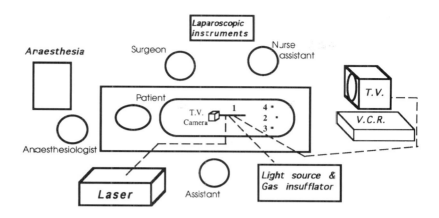

Figure 5.9 Suggested optimal setup for a laparoscopic operating room (for pelvic surgery). All members of the surgical team can easily watch a single television monitor, located at the patient's caudal side. Points 1–4 represent trocar puncture sites.

influencing accessories design, beam geometry and safety measures is required. The availability of several delivery systems provoked its use in other areas like general surgery, thoracoscopy and arthroscopy, and it is expected that surgeons from various disciplines will use similar instruments and further modify them according to specific needs.

'Combo' laser units, that combine more than one wavelength, are available on the market, and will probably be more commonly used in the future. Present combinations like Nd:YAG + KTP; CO_2 + Nd:YAG and Nd:YAG 1060 + 1320 nm are some of the experimental prototypes.

In the last decade, several segments of infertility treatment have moved from the human body into the 'Petri dish' and this process has provoked the developments of dedicated instrumentation. The potential role of lasers in gamete micromanipulation is currently being assessed (Palanker et al., 1991; Tadir et al., 1991) and discussed in Chapter 48.

Acknowledgements

This work was supported by grants NIH PRO 1192, ONRN 00014-91-C-0134 and DOE DE-FG03-91 ER 61227.

References

Baggish MS & ElBakrey MM (1986) A flexible CO_2 laser fiber for operative laparoscopy. *Fertility and Sterility* **46**: 16.

Baggish MS, Sze E, Badawy S & Choe J (1988) Carbon dioxide laser laparoscopy by means of 3.0 mm diameter rigid wave guide. *Fertility and Sterility* **50**: 419.

Beuthan J, Muller G, Schaldach B & Zur Ch (1991) Fiber design for interstitial laser treatment. *The International Society for Optical Engineering (SPIE)* **1420**: 234–241.

Bruhat M, Mage C & Manhes M (1979) Use of the CO_2 laser via laparoscopy. In Kaplan I (ed.) *Laser Surgery III, Proceedings of the Third International Society for Laser Surgery*, pp. 274–276. Tel-Aviv: Ot-Paz.

Daikyzono S & Joffe SN (1985) Artificial sapphire probe for contact photocoagulation and tissue vaporization with the Nd:YAG laser. *Medical Instruments* **19**: 173–178.

DeCherney AH (1985) The leader of the band is tired. *Fertility and Sterility* **44** 299.

Gannot I, Dror R, Dahan N & Croitoru N (1992) Improved plastic hollow fibers for CO_2 laser radiation transmission for possible endoscopic use. *The International Society for Optical Engineering (SPIE), Proceedings*, **1649**: in press.

Johnson DE & Cromeens DM (1992) Use of holmium YAG laser in urology. *The International Society for Optical Engineering (SPIE), Proceedings* **1649**: in press.

Jolez FA, Bleier AR, Jakab P et al. (1988) MR imaging of laser–tissue interaction. *Radiology* **168 (1)**: 249–253.

Katzir A & Arieli A (1982) Long wavelength infrared optical fibers. *Journal of Non-Crystalline Solids* **47**: 149–158.

Kubo U, Hashishin Y, Tanaka H & Mochizuki T (1992) Development of optical fiber for medical Er,YAG laser. *The International Society for Optical Engineering (SPIE), Proceedings* **1649**: in press.

Levi M (1992) Hollow flexible fibers for medical use. *SPIE, Proceedings* **1649**: in press.

Palanker D, Ohad S, Lewis A et al. (1991) Technique for cellular microsurgery using the 193 nm Excimer laser. *Lasers in Surgery and Medicine* **11**: 580–586.

Sutton CJG & Macdonald R (1990) Laser laparoscopic adhesiolysis. *Journal of Gynecological Surgery* **6 (3)**: 155–160.

Tadir Y, Ovadia J, Zukerman Z et al. (1981) Laparoscopic application of CO_2 laser. In Atsumi K & Nimsakul N (eds) *Laser Tokyo 81*, pp 13–27. Tokyo: Inter Group Corp.

Tadir Y, Kaplan I, Zukerman Z et al. (1984) New instrumentation and technique for laparoscopic carbon dioxide laser operations: a preliminary report. *Obstetrics and Gynecology* **63**: 582–585.

Tadir Y, Kaplan I, Zukerman Z & Ovadia J (1986) Effective CO_2 laser power on tissue in endoscopic surgery. *Fertility and Sterility* **45 (4)**: 492–495.

Tadir Y, Karni Z, Fisch B & Ovadia J (1988) Transmission of Nd:YAG laser via fluids. *Colposcopy and Gynecologic Laser Surgery* **4**: 107–110.

Tadir Y, Karni Z, Fisch B *et al.* (1989) Tissue effects of a new laparoscopic carbon dioxide laser probe. *Fertility and Sterility* **51**: 1046–1049.

Tadir Y, Wright WH, Vafa O *et al.* (1991) Micromanipulation of gametes using laser microbeams. *Human Reproduction* **6**: 1011–1016.

6

Electrosurgery

ROGER ODELL

Electroscope Inc., Boulder, Colorado, USA

The use of high-frequency electrical energy for surgical application dates back nearly a century. Electrosurgery is the generation and delivery of radiofrequency current between an active electrode and a dispersive electrode in order to elevate the tissue temperature for the purpose of cutting, fulguration and desiccation. In contrast to electrocautery, the electric current actually passes through the tissue. Harvey W. Cushing, MD with the assistance of William T. Bovie, PhD was the first surgeon to document the principles in depth regarding both the art as well as the biophysics pertaining to electrosurgery. These early documents detailed his appreciation of Dr Bovie's device and his encouragement regarding the versatility of this energy source. It truly changed the course of neurosurgery and other surgeons' views during his practising years for the potential uses of electrosurgical energy. The intent of this chapter is to highlight the practical application of the three modalities and how to maximize their intended uses. With the rapid shift to minimally invasive surgical technique, a detailed discussion regarding how the electrosurgical energy is delivered will be covered as well as the pitfalls associated with laparoscopy.

Temperature and Tissue

Energy cannot be created or destroyed, but it can be converted from one form to another. In electrosurgery electrosurgical current is converted into heat in the tissue for the purpose of vaporizing/cutting and coagulation. The principles are quite similar to those of laser energy when converted to heat within the tissue.

At or above 44°C tissue necrosis starts. At or above 70°C coagulation begins where collagen is denatured and the clotting mechanism is activated. At or above 90°C tissue desiccation begins where the tissue is dehydrated. At or above 100°C vaporization occurs where the tissue is converted into a vapour. At or above 200°C carbonization starts; this black eschar can only occur from fulguration.

How Electrical Energy Affects Tissue Temperature

The three electrical properties that cause temperature rise are as follows.

- Current = I
- Voltage = V
- Resistance (impedance) = R

To help overcome the electrical energy terms and meanings a direct analogy to water or hydraulics energy source will be made. The following water tower in Figure 6.1 presents a hydraulic energy source for the purpose of performing work. Figure 6.2 shows an equivalent electrosurgical tower with the electrical terms, current, voltage, and resistance inserted. This direct relationship is important in overcoming the mystique of electrosurgical units modalities.

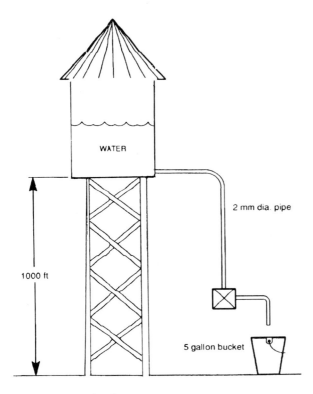

Figure 6.1 Hydraulic energy source.

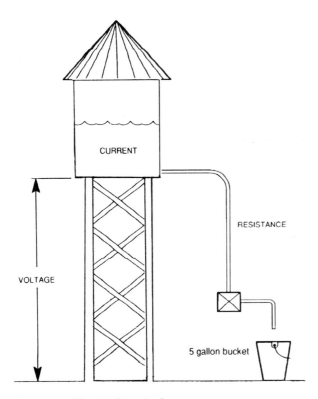

Figure 6.2 Electrical equivalents terms.

Ohm's law, $I = V/R$ shows the relationship between the properties of electrosurgical energy.

Power Formula

Energy in wattage, $W = V \times I$ is valuable in understanding how the three modalities waveforms, cut, fulgurate and desiccate, are compared in performing various therapeutic effects. The ratio of the voltage to current of the electrosurgical waveforms is what is primarily responsible for the effects to tissue observed when time and electrode size are kept equal.

Power Density

Power density = (current density) squared × resistivity. Power density is the relationship of the size of the active electrode in contact with the tissue, and the effect on the tissue at a given energy setting. In non-contact modalities, i.e. cutting and fulgurating, this would be equivalent to the sparking area between the active electrode and the tissue. Only when desiccating is the exact surface area of the electrode in contact with the tissue of importance when calculating power density. During fulguration and cutting the electrode is not in contact, therefore the power density can only be approximated.

In general, the larger the electrode surface area the lower the power density, the smaller the electrode surface area the higher the power density.

Time

The time element is the primary component determining the depth and degree of tissue necrosis at a given energy setting. Many other components contribute to this discussion, but time is important as will be demonstrated in the following sections.

Cut – Fulgurate – Desiccate

The following are the three distinct therapeutic effects to tissue, that electrosurgical energy has been reduced to in practice. Unfortunately most electrosurgical units are labelled simply by two modes, 'cut' and 'coag'. These terms do not help in the present confusion pertaining to the optimal use of the energy.

Cut

A high current, low voltage (continuous) waveform elevates the tissue's temperature, rapidly producing vaporization or division of tissue with the least effect on coagulation (haemostasis) to the walls of the incision—see Figure 6.3, cutting waveform with electrosurgical unit (ESU) set at 50 W. During optimal electrosurgical cutting the current travels through a steam bubble between the active electrode and the tissue. Therefore it is important to recognize that electrosurgical cutting is a *non-contact* means of dissection. The electrode floats through the tissue and there is very little tactile response transmitted to the surgeon's hand. The continuous waveform is analogous to the garden valve shown in Figure 6.1, having a constant even flow of water being delivered. Due to the constant flow of current and the lowest possible voltage to dissect, the width and depth of necrosis to the walls of the incision are minimal. Therefore the ratio of high current to low voltage within the waveform produces less necrosis. If the electrode is allowed to remain stationary or is slowed, the maximum temperature attained is increased as well as the width of thermal damage to the tissue.

Blend 1, 2, and 3

With a ratio modification of the cutting waveform (i.e. changing the current, voltage product) by interrupting current and increasing the voltage, the waveform becomes non-continuous with a train of packets of energy consisting of higher voltage and reduced current per time. Total energy remains the same, the ratio of voltage and current are modified to increase haemostasis during dissection with electrosurgical current—see Figure 6.4, Blend 1, 2, and 3 with voltage current ratio shown. This would be analogous to the garden valve pulsing the water, with an increased height to the water tower to make up for the reduction of hydraulic energy, as a result of reducing the time that the water was allowed to flow. In utilizing the blend modes as well the electrode should float through the tissue. The blend waveforms will require a longer period of time to dissect the same length of incision as compared to the cutting waveform. This is due to the interrupted delivery of current at the same power setting. With this increased time comes an increase in thermal spread from the voltage component of the blend waveform. This increased thermal spread improves coagulation of small vessels while dissecting. When needed these blend modes can be a very valuable option in controlling bleeding as needed when dissecting.

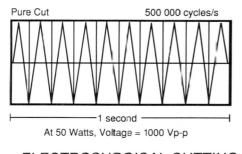

Pure Cut 500 000 cycles/s

├──── 1 second ────┤

At 50 Watts, Voltage = 1000 Vp-p

ELECTROSURGICAL CUTTING

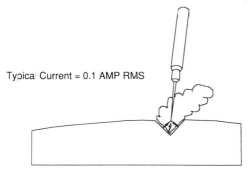

Typical Current = 0.1 AMP RMS

Figure 6.3 Electrosurgical cutting waveform. 'Electrode not in contact with tissue.'

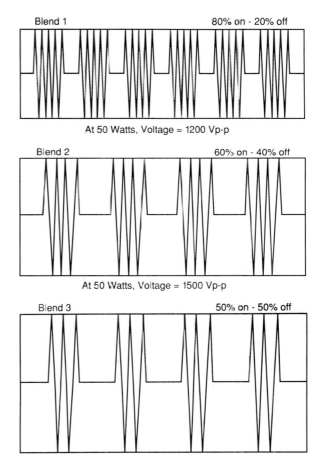

Blend 1 80% on - 20% off

At 50 Watts, Voltage = 1200 Vp-p

Blend 2 60% on - 40% off

At 50 Watts, Voltage = 1500 Vp-p

Blend 3 50% on - 50% off

At 50 Watts, Voltage = 2000 Vp-p

Figure 6.4 Blend 1, Blend 2 and Blend 3 waveforms.

On the other hand, if used and not needed the increase in the width of necrosis may result in a higher postoperative infection level, as a direct result of the increased amount of tissue necrosis. Also the amount of smoke plume will be increased in laparoscopy using high blend or coagulation modes. Blend 1 has slightly increased haemostasis, blend 2 moderate, with blend 3 showing a marked increase in haemostasis while dissecting.

When dissecting tissue with a cut or blended mode the ESU should be activated first before the electrode touches the tissue. A feathering or light stroking similar to when painting with a two bristle paint brush for touch-up or fine detail work needs to be simulated. This will allow for the maximum power density as the electrode approaches the tissue just before contact. This will help initialize vaporization or dissection of tissue. In theory and in practice with optimum technique and control setting, the force required to dissect tissue would be zero grams of pressure between the electrode and the tissue.

Fulgurate

A high voltage, low current non-continuous waveform (highly damped) is designed to coagulate by means of spraying long electrical sparks to the tissue—see Figure 6.5, coagulation (fulguration) waveform set at 50 W. The most common use of fulguration is when coagulation is needed in an area that is oozing such as in a capillary or arteriole bed, where a discrete bleeder cannot be identified. The benefit of fulguration is its ability to arrest oozing emanating from a large area in a most efficient manner. Cardiovascular, urological and general surgeons have relied on fulguration for their most demanding applications, i.e. hepatic resections, bleeding from a bladder tumour resection and surface bleeding on the heart. With fulguration a very superficial eschar is produced, therefore the depth of necrosis is minimal as a result of the defocusing of the power density. By drawing the electrode away from the tissue, the power density goes down. A great deal of the energy is lost in the air that the current passes through. Fulguration as well as electrosurgical cutting are non-contact modalities. Fulguration can be initiated in two ways:

1. By very slowly approaching the tissue until a spark jumps to the tissue whereupon a raining effect of sparks will be maintained until such time the electrode is withdrawn or the tissue is carbonized to the point where the sparks cease.

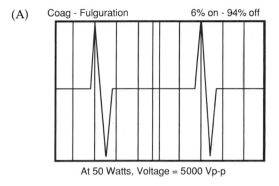

(A) Coag - Fulguration   6% on - 94% off

At 50 Watts, Voltage = 5000 Vp-p

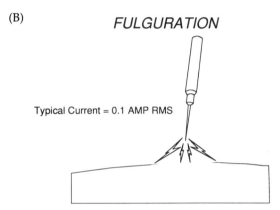

(B)   *FULGURATION*

Typical Current = 0.1 AMP RMS

Figure 6.5 Fulguration. 'Electrode not in contact with tissue.'

2. Bouncing the electrode off the tissue will result in a raining effect of sparks to the tissue without the painstaking effort of approaching the tissue until a spark jumps without touching.

Electrosurgical fulguration is the most effective means of arresting this form of bleeding.

Desiccation

Any waveform will desiccate due to the electrode being in contact with the tissue for the first time—see Figure 6.6. Regardless of the current voltage ratio with the electrode in contact with

DESICCATION

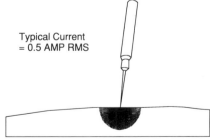

Typical Current
= 0.5 AMP RMS

Figure 6.6 Desiccation. 'Electrode in contact with tissue' (no sparking between electrode and tissue).

the tissue, the magnitude of energy in watts is of the greatest importance. Desiccation is another form of coagulation. Most surgeons do not make a distinction between fulguration and desiccation, but refer to both as coagulation. The application of electrosurgical current by means of direct contact with the tissue will now result in all of the energy set on the ESU being converted into heat within the tissue. By contrast, in both cutting and fulgurating mode a significant amount of the electrical energy converted to heat went into heating up the atmosphere or air/CO_2 between the electrode and the tissue. Therefore with contact coagulation/desiccation the increased energy delivered into the tissue results in deep necrosis, as deep as it is wide, as observed on the surface where the electrode makes contact (see Figure 6.6).

The most common application of desiccation is when a discrete bleeder is encountered and a haemostat is introduced to occlude the vessel first by mechanical pressure, then the electrosurgical energy is applied to the body of the haemostat. In this way the current must pass through the haemostat into the tissue grasped by the jaws and back to the patient return electrode. The coaptation of vessels was documented (Sigel and Dunn, 1965) as producing a collagen chain reaction resulting in a fibrous bonding of the dehydrated denatured cells of the endothelium. Because the electrode is in good electrical contact with the tissue the voltage current ratio is not nearly as important as in cutting and fulgurating. In practical terms the cut/blend waveforms are superior for this application over the fulguration waveform when desiccation is desired. The primary reason is the fulguration waveform will tend to spark through the coagulated tissue, resulting in voids in the bonding to the end of the vessel. Also when sparks occur at the electrode in contact or near contact the metal in the electrode will heat up rapidly, causing the tissue to adhere to the electrode when drawn off the target site. Bleeding will continue each time the eschar is pulled off due to adhesion from heat within the electrode.

In bipolar desiccation, the waveform plays a far more important role. Today, for the most part, the manufacturers have incorporated a continuous low voltage, high current waveform in the bipolar output to maximize the effect on desiccation. With the older models, the manufacturer allowed the surgeon to select either a continuous cut, blend or fulguration waveform when bipolar desiccation was needed. The lack of understanding on the physician's part, in combination with the literature not being clear on the tissue effect when bipolar desiccation was performed with these waveforms,

led to a number of associated documented (Soderstrom, 1982) problems. Therefore at this time the generally accepted waveform for bipolar desiccation is a continuous low voltage, high current waveform. The author recommends, when bipolar desiccation is critical, that a newer model ESU with a dedicated continuous bipolar waveform be used. If one must use an ESU that allows you to select, both cut/blend, fulguration and bipolar currents, it is best to start with the pure cut (continuous) waveform for best results. When performing desiccation, patience is the key to good results. Typically the power density is much lower when desiccating. The physical size of the active electrodes is therefore larger. The larger electrode or contact area to tissue will require longer activation times to attain the desired therapeutic effect. If higher energy is introduced to speed up the desiccation process, this will most likely be counter-productive. Higher energy levels will increase the temperature to the tissue adjacent to the electrode/s, potentially forcing the current to spark through the necrosis, resulting in fulguration rather than desiccation. Fulguration or sparking immediately stops the deep heating process and starts to carbonize the surface of the tissue only. Therefore when sparking is observed during desiccation, it is wise to stop and reduce the power or pulse the current by keying on and off the ESU to overcome this natural tendency of the electrosurgical energy. Sparking is not needed or wanted when desiccating. It causes tissue sticking and creates uneven necrosis and may compromise the intent to coapt the vessel. To help assist the surgeon when desiccating an ammeter (Model EPM-1 ammeter, Electroscope, Inc., Boulder, CO, USA) may be used to control the amount of current as well as determine end point coagulation/desiccation. This will help confirm the visual effect seen by the surgeon. The ammeter will only show current flow when the tissue still contains electrolytic fluid. Total or complete desiccation occurs after dehydration has taken place.

Inherent Risks

Since the inception of monopolar electrosurgery, there have been three potential sites for patient burns due to the presence of electrosurgical current—one intended, two unintended. The intended site is at the active electrode where the unit is used to cut, fulgurate or desiccate the tissue in surgery. Due to its design, the active electrode has a high power density to heat tissue rapidly. If not tended this electrode can burn the patient severely if not kept in control at all times. Therefore the author strongly recommends that the active electrode when not in use be stored in an insulated holster or tray.

There are two unintended sites, the first is a consequence of current division. Current division to alternate ground points to the patient can only occur on ground referenced electrosurgical units. Secondly, the patient may be burned due to a fault condition at the site of the patient return electrode, i.e. partial detachment or manufacturing defect that forces the current returning to the ESU via a high current density. The patient return electrode (ground plate) has approximately a surface area of 20 square inches or larger when properly applied. Therefore very little temperature rise occurs at this site under normal conditions. Both of these potential burns sites have been overcome by improved design within the newer electrosurgical units developed in the last two decades. These safety circuits or features are available on most units sold within the past 10 years. The two major advancements in overcoming these risks are as follows.

Isolated Electrosurgical Outputs

Isolated electrosurgical units were introduced in the early 1970s. The primary purpose of their introduction was the prevention of alternate ground site burns due to current division. Today the number of alternate site burns as a direct result of current division is essentially zero with the introduction of isolated ESUs. There is a small percentage of hospitals that use ground reference ESUs. Therefore it would be wise to qualify the type of ESU that is in service at your hospital, regarding the type of output.

Contact Quality Monitors

Contact quality monitoring circuits were introduced in the early 1980s. The primary purpose of their introduction was to prevent burns at the patient return electrode site. The contact quality monitor incorporated a dual section patient return electrode and circuit for the purpose of evaluating the total impedance of the patient return electrode during surgery. Therefore during the course of surgery if the patient return electrode became compromised the contact quality circuit would inhibit the electrosurgical generator output based on this dual section patient return electrode and circuit combination. This feature has essentially eliminated the secondary unintended patient burns—those that appear at the site of the patient return electrode.

These two technological advancements have truly reduced the potential for patient burns while performing classical open electrosurgical procedures. These features are now found on the major manufacturers of electrosurgical units such as Apen (Denver, Colorado), Birtcher (Irvine, California) and Valleylab (Boulder, Colorado).

Laparoscopic Issues

The use of electrosurgery (Rioux, 1973) in laparoscopic surgery has been used by gynaecologists for the past two decades. With the recent flurry of interest in laparoscopy for general, urological and other surgical disciplines a major question of contention is whether electrosurgical energy can be safely used in laparoscopy. The purpose of this section is to address the real issues pertaining to its safe use in laparoscopy, in a similar fashion to the potential hazards discussed previously regarding the general use of electrosurgery in open surgery. Additionally, options available to help minimize or eliminate the potential of unintended burns within the peritoneal cavity during laparoscopic surgery will be described.

There are two potential hazards in the use of electrosurgical energy during laparoscopy. They are a direct result of two factors:

1. How access is obtained to the peritoneal cavity through the trocar cannulas; and
2. The laparoscope views less than 10% of the total electrosurgical probe.

In passing the electrosurgical active electrode through these access channels and viewed in such a fashion, the following describes the potential for unintended burns.

Most laparoscopic accessories are approximately 35 cm long. The laparoscopic images viewed on the monitor shows a small portion, typically less than 5 cm of the distal end of the device. Therefore the active electrode used for the delivery of the electrosurgical energy has insulation covering most of the electrode. Unfortunately 90% or more of this insulated portion of the electrode is out of the viewing image seen on the monitor. Therefore if a breakdown of the insulation occurs on the shaft of the electrode, out of view from the operator, a severe burn may occur on the bowel or other organs near or touching the electrode at this site, see Figure 6.7. These burns

(a)

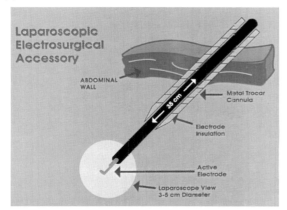

(a)

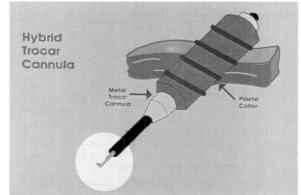

(b)

DIRECTLY COUPLED ENERGY

• Insulation Breakdown
• Exposed Active Tip

(b)

CAPACITIVELY COUPLED ENERGY

• Metal Cannula
• Laparoscope Single, Multiple Puncture(s)

(c)

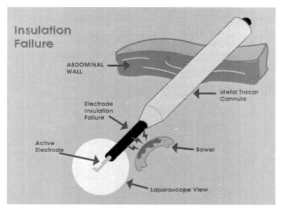

(c)

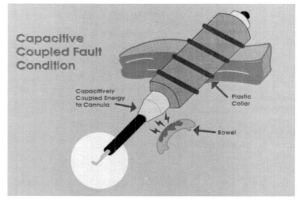

Figure 6.7 (a) Full view of electrosurgical accessory into the peritoneal cavity. (c) Full view of electrosurgical accessory with insulation failure.

Figure 6.8 (a) Hybrid trocar cannula that blocks the capacitive current from the abdominal wall. (c) Capacitive coupling with dangerous stray pathway back to patient return electrode.

may not be noticed during the course of surgery and may result in severe postoperative complications. It is most important to examine or have your biomedical staff set up a routine inspection of these electrodes periodically.

The second hazard that exists is one of capacitively coupled energy into other metal laparoscopic instruments or trocar cannulae. The principle of how capacitance occurs requires a degree of understanding of electrical physics beyond the scope of this chapter. The bottom line is that 5–40% of the power level that the

electrosurgical unit is set on to deliver, can be coupled or transferred into the (10 cm) trocar cannula. This energy in itself may not be dangerous, providing it is allowed to pass through a low power density pathway such as the all-metal (conductive) trocar cannula inserted into the abdominal wall and returned to the patient return electrode.

The problem arises when this energy is allowed or made to pass through a high power density pathway (see Figure 6.8). This can happen for example with the part plastic (non-conductive) and

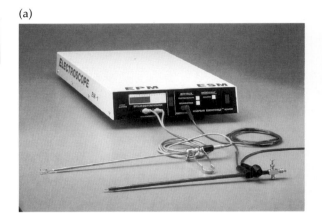

(a)

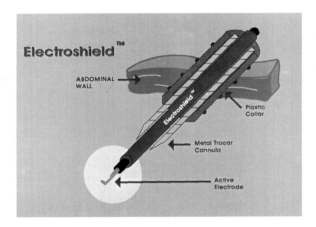

Figure 6.9 Electroshield^R: a sheath that surrounds existing laparoscopic electrosurgical instruments.

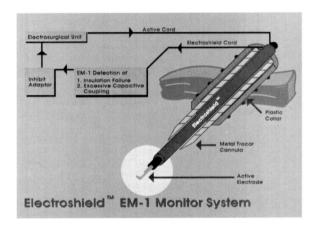

Figure 6.10 Electroshield^R monitoring system: dynamically detects any insulation faults and shields against capacitive coupling.

(b)

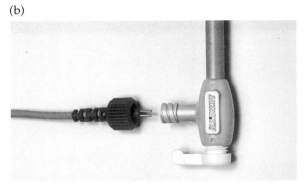

Figure 6.11 (a) Electroshield^R Monitoring System 2 (EM-2). (b) Electro-shield^R cable connection.

part metal (conductive) trocar cannulas on the market. Some trocar manufacturers supply a plastic thread to the metal cannula tube to help hold the cannula in the abdominal wall when the laparoscopic electrode is positioned in and out of the cannula port (see Figure 6.8). To avoid this hazard the author strongly recommends that the electrosurgical active laparoscopic electrode is passed through an all-metal or all-plastic trocar cannula.

Capacitive coupling to a lesser degree can occur with crossing another laparoscopic instrument with the electrosurgical laparoscopic electrode within the peritoneal cavity, i.e. atraumatic grasper etc. The energy transfer to these instruments can range from 1 to 10% of the power set on the electrosurgical unit. Some caution should be taken under this condition, especially during long activation times.

The issue of capacitive coupling was first detected in performing operative, single-puncture laparoscopic procedures (Corson, 1974; Engel, 1975). These laparoscopes have an operating channel (30–40 cm long) to pass various instruments through. It was observed that when a plastic 10–12 mm cannula was used to pass the operating laparoscope through, that the distal end of the metal laparoscope could deliver a portion of the power (40–80%) set on the ESU, and burns to adjacent tissue were documented. Therefore during single puncture operative laparoscopy where electrosurgery may be used, only all-metal trocar cannulae should be used to pass both the laparoscope and electrosurgical electrode into the peritoneal cavity. There was a strong recommendation made to this effect by the FDA in the late 1970s.

The all-metal trocar cannula is also a benefit in multiple-puncture laparoscopic procedures, in the event of the active electrode accidentally touching the end of the metal laparoscope during activation. The metal trocar cannula will allow this energy to pass safely into the abdominal wall via a low power density pathway. If a plastic cannula were used, the current may exit to the bowel or other organs touching the laparoscope, out of view of the monitor. This is due to the plastic cannula blocking the directly coupled energy from safely being passed into the abdominal wall and back to the patient return electrode.

Electroscope, Inc. of Boulder, CO, USA has recently released a proprietary technology consisting of the following: Electroshield ™/EM-1 Monitoring System that protects against both of these primary hazards while performing laparoscopic application of electrosurgical energy. The Electroshield system features a reusable shield (see Figure 6.9) that surrounds 'existing' dissecting and coagulating laparoscopic electrodes. The Electroshield Monitor (EM-1) dynamically detects (see Figure 6.10) any insulation faults and shields against capacitive coupling. If an unsafe condition exists, the Electroshield system (Figure 6.11) automatically deactivates the generator before a burn can occur. With this technological advancement, electrosurgical energy can be used in laparoscopy, with the same efficacy and safety considerations as in classical open surgical procedures.

Summary

Electrosurgical energy has by far the most diverse capabilities as compared with other energy sources. The technological advancements in performance and safety have positioned this device as one of the more useful tools in a surgeon's armamentarium. As with any surgical tool or energy source, education and skill are required. This introduction to the principles of the biophysics of electrical energy on tissue and the safety considerations is an attempt to begin to further our understanding of this powerful surgical tool.

References

Corson SL (1974) Electrosurgical hazards in laparoscopy. *Journal of the American Medical Association* **227 (11)**: 1261.

Engel T (1975) Electrosurgical dynamics of laparoscopic sterilization. *Journal of Reproductive Medicine* **15**: no. 1.

Sigel B & Dunn MR (1965) The mechanism of blood vessel closure by high frequency electrocoagulation. *Surgery, Gynecology and Obstetrics* **121**: 823–831.

Rioux JE (1973) Laparoscopic tubal sterilization: sparking and its control. *La vie médicale au Canada français* **2**: 760–766.

Soderstrom RM (1982) Hazards of laparoscopic sterilization. *Gynecology and Obstetrics*, Ch 24, pp. 1–6. Harper & Row.

7

Tissue Effects of Different Lasers and Electrodiathermy

JÖRG KECKSTEIN

Department of Obstetrics and Gynaecology, University of Ulm, Germany

Introduction

In surgery great importance has always been attached to the techniques of incision, preparation and haemostasis. With the advent of endoscopic operations most surgical techniques required either modification or complete change. A profound knowledge of the interaction between biological tissue and implements used is of vital importance for achieving optimal results.

The method most commonly practised in surgical medicine is that of putting to use operative-therapeutic heat to destroy or coagulate tissue. Table 7.1 shows the various incision and coagulation procedures available for biological tissue.

While the scalpel is still the most inexpensive and most commonly used instrument for the separation of tissue, its use in conjunction with endoscopic instruments is rather limited.

Bleeding control during cutting affords a good overall view of the operational site and conse-

quently reduces operating time. Here the laser systems and high-frequency (HF) surgery come into their own. The tissue changes brought about by these instruments are chiefly due to thermal effects. In Table 7.2 the correlation of tissue effect and temperature is demonstrated.

Electrodiathermy

The term 'diathermy' is often used in connection with HF surgery and is in this context a regrettable misnomer. In actual fact, diathermy stands for the application of extremely high-frequency

Table 7.1 Different instruments for incision used in endoscopic surgery

Scalpel
Electric blade (HF surgery)
Laser
Ultrasound dissector
Jet of liquid
Plasma scalpel
Microwave scalpel
HF-controlled rare-gas jet

Table 7.2 Thermal tissue effect in relation to different temperatures

Temperature (°C)	Tissue effect
37–43	Heating of the tissue
43–45	Retraction
> 50	Reduction of enzyme activity
45–60	Denaturation of protein coagulation
90–100	Drying of tissue
> 100	Boiling point of water, destruction of cell membrane
> 150	Carbonization
> 300	Vaporization
> 500	Burning

alternating current (>1 GHz) to yield heating of entire body parts. By contrast, the term 'HF surgery' applies to alternating current whose frequency range starts at 300 kHz and is used for incision and coagulation.

Electric current renders living tissue electrically conductive, the degree of conductivity depending on the electrolyte content. When electrical current passes through living tissue, three qualitatively different endogenous effects can be observed:

1. electrolytic effect,
2. stimulation of nerves and muscles,
3. thermic effect.

Cutting with HF surgical instruments requires the presence of high voltage (peak voltage of approximately 200 V) between electrode and tissue. Such high frequency excludes stimulation of nerves and muscles likely to interfere with the surgical procedure. It is produced by a small active electrode whose outgoing current is highly concentrated on tissue contact but is then dispersed in the body, eventually rendering the electrode quasi-neutral. This means that an effect is only produced at the point of entry. The resulting electric arcs (Figure 7.1) are like microscopic flashes and appear when electrode and tissue come within close proximity of each other. If the voltage is below 200 V the tissue cannot be cut.

In addition to the cutting effect, a variable coagulation effect (Figure 7.1) is produced along the incision line, both these depending on parameters such as peak voltage, HF frequency, modulation, cutting and coagulation speed, shape of electrode, and tissue.

Experimental studies showed a close association between *peak voltage* and coagulation zone. The correlation between the depth of coagulation and voltage is demonstrated in Figure 7.2. Low-voltage

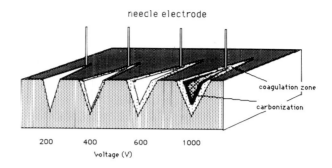

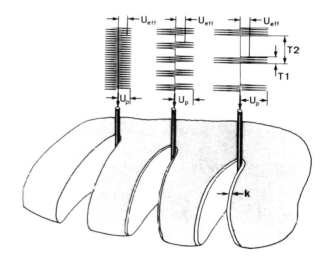

Figure 7.2 Tissue effect of HF surgery. Correlation between intensity of voltage and coagulation effect. A relatively low peak voltage of 200 V is used to produce cuts with small necrosis zones.

Figure 7.3 Different tissue effects depending on different voltages and modulation. The depth of the coagulation effect increases with increasing peak value U_p. Some high-frequency surgical equipment offers the option to modulate electric current enabling the surgeon to determine the quality of the cut. (Published by kind permission of G. Farin, Erbe, Tübingen.)

current produces incisions with little coagulation effect, while high voltages create incisions with broader coagulation zones (Figure 7.2).

The *frequency* of HF current ranges between 400 and 40 000 kHz and is produced by a tube generator and a spark generator. For cutting, unmodulated high-frequency current (Figure 7.3) is produced by the tube generator. The spark generator provides amplitude-modulated HF voltages yielding a greater coagulation effect (Figure 7.3). A combination of the different HF *voltage modulations* permits tissue effects to be varied.

Another factor influencing tissue effect is the *cutting speed* of the electrode. When the electrode

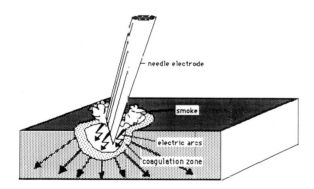

Figure 7.1 Incision with HF current. A cut is produced when a peak voltage of >200 V between electrode and the tissue is reached, resulting in vaporization of the tissue.

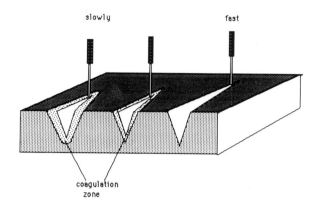

Figure 7.4 Tissue effect of HF surgery in relation to the cutting rate.

is moved at high speed, there is little coagulation effect (Figure 7.4). Slowing down the rate increases the coagulation effect.

The *shape* of the cutting electrodes is of decisive influence on tissue effect. The thicker the electrode is, the deeper is the coagulation zone. Thin-needle electrodes, used in microsurgery, or wire loops have poorer coagulation properties than knife- or ball-shaped electrodes (Figure 7.5). Knife-shaped electrodes permit very smooth incisions but create a larger coagulation border. When the electrode is used to aid coagulation its broad end is pressed against the incision surface.

Coagulation

Biological tissue to be coagulated requires a temperature build-up of 70°C. Table 7.2 shows

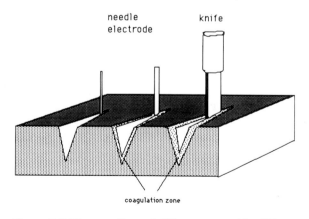

Figure 7.5 Tissue effect of HF surgery with different shapes of electrode: small coagulation zone with needle electrode; large coagulation zone with thick blades.

the different tissue effects in relation to temperature.

With high-frequency electric alternating current used for heating biological tissue, tissue temperature rises in proportion to tissue resistance. A temperature increase beyond 70°C may trigger additional problems. Dehydration, vaporization, or carbonization may interfere with the coagulation effect and thus hamper the determination of the size of the coagulation zone. The lack of homogeneity of the tissue's electrical and thermal properties causes the temperature to rise at varying rates, rendering coagulation effect control quite difficult. The coagulation of tissue is a dynamic process and presents the surgeon attempting to obtain a specific tissue effect with a variety of complex problems.

The size of the coagulation zone can be determined by the type of technique applied and by the rate of coagulation. There are three different coagulation modes (Figure 7.6 a–c):

1. soft coagulation,
2. forced coagulation,
3. spray coagulation.

Soft coagulation (Figure 7.6a) refers to voltages below 200 V. The electrodes are brought into direct contact with the tissue. Unmodulated HF voltages with absence of electric arcs exclude tissue vaporization or carbonization. The tissue is heated gradually according to coagulation time and electric resistance of the tissue. Because of the low voltage the tissue does not become carbonized.

Forced coagulation (Figure 7.6b) uses small electrodes and is characterized by electric arcs generated between coagulation electrode and tissue to obtain deeper coagulation. This specific mode requires voltages of >500 V. HF current needs to be modulated and voltages must not be too high as this creates a cutting effect.

HF voltages with peak values of a few kilovolts are recommended for *spray coagulation* (Figure 7.6c). With this technique, especially used for surface coagulation, long electric arcs produced between electrode and tissue make direct contact superfluous.

Monopolar versus Bipolar HF Surgery

Density distribution of the HF current is chiefly determined by the technique applied. Totally different results are achieved when using monopolar as opposed to bipolar HF current.

The size of a coagulum produced by the

Figure 7.6 Coagulation modes with different techniques and electrodes. Each technique has a different peak voltage and modulation of the HF current. a, Soft coagulation; b, forced coagulation; c, spray coagulation. (Published by kind permission of G. Farin, Erbe, Tübingen.)

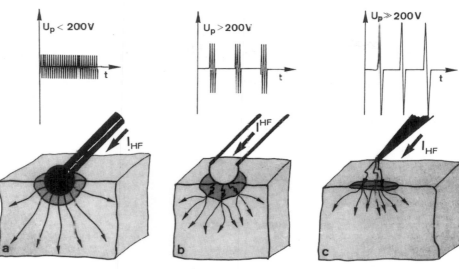

Figure 7.7 Tissue effect of monopolar and bipolar HF coagulation with different application techniques. A–C depict monopolar coagulation with ball electrode and thin-needle electrode for interstitial coagulation. and coagulation of a vessel by forceps. In bipolar (D–F) coagulation the current flow between the two electrodes affords a better control of the coagulation effect. K, coagulation zone, I, current. (Published by kind permission of G. Farin, Erbe, Tübingen.)

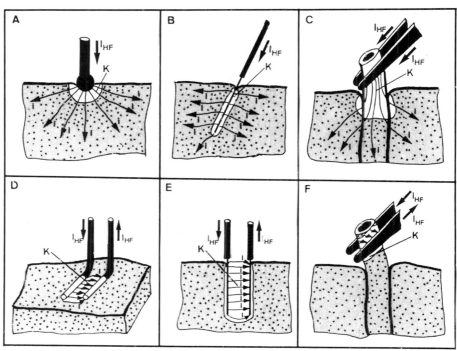

monopolar and bipolar technique is depicted in Figure 7.7 (A–F).

Laser

In the field of medicine the CO_2 laser, the Nd:YAG, argon, KTP, and Dye lasers have been in use for some time now and have proved worthwhile, whereas the excimer laser, so far chiefly used in research, is only just beginning to gain ground in the medical field

Table 7.3 and Figure 7.8 show the emission wavelengths of lasers used in medicine. The aiming beam of the individual types of invisible lasers is the helium–neon (He–Ne) laser. Each of

these lasers has distinctive properties which yield different tissue effects and thus allow specific applications.

We carried out a number of experimental *in vitro* studies to assess and compare CO_2, argon, and Nd:YAG laser performance, testing the cutting and coagulation effect on the extirpated uteri of pigs. Fibres of 600 μm diameter were chosen. To ensure uniform experimental conditions with regard to tissue tension and cutting velocity, equal-length strips of material were stretched on a portable cart and secured by weights. The laser guide was fixed on a support and the tissue moved with a speed of 2.5 cm per second (Figure 7.9).

Criteria for effect evaluation were vaporization depth and coagulation of the cut borders. Results are shown in Figures 7.13–7.17 (see later).

Figure 7.8 Different tissue effects of CO_2, Nd:YAG and argon lasers.

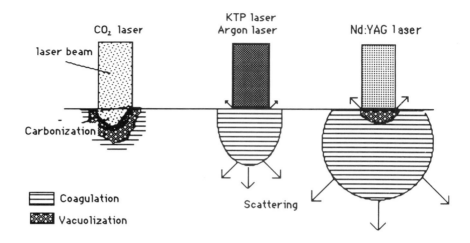

Table 7.3 Different wavelengths of laser systems used in endoscopic surgery

System	Wavelength
CO_2 laser	10.60 μm
Nd:YAG laser	1.06 μm or 1.32 μm
Argon laser	488/514 nm
KTP laser	530 nm

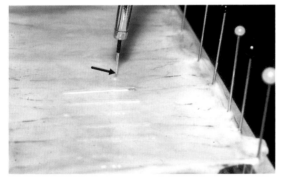

Figure 7.9 Experimental study of tissue effect with different laser systems. The picture shows a bare fibre (arrow) for the use of Nd:YAG laser in non-contact technique.

Laser systems

CO_2 LASER

The coherent monochromatic CO_2 laser beam can be accurately focused through an optical lens system. The high-energy laser beam passes through air and is absorbed as it hits liquid or solid objects. It can thus be used for precise surgical work such as tissue incision, vaporization, and coagulation. Body tissue with a water content of 80–90% absorbs the laser energy very rapidly.

The tissue is incised by heating intracellular and extracellular water to boiling point, resulting in the formation of steam. The energy of a continuously emitted CO_2 laser beam creates an incision by tissue vaporization. This makes the laser eminently suitable for surgery. Some of the debris is carbonized as it passes through the beam, some ignites and burns, thus creating the 'laser plume'.

The defocused laser beam has low-energy density and causes a rapid rise of tissue temperature, with gradual fluid vaporization, dehydration and carbonization.

Histological examination of sections derived from laser wounds of various organs (Figure 7.10) has shown that cellular damage occurs within a range of 500 μm from laser impact. The depth of thermal necrosis is, however, generally below 100 μm. With normal blood flow, veins and arteries up to 0.5 mm vascular diameter can be sealed by laser. The CO_2 laser has been the subject of many studies investigating the tissue effects of the laser beam (Bellina et al., 1984; Badaway et al., 1986; Baggish and ElBakry, 1986; Filmar et al., 1986; McKenzie, 1986; Barbot et al., 1987; Luciano et al., 1987; Puolakkainen et al., 1987; Keckstein, 1990).

Our experiments showed that with increasing power the vaporization effect intensified whereas the coagulation effect weakened (Keckstein, 1990). Various authors report a reduced rate of tissue necrosis when using the CO_2 laser in superpulse mode (Badaway et al., 1986; Baggish and ElBakry, 1986; Luciano et al., 1987; Keckstein, 1990). This is attributable to the interval between each laser pulse which eliminates the constant tissue heating experienced with the continuous mode.

A recent development in CO_2 laser technology is the 'ultrapulse' closed facility. In this mode the laser beam is delivered as very high pulse energy

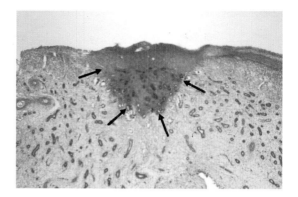

Figure 7.11 Tissue effect of Nd:YAG laser. The section demonstrates a deep coagulation effect (arrows) without any vaporization effect.

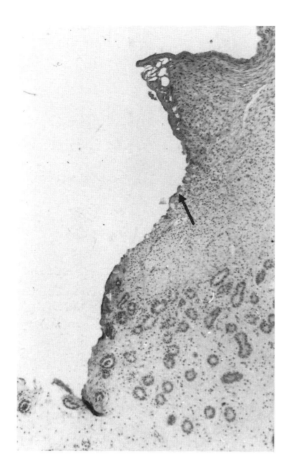

Figure 7.10 Incision with the CO_2 laser. The depth of thermal necrosis is <100 μm (arrow).

bursts of up to 250 mJ and average powers of 950 mW. The advantage of this mode is char free, extremely precise cutting with minimal thermal damage to surrounding tissue even at spot sizes of up to 3 mm in diameter. Although this laser unit has been available in the United States for some time, it has only recently become commercially available in Europe and represents the state of the art technology in CO_2 laser surgery (Coherent, Palo Alto, California, USA; Coherent, Cambridge, UK).

THE ND:YAG LASER

In contrast to the CO_2 laser, the beam of the Nd:YAG laser has a greater depth of tissue penetration, yielding totally different tissue effects (Figures 7.8 and 7.11). The amount of energy available does not, usually, suffice for instant tissue vaporization. Thus, brief laser application only produces coagulation (Figure 7.11). With increasing time of application, tissue temperature rises to approximately 100°C. The ensuing tissue dehydration impairs heat conduction, causing a further rise in temperature. Once the laser-treated

surface is dry and begins to carbonize, the absorption properties of the tissue change. The result is a vaporization effect.

Thanks to its great depth of tissue penetration the Nd:YAG laser beam is capable of coagulating, shrinking, and hence sealing blood vessels of up to 5 mm diameter.

ARGON LASER/KTP LASER

The depth of penetration of the argon laser lies between 0.5 and 2.5 mm. Its applicability ranges between that of the CO_2 laser and the Nd:YAG laser. The KTP laser has a wave length similar to the argon laser and is equivalent to the argon laser in terms of practicability.

The argon laser produces a blue light and is a mixture of different wave lengths between 488 and 515 nm. The KTP 532 laser is essentially Nd:YAG laser energy which is passed through a potassium-titanyl-phosphate crystal, effectively halving the wavelength so that emerald green light at 532 nm emerges from the laser generator. One advantage of this laser is that at a flick of a switch a mirror is interposed which stops the Nd:YAG laser energy from hitting the crystal and allows it to come out as pure Nd:YAG energy, effectively giving two lasers for the price of one.

Although these lasers have very similar wave-lengths, it is obvious on using them clinically that the argon laser is more effective as a photocoagulating laser, whereas the KTP laser is a very effective cutting instrument, especially using a 300 μm fibre, and if the fibre is withdrawn from the tissue it acts as a very effective coagulator. The argon laser seems to be less effective at cutting, possibly because of the lower power at which it works, but also because the end of the fibre burns off during cutting. Continuous measurements of the loss of laser power at the fibre tip during cutting show a nearly exponential decrease of power output with length of cut; after 50 cm only 10% of the laser power exits from the fibre tip. Correspondingly the cutting efficiency is reduced to 30% but without any influence on the coagulation zone (Keckstein *et al.*, 1988). The KTP 532 laser is particularly suitable for dealing with advanced endometriosis, especially ovarian endometriomas, and is also useful for dealing with haemorrhagic ovarian cyst or ectopic pregnancies.

Laser Techniques

LASER APPLICATION IN CONTACT AND
NON-CONTACT TECHNIQUE
ARGON VERSUS Nd:YAG LASER

The use of Nd:YAG (Keckstein *et al.*, 1987; Wallwiener *et al.*, 1987; Grochmal, 1988; Kojiama *et al.*, 1988; Daniell, 1989; Keckstein, 1990) and argon lasers (Bellina *et al.*, 1983; Keye and Dixon, 1983; Keckstein *et al.*, 1988; Keckstein, 1990) for endoscopic operations has been described by a number of authors. The poor cutting properties of the Nd:YAG laser were overcome by using sapphire tips or by adapting the bare-fibre technique.

We carried out *in vitro* studies to examine the tissue effects produced by Nd:YAG and argon lasers both in contact and non-contact technique (Figure 7.12). Measurements obtained for the individual lasers and techniques showed cutting depth and coagulation to be a function of laser power and energy density (Figures 7.13–7.17).

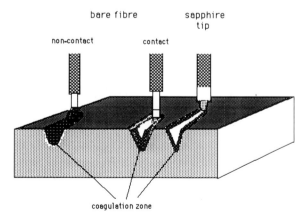

Figure 7.12 Application modes of 'fibre-lasers': bare-fibre technique in non-contact mode, bare fibre in contact mode, sapphire tips.

NON-CONTACT TECHNIQUE

With the non-contact technique (Figures 7.13 and 7.14), the Nd:YAG laser only produces deep and wide tissue coagulation. Increasing laser power enlarges the coagulation zone. The argon laser, too, at low power produces a coagulation effect only. With increased power, however, the argon laser, unlike the Nd:YAG laser, can reach the same vaporization depth as that attained with the contact techique (Figures 7.15 and 7.16). Power increase results in a clear increase of cutting depth, with only minor broadening of the coagulation zone. At 10 W the coagulation zone amounts to 70% of the cutting depth, and at 15 W it is 50% of the cutting depth.

CONTACT TECHNIQUES—Nd:YAG

Sapphire Tips versus 'Bare Fibre'

With both techniques (Figures 7.13–7.16), the Nd:YAG laser produces tissue vaporization. Histological tissue preparation and measurement of the cuts showed that, on average, the use of the bare-fibre technique (Figure 7.13) produced a 30% deeper cut than sapphire tips (Figure 7.16). With either technique cutting depth and coagulation increased with rising power.

Sapphire Tips

Sapphire tips (Figure 7.17) have been widely used and their specifications and limitations are well known. The role of the laser light in connection with such probes is still a point of debate. It is obvious that heating of the tip enhances cutting efficacy. A new tip with an optically clean surface does not cut at all, it must first be immersed in blood or other biological matter to absorb enough laser light. Heat will therefore not only be generated at the end of the tip but also in part of the probe. The heat absorbed by the tissue in the cutting process must be regenerated by the laser light. Only a small amount of laser light is transmitted directly to the tissue, contributing to coagulation.

Any cutting and coagulation achieved with sapphire tips is thus chiefly attributable to a heating effect.

Bare Fibre
This technique presents totally different results. Histological tissue preparation and measurement of the cuts generally showed greater depth of incision, compared with that realized with sapphire tips (Figures 7.15 and 7.16). Moreover,

Figure 7.13 Coagulation versus vaporization. Argon laser radiation with bare fibre in non-contact technique.

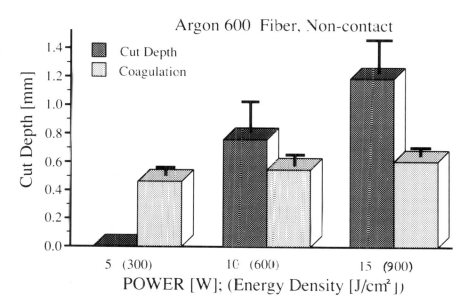

Figure 7.14 Coagulation versus vaporization. Nd:YAG laser radiation with bare fibre in non-contact technique.

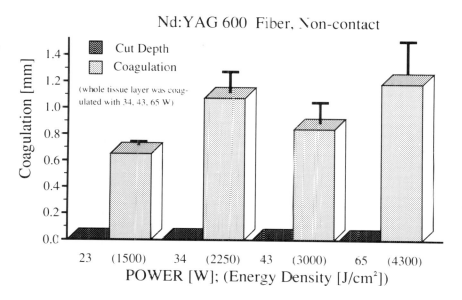

Figure 7.15 Coagulation versus vaporization. Argon and Nd:YAG laser application with the bare fibre (0.6 mm) in contact technique.

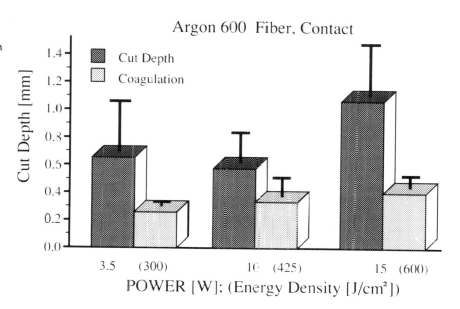

Figure 7.16 Coagulation versus vaporization. Argon and Nd:YAG laser application with the bare fibre (0.6 mm) in contact technique.

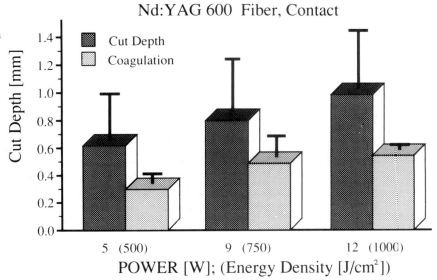

Figure 7.17 Coagulation versus vaporization. Use of sapphire tips with the Nd:YAG laser.

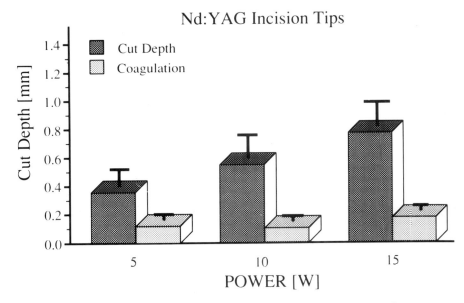

the depth of necrosis exceeded incision depth. This is due to the fact that, with the bare-fibre technique, a far higher proportion of laser light penetrates into the tissue, compared with the conically shaped contact probes.

The use of the bare-fibre technique may cause various technical problems. High power densities on the very end of the quartz fibres produce high temperatures which result in a good vaporization effect. During the vaporization process, tissue debris may stick to the fibre surface causing a change in transmission properties. The high absorption rate of the laser light within the fibre or on the surface then leads to rapid temperature increase of up to 800 or 1000°C. While this may diminish the laser light transmission rate into the tissue and thus enhance thermal tissue effect, the laser fibre may be damaged by such high temperatures and by the change in transmission characteristics. A highly contaminated

or destroyed fibre surface, however, rules out any subsequent non-contact procedure.

Using a constant temperature control at the fibre tissue interface, the Fibertom (MBB) protects the laser fibre against rapid destruction. During vaporization, visible light is produced which correlates with the temperatures at the fibre end. This allows temperature control by way of a feedback system with integrated microprocessors, regulating laser output in accordance with the visible light (temperatures) produced during laser application. The visible light is kept at constant intensity according to the control parameters (power and reference value). Alteration of these parameters leads to varying tissue effects. The system's advantages are:

- protection of the optical fibre through temperature control
- possibility of combined procedures (non-contact/contact)

- no need for a cooling system (saline, gas) for fibre protection
- controllable coagulation and vaporization effect.

Our experimental studies on uteri showed vaporization depths of between 0.4 and 0.9 mm and coagulation zones of between 0.2 and 0.6 mm. The fibre surface was controlled by alternating non-contact with contact mode laser use. Thanks to the feedback control system the laser fibre can be used two to three times longer than conventional Nd:YAG laser systems. The fibres are, unfortunately, not totally invulnerable to surface destruction.

In summary, it can be said that the Nd:YAG laser is well suited as a cutting instrument in contact technique, using either sapphire tips or bare fibres. Sapphire tips yield a smaller coagulation zone. Comparing argon with Nd:YAG lasers, using the bare-fibre technique, the argon laser produces a 10% greater depth of vaporization which is not significant. This effect is not dependent on energy density. Coagulation zone width follows the same pattern as cutting depth in that it is only power dependent at a certain cutting speed and unaffected by fibre diameter. Comparing the contact versus non-contact mode of the different laser systems, the former produces a smaller coagulation zone in the incisions.

Summary

Heat generation for operative and therapeutic destruction or coagulation of biological tissue can be achieved by either electrodiathermy or medical laser systems. The effect these methods produce varies according to the amount of energy applied. Electrodiathermy is a very versatile cutting and coagulation method. Tissue effect is, however, dependent on variables such as peak voltage, HF frequency, modulation, cutting and coagulation speed, shape of electrode and type of tissue. The laser systems currently available are well suited to coagulation and/or cutting of tissue in non-contact technique. The Nd:YAG or KTP lasers can also be put to a multitude of uses when applied in contact technique.

References

Badaway SZA, ElBakry MM, Baggish MS & Choe JK (1986) Pulsed CO_2 laser versus conventional microsurgical anastomosis of the rat uterine horn. *Fertility and Sterility* **46**: 127–131.

Baggish MS & ElBakry MM (1986) Comparison of electronically superpulsed and continuous-wave CO_2 laser on the rat uterine horn. *Fertility and Sterility* **45**: 120–127.

Barbot J, Parent B, Dubuisson JB & Aubriot FX (1987) A clinical study of the CO_2 laser and electrosurgery for adhesiolysis in 172 cases followed by early second-look laparoscopy. *Fertility and Sterility* **48**: 140–142.

Bellina J, Fisher Ross L, Holmquist N, Voros J & Moorehead M (1983) Linear and nonlinear effect of the argon laser on a fallopian tube animal model. *Lasers in Surgery and Medicine* **2**: 343–355.

Bellina JH, Hemmings R, Voros J & Ross LF (1984) Carbon dioxide laser and electrosurgical wound study with an animal model: a comparison of damage and healing patterns in peritoneal tissue. *American Journal of Obstetrics and Gynecology* **148**: 327–334.

Daniell J (1989) Fiberoptic laser laparoscopy; In Sutton C (ed.) *Laparoscopic Surgery*, pp. 545–562. London: Baillière.

Farin G (1990) *Principles of High Frequency Surgery*, 12 pp. Tübingen: Erbe Elektromedizin.

Filmar S, Gomel V & McComb P (1986) The effectiveness of CO_2 laser and electrosurgery in adhesiolysis: a comparative study. *Fertility and Sterility* **45**: 407–411.

Grochmal S (1988) Contact Nd:YAG superior to CO_2 for treatment of ovarian disease. *Laser Practice Report* **3**: 1S–2S.

Keckstein J (1990) *Laser in der operativen Pelviskopie. In vitro, tierexperimentelle und klinische Studien über Gewebereaktionen und Applikationsarten von CO_2-, Nd:YAG- und Argon-Laser für endoskopische Operationen.* Habilitationsschrift [Postdoctoral thesis], Ulm.

Keckstein J, Finger A & Steiner R (1988) Laser application in contact- and non-contact procedures; sapphire tips in comparison to 'bare-fiber' argon laser in comparison to Nd:YAG laser. *Lasers in Surgery and Medicine* **4**: 158–162.

Keckstein J, Wolf A & Steiner R (1987) The use of contact laser probe in gynecological endoscopy. *Proceedings of the 7th Congress International Society for Laser Surgery and Medicine*, Munich, pp. 267–272.

Keye W & Dixon J (1983) Photocoagulation of endometriosis by the argon laser through the laparoscope. *Obstetrics and Gynecology* **62**: 383–386.

Kojiama E, Yanagigori A, Yuda K & Hirakawa S (1988) Nd:YAG laser endoscopy. *Journal of Reproductive Medicine* **33**: 907–911.

Luciano AA, Whitman G, Maier DB, Randolph J & Maenza R (1987) A comparison of thermal injury, healing patterns, and postoperative adhesion formation following CO_2 laser and electromicrosurgery. *Fertility and Sterility* **48**: 1025–1029.

McKenzie AL (1986) A three-zone model of soft tissue

damage by a CO_2 laser. *Physics in Medicine and Biology* **31**: 967–983.

Puolakkainen P, Brackett K, Sankar NY, Joffe S & Schröder T (1987) Effects of electrocautery, CO_2 laser, and contact Nd:YAG laser scalpel in the healing of intestinal incision. *Lasers in Surgery and Medicine* **7**: 507–511.

Wallwiener D, Morawski A, Plantener G & Bastert G (1987) Ist die Adhäsiolyse mittels Nd:YAG-Laser eine Alternative zur CO_2-Laser-Adhäsiolyse? *Lasers in Surgery and Medicine* **3**: 142–147.

8

Laparoscopic Use of the Argon Beam Coagulator

JAMES F. DANIELL

2222 State Street, Nashville, Tennessee, USA

Introduction

Over the years, many methods have been used
for laparoscopic surgery, including blunt traction,
scissors, forceps, and electrosurgical energy by
both unipolar and bipolar methods (Murphy,
1987). This last decade, various lasers have been
used, including the CO_2 (Daniell, 1985), argon
(Keye and Dixon, 1983), KTP (Daniell *et al.*,
1986) and the Nd:YAG laser. Newer mechanical
methods for laparoscopic surgery also include
permanent clips, laparoscopic suturing techniques, and mechanical stapling devices (Daniell
et al., 1991). The advantages and disadvantages
of all these types of operative laparoscopic
procedures are discussed in this book. This
chapter reviews our initial investigations of the
newest form of electrosurgical energy to be
used laparoscopically, the argon beam coagulator
(ABC).

Method of Action of the Argon Beam Coagulator

The argon beam coagulator allows a jet of argon
gas to carry electrons from a unipolar electrode
through space, to impact on tissue which is
appropriately grounded, delivering electrosurgical
energy as standard unipolar cautery. However,
this energy is delivered in a no-touch technique
through a plume of argon gas so that no smoke
develops with the coagulation. In addition, the

plume of argon gas that sprays around the needle
electrode and conducts the electrical energy
through space has a blast effect on the tissue
before impact. Thus, fluids such as blood or
irrigation fluids will be momentarily blown away
from the tissues to allow the electrosurgical energy
to impact on the actual bleeding site instead of
coagulating the protein in overlying blood. The
flow rates of argon gas can be varied, and as of
this writing, the minimal volume of gas used to
deliver the argon beam to tissue is 4 litres per
minute. The spot diameter of the argon gas that
delivers the beam can vary, and power settings
of 40–150 W are available for clinical use. The
electrosurgical principles of this system are the
same as unipolar coagulation, the only difference
being that electrons flow from a needle electrode
through space to the tissue, carried by argon gas.
The distance that these electrons arc to tissue
depends on the diameter of the plume, the
wattage being delivered from the electrosurgical
unit, and the conductivity of the tissue. Tissue
effects are the same as with unipolar cautery
histologically. Animal studies have shown that
thermal necrosis at 40 W will extend to 2–3 mm
(Rusch *et al.*, 1990). The diameter of the impact
site varies with the diameter of the nozzle that
carries the cone of argon gas to the tissue. This
diameter expands as the tip of the nozzle is held
further away from the tissue impact site. In our
preliminary animal studies including both pigs
and rabbits, energy will pass a distance of 1 cm
at laparoscopy, with power settings up to 100 W.
Early histological investigations of the effects of
laparoscopic use of the argon beam coagulator in

both pigs and rabbits demonstrate thermal damage to tissue similar to that seen with unipolar electrosurgery at the same wattage (Bard Electro Medical Systems, 1988).

Investigations of the argon beam coagulator have begun at open surgery in several specialties, including head and neck surgery (Ward *et al.*, 1989), thoracic surgery (Rusch *et al.*, 1990) and gynaecology (Brand and Pearlman, 1990). All investigators have been impressed with the rapidity with which bleeding can be controlled in a non-contact method, compared to other methods for haemostasis at surgery.

Early Animal Investigations of the Argon Beam Coagulator for Laparoscopy

The first laparoscopic investigation of the ABC was begun at Centennial Medical Center in Nashville, Tennessee, in February, 1991 (Daniell *et al.*, 1992). Using anaesthetized pigs undergoing laparoscopic cholecystectomy in training courses in laparoscopic techniques for surgeons, the ABC was used with a prototype 10 mm diameter probe. This probe contained a needle electrode slightly recessed from its tip to provide the electrosurgical spark. The diameter of the probe tip through which the argon gas flowed around the needle electrode was 3 mm. During laparoscopic cholecystectomy in the pigs, the ABC probe was placed through an accessory 10 mm port, and used to coagulate the liver bed, both prior to any bleeding and after intentional or accidental bleeding had occurred from the bed of the liver during manipulations at laparoscopic cholecystectomy. The pigs underwent general anaesthesia with a pulse oximeter being used to monitor oxygen changes. An anaesthesiologist and veterinarian were present for careful observations in this initial series of five pigs. All pigs survived the laparoscopic cholecystectomy with use of the ABC with no detectable physiological changes under anaesthesia. Flow rates of argon were regulated at 4 litres per minute with simultaneous evacuation of the pneumoperitoneum and argon gas that was used to deliver the electrosurgical effect to the tissue in the pigs. After successfully using the ABC in the pig model with no evidence of immediate or delayed complications, Investigational Review Board approval was obtained at Centennial Medical Center for early clinical trials of the ABC laparoscopically in humans, in both general surgery and gynaecology.

Modifications of the Argon Beam Coagulator for Laparoscopic Use

The initial prototype probe for laparoscopic use of the ABC was made of plastic, 10 mm in diameter, and attached to the electrosurgical generator by a tube, approximately 15 feet long. The tip of the disposable probe was coned down to 3 mm in diameter (Figure 8.1). Inside this tip was a standard unipolar needle electrode, which was recessed from the surface of the opening of the cone by approximately 2 mm. Thus, if this probe was touched to the tissue, there would be no tissue contact with the unipolar electrode. The initial 10 mm probe was disposable and somewhat flimsy, because it was made of plastic. Particularly, the attachment of the tubing to the probe was weak and would occasionally separate with manipulations at laparoscopy. This resulted in instantaneous cessation of coagulation, since the argon gas would leak and not deliver a flow of gas to the needle electrode in the tip of the probe.

We are presently continuing clinical trials and evaluating modified delivery probes. The next system planned for evaluation is a 10 mm probe, which has a 2 mm port for irrigation or delivery of a needle electrode which can be advanced when needed from the end of the probe for direct use. This probe is still 10 mm in diameter and thus is somewhat cumbersome. In the future, the manufacturer plans to develop and market 5 mm probes with varying diameter tips and probes that can be angled for more effective delivery to the tissue. We have not yet had a chance to

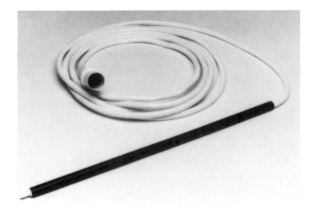

Figure 8.1 The 10 mm prototype disposable probe for laparoscopic use of the argon beam coagulator is shown here. Argon gas from the ABC flows through the instrument at 4 litres per minute during coagulation. The white tip of the probe delivers an argon beam 3 mm in diameter for non-touching unipolar coagulation.

evaluate any of these planned new probes for laparoscopy.

Techniques of Laparoscopic Use of the Argon Beam Coagulator

The ABC is electrosurgical energy, and all the standard safety precautions must be followed, such as proper grounding of the patient, correct setting of the desired wattage, and isolation of the unit to minimize electrical problems. At present, for laparoscopy, the ABC must be introduced through an accessory probe. Thus, most laparoscopies require at least three probes, one for the optical channel, one for an accessory probe for manipulation, and a third probe to deliver the argon beam. Before the ABC is fired, it is important to anticipate and prepare for management of the sudden burst of argon gas which will be flowing intraperitoneally through the probe. At present, this flow is 4 litres per minute. It is best to use a high-flow automatic insufflator that shuts off when the intraperitoneal pressure is greater than 20 mmHg. Just before firing the ABC, we place a 5 mm suction irrigation probe close to the point of impact, and aspirate, using a PumpVac II disposable suction irrigation system for laparoscopy (Marlow Medical, Willoughby, OH, USA). Thus, by actively suctioning as the ABC is fired, we rapidly remove the argon gas from the intraperitoneal cavity and vent it straight into the wall suction system of the operating room. This eliminates accumulation of argon gas in the room, rapidly removes it from the intraperitoneal environment, and helps reduce intraperitoneal pressure. We have recommended to the manufacturer that they consider developing an argon beam probe that has an automatic pop-off valve that will vent off excessive argon gas or stop firing automatically if intraperitoneal pressure exceeds 20 mmHg. At present, such a probe has not yet been clinically evaluated, either in animals or humans. Because of this potential for sudden increased intraperitoneal pressure, the anaesthesiologist should always be alerted before the ABC is to be fired laparoscopically. To date, in over 80 cases in patients, we have noted no physiological changes under anaesthesia that we can relate to the laparoscopic use of argon gas. However, this remains a constant concern for us in our ongoing clinical trial evaluations.

Electrosurgical energy is invisible, but as electrons flow through the argon gas, there is an arcing effect which is visible. This is similar to the glow seen with neon lights. This gives the operator the ability to see the diameter of the beam when firing laparoscopically. There is a total lack of smoke with coagulation because argon gas completely surrounds the impact site. This allows excellent visibility of tissue effects at laparoscopy compared to other forms of electrosurgery or various lasers. Our method of use is to touch the tip of the probe to the planned impact site, back away 2 or 3 mm, and then activate the ABC while instantaneously suctioning. We then adjust the distance from the tip of the probe to the tissue, depending on the tissue effects that we see visually. The 4 litre per minute plume of argon gas begins to flow just before the needle electrode is energized. Thus, blood or irrigation fluids are blown away from the impact site, allowing rapid haemostasis by direct coagulation to exposed vessels. Since the spot size is never smaller than 3 mm, fine cutting is impossible with this form of electrosurgical energy. However, for haemostasis and blunt dissection with coagulation, we have found the ABC to be rapid and effective. After firing the ABC, fresh CO_2 infused via the high flow insufflator rapidly washes out the residual intraperitoneal argon gas. After the procedure, the disposable probe is sent to our laboratory for use in animal investigations and cannot be re-used in humans.

Early Clinical Use of the Argon Beam Coagulator at Laparoscopy in Humans

Our initial clinical trials of the ABC were to evaluate its safety at laparoscopy and its effectiveness for haemostasis. This first series of patients has been reported (Daniell et al., 1992). In this group of 20 patients, we were able successfully to accomplish haemostasis with the ABC following adhesiolysis, myomectomy, cholecystectomy, and endometriosis ablation. After becoming comfortable with laparoscopic use of the ABC and its tissue effects, we began to use its coagulation effects as primary therapy for endometriosis, myomectomy, uterosacral ligament transection, and presacral neurectomy (Table 8.1). For uterosacral ligament transection with the ABC, a third probe is always needed, so that traction can be placed on the ligament. With such traction, the 3 mm diameter spot of the ABC will successfully coagulate and haemostatically separate the uterosacral ligaments. If there is not tissue traction, coagulation only occurs without

Table 8.1 Laparoscopic use of the argon beam coagulator—early clinical evaluation (20 patients)*

Coagulation of endometriosis	14
Uterosacral nerve ablation	10
Presacral neurectomy	3
Myomectomy	1
Excision of ovarian fibroma	1
Conservative surgery for ectopic	1

* Multiple procedures were performed on certain patients

adequate separation. For myomectomy, we have found the ABC to be an excellent laparoscopic adjuvant to our dissection techniques because of the smoke that is generated with other forms of dissection in the myometrium, and the potential for bleeding from this operation.

Laparoscopic Presacral Neurectomy with the Argon Beam Coagulator

Recently, laparoscopic presacral neurectomy has been reported to successfully treat certain forms of midline pelvic pain (Perez, 1990). We have performed this procedure in the past, as initially described, but had problems with bleeding retroperitoneally that prolongs the operation and frightens the operator. With the availability of the ABC, we have now been able to perform five laparoscopic presacral neurectomies with no complications. Our technique is to identify the retroperitoneal structures, open the retroperitoneal space with a needle electrode, and then instead of dissecting the nerve bundles, and isolating and coagulating the vessels, we use the ABC at a setting of 80 W. Using the periosteum as a backstop, we slowly pass the ABC probe transversely across the presacral area, being careful to stay above the sacral promontory and medial to the right ureter and the vessels of the left colonic mesentery. With this technique, we are able to coagulate and separate the presacral nerves along with its associated fat and vessels. In these five cases of laparoscopic presacral neurectomy with the ABC, we have had no bleeding or other surgical complications. In early follow-up, all patients have reported subjective reduction in their pelvic pain. However, longer follow-up in greater numbers of patients is needed before any meaningful conclusions can be drawn concerning the effectiveness of this new method for performing an old operation.

Laparoscopic Treatment of Endometriosis

There is a long history of effective laparoscopic treatment of endometriosis, for both pain relief and enhancement of fertility using electrosurgical energy (Daniell and Christianson, 1981; Murphy et al., 1991). Recently, lasers of various types have become popular for laparoscopic treatment of endometriosis (Daniell and Brown, 1982; Feste, 1985; Martin, 1985; Diamond et al., 1987; Daniell et al., 1991b). After over 10 years' experience with lasers for laparoscopic endometriosis treatment, we are now returning to electrosurgical energy for most of our laparoscopic endometriosis treatment. The ease with which the ABC allows us to rapidly coagulate endometriosis without smoke production and with excellent visible observation of the tissue is impressive. It is still too soon to conclude that the ABC will replace surgical lasers or conventional electrosurgical techniques for endometriosis ablation via laparoscopy. However, our early results in 20 patients are promising.

For laparoscopic treatment of endometriosis with the ABC, a setting of 60–80 W is used and the probe held 3–5 mm away from the implant. With firing, the tissue coagulation effects can be clearly seen, since no smoke occurs and the probe is not touching the tissues. Each area is ablated with adjacent peritoneal edges coagulated for 2–3 mm. The jet of argon gas blows blood and debris away from the impact site and allows haemostatic coagulation within a 3 mm spot diameter. We have thus been able to treat 90% of all implants with this simple rapid method of coagulation. Actual operating time with the ABC is reduced compared to surgical lasers or contact cautery due to less smoke generation, reduced bleeding, and unnecessary delays for reinsufflation. This shortens anaesthesia time, reduces operator fatigue, and thus benefits all parties involved.

Much more information is needed on tissue effects of the ABC on endometrial implants at both open and laparoscopic surgery. In addition, the physiological effects and potential risks (if any) of inert argon gas flowing intraperitoneally during ABC firing must be carefully studied. If it is shown that the ABC is safe and effective long-term therapy, this new emerging technology for controlled laparoscopic tissue ablation may become the treatment of choice for endometriosis.

Laparoscopic Myomectomy

Symptomatic uterine fibroids are common in many women who wish pregnancy or to avoid major surgery or hysterectomy. Laparoscopic myomectomy thus is becoming more commonplace in this era of aggressive endoscopic surgery (Gurley and Daniell, 1991). Present techniques combine preoperative suppression of growth, atraumatic dissection, effective haemostasis, myometrial closure, and removal of portions of the myoma by morcellation or colpotomy. Obtaining haemostasis during myomectomy can be tedious and difficult at laparoscopy. Since the availability of the ABC for laparoscopic evaluation in our practice, we have been impressed with its ability to accomplish rapid haemostasis during dissection in the myometrium. Blood loss is reduced and the operation proceeds more easily when the ABC is used to bluntly dissect the fibrous myoma from the vascular myometrium. We now consider the ABC to be our primary method for dissection for both open and laparoscopic myomectomy.

Laparoscopic Enterolysis

Laparoscopic lysis of adhesions to bowel is becoming a common operation (Daniell, 1989; Sutton and MacDonald, 1990). Usually, blunt or sharp dissection are satisfactory, but often, significant bleeding can occur. This can often be managed with many techniques, including mechanical, electrosurgical, or with lasers. Occasionally, laparotomy is the only recourse to successful and safe control of some of these events. The ABC is especially effective for accomplishing haemostasis in oozing areas when actual vessels are difficult to identify and control. Omental bleeding can be controlled with 60–80 W of power with the ABC without smoke production by merely passing the probe slowly over the bleeding area from a distance of 3–4 mm. The plume of argon gas that blows over the clots allows the electrons to impact on the actual vessels for coagulation. Since this is all done with a non-touching technique, the resulting coagulum is not dislodged as often occurs with unipolar or even bipolar coagulation. No smoke occurs, so operator control is excellent. The depth of tissue coagulation is safely limited to 2–3 mm and irrigation is possible while firing the ABC, since the first jet of argon gas blows the fluids off the tissue prior

to actual coagulation. This gives the laparoscopist a valuable new tool for attempts at safe, effective adhesiolysis.

The Future of the ABC for Laparoscopy

The ABC should become a valuable tool for certain laparoscopic procedures. In our early evaluations, it has proved to be a safe and simple system to deliver laparoscopically. If other laparoscopists find the system as effective for haemostasis and coagulation as we have, it should become commonly used for many laparoscopic operations. All surgeons and operating room personnel are already experienced in the safe use of electrosurgical energy. Thus, introduction of the ABC does not entail extensive new orientation. The ABC can be a very cost-effective addition to the operating room, since it provides a combined unipolar, bipolar, and argon beam coagulation system. It can then be used by many surgical

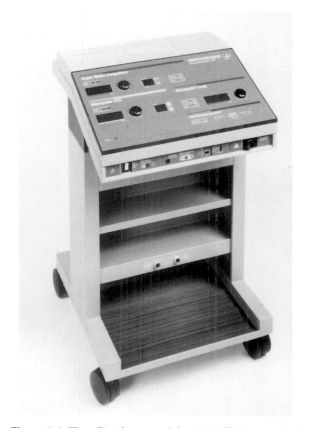

Figure 8.2 The Birtcher model 6400 Electrosurgical Generator—ABC is seen in this photograph. It can be used for standard unipolar cutting or coagulation or for argon beam coagulation. The power for each mode of use is monitored by a digital readout system.

disciplines. At present, these multiple use top of the line electrosurgical generators cost under $15,000.00 in the USA (Figure 8.2). This combination of reduced capital costs to the hospital and shortened operating time should translate into significant savings to all patients in the health care system. Particularly in this era of patient awareness of minimally invasive surgery and spiralling health care costs, we should all consider cost containment in health care delivery.

In our opinion, the ABC with an effective delivery system for laparoscopic surgery may possibly have as much impact in the 1990s as lasers have had over the last decade. In our hands, we have found it useful for many laparoscopic procedures without complications. It reduces operating times, and eliminates excessive intra-peritoneal smoke, while increasing our confidence levels when faced with potential or actual bleeding episodes during laparoscopic manipulations.

Much further evaluation of the ABC is needed in animal models and clinically at both laparotomy and laparoscopy before its true role in surgery is clear. However, all operative laparoscopists should become familiar with the effects of the ABC at laparotomy and consider exploring its potential for assisting at operative laparoscopy. Only time and careful future investigations will be able to determine the true benefits of the ABC for laparoscopic surgery.

References

Bard Electro Medical Systems (1988) *System 6000 argon beam coagulator tissue effects*. Technical document. Englewood, Colorado: Bard Electro Medical Systems, Inc.

Brand E & Pearlman N (1990) Electrosurgical debulking of ovarian cancer: a new technique using the argon beam coagulator. *Gynecologic Oncology* **39**: 115.

Daniell JF (1985) The role of lasers in infertility surgery. *Fertility and Sterility* **45**: 815.

Daniell JF (1989) Laparoscopic enterolysis for chronic abdominal pain. *Journal of Gynecologic Surgery* **5**: 61–66.

Daniell JF & Brown DH (1982) Carbon dioxide laser laparoscopy: initial experience in experimental animals and humans. *Obstetrics and Gynecology* **59**: 761.

Daniell JF & Christianson C (1981) Combined laparoscopic surgery and Danazol therapy for pelvic endometriosis. *Fertility and Sterility* **35**: 521.

Daniell JF, Miller SW & Tosh R (1986) Initial evaluation of the use of the potassium-titanyl-phosphate (KTP/532) laser in gynecologic laparoscopy. *Fertility and Sterility* **46**: 373.

Daniell JF, Gurley LD & Chambers JF (1991a) The use of an automatic stapling device for laparoscopic appendectomy. *Obstetrics and Gynecology* **78**: 721.

Daniell JF, Gurley LD & Kurtz B (1991b) Laser laparoscopic management of large endometriomas. *Fertility and Sterility* **55**: 692.

Daniell JF, Fisher B & Alexander W (1992) Laparoscopic evaluation of the argon beam coagulator—initial report. *Journal of Reproductive Medicine* (in press).

Diamond MP, Boyers, SP, Lavy G et al. (1987) Endoscopic use of the potassium-titanyl-phosphate 532 laser in gynecologic surgery. *Colposcopy and Gynecologic Laser Surgery* **3**: 213.

Feste JR (1985) Laser laparoscopy: a new modality. *Journal of Reproductive Medicine* **30**: 413.

Gurley L & Daniell JF (1991) Laparoscopic management of clinically significant symptomatic uterine fibroids. *Journal of Gynecologic Surgery* **7**: 37–40.

Keye WR & Dixon J (1983) Photocoagulation of endometriosis by the argon laser through the laparoscope. *Obstetrics and Gynecology* **62**: 383.

Martin DC (1985) CO_2 laser laparoscopy for the treatment of endometriosis associated with infertility. *Journal of Reproductive Medicine* **30**: 409.

Murphy AA (1987) Operative laparoscopy. *Fertility and Sterility* **47**: 6.

Murphy AA, Schlaff WD, Hassiakos D et al. (1991) Laparoscopic cautery in the treatment of endometriosis-related infertility. *Fertility and Sterility* **55**: 246.

Perez JJ (1990) Laparoscopic presacral neurectomy. *Journal of Reproductive Medicine* **35**: 625–630.

Rusch VW, Schmidt R, Yoshimi S & Fujimura Y (1990) Use of the argon beam electrocoagulator for performing pulmonary wedge resections. *Annals of Thoracic Surgery* **49**: 287.

Sutton C & MacDonald R (1990) Laser laparoscopic adhesiolysis. *Journal of Gynecologic Surgery* **6**: 155–159.

Ward PH, Castro DJ & Ward S (1989) The argon beam coagulator—a significant new contribution to radical head and neck surgery. *Archives of Otolaryngology—Head and Neck Surgery* **115**: 921.

9

New Developments in Equipment for Insufflation and Smoke Evacuation

ADOLF GALLINAT

Altonaer Strasse 59, Hamburg, Germany

According to an estimation of Semm (1990) about 80% of all benign gynaecological diseases can be managed laparoscopically. If hysteroscopic indications are added the overall rate will probably reach 90% or more. To manage all these kinds of indications, special equipment is required to insufflate and distend body cavities and to remove the smoke and debris generated by endoscopic laser surgery.

Laparoscopy

There are several laser types in use in the field of gynaecological surgery (Table 9.1); all these lasers can also be used in gynaecological endoscopy. The various laser types differ in their wavelength. This implies the different physical behaviour as well as their biophysical reaction seen as tissue effect. High laser energy impacting on tissue causes smoke generation and vision is inevitably obscured for a short time (Figure 9.1).

The physical interaction between lasers and living tissue will result in a vaporization or coagulation effect. The most popular laser in the field of gynaecological surgery is the CO_2 laser. Its exclusive vaporization effect results in high smoke generation. But even the most coagulating laser types, as well as electrosurgical techniques, produce sufficient smoke to disrupt vision.

Smoke evacuation during laparoscopic surgery is technically not a problem even when the CO_2 laser is used, which means there might be very large amounts of smoke generated. Working with a filling volume of the abdomen at laparoscopy of between 3 and 5 litres per minute, there are different techniques in use.

Table 9.1 Laser types in gynaecological endoscopy

Laparoscopy	CO_2 laser
	Nd:YAG laser
	KTP
	Argon
	(Holmium)
Hysteroscopy	Nd:YAG laser
	KTP
	Argon

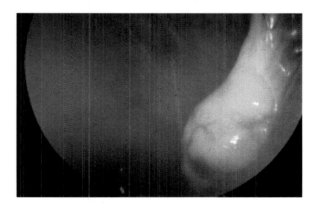

Figure 9.1 Smoke development under CO_2 laser excision of a field of endometriosis in the right fossa ovarica.

Chimney System

The most simple is to introduce, via an additional puncture, a tube through which the smoke can escape. Due to the higher intra-abdominal pressure, the smoke containing gas is expelled via the tube. Using this simple system, the view cannot always be kept clear; thus there are some stoppages especially during treatment of bigger tissue masses. With the insufflation machine, simultaneously about the same amount of gas that is lost must be replaced. A major disadvantage of this simple and relatively inefficient working system is that the smoke containing gas is released to the surrounding environment.

Endo-irrigation Unit

More efficient smoke evacuation is achieved by using the endo-irrigation unit for smoke aspiration. This unit is required for modern laparoscopic surgery anyway. The smoke is aspirated directly at the area of the laser target. The volume cleared by active aspiration is much higher and thus the method is more effective. For CO_2 replacement, higher amounts of CO_2 should be available via the insufflation apparatus to prevent collapse of the pneumoperitoneum.

There have been several attempts to keep the distending intra-abdominal gas volume automatically constant. Pressure controlled CO_2 delivery machines lead to failure in this automatic CO_2 replacement due to the influence of anaesthesia on the intra-abdominal pressure. Within limits, intra-abdominal pressure depends more on the quality of anaesthesia than on the volume of gas filling the abdomen. Therefore, an assistant should

watch that gas loss and CO_2 replacement in these two methods is within the same range.

Continuous Smoke Evacuation System

For frequent laparoscopic laser surgery a special insufflation apparatus was developed (Figure 9.2). Normal CO_2 insufflation is started under flow and pressure controlled conditions. Having ensured the intra-abdominal position of the tip of the Veress needle is correct, insufflation can be continued with high flow of about 4 litres CO_2 per minute. This is an acceptable compromise between the wish of the surgeon to establish pneumoperitoneum without wasting time, and to avoid cardiac arrhythmias. Starting directly with a high insufflation rate, the sudden pressure change results in unintentional stimulation receptors, leading to cardiac arrhythmias (Lindemann *et al.*, 1976). For safety reasons, therefore, insufflation in this apparatus can only be started when the right insufflation button is pushed. Afterwards insufflation might be accelerated by pushing the middle button, achieving high flow. The integrated endo-irrigation unit is situated on one side of the insufflator with the continuous CO_2 smoke evacuation system via a microfilter on the other. Having established the normal pneumoperitoneum at the beginning of surgery, the intra-abdominal smoke containing CO_2 gas is aspirated, cleared via the microfilter and the same amount of CO_2 which is aspirated is replaced simultaneously. This aspiration is started with the third, left button. The clearance volume is 4 litres per minute. Thus the whole intra-abdominal CO_2 is exchanged completely every minute. In this closed circulating system the volume of aspirated CO_2

Figure 9.2 Laser-endosurgical insufflator and irrigator (R. Wolf Co., Knittlingen, Germany). A modern insufflation apparatus with integrated endo-irrigation unit and smoke evacuation system.

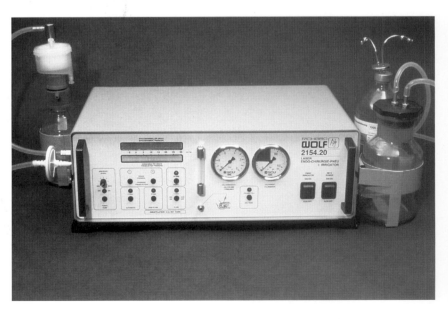

is replaced exactly. There is no gas loss or gas overload which makes the operation easier for the surgeon. The smoke containing CO_2 gas is filtered and not released to the surrounding atmosphere. The insufflator offers the most effective smoke evacuation system. This apparatus combines all the requirements for advanced laparoscopic surgery:

1. efficient insufflation system,
2. endo-irrigation unit,
3. smoke evacuation system.

Permanent high-flow gas spillage could theoretically lead to desiccation of the peritoneum which must be avoided. But continuous endo-irrigation, which is anyway essential to remove carbon particles generated by laser treatment, leads to moistening and prevents desiccation. After operation an additional amount of ascites develops caused by the irritant effect of carbonic acid.

High-flow gas spillage can also lead to body cooling. This is prevented by high volumes of Ringer's lactate solution which we use for irrigation. The irrigation solution is used at either body temperature or a temperature of about 42°C to achieve an additional mild haemostasis by this temperature effect.

As the pouch of Douglas is mostly filled with Ringer's lactate solution which is used in this area as a backstop to absorb CO_2 laser energy, intra-abdominal moisture content is high so that there is no fear of desiccation or cooling of tissues. An alternative smoke evacuator—the 'Bedford' is illustrated in Figure 9.3.

Table 9.2 CO_2 hysteroscopy

1 Physiological gas
2 No allergic reaction
3 Best visibility
4 Clean and fast operation

Metromat

1 No side-effects
2 No fear of gas embolism
3 No change in blood gas analysis
4 Unlimited time of surgery

Hysteroscopy

For hysteroscopic distension, CO_2 gas as well as fluids can be used. The use of CO_2 has many advantages and especially for diagnostic purposes this is the preferable distension medium (Table 9.2) (Lindemann *et al.*, 1979). In contrast, for surgical hysteroscopy more and more groups are using a liquid distension medium (Table 9.3) (Donnez, 1989).

Using the Nd:YAG laser several kinds of distension medium can be used. We normally

Table 9.3 Liquid distension for hysteroscopy

No smoke

Automatically washes out blood and mucus (continuous flow system, Wamsteker, de Blok)

Figure 9.3 The 'Bedford' smoke evacuator for laparoscopic surgery. (Courtesy of Litechnica Ltd, Manchester, UK.)

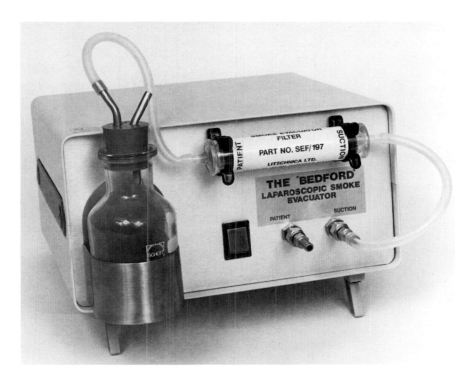

prefer the CO_2 as the distension medium for hysteroscopy. In contrast to the use of the resectoscope or the roller ball when liquid distension is required, we feel that CO_2 is the ideal distension medium for intrauterine Nd:YAG laser surgery (Gallinat, 1992). Using CO_2 distension medium in a long intrauterine surgical case, fluid overload and electrolyte imbalance are avoided and there is no intra-abdominal spillage. The YAG laser treatment is much more effective in a gaseous medium but it is essential that only CO_2 is used in an insufflator especially designed for hysteroscopy. On no account should air, nitrogen or nitrous oxide be used as this has led to several cases of fatal gas embolism (Baggish and Daniell, 1989).

Due to the physical characteristics of the Nd:YAG laser up to an output of approximately 30 W the coagulating effect predominates and only small amounts of smoke are developed, which hardly obscures the view. However, at higher outputs, a considerable amount of smoke is generated hindering the view until it has been cleared again by the continuous CO_2 insufflation. To avoid this inconvenience when vaporizing large submucous fibroids or broad septae, a smoke evacuator for continuous gas circulation has been constructed. Essential to the development of such a machine is the fact that the CO_2 insufflation is not allowed to exceed 100 ml/min (Lindemann and Gallinat, 1976). Under normal utero-tubal conditions the CO_2 flow is about 40–60 ml/min. The smoke generated by hysteroscopic YAG laser treatment is aspirated by the new smoke evacuator. Under pressure and flow control conditions this new machine at the same time clears the smoke by suction via microfilter and simultaneously replaces the CO_2, preventing a collapse of the pneumometra (Figure 9.4). That means the gas insufflation from the Metromat takes place within fixed physiological limits while at the same time the intrauterine gas volume is cleared from the smoke by the new apparatus. In this new machine these two completely different systems are separated and thus there is no interference of the smoke evacuator with the CO_2 gas insufflator (Gallinat *et al.*, 1991). Figure 9.5 shows the Metromat CO_2 gas insufflation apparatus on top of which is the prototype of the new smoke evacuator. For intrauterine laser surgery we use a coated Teflon probe with an internal diameter of the quartz glass fibre of 0.6 mm. The carbon dioxide is insufflated via the laser probe. The gas is delivered at the same place where the smoke is produced by tissue vaporization. The smoke is blown aside and visibility remains clear (Figure 9.6). While laser

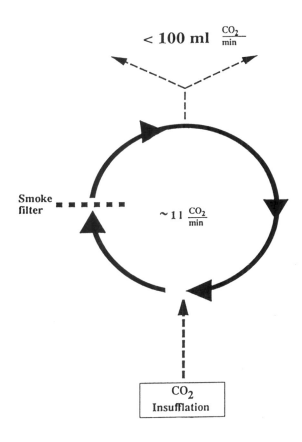

Figure 9.4 Principle of smoke evacuation.

surgery continues the distending CO_2 of the pneumometra is cleared by the smoke evacuator. The smoke containing gas is aspirated via the working channel of the hysteroscope and reinsufflated via the laser probe. The newly developed smoke evacuator is an added advantage and the operating time is reduced dramatically without increasing the risk compared with conventional CO_2 diagnostic hysteroscopy.

The main indication for hysteroscopic laser surgery is endometrial ablation with the YAG laser and treatment using a CO_2 distension medium has many advantages as certified by our excellent results (Table 9.4). We have performed 145 operations with no complications during hysteroscopic surgery or during the immediate post-operative period. All operations were performed on an out-patient basis and the patients were able to leave the department after 2–3 hours. While the removal of synechiae or smaller myomata is no problem, the extirpation of large myomata can be very time consuming. In these cases, Nd:YAG laser treatment has to be compared with the use of the resectoscope (Gallinat, 1992; Wamsteker, 1992).

Figure 9.5 Metromat: modern hysteroscope CO_2 insufflation apparatus. On top the new developed smoke evacuator. Metromat (R. Wolf Co., Knittlingen, Germany).

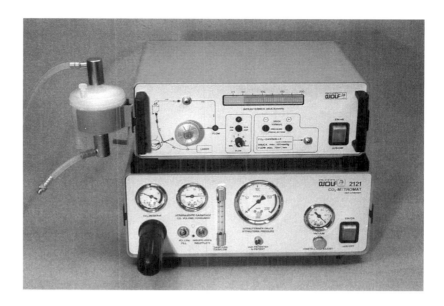

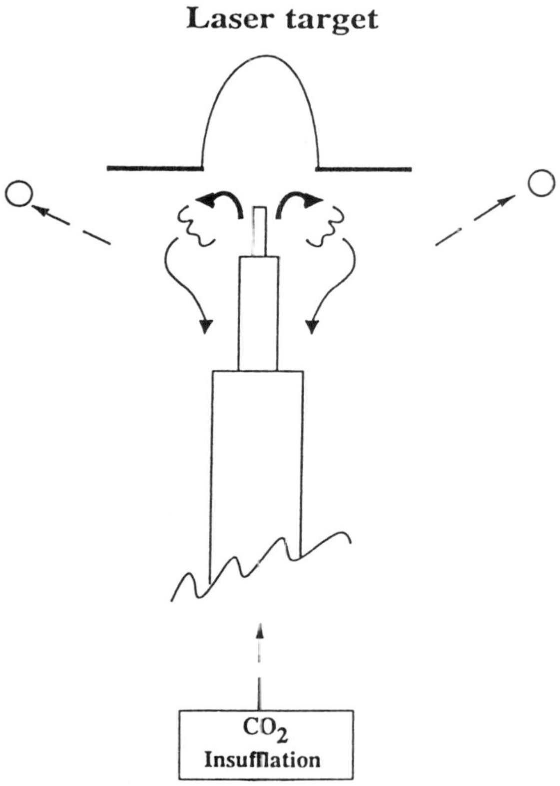

Laser target

Figure 9.6 Smoke evacuation (hysteroscopic Nd:YAG laser surgery).

New Developments

Regardless of whether the removal of myomata is by laparoscopy or hysteroscopy it is not only the smoke problem which might prolong the endoscopic procedure. Even if pretreatment with LHRH analogues reduces the bleeding, sometimes the removal of the myoma is very time consuming. Therefore, we have developed a new approach to the treatment of big masses. This new development has been made possible by modern electro-surgical techniques, using a microcomputer-assisted electro-technique as shown in the new apparatus 'ACC 450' (Figure 9.7), employing high power coagulation and continuous measurement of tissue resistance. After adequate tissue coagulation this generator stops automatically, which means there is no risk of overcoagulation or carbonization. The laparoscopic view (Figure 9.8) shows a special bipolar needle for puncturing subserosal or intramural myomata. After several punctures the capsule of the myoma and the nourishing vessels as well as the centre of the myoma are coagulated. The coagulation of the whole myoma performed by several punctures takes only a few seconds for each puncture. Using this treatment the myoma becomes ischaemic and

Table 9.4 Endometrial ablation (Nd:YAG laser)

	Goldrath	Gallinat/Lueken	Loffer	Donnez
No. operations	215	145	60	50
Amenorrhoea	103 (48%)	32 (22%)	11 (20%)	17 (34%)
Hypomenorrhoea	103 (48%)	104 (71.7%)	27 (49%)	30 (60%)
Total	(96%)	(93.7%)	(69%)	(94%)

Figure 9.7 ACC 450:
Microprocessor assisted
electrogenerator.

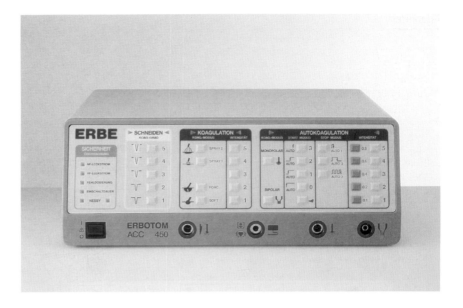

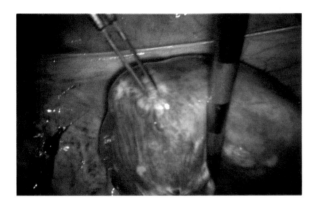

Figure 9.8 Puncture of an intramural myoma with a
special bipolar needle.

treatment are very quick operation, no bleeding
and no smoke generation.

The proximal part of the bipolar needle has an
insulated area. This insulation of the surface
perimetrium ensures that there is no damaged
area.

For hysteroscopy the same approach is used.
At the moment we have to use a unipolar needle
to puncture the base of the myoma as in Figure
9.10. Coagulation is rapid and while the needle
is inserted into the mass of the myoma near the
capsula there is no smoke generation, ensuring
good vision.

the coagulated tissue is clearly delineated from
the normal uterine muscle (Figure 9.9). The
gradual disappearance of the myoma can be
followed sequentially in the following weeks by
serial ultrasound examination. Advantages of this

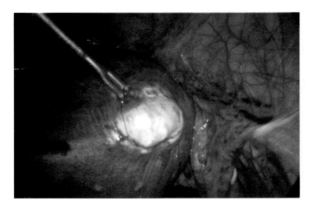

Figure 9.9 After several punctures, especially of the
base, the myoma is completely coagulated
and shrinks.

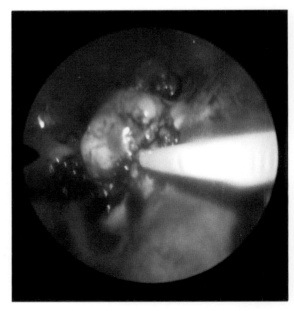

Figure 9.10 Hysteroscopic treatment of a submucous
myoma solely by coagulation using modern
electrotechnique.

References

Baggish MJ & Daniell JF (1989) Death caused by air embolism associated with neodymium:YAG laser surgery and artificial sapphire tips. *American Journal of Obstetrics and Gynecology* **161**: 877–878.

Donnez J (1989) Instrumentation. In Donnez J (ed.) *Laser Operative Laparoscopy and Hysteroscopy*, pp. 207–221. Leuven: Nauwelaerts Printing.

Gallinat A (1992) Treatment of submucous myomata by the use of the Nd:YAG laser. In Lewis BV & Magos AL (eds) *Endometrial Ablation*, in press. Edinburgh: Churchill Livingstone.

Gallinat A, Lueken RP & Moeller CP (1991) A smoke evacuator for intrauterine YAG-laser surgery using the CO_2 hysteroscopy. In Valle RF, Esposito JM & Phillips JM (eds) *Proceedings of the World Congress of Gynecologic Endoscopy*, pp. 153–155. AAGL 18th Annual Meeting, Washington DC.

Lindemann HJ & Gallinat A (1976) Physikalische und physiologische Grundlagen der CO_2 Hysteroskopie. *Geburtshilfe Frauenheilkunde* **36**: 729.

Lindemann HJ, Gallinat A & Lueken RP (1979) Metromat—new instrument for producing pneumometra. *Journal of Reproductive Medicine* **23**: 73.

Lindemann HJ, Mohr J, Gallinat A et al. (1976) Der Einfluss von CO_2 Gas waehrend der Hysteroskopie. *Geburtshilfe Frauenheilkunde* **36**: 153.

Semm K (1990) Bericht über die Arbeitsgemeinschaft gynäkologische und geburtshilfliche Endoskopie in der Deutschen Gesellschaft für Geburtshilfe und Gynäkologie. *Endometriose* No. 3:78.

Wamsteker K (1992) Treatment of submucous myomata by the use of the resectoscope. In Lewis BV & Magos AL (eds) *Endometrial Ablation*, in press. Edinburgh: Churchill Livingstone.

10

Clinical Results of Laser and Electrosurgery

TOGAS TULANDI

Division of Reproductive Endocrinology and Infertility, McGill University, Canada

Surgical Modalities

The basic physics of electrodiathermy, laser and their tissue effects are already discussed in Chapter 7. In short, coagulating current causes cellular dehydration and its main effect is haemostatic. It is a current that is interrupted with periods of electrical inactivity. Cutting current is a continuous current which causes explosion of the cell membrane due to intense heat generated within the tissue itself. A blend between cutting and coagulation currents is called blended current.

With endocoagulation (Semm, 1977) the mechanism by which this is achieved is completely different from the above. It still requires electricity to produce heat, but it coagulates by direct application of heat to the tissue. Electrical current passes through the element at the tip of the Teflon-coated probe, generating heat up to 120°C. It is safer than electrodiathermy because it eliminates a high frequency of electrical current in the abdominal cavity. However, it can only coagulate superficially. A laser works by a similar mechanism to that of cutting current; it 'boils' the intracellular water above 100°C. It can also be made to mimic electrocoagulation.

Studies in the early 1980s suggest that the use of carbon dioxide (CO_2) laser is associated with minimal tissue damage (Baggish and Chong, 1981), minimal scar formation and rapid healing (Bellina, 1981). Recent studies disproved that laser produces less tissue damage than other surgical modalities. Luciano *et al.* (1987) reported that in their rabbit model, there were no differences in the depth of thermal damage and in postoperative adhesion formation between the CO_2 laser and electrocautery. Filmar *et al.* (1989a, b), on the other hand, demonstrated that the use of the CO_2 laser on the rat's uterine horn produces more tissue necrosis and more extensive foreign body reaction than the use of microscissors. But, the use of laser is associated with less particulate carbon when compared to electrosurgery. Other studies suggest that the use of superpulse and ultrapulse CO_2 lasers produces a localized thermal necrosis without lateral spread. Other lasers such as neodymium yttrium–aluminium–garnet (Nd:YAG) laser and potassium–titanyl–phosphate (KTP) produce more tissue necrosis than that of the CO_2 laser.

It was initially believed that the results of surgery with lasers are superior to those of conventional techniques, but in randomized clinical studies comparing reproductive surgery using laser and electrodiathermy by laparotomy, similar results are found (Tulandi and Vilos, 1985; Tulandi, 1986). The degree of post-surgical adhesion is also comparable (Tulandi, 1987). It seems that there is little advantage of using lasers for reproductive surgery by laparotomy. Its use by laparoscopy, however, offers some benefits including less risk of electrical injury. Also, its tissue impact can be more controlled and predictable. The use of lasers is more precise and may be safer, but it requires a laser machine which is expensive.

Electrical current, especially the unipolar cautery, can damage vital structures such as intestines and larger areas of thermal damage might not be recognized at the time of surgery. The newer generators, however, are safer than the original spark gap generators. The use of unipolar needle cautery of short duration with blended current further reduces the risk of electrical injury. Regardless of the surgical modalities, the skill and experience of the endoscopist is probably the most important factor.

Laparoscopic Salpingo-ovariolysis

Liberation of adhesions can be done with laparoscopic scissors, electrodiathermy or with lasers. Previous studies on salpingo-ovariolysis by laparotomy suggest that the use of electrodiathermy or CO_2 laser produces similar results. The reproductive outcome after salpingo-ovariolysis using laparoscopic scissors, electrodiathermy and lasers is given in Table 10.1. It appears that comparable results are produced, regardless of surgical modality.

Terminal Salpingostomy

Terminal salpingostomy is reconstructive surgery for hydrosalpinx or terminal tubal occlusion. In the presence of periadnexal adhesions, these should be first freed by laser (power density, 5000–10 000 W/cm^2) or with needle point unipolar electrodiathermy and blended current. The tube is distended by chromopertubation using a dilute solution of methylene blue dye. The 'central dimple' of the occluded fimbrial end is then identified and is entered using laser or electrocaut-

ery needle. Terminal salpingostomy is performed by radial incisions of the hydrosalpinx along the relatively avascular white lines. The incision is done using the same power as described above. To maintain the eversion of the neo-ostium, the mucosal flap can be everted without tension by a few interrupted sutures of 6/0 or 8/0 polyglactin (Vicryl®, Ethicon, Inc., Somerville, NJ, USA) or easier with laser or with electrocoagulation. Laser eversion is done by defocusing the CO_2 laser and directing the beam 0.5 cm along the margin of the flap. Retraction of the mucosal flap creates an eversion. This can also be accomplished by using a light electrocoagulation using a bipolar cautery or an endocoagulator. The same principle can be applied using other lasers.

Terminal salpingostomy can be done by laparotomy or by laparoscopy. Although there is no randomized study comparing the two techniques, the results appear to be comparable. One of the factors that might affect the results is the degree of tubal damage (Donnez and Casanas-Roux, 1986; DeBruyne et al., 1989; Schlaff et al., 1990). Laparoscopic salpingostomy can be done as an extension of a diagnostic laparoscopy.

The reproductive outcome after laparoscopic salpingostomy is depicted in Table 10.2. The small number of patients in some of the studies, the variation in follow-up time and the different surgeons make it difficult to evaluate the efficacy of these various techniques. Nevertheless, it seems that salpingostomy using laparoscopic scissors, laser or electrodiathermy produces comparable results. This is in agreement with previous randomized studies comparing the results of laser surgery and electrosurgery by laparotomy (Tulandi and Vilos, 1985). Currently, there is no randomized study comparing the results of laparoscopic salpingostomy using these different techniques. However, this might be unnecessary,

Table 10.1 Reproductive outcome after laparoscopic salpingo-ovariolysis using cold instrument, laser or electrodiathermy

Technique	Authors	No.	Follow-up (years)	Intrauterine pregnancy (%)	Ectopic pregnancy (%)	Total pregnancy (%)
Scissors	Gomel (1983)	92	1	62.0	5.4	67.4
Scissors	Fayez (1983)	50	2	56.0	4.0	60.0
Electro-diathermy	Mettler et al. (1979)	44	1–6	NA	NA	29.5
Electro-diathermy	Bruhat et al. (1983)	93	1	51.6	7.5	59.1
CO_2 laser	Donnez et al. (1989)	186	1½	NA	NA	58.0

Table 10.2 Reproductive outcome after laparoscopic salpingostomy using cold instrument, laser or electrodiathermy

Technique	Authors	No.	Follow-up (years)	Intrauterine pregnancy (%)	Ectopic pregnancy (%)	Total pregnancy (%)
Scissors	Gomel (1977)	9	1	44.4	0	44.4
Scissors	Mettler et al. (1979)	36	1–6	NA	NA	26.0
Scissors	Fayez (1983)	19	2	0	10.0	10.0
CO$_2$ laser	Daniell & Herbert (1984)	21	1–1$\frac{1}{2}$	19.0	5.0	24.0
CO$_2$ laser	Donnez et al. (1989)	25	1$\frac{1}{2}$	NA	NA	20.0
Combined	Dubuisson et al. (1990)	34	1$\frac{1}{2}$	29.4	2.9	32.4

because the results of terminal salpingostomy are generally poor. Patients with bilateral hydrosalpinx are better candidates for *in vitro* fertilization than for salpingostomy by laparotomy. Laparoscopic salpingostomy is still a viable alternative for selected patients who do not wish to undergo *in vitro* fertilization or for those who are found to have hydrosalpinx on screening laparoscopy.

Endometriosis

Several studies have shown that the results of conservative surgical treatment of endometriosis by laparoscopy is similar if not superior to that after laparotomy (Olive and Martin, 1987; Nezhat *et al.*, 1989). It is associated with high fecundity rate even in advanced diseases and there is a trend of increased early pregnancy rates (Adamson *et al.*, 1988). Conservative surgical treatment of endometriosis can be achieved by liberating the adhesions, ablation of endometriotic implants, ablation of endometrioma and segmental ablation of uterosacral ligaments.

Endometriotic implants can be coagulated with electrocautery, endocoagulator or vaporized with laser. Some reproductive surgeons also advocated excision of the lesion (Martin and van der Zwaag, 1987). It is still not clear whether excision is better than ablation only.

In 1986, Seiler *et al.* compared the effects of medical treatment with danazol and laparoscopic electrocoagulation of moderate endometriosis and found that there is no difference between the pregnancy rate in the danazol group (39%) and the electrosurgery group (44%) at 7 months

follow-up. Others have reported good pregnancy rates after electrocoagulation of endometriosis (Murphy *et al.*, 1991; Tulandi and Mouchawar, 1991). The procedure is done by ablating the endometriotic implants with bipolar cautery. Deep implants have to be eliminated by unipolar cautery which has deeper penetration. Due to the potential risk of electrical injury with unipolar cautery, some reproductive surgeons prefer using laser (Olive and Martin, 1987; Nezhat *et al.*, 1989; Sutton and Hill, 1990). Olive and Martin (1987) found that the use of CO$_2$ lasers is as effective as other forms of conventional treatment. The occurrence of pregnancy is independent of the stages of the endometriosis (Figure 10.1) and directly related to the duration of infertility. In a non-randomized study, Adamson *et al.* (1988) reported that the 6 and 12 months estimated cumulative pregnancy rates after laparoscopic laser treatment of endometriosis were 32% and 55% versus 17% and 43% after conventional treatment with danazol or LHRH analogue. Although the pregnancy rates after laser treatment are not significantly higher than after conventional treatment, there is a trend of increased early pregnancy rates after laser treatment. The results of laparoscopic treatment of endometriosis using electrocautery and laser are shown in Table 10.3. It appears that the overall pregnancy rate after laser surgery is similar to that after electrosurgery.

One study recently showed that laparoscopic laser treatment is superior to laparoscopic treatment of stage I and II endometriosis with electrocautery (Paulson *et al.*, 1991). The study, however, is retrospective in nature with the non-laser group serving as a historical control (patients undergoing non-laser treatment in previous years). Other lasers including argon laser, Nd:YAG

Figure 10.1 Cumulative pregnancy rates (life table analysis) of women with minimal (stage I, ...), mild (stage II, ----) and moderate (stage III, ———) endometriosis after laparoscopic surgery with CO_2 laser. (Adapted from Olive and Martin, 1987. Reproduced with permission of the Publisher, The American Fertility Society.)

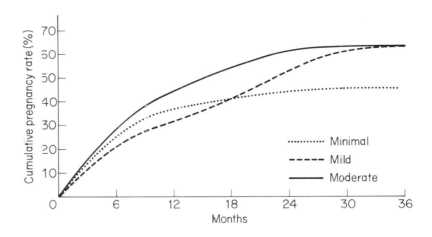

Table 10.3 Pregnancy rates after laparoscopic treatment of endometriosis by electrocoagulation and by laser

Technique	No. of pregnancies/no. treated				
	Minimal	Mild	Moderate	Severe	Combined
Electrocoagulation	28/44 (64%)	110/210 (52%)	24/67 (36%)	4/8 (50%)	214/412 (52%)
CO_2 laser	329/553 (59%)	230/397 (58%)	94/162 (58%)	37/58 (64%)	690/1170 (59%)

Adapted from Cook and Rock (1991). Reproduced with permission of the Publisher, The American Fertility Society.

laser and KTP laser have also been used (Lomano, 1985; Daniell et al., 1986; Keye et al., 1987). Argon lasers can selectively vaporize pigmented lesions while preserving normal surrounding tissue. The overall pregnancy rate after treatment of endometriosis with argon lasers is 33.9% (Keye et al., 1987). It appears that electrosurgery is as effective as laser surgery.

Treatment versus No Treatment

Many authors reported the occurrence of pregnancy after laparoscopic treatment of endometriosis. However, most of the studies have no untreated controls and the success of the procedure is frequently reported as crude pregnancy rates. Also, pregnancy often occurs among women with endometriosis independent of treatment. In a non-randomized study, Tulandi and Mouchawar (1991) recently found that laparoscopic coagulation of minimal and mild endometriosis (stage I and II, Revised American Fertility Society Classification) is superior to no treatment. In a randomized study, Nowroozi et al. (1987) reported that the pregnancy rate after cauterization of mild endometriosis (60.9%) is significantly higher than that after expectant management (18 5%). It suggests that ablation of endometriosis improves the pregnancy rate.

Laparoscopic Uterine Nerve Ablation (LUNA)

Laparoscopy is an effective tool in the evaluation of pelvic pain. In selected cases it can also be therapeutic. In the presence of endometriosis, ablation of endometriosis and lysis of adhesions can be done with lasers or electrosurgically. It appears that adhesions that restrict the mobility of pelvic organs, especially those involving the parietal peritoneum and intestines are most likely to cause pain. In women who complain of pelvic pain, ablation of the nerve fibres in the uterosacral ligaments can be performed. The uterosacral ligaments are coagulated or vaporized close to its insertion to the cervix and then transected (Feste, 1985; Lichten and Bombard, 1987). The effect is similar to anaesthesia with a paracervical block. Approximately 70% of patients with pelvic pain will experience pain relief. It seems that its efficacy is equivalent to that after presacral neurectomy. Uterosacral ligament transection in conjunction with presacral neurectomy does not produce additional pain relief (Lee et al., 1986).

Laparoscopic Treatment of Polycystic Ovarian Syndrome

Several authors have reported the treatment of polycystic ovarian syndrome by laparoscopy.

The procedure can be done electrosurgically by creating eight holes of 3 mm in diameter and 2–4 mm in depth on the ovarian surface with a unipolar cautery (Gjönnaess, 1984) or by cauterizing the polycystic follicles and removing the thickened capsule overlying the follicles (Sumioki et al., 1988). Hormonal changes after this procedure are similar to those after ovarian wedge resection (Greenblatt and Casper, 1987; Sumioki et al., 1988). Regular menstrual cycles and ovulation are established in about 90% of patients and conception occurs in 70% of patients. Various lasers have also been used to treat polycystic ovaries. This is done by vaporizing all follicles and drilling craters in the ovarian stroma. Daniell and Miller (1989) reported that ovulation occurred in 71% of patients so treated and 56% of patients conceived within 6 months of the procedure.

Summary

Numerous studies on the success of reproductive surgery are published in the literature. The majority are the personal experiences of one or several surgeons and the results are often complicated by many variables including surgeon's experience and the presence of other infertility factors. Success is often reported as crude pregnancy rate with different durations of follow-up and few studies rely on life table analysis. Without a randomized trial, it is difficult to evaluate the efficacy of a particular procedure with certainty. Nevertheless, in the hands of trained laparoscopists, operative laparoscopy is effective whether using cautery, endocoagulation or laser energy. The surgeon's experience and preference and proper patient selection play a more important role.

References

Adamson GD, Lu J & Subak LL (1988) Laparoscopic CO_2 laser vaporization of endometriosis compared with traditional treatments. Fertility and Sterility 50: 704–710.

Baggish MS & Chong AP (1981) Carbon dioxide laser microsurgery of the uterine tube. Obstetrics and Gynecology 58: 111–116.

Bellina JH (1981) Reconstructive microsurgery of the fallopian tube with the carbon dioxide laser. Procedure and preliminary results. Reproduction 5: 1–8.

Bruhat MA, Mage G, Manhes H et al. (1983) Laparoscopic procedures to promote fertility ovariolysis and salpingolysis: results of 93 selected cases. Acta Europaea Fertilitatis 14: 113.

Cook AS & Rock JA (1991) The role of laparoscopy in the treatment of endometriosis. Fertility and Sterility 55: 663–680.

Daniell JF & Herbert CM (1984) Laparoscopic salpingostomy utilizing the CO_2 laser. Fertility and Sterility 41: 558–563.

Daniell JF & Miller W (1989) Polycystic ovaries treated by laparoscopic laser vaporization. Fertility and Sterility 51: 232–236.

Daniell JF, Miller W & Tosh R (1986) Initial evaluation of the use of the potassium–titanyl–phosphate (KTP/532) laser in gynecologic laparoscopy. Fertility and Sterility 46: 373.

DeBruyne, Puttemans P, Boeckx W & Brosens I (1989) The clinical value of salpingoscopy in tubal infertility. Fertility and Sterility 51: 339–340.

Donnez J & Casanas-Roux F (1986) Prognostic factors in fimbrial microsurgery. Fertility and Sterility 46: 200–204.

Donnez J, Nisolle M & Casanas-Roux F (1989) CO_2 laser laparoscopy in infertile women with adnexal adhesions and women with tubal occlusion. Journal of Gynecologic Surgery 5: 47–53.

Dubuisson JB, De Jolinière JB, Aubriot FX et al. (1990) Terminal tuboplasties by laparoscope: 65 consecutive cases; Fertility and Sterility 54: 401–403.

Fayez JA (1983) An assessment of the role of operative laparoscopy in tuboplasty. Fertility and Sterility 39: 476–479.

Feste JR (1985) Laser laparoscopy, a new modality. Journal of Reproductive Medicine 30: 413–417.

Filmar S, Jetha N, McComb P & Gomel V (1989a) A comparative histologic study on the healing process after tissue transection. I. Carbon dioxide laser and electromicrosurgery. American Journal of Obstetrics and Gynecology 160: 1062–1067.

Filmar S, Jetha N, McComb P & Gomel V (1989b) A comparative histologic study on the healing process after tissue transection. II. Carbon dioxide laser and surgical microscissors. American Journal of Obstetrics and Gynecology 160: 1068–1072.

Gjönnaess H (1984) Polycystic ovarian syndrome treated by ovarian electrocautery through the laparoscope. Fertility and Sterility 41: 20–25.

Gomel V (1977) Salpingostomy by laparoscopy. Journal of Reproductive Medicine 18: 265–268.

Gomel V (1983) Salpingoovariolysis by laparoscopy in infertility. Fertility and Sterility 40: 607–611.

Greenblatt E & Casper RF (1987) Endocrine changes after laparoscopic ovarian cautery in polycystic ovarian syndrome. American Journal of Obstetrics and Gynecology 156: 279–285.

Keye WR, Hanso LW, Astin M et al. (1987) Argon laser therapy of endometriosis: a review of 92 consecutive patients. Fertility and Sterility 47: 208–212.

Lee RB, Stone K & Magelssen et al. (1986) Presacral neurectomy for chronic pelvic pain. Obstetrics and Gynecology 68: 517–521.

Lichten EM & Bombard J (1987) Surgical treatment of primary dysmenorrhea with laparoscopic uterine nerve ablation. Journal of Reproductive Medicine 32: 37–41.

Lomano JM (1985) Photocoagulation of early pelvic endometriosis with the Nd:YAG laser through the laparoscope. *Journal of Reproductive Medicine* **30**: 77–81.

Luciano AL, Whitman G, Maier DB *et al.* (1987) Comparison of thermal injury, healing patterns and postoperative adhesion formation following CO_2 laser and electromicrosurgery. *Fertility and Sterility* **48**: 1025–1029.

Martin D & van der Zwaag R (1987) Excisional techniques for endometriosis with the CO_2 laser laparoscope. *Journal of Reproductive Medicine* **32**: 753–758.

Mettler L, Giesel H & Semm K (1979) Treatment of female infertility due to tubal obstruction by operative laparoscopy. *Fertility and Sterility* **32**: 384–388.

Murphy AA, Schlaff WD, Hassiakos D *et al.* (1991) Laparoscopic cautery in the treatment of endometriosis infertility. *Fertility and Sterility* **55**: 246–251.

Nezhat C, Crowgey S & Nezhat F (1989) Videolaseroscopy for the treatment of endometriosis associated infertility. *Fertility and Sterility* **51**: 237–240.

Nowroozi K, Chase JS, Check JH & Wu CH (1987) The importance of laparoscopic coagulation of mild endometriosis in infertile women. *International Journal of Fertility* **32**: 442–444.

Olive DL & Martin DC (1987) Treatment of endometriosis-associated infertility with CO_2 laser laparoscopy: the use of one and two-parameter exponential models. *Fertility and Sterility* **48**: 18–23.

Paulson JD, Asmar P & Saffa DS (1991) Mild and moderate endometriosis. Comparison of treatment modalities for infertile couples. *Journal of Reproductive Medicine* **36**: 151–155.

Schlaff WD, Hassiakos DK, Damewood MD & Rock J (1990) Neosalpingostomy for distal tubal obstruction. Prognostic factors and impact of surgical technique. *Fertility and Sterility* **54**: 984–990.

Seiler JC, Gitwani G & Ballard L (1986) Laparoscopic cauterization of endometriosis for infertility: a controlled study. *Fertility and Sterility* **46**: 1098–1100.

Semm K (1977) The laparoscopic instrumentation. In *Atlas of Gynecologic Laparoscopy and Hysteroscopy*, p 30. Philadelphia: W.B. Saunders & Co.

Sumioki H, Utsunomyiya T, Matsuoka K *et al.* (1988) The effect of laparoscopic multiple punch resection of the ovary on the hypothalamo-pituitary axis in polycystic ovary syndrome. *Fertility and Sterility* **50**: 567–572.

Sutton C & Hill D (1990) Laser laparoscopy in the treatment of endometriosis. A 5 year study. *British Journal of Obstetrics and Gynaecology* **97**: 181–185.

Tulandi T (1986) Salpingo-ovariolysis: a comparison between laser surgery and electrosurgery. *Fertility and Sterility* **45**: 489–491.

Tulandi T (1987) Adhesion reformation after reproductive surgery with or without the carbon dioxide laser. *Fertility and Sterility* **47**: 704–706.

Tulandi T & Mouchawar M (1991) Treatment-dependent and treatment-independent pregnancy among women with minimal and mild endometriosis. *Fertility and Sterility* **56**: 790–791.

Tulandi T & Vilos GA (1985) A comparison between laser surgery and electrosurgery for bilateral hydrosalpinx: a 2 year follow-up. *Fertility and Sterility* **44**: 846–848.

11

Laser Neosalpingostomy and Fimbrioplasty

J.B. DUBUISSON, J. BOUQUET DE JOLINIÈRE AND L. MANDELBROT

Clinique Universitaire Port Royal, Paris, France

With progress in operative laparoscopy, fimbrioplasty and neosalpingostomy may be performed employing microsurgical conditions. This may be attributed to the development of appropriate atraumatic instrumentation, high-resolution optical devices, and the carbon dioxide laser. Laparoscopy provides easy access to the pelvis and allows for the diagnosis and treatment of a wide variety of pathologies: ectopic pregnancy, ovarian cyst, endometriosis and myomas. Laparoscopic salpingo-ovariolysis is also a widely performed procedure giving well established results (Bruhat *et al.*, 1983; Gomel, 1983).

Immediate opening of hydrosalpinges allows for precise evaluation of the tubal mucosa, thereby establishing the prognosis. In cases with a severely altered mucosa, *in vitro* fertilization may then be considered as the treatment of choice. When the mucosa is satisfactory, laparoscopic fimbrioplasty or neosalpingostomy may be performed immediately. Within 1 year after one of these procedures, a pregnancy is generally achieved in one of three patients.

In this chapter, laparoscopic techniques for distal tubal pathology are described and the results discussed, compared with the results obtained with microsurgery by laparotomy.

Anatomy of the Distal Fallopian Tube

Precise knowledge of the anatomy and physiology of the fallopian tube is needed to understand the mechanisms of each case of tubal infertility and to establish its prognosis. Operative strategy must be adopted to avoid an inappropriate reconstructive procedure. The distal portion of the tube will be detailed, since it is amenable to laparoscopic surgery. The narrow isthmus and the interstitial portion will not be described here, since they cannot at present be repaired laparoscopically. They must still be treated using classical microsurgical techniques.

The ampulla, the next most lateral portion of the tube, is elastic and sinuous. Its length is 5–8 cm. Its diameter increases distally, reaching 1–2 cm at its extremity. Its thin wall allows it to be distended readily by fluids. The distal portion, or infundibulum, measures 2–3 cm long. It is funnel-shaped, opening into the peritoneal cavity by the abdominal ostium, which is surrounded by 12–15 mobile fimbriae. The internal diameter of the ostium is 2 mm, but is distensible. Microscopic studies have shown that the fimbriae are continuous with complex longitudinal branching folds. The ampulla includes three to five principal folds. The columnar mucosal epithelium, or endosalpinx, consists of secretory and ciliated cells.

Pathology of the Distal Fallopian Tube

Lesions of the distal tube are most often secondary to pelvic inflammatory disease. Other causes of distal tubal pathology include tuberculosis, schistosomiasis, endometriosis and congenital anomalies (De Brux, 1982). The two degrees of obstruction are: partial stenosis with some degree of tuboperitoneal permeability and total obstruction with hydrosalpinx.

Four principal anatomical problems may be observed in partial obstruction:

1. adhesions encapsulate the fimbrial extremity.
2. adhesions glue the fimbriae together and may extend into the ampulla.
3. a retracted peritoneal ring strangulates the distal tube.
4. less frequently, adhesions affect the ostium itself, resulting in ampullar dilatation with normal fimbriae. Under high-pressure chromopertubation, permeability is demonstrated.
5. histological evidence of chronic salpingitis may sometimes be observed on the ampulla and infundibulum. In cases with glued fimbriae, more severe lesions of follicular salpingitis are not infrequent.

The anatomical aspects of hydrosalpinges are related to the degree of damage to the mucosa and tubal wall.

Hydrosalpinx simplex is a moderately dilated ampulla containing clear yellow fluid. The tubal wall is thinned and there is atrophy of the mucosa. Mucosal folds may be decreased or absent. The epithelium is usually altered with flattened cells and a marked reduction in the number of ciliae.

In follicular hydrosalpinx, the lumen is divided by adhesions forming septa, which terminate on fimbrial adhesions. This is the most advanced stage of follicular or alveolar salpingitis. The epithelium is often hypertrophic, the cells retaining their morphological characteristics and ciliae.

Hydrosalpinx with pachysalpinx is characterized by a thickened tubal wall with local sclerosis (fibrosis) replacing smooth muscle fibres.

Inflammatory hydrosalpinges show lymphoplasmocytic infiltration and tubal wall oedema.

Preoperative Evaluation

All possible male and female factors for infertility should always be investigated. Spermocytogram, post-coital testing, temperature charts, hormone assays and testing for infections, including *Neisseria gonorrhoea* and *Chlamydia trachomatis* must be systematic.

Hysterosalpingography (HSG) remains indispensable in the work-up of tubal infertility. It gives information on the patency of each tube, the location of obstruction or stenosis in relation to the abdominal ostium and on the quality of the tubal mucosa. Mucosal folds appear rarely and are thickened or even absent in atrophic forms. Intratubal adhesions resulting in disorganized bands, giving a honeycomb aspect, are observed in follicular hydrosalpinges. Whenever HSG shows signs of disease of the ampulla or infundibulum or altered permeability and/or dispersion of the contrast medium in the peritoneal cavity, laparoscopy is necessary to complement the diagnosis and establish a prognosis. Laparoscopic surgery should always be considered whenever a diagnostic laparoscopy is performed.

Diagnostic laparoscopy always precedes laparoscopic surgery. It explores completely the pelvis and the entire abdominal cavity. An intrauterine cannula allows for mobilizing the uterus, which is anteverted for a better view of the fallopian tubes and pelvic anatomy. Chromopertubation is performed using methylene blue dye.

Selection of patients for laparoscopic surgery is difficult. Considerable experience is required to choose the appropriate strategy between two extremes. Rigorous selection for surgery increases the likelihood of success, but excludes the majority of patients. Wide selection criteria give a chance to most patients, but lead to mediocre overall results.

Prognostic Factors

Age is important, since fertility decreases notably after 38 years. Some aetiological factors carry a poor prognosis; for instance, tuberculosis and schistosomiasis are contraindications to surgery. Severe tubal disease is also a contraindication: follicular hydrosalpinges, rigid thick-walled tubes, bifocal lesions associating proximal and distal lesions. Treatment must be delayed whenever there is evidence of ongoing inflammatory disease.

The tubal operability score determines the severity of distal tubal disease (Mage and Bruhat, 1987). It is based on three factors (Table 11.1). First, distal obstruction is defined as partial (2 points) or complete (5 points). Secondly, the ampullary mucosa is rated as having normal folds (0 point), some more or less regular folds (5 points) or complete atrophy or a honeycomb follicular salpingitis (10 points). The tubal wall is rated as normal (0 point), thin (5 points) or thickened (10 points). The sum of the three factors places the patient in one of four stages, from the least to the more severe prognostic group. The best indications for laparoscopic surgery are

Table 11.1 Tubal scoring system

Tubal patency	Ampullar mucosa	Ampullar wall (laparoscopy)
0 Normal	0 Normal folds	0 Normal
2 Partial occlusion (phimosis)		
5 Total occlusion (hydrosalpinx)	5 Decreased folds	5 Thin
10	10 No fold or honeycomb	10 Thick or rigid

stages I and II. Stage IV is an indication for IVF. Stage III patients may be oriented towards either surgery or IVF. Severe adhesions and/or evolving lesions are arguments for IVF.

Contraindications to laparoscopic surgery must be respected. Classical absolute contraindications are cardiovascular and arrhythmic diseases and uncorrected disorders of haemostasis. Some contraindications are relative, depending on the operator's experience, such as several previous laparotomies or obesity.

Instrumentation

Pneumoperitoneum is performed through a 7–12 cm long needle (Veress needle, Storz-France) by an electronic CO_2 Pneumoperitoneum Apparatus with simultaneous measurement of the static and insufflation pressure, insufflation rate, gas flow and actual volume (Storz-France).

The straight Forward 0° endoscope is most often used. With the Forward-Oblique endoscope 30°, a larger area can be observed by rotating the instrument. We generally use a 10 mm diameter endoscope. A single puncture operating laparoscope is used for CO_2 laser surgery: a 6 mm instrument channel for the CO_2 laser is associated with a straight Forward 0° endoscope with an eyepiece. Trocar size is 11 mm. Endoscopes are adapted to a cold light fountain (250 W halogen lamp) and to a video camera with a high-resolution monitor.

Operating instruments are atraumatic scissors, atraumatic grasping forceps and the material for irrigation and aspiration (Triton, Micro-France, Bourbon l'Archambault, France; Aquapurator, Storz-France, Paris, France). For coagulation, a bipolar coagulating forceps or a probe for thermocoagulation are used. All the instruments are introduced through two or three 5 mm

suprapubic trocar sheaths. CO_2 laser surgery is generally performed using a single puncture operating laparoscope. A uterine grasping forceps (Storz-France) is used for manipulation of the uterus during the operative procedure and a Cohen uterine cannula for chromopertubation with methylene blue dye.

Operating Technique

In the lithotomy position, the bladder is emptied and an intrauterine cannula is placed for chromopertubation. In the Trendelenburg's position, laparoscopy is performed transumbilically under general anaesthesia with intubation. The uterus is then anteverted, permitting a better visualization of the tubes and the ovaries.

Before distal tuboplasty, meticulous excision of all adhesions from the ovary and the tube are performed to re-establish mobility of the ampulla and of the fimbria ovarica. Velamentous adhesions or adhesions encapsulating fimbria or ovary are excised using scissors exclusively. Vascularized adhesions may require bipolar coagulation before excision. Dense adhesions are excised using the CO_2 laser, especially those gluing the ampulla to the ovary or ovary to the uterus. However, some authors (Donnez *et al.*, 1989; Macdonald and Sutton, 1992) systematically use the CO_2 laser, even when adhesions are thin and velamentous.

FIMBRIOPLASTY

All the operative distal tuboplasty techniques are performed with a 'microsurgical approach': magnification with the laparoscope, atraumatic dissection, irrigation with warm saline solution. After chromopertubation, adhesions encapsulating the fimbriae are incised or excised using fine scissors. Constrictive fibrotic bands are incised using scissors. Agglutinated fimbriae are dilated with atraumatic forceps introduced into the ostium closed and then withdrawn opened. The procedure is repeated several times. The same procedure is performed for the treatment of phimosis of the ostium. The fimbria is then irrigated until haemostasis is completed.

NEOSALPINGOSTOMY (Figure 11.1)

Laparoscopic correction was described more than a decade ago by Gomel (1977) and Mettler *et al.* (1979). Initially, neosalpingostomy by laparoscopy was largely reserved for patients in whom prior neosalpingostomy by laparotomy had failed. Now, initial neosalpingostomy is performed by

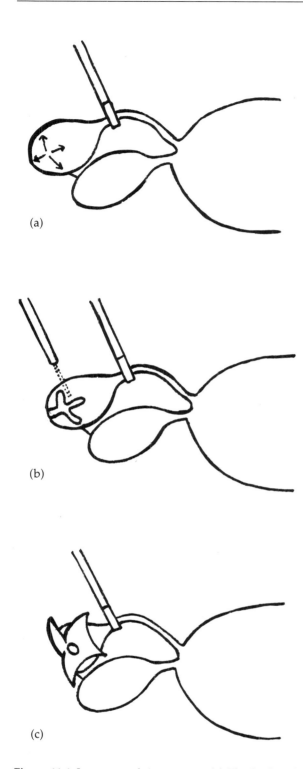

(a)

(b)

(c)

Figure 11.1 Laser neosalpingostomy. (a) The hydrosalpinx is incised at the thinnest point in the tubal wall (scissors or CO_2 laser). (b) After enlargement of the opening, eversion of the edges is obtained by retracting the distal serosa (CO_2 laser or coagulation). (c) Final result.

laparoscopy. A prerequisite is adhesiolysis to free the hydrosalpinx and infundibulo-ovarian ligament. The fallopian tube is then dilated by transcervical chromopertubation. The fimbriated end of the dilated ampulla is immobilized and well oriented. It is then incised at the thinnest point in the tubal wall. The incision may be performed with scissors or with the CO_2 laser. The laser is set on continuous mode (40 W) with a focused beam to cut the tube. Salpingoscopy with the laparoscope of the distal end of the ampulla checks the quality of the mucosa and the possibility of performing a neosalpingostomy. Severe chronic lesions of follicular salpingitis or thick-walled ampulla are a contraindication to completing the neosalpingostomy. A laparoscopic salpingectomy may be more appropriate in this situation and should have been discussed previously with the patient. If a neosalpingostomy is decided upon, the opening of the hydrosalpinx is enlarged toward the ovary to form a new fimbria ovarica, using scissors or CO_2 laser. The enlargement may be completed by applying careful divergent traction with atraumatic forceps which is limited to the scarred areas. When the tube has been sufficiently opened to create a neo-ostium, eversion of the edges is obtained by retracting the distal serosa. Retraction is obtained using thermocoagulation, bipolar coagulation or defocused CO_2 laser beam with a reduced power (4–5 W). Eversion is achieved when coagulation produces blanching of the serosa. At the end of the procedure, the peritoneal cavity is irrigated with Ringer's lactate solution. Prophylactic antibiotics (cyclins) are generally administered for 1 or 2 weeks.

Discussion

Microsurgery by laparotomy has been the treatment of choice of tubal sterility except in cases of severe disease, for which *in vitro* fertilization is indicated. In Gomel's series (Gomel, 1978), 89 microsurgical neosalpingostomies by laparotomy were followed for more than 1 year; 30 patients (33.7%) achieved one or more pregnancies, 28 (31.5%) had one or more live births and 8 (9%) had ectopic pregnancies. In our series of 76 microsurgical neosalpingostomies with a follow-up of >2 years, 28 patients (36.8%) achieved one or more pregnancies and 17 (2.3%) had ectopic pregnancies (Dubuisson *et al.*, 1985).

The outcome after laparoscopic distal tuboplasty was disappointing in early reports (Fayez, 1983).

Table 11.2 Results of fimbrioplasty by laparoscopy

Author	Total patients	IUP	EP
Gomel (1983)	40	20 (50%)	2 (5%)
Dubuisson *et al.* (1990)	31	8 (25.8%)	3+1 (12.9%)

IUP, intrauterine pregnancy; EP, ectopic pregnancy.

More recently, several authors have reported encouraging results after such procedures (Gomel, 1977; Daniell and Herbert, 1984; Donnez *et al.*, 1989). In a series of 62 neosalpingostomies, Bruhat *et al.* (1989) obtained 17 intrauterine pregnancies (27.4%). In our published series where outcome was evaluated at 18 months postoperation, we have observed an intrauterine pregnancy rate of 29.4%. In the absence of randomized clinical trials in large populations, laparoscopic and laparotomic microsurgical approaches cannot be compared directly. However, at present operative laparoscopy appears to give results almost as good as those of microsurgery. This improvement can be attributed to the development of atraumatic instruments adapted for laparoscopic surgery and also to the use of the CO_2 laser. With a 10 mm diameter laparoscope, the magnification is estimated at three times when the tip of the endoscope is placed 1 cm from the fimbria. Such magnification is sufficient for performing fimbrioplasty or neosalpingostomy. For eversion of neosalpingostomy, the laparoscopic technique using the CO_2 laser or bipolar or thermocoagulation achieves results anatomically comparable with those obtained by microsurgery (Tables 11.2 and 11.3).

Laparoscopic surgery offers greater comfort to patients. There is a minimum of postoperative pain, ileus and venous stasis. Feeding can be typically resumed the same day and women can walk normally by the next day. Laparoscopic surgery is also more economical, with shorter operations and hospital stays than laparotomy. Laparoscopic procedures limit the risk of postoperative adhesions (Lundorff *et al.*, 1991). Complications may be avoided in most cases by careful patient selection and use of appropriate instrumentation. Nevertheless, operative laparoscopy requires a laparoscopist well trained in endoscopic procedures and tubal surgery.

Conclusion

Actual results and greater comfort to patients suggest that operative laparoscopy can definitely replace microsurgery by laparotomy in the management of distal tubal lesions. Furthermore, the major advantage of laparoscopic techniques is their availability at the time of diagnostic laparoscopy. Immediate opening of hydrosalpinges allows for precise evaluation of the tubal mucosa, thereby establishing a realistic prognosis. In cases with a severely damaged mucosa, *in vitro* fertilization should be considered as an alternative.

Table 11.3 Results of salpingostomy

Author	Total patients	IUP	EP
Gomel (1977)	9	4	0
Daniell & Herbert (1984)	22	4	1
Bruhat *et al.* (1989)	68	17 (25%)	5 (7%)
Dubuisson *et al.* (1990)	34	10 (29%)	1

IUP, intrauterine pregnancy; EP, ectopic pregnancy.

References

Bruhat MA, Mage G & Manhes H (1983) Laparoscopic procedures to promote fertility, ovariolysis and salpingolysis. Results of 93 selected cases. *Acta Europea Fertilitatis* **14**: 113–115.

Bruhat MA, Dubuisson JB & Pouly JL (1989) La coeliochirurgie. In *Encyclopédie Medicochirurgicale, Techniques chirurgicales, Urologie-gynécologie* 41515,6-1989, 38 p: Paris, Encyclopédie Medico-chirurgicale.

Daniell JF & Herbert CM (1984) Laparoscopic salpingostomy utilizing the CO_2 laser. *Fertility and Sterility* **41**: 558–563.

De Brux J (1982) Les trompes. In de Brux J (ed) *Histopathologie Gynécologique*, pp 257–298. Paris: Masson.

Donnez J, Nisolle M & Casanas-Roux F (1989) CO_2 laser laparoscopy in infertile women with adnexal adhesions and women with tubal occlusion. *Journal of Gynecologic Surgery* **5**: 47–53.

Dubuisson JB, Aubriot FX & Barbot J (1985) Traitement microchirurgical des lésions tubo-péritonéales. I Résultats des plasties distales. *Journal de Gynécologie-Obstétrique et de Biologie de la Réproduction* **14**: 641–645.

Dubuisson JB, Bouquet de Jolinière J & Aubriot FX (1990) Terminal tuboplasties by laparoscopy: 65 consecutive cases. *Fertility and Sterility* **54**: 401–403.

Fayez JA (1983) An assessment of the role of operative

laparoscopy in tuboplasty. *Fertility and Sterility* **4**: 476–479.

Gomel V (1977) Salpingostomy by laparoscopy. *Journal of Reproductive Medicine* **18**: 265–267.

Gomel V (1978) Salpingostomy by microsurgery. *Fertility and Sterility* **29**: 380–385.

Gomel V (1983) Salpingo-ovariolysis by laparoscopy in infertility. *Fertility and Sterility* **40**: 607–611.

Lundorff P, Hahlin M, Kiallfelt B *et al.* (1991) Adhesion formation after laparoscopic surgery in tubal pregnancy: a randomized trial versus laparotomy. *Fertility and Sterility* **55 (6)**: 911–915.

Macdonald R & Sutton CJG (1992) Adhesions and laser laparoscopic adhesiolysis. Chapter 5. In Sutton CJG (ed) *Lasers in Gynaecology*, pp 95–118. London: Chapman & Hall Medical.

Mage G & Bruhat MA (1987) Score d'opérabilité tubaire. In Masson (ed) *La Part de l'Homme et la Part de la Femme dans la Stérilité*, pp 93–96. Paris: Masson.

Mettler L, Giesel H & Semm K (1979) Treatment of female infertility due to tubal obstruction by operative laparoscopy. *Fertility and Sterility* **32**: 384–388.

Wolfe WM & Yussman MA (1989) The use of endothermal coagulation for the endoscopic management of bilateral saccular hydrosalpinx. *Journal of Gynecologic Surgery* **5**: 105–108.

12

Non-laser Fertility-promoting Procedures

VICTOR GOMEL* AND MALCOLM G. MUNRO‡

Department of Obstetrics and Gynecology, Faculty of Medicine, *University of British Columbia, Vancouver, BC, Canada
‡University of California, Los Angeles, California, USA

Introduction

Laparoscopy was introduced into gynaecology primarily as a diagnostic tool. Its dissemination among gynaecologists of the English-speaking world was largely because of its application to the performance of tubal sterilization. The enthusiasm for laparoscopic sterilization did not initially extend to other operative procedures. However, in recent years, laparoscopy has gained universal acceptance as an operative modality (Gomel, 1989). This was, however, slow in coming and many of the techniques were developed in the 1970s by a handful of workers (Gomel, 1975, 1977; Mettler et al., 1979). Laparoscopic procedures to promote fertility in women were amongst the first to be reported.

This chapter will review periadnexal adhesive disease, distal tubal occlusion, and discuss, in detail, the techniques of laparoscopically directed salpingo-ovariolysis, fimbrioplasty and salpingostomy.

Periadnexal Adhesive Disease

Pelvic and especially periadnexal adhesions are usually secondary to pelvic inflammatory disease (PID). Another infectious cause is acute ruptured appendicitis. Adhesions resulting from operative procedures can be extensive and are usually more cohesive and dense in nature than are adhesions

due to PID. Adhesions associated with endometriosis are usually encountered in the more extensive stages of this disease.

While periadnexal adhesions usually accompany other occlusive tubal conditions, they may be present in the absence of any apparent tubal disease. In such instances, adhesions, by enveloping the fimbriated end of the tube, the ovary or both, may prevent the transport of the oocyte into the fallopian tube. In other instances, adhesions, even localized, may distort the normal anatomical relationship between the tube and ovary, and thus impair fimbrial ovum pickup.

Adhesions are composed largely of connective tissue and contain a variable degree of vascularity. Consequently, the appearance of adhesions covers a spectrum ranging from those that are filmy or thick and relatively avascular, to those that are richly supplied with blood vessels. Adhesions may also vary in their cohesiveness, that is, the amount of space that exists between the structures abnormally joined and the density of the adhesive process. Highly cohesive adhesions leave virtually no space, or 'slack', between the abnormally attached structures; this adhesive process is usually very dense. 'Fatty adhesions' are, in fact, omentum or appendicae epiploica that have adhered to an organ or the parietal peritoneum.

Salpingitis may also cause varying degrees of distal tubal occlusion. Agglutination of the fimbriae may produce phimosis of the distal tubal opening which may or may not be covered by fibrous scar tissue. In other instances the distal tube may be totally occluded (hydrosalpinx) in which case the ampulla exhibits varying degrees of dilatation. Such distal tubal occlusions are usually associated with periadnexal adhesions.

Instruments

Modalities for Cutting

Transection via laparoscopy may be accomplished with scissors, electrosurgery, or laser energy.

SCISSORS

Laparoscopic scissors are used principally to effect mechanical division, even when they possess electrosurgical capability. Since the introduction of laparoscopic techniques, scissors have been our cutting instrument of choice in salpingo-ovariolysis and other fertility-promoting procedures of the oviduct. Although laparoscopic scissors are now available in a number of models, the most important characteristic required is their ability to cut effectively, an attribute that is frequently elusive. Indeed, the maintenance of scissors is difficult. This partially relates to the disproportionate ratio between the length and calibre of the instrument which largely negates any beneficial effect yielded by sharpening. These characteristics led to the development of disposable scissors. We are, in general, philosophically opposed to the use of disposable instruments because of cost/benefit considerations. However, we believe that because of the difficulties associated with their maintenance in good working order, that a strong argument can be made in favour of disposable or re-usable disposable scissors.

The hooked scissors provide certain advantages. They allow the operator to lift an adhesion away from adjacent tissue before cutting it; the pointed tip provides ease of entry into the fallopian tube. It is important, however, to select a type of hooked scissors, the points of which do not overlap when the jaws are closed. Overlap of the pointed tip(s) may be dangerous when the scissors are employed in retraction, dissection or left unattended within the peritoneal cavity.

Laparoscopic operative instruments must be improved. This is largely a matter of engineering and undoubtedly more functional instruments will be available in the foreseeable future.

ELECTROSURGICAL INSTRUMENTS

A sound knowledge of the principles and bio-effects of electrosurgery is mandatory for the use of this modality. Effective cutting is ideally achieved with the use of non-modulated monopolar current (cutting mode) and a fine-pointed electrode. The 'coagulating' mode is used selectively to achieve haemostasis. Blended current provides a thermal coagulating effect along with the cutting action. In adhesiolysis we employ electrosurgery principally to coagulate blood vessels encountered along the line of mechanical transection, or to stop persistent bleeders at the end of the procedure. Bipolar current with compatible electrodes may also be employed for coagulation of blood vessels.

During the late 1970s concerns were raised regarding the use of monopolar current at laparoscopy because of the risk of inadvertent thermal injury to adjacent organs. However, with the production of improved electrosurgical generators and instruments and a better understanding of the principles of electrosurgery, properly employed monopolar surgical techniques should not cause a greater rate of injury than other modalities.

LASERS

Of the four lasers that have been employed in the pelvis for cutting purposes (CO_2, KTP, argon, and Nd:YAG) the CO_2 laser has been the most popular. The CO_2 laser is usually used as a laser beam; because of the properties of CO_2 laser energy, it cannot be effectively propagated along a flexible fibre. Consequently, at present, the light beam must be guided into the peritoneal cavity through a straight, hollow tube (wave guide) which, in some instances, limits direction of effective delivery.

With the other three lasers, the energy may be propagated along a quartz fibre which may be bent to direct the beam as necessary. The argon and KTP lasers as well as sapphire tips attached to the fibre of the Nd:YAG laser allow the surgeon to operate in contact with tissue. However, this system causes greater thermal damage.

The argon laser has the following disadvantage; its operation requires water cooling, necessitating the installation of new plumbing into the operating rooms. The KTP laser is now available in an air-cooled version which avoids this problem. With the available generators the cutting action of argon and KTP lasers is associated with greater adjacent thermal injury than experienced with the CO_2 laser.

Other Instruments

The other important instruments used in the performance of fertility promoting procedures include probes, grasping instruments, irrigation and suction devices, and on occasion needle holders. These are available in different calibres, usually 3 mm and 5 mm. Grasping instruments are manufactured in different lengths, and with a variety of jaw and handle designs. The suction irrigation device permits effective lavage of the pelvis. In addition, it may be used for dissection by introducing an isotonic solution under pressure (hydrodissection). For the purposes of irrigation and pelvic lavage we employ heparinized lactated Ringer's solution.

Investigation

In addition to appropriate history and physical examination of the couple, preliminary investigation must include semen analysis and determination of the ovulatory status of the woman. Hysterosalpingography (HSG) and laparoscopy are complementary methods of assessing tubal and peritoneal causes of infertility. Hysterosalpingography should be the initial investigation for uterine, tubal and peritoneal factors. It is our opinion that a properly performed HSG can be of inestimable value, while a poorly performed HSG is of little value to the physician and an unnecessary source of discomfort to the patient. The advantages of the initial HSG include:

1. identification of uterine anomalies and intra-uterine lesions;
2. identification of cornual occlusion and/or non-occlusive proximal tubal disease;
3. identification of distal occlusion and assessment of intratubal architecture which is of prognostic significance.

The preceding information is of great value in deciding whether or not to perform corrective surgery at the time of the initial diagnostic laparoscopy (Gomel et al., 1986). Corrective surgery for distal tubal disease carries a better prognosis in the presence of relatively normal intratubal architecture. Prior HSG demonstrating a normal uterine architecture and tubal patency will encourage the surgeon who discovers periadnexal adhesive disease to proceed with immediate salpingo-ovariolysis. In addition, such information will enable the surgeon to request appropriate operating room time for the procedure.

Surgical Technique

The patient is placed in the modified lithotomy position which allows ready access to the genital tract from below. A rigid uterine cannula is attached to the cervix by means of a tenaculum. In addition to providing the means to perform intraoperative chromopertubation, the rigid cannula enables the manipulation of the uterus during the operative procedure. Manipulation of the uterus enhances pelvic exposure and permits the immobilization of the adnexal structure to be operated on and thus facilitates the procedure.

Operative laparoscopy requires the use of a multiple puncture technique. We normally employ a 7 mm laparoscope inserted intra-umbilically. Additional punctures are usually placed suprapubically in the midline and at McBurney's point. When circumstances necessitate an additional entry site, it is placed over the left lower quadrant. The separation of the visual and operative axes provided by this technique allows better depth perception, recognizing the loss of binocular vision at laparoscopy. The procedure is performed by viewing a good quality television monitor, thus appropriate interaction between the surgeon, assistant and Operating Room personnel is achieved. We normally locate the television monitor at the caudal end of the operating table. Such placement permits all those involved with the case to have a clear view of the screen.

Fertility-promoting Procedures

The fertility-promoting procedures of proven value include:

1. salpingo-ovariolysis,
2. fimbrioplasty, and
3. salpingostomy.

Although there have been a number of reports of laparoscopic tubotubal anastomosis, this approach at present must be viewed as experimental. Our scepticism in this regard results from the following observations. The ideal application of reconstructive microsurgery in gynaecology is tubotubal anastomosis; it permits meticulous opposition of tissue planes and the reconstruction of a tube that is almost normal, albeit shortened. It yields excellent results (reported live birth rates vary between 60 and 80%).

GENERAL PRINCIPLES

Microsurgery represents the gold standard of reconstructive surgery in gynaecology. When such procedures are undertaken laparoscopically it is necessary to emulate microsurgical principles. Infertility microsurgery is a discipline that uses magnification integrated with the philosophy of tissue care designed to minimize trauma (Gomel, 1983a). Peritoneal trauma, whether mechanical, thermal or chemical, elicits an inflammatory reaction. This inflammatory exudate contains fibrinogen, which is transformed into fibrin. Fibrin deposition and fibroblastic proliferation are the basis for adhesion formation.

With proper positioning of the patient and appropriate distension of the peritoneal cavity, excellent exposure can be obtained at laparoscopy. The ability to bring the laparoscope into the vicinity of the area of interest may render exposure even better than that at laparotomy. In addition, the laparoscope provides a degree of magnification.

Since the procedure is carried out within a closed abdomen, in normal conditions desiccation of the peritoneal surfaces is largely prevented. This protective effect of operative laparoscopy may be eliminated by continuous insufflation of high volumes of CO_2 required for the elimination of smoke (plume) generated by the intraperitoneal use of laser energy.

As in microsurgery few instruments are used during operative laparoscopy. However, the refinement that has been possible in microsurgical instruments is lacking in the laparoscopic instruments currently in use. Furthermore, the length of these instruments with the cannula acting as a fulcrum increases exponentially the force applied to the tissue. This generates unnecessary tissue trauma. Undoubtedly many of these problems, which are largely technical, will be partly eliminated with the development of improved instruments. Another limitation is related to optics. In view of the monocular vision at laparoscopy, the depth perception is significantly decreased. An additional limitation relates to the angle of approaching the tissue under reconstruction. This limitation may be partly overcome by mobilization of the uterus and adnexal regions as well as the use of the uterus to immobilize the adnexa in an appropriate position. Access to a specific area may also be improved by the introduction of rectal or vaginal probes and variations in the horizontal and lateral tilt of the operating table.

Laparoscopy permits intraoperative irrigation and thorough pelvic lavage at the end of the procedure. In addition, when appropriate, dissection of tissues can be achieved by introducing irrigation fluid under pressure (hydrodissection).

Despite the development of relatively fine electrodes (both monopolar and bipolar), laparo-scopic haemostasis remains relatively crude in comparison to microsurgery. Fortunately, most bleeders encountered during fertility-promoting procedures cease spontaneously and on occasion, the use of a very dilute vasopressin solution may be sufficient to overcome the problem.

Another limitation of operative laparoscopy in comparison to microsurgery lies with the precise alignment and approximation of tissue planes. Despite the development of needle holders and suturing techniques, including intra-abdominal suturing techniques (which is our preference), laparoscopic suturing is awkward and more time consuming. In view of this limitation and since one invariably uses suture material of larger calibre than that used in microsurgery, the tendency is to apply fewer sutures in operative laparoscopy.

SALPINGO-OVARIOLYSIS

Patients with prior abdominal surgery frequently exhibit adhesions between the omentum and anterior abdominal wall. If such adhesions limit pelvic visualization it is necessary to remove them first. Adhesiolysis in this instance should be carried out at the level of the parietal peritoneum. Whereas the omentum is a fatty organ, at its site of adherence to the parietal peritoneum the adhesive process may be relatively velamentous. Successful lysis of these adhesions will be dependent upon the optimal exposure of the dissection plane. This is accomplished by retraction of the omentum. If the adhesive process is relatively velamentous it will lend itself to mechanical division with laparoscopic scissors. When the adhesive process is more cohesive it will be necessary to carry out dissection along the appropriate plane. The process is not different from that which is carried out at laparotomy.

The first step in salpingo-ovariolysis is to assess the type and extent of the adhesive process and the structures involved. One of the clear prerequisites of surgery is the recognition of structures, especially when the anatomy is distorted. Adherence to this principle reduces unnecessary trauma and avoids complications. Section of adhesions should ideally be performed along the organ that requires to be freed. Furthermore, adhesiolysis should be carried out one layer at a time, keeping in mind that what superficially appears to be a single layer of adhesion is usually composed of two. Adhesiolysis should be commenced in a well exposed area near the optic. Division must be effected parallel to the affected organ, keeping slightly away from the serosa. This is especially important when

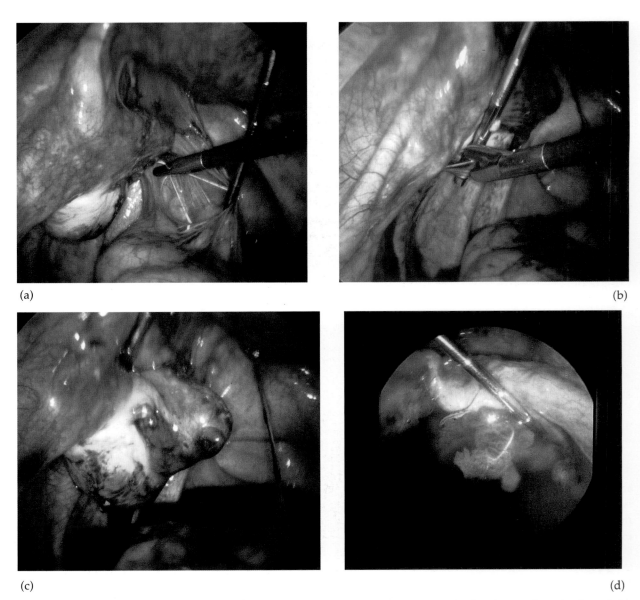

(a)

(b)

(c)

(d)

Figure 12.1 Salpingo-ovariolysis. Adhesions encapsulate the distal half of the tube, binding it deep in the cul de sac and extend to bowel loops. (a) Adhesions are exposed and divided one layer at the time remaining close and parallel to the tube. (b) An adhesion fixing the ovary is isolated and divided. (c) The tube and ovary have been completely freed of adhesions and fimbrial ovarian relationship restored to normal. The dye solution escapes freely. (d) Pelvic lavage completes the procedure. The fimbriae open up within the lavage solution. From Gomel (1983a), with permission from Little, Brown and Company, Boston.

adhesiolysis is performed with electrosurgery or laser energy since with both of these modalities lateral spread of the thermal energy occurs.

Effective and safe adhesiolysis requires:

1. recognition of what lies behind the adhesion,
2. retraction of the adhesion with a probe or traction with grasping forceps applied to the adhesion and not to the target organ.

A small incision is made to elucidate what is behind the adhesion and whether the adhesion is composed of two rather than one layer. Division is accomplished parallel to the organ as indicated earlier. Shallow adhesions are simply divided.

Broad adhesions should be removed by dividing them at their outer margin in a similar fashion. Such adhesions are then removed through one of the portals of entry.

We prefer mechanical division of adhesions using laparoscopic scissors and use electrocoagulation only when significant vessels cross the line of section.

Adhesions encountered secondary to pelvic inflammatory disease are usually relatively avascular and readily amenable to mechanical section or excision. Fatty adhesions are usually those related to the omentum or appendicae epiploicae. When such adhesions are put on the stretch it will usually be possible to visualize a relatively avascular or filmy attachment where the omentum or appendicae epiploicae meet the serosa of the organ to which they are attached. If the adhesive process is cohesive one should refrain from using any type of thermal energy. It is necessary to make a small incision at the edge of such adhesions and develop a dissection plane either by spreading the jaws of the scissors and/or using hydrodissection.

The procedure is completed with a thorough pelvic lavage. This process, in addition to removing blood and debris from the pelvis, enables the visualization of persistent bleeders. These are individually electrocoagulated using an appropriate unipolar or bipolar electrode.

With all fertility-promoting procedures at the close of the operation we leave 150–200 ml of lactated Ringer's solution containing 500 mg of hydrocortisone succinate in the pelvis.

FIMBRIOPLASTY

Fimbrioplasty refers to the reconstruction of existent fimbriae in a partially or totally occluded oviduct. In the majority of such cases periadnexal adhesions are also present in which case salpingo-ovariolysis is carried out first. Stenosis or obstruction of the distal tube may be the result of agglutination of the fimbriae. As a result the terminal end of the tube may have a phimotic appearance with a degree of patency. Transcervical chromopertubation will distend the ampulla prior to the escape of the dye solution. In other instances, the agglutinated fimbriated end is also covered by a fibrous layer that may cause complete occlusion at the site. Less frequently the stenosis is located at the level of the abdominal tubal ostium located at the apex of the infundibulum (prefimbrial phimosis). When the fimbriated end is covered by a fibrous layer, it will be necessary to incise or excise this layer in order to expose the agglutinated fimbriae. This can be accomplished using laparoscopic scissors or laser energy. To deagglutinate the fimbriae a closed 3 mm alligator forceps is introduced into the fallopian tube through the phimotic opening. The jaws of the forceps are opened within the tube and the forceps withdrawn with the jaws in the open position. This procedure is repeated several times, varying the direction of the jaws, until satisfactory fimbrial deagglutination is obtained. With gentle manipulation bleeding is seldom encountered.

Prefimbrial phimosis is best corrected by placing an incision over the antemesosalpingial edge of the fallopian tube from the fimbriated end into the distal ampulla in order to get beyond the stenotic site. The tube is immobilized and if possible a narrow plastic or Teflon probe is introduced through the fimbriated end into the ampulla. Using electrosurgery and a needle electrode the incision is commenced at the fimbriated end of the tube and extended into the distal ampulla beyond the site of stenosis. Bleeders on the incisional edges are individually electrocoagulated. A thorough pelvic lavage is then carried out.

SALPINGOSTOMY (NEOSALPINGOSTOMY)

Laparoscopic neosalpingostomy was first reported from Vancouver (Gomel, 1977). Although initially mainly employed as an iterative procedure, laparoscopic salpingostomy is gaining wide acceptance for correction of distal tubal occlusion (hydrosalpinx) as the primary approach. This is the result of improvement in techniques, the availability of *in vitro* fertilization and embryo transfer as a therapeutic alternative, and the recognition of the factors that affect the surgical outcome. These factors are largely inherent to the status of the fallopian tube at the time of surgery.

Since periadnexal adhesions coexist with most cases of hydrosalpinx, salpingo-ovariolysis constitutes the first phase of the procedure. The next step is a thorough assessment of the distal tube and its relationship with the ovary. It is imperative to determine whether or not the occluded distal tube is free. When the distal tube is free the tubo-ovarian ligament is readily visible. In some instances the terminal end of the tube is adherent to the ovary, in which case the tubo-ovarian ligament is not in view. When the distal tube is adherent to the ovary it is necessary to free the tube from the ovary prior to performing a neosalpingostomy.

The salpingostomy technique employed attempts to imitate the proven microsurgical approach (Gomel, 1978). The tube is distended by transcervical chromopertubation. This confirms patency of the proximal tube up to the distal occlusion site. It also facilitates identification of the scars at the terminal end of the tube, that usually extend from a central dimple in a cartwheel configuration. The central dimple is entered with the pointed tips of the scissors (or electrosurgically using a needle electrode). The first incision is carried out towards the ovary to form a new fimbria ovarica. Once thus entered it becomes possible to view the tube from within and to fashion additional incisions along the circumference of the tube over avascular regions (over the scarred areas). This is achieved by grasping the tube at the edge of the initial incision, retracting the tube and folding it slightly backward. Additional incisions are then placed appropriately using the scissors (or needle electrode). Viewing the tube from within will permit these incisions to be made along the circumference of the tube over avascular regions, avoiding transection of the vascular mucosal folds; preservation of these folds is essential to maintain the ovum-capturing potential of the oviduct.

Once a satisfactory neostomy is obtained it is possible to achieve eversion of the edges by the application of two or three 5-0 or 6-0 Vicryl sutures. However, there is no evidence to suggest that suturing improves the outcome. Eversion of the tubal edges can also be accomplished by gentle electrocoagulation of the serosa. The desiccation caused by mild electrocoagulation results in retraction of the affected serosa and eversion of the edges. The same result can be obtained by the use of a defocused CO_2 laser beam at low power density.

Once the tube is entered in the region of the central dimple it is possible to inspect the ampullary epithelium using a rigid or preferably flexible hysteroscope introduced through one of the portals of entry. Distending the tube with lactated Ringer's solution, it is possible to inspect most of the ampullary portion of the tube. In the face of extensive endosalpingial damage there may be an argument in favour of performing a salpingectomy. However, short of extensive intertubal adhesions, there may be an argument to complete the salpingostomy since the mucosa may regenerate and since intrauterine pregnancies have occurred in the face of apparently severely damaged oviducts. The information provided by the tuboscopy may influence the decision to proceed with IVF sooner rather than later.

Results

There is a paucity of data analysing the relationship of adhesions to pain and/or the impact of adhesiolysis on such symptoms. Consequently, we will review only the data relating to therapy of adnexal adhesive disease and infertility.

For any type of infertility therapy, the results of clinical investigation may be presented and interpreted in a number of ways. When infertility is presumed or known to be secondary to tubal disease, patency and total pregnancy rates are often suggested or reported as appropriate measures of outcome. However, patency does not equal conception, many gestations are ectopic in

location and not all intrauterine pregnancies result in a living baby. Consequently, for the patient and her physician, the only acceptable target is the successful delivery of a healthy baby.

Critical evaluation of the impact of laparoscopic procedures requires distinction between pregnancies that are clearly the result of surgery from those that occur despite such intervention. When surgery is performed on women in whom infertility is secondary to tubal disease that completely occludes both oviducts, subsequent pregnancies may be appropriately attributed to the procedure. However, when there is pre-existing unilateral or bilateral patency, even 'partial' in nature, pregnancy could occur without surgery. Consequently, studies evaluating the effect of laparoscopically directed tubal surgery on women with pre-existing tubal patency that do not have control groups, can overestimate the therapeutic effects of the intervention.

Salpingo-ovariolysis

Gomel (1975) provided the initial report on laparoscopic salpingo-ovariolysis and fimbrioplasty. Fourteen patients achieved one or more intrauterine pregnancies. Among the 24 patients followed for a year or more the intrauterine pregnancy rate was 59%.

In 1979 Semm's group from Kiel reported (Mettler *et al.*, 1979) on salpingolysis and ovariolysis. The total pregnancy rates were 38 and 21% respectively. However, the location and outcome of these pregnancies was not stated.

Gomel (1983b) reported a series of 92 patients who underwent laparoscopic salpingo-ovariolysis. Thirteen of these had moderate while 79 had severe periadnexal adhesions and all had experienced at least 20 months of infertility. After a follow-up period of at least 9 months 57 (62%) had conceived, 54 (59%) with an intrauterine pregnancy. Half of these women conceived within 6 months of surgery. Following this report four additional patients delivered healthy infants.

Corroborative outcomes were reported by Fayez (1983) and Bruhat *et al.* (1983). They attained intrauterine pregnancies in 56% of 50 and 52% of 93 patients respectively.

We must draw attention to the ectopic gestation rates in the preceding reports which ranged between 4 and 7.5% of operated patients. These rates suggest that periadnexal disease is not an isolated entity and that, in a proportion of cases, it is associated with significant damage of the tubal endothelium.

Fimbrioplasty

Relatively few investigators separately classify and report cases where fimbrioplasty is performed. Among 40 patients reported by Gomel (1983c), 19 (47.5%) had successful deliveries and two had ectopic gestations.

The Kiel group (Mettler *et al.*, 1979) reported a 31% pregnancy rate, although again, the location and outcome of these pregnancies was not revealed.

More recently, Dubuisson *et al.* (1990) reported intrauterine and ectopic pregnancy rates of 25.8 and 12.9% respectively, in 31 women followed for 18 months. Surprisingly, these results were inferior to those yielded by their salpingostomy group. No patient conceived between 12 and 18 months.

Salpingostomy

Laparoscopic salpingostomy was initially reported by Gomel in 1977; four of nine patients conceived, all with successful pregnancies. Of note is that eight of these women had previous conventional salpingostomy via laparotomy with subsequent reocclusion of the tube(s).

Mettler *et al.* (1979) reported 10 pregnancies among 38 patients after laparoscopic salpingostomy with the use of thermal coagulation. The location and outcome of these pregnancies were not specified. Daniell and Herbert (1984) reported on 22 patients in whom salpingostomy was performed using CO_2 laser via laparoscopy. Four patients achieved intrauterine pregnancies, one of which was aborted; one patient had a tubal pregnancy.

Dubuisson *et al.* (1990) reported 10 uterine pregnancies (32.4%) and only one tubal pregnancy among 34 patients after laparoscopic salpingostomy.

McComb and Paleologou (1991) reported five term pregnancies in 22 patients followed for more than one year. One patient had an ectopic gestation.

Bruhat *et al.* (1989) reported intrauterine pregnancies in 17 (27.4%) of 62 patients. These authors classified their patients into four groups. The fallopian tubes in the most favourable group are described as having 'partial occlusion (phimotic tube)'. This group, which yields the best outcome, is in effect a fimbrioplasty group.

Conclusions

Pelvic and periadnexal adhesions arise as a result of an inflammatory process secondary to infection, endometriosis, and physical or chemical trauma. They are most frequently encountered in association with infertility or pelvic pain. With appropriate planning, case selection, instruments and technique, periadnexal and pelvic adhesions and distal tubal occlusion can be treated laparoscopically in a safe and effective manner. The results obtained by laparoscopically directed salpingo-ovariolysis and fimbrioplasty approach or equal those obtained by microsurgery. The advantages afforded by the described procedures that can be performed at the time of the initial diagnostic laparoscopy are evident.

The results afforded by laparoscopic salpingostomy appear to be lower than those yielded by microsurgery. However, the principal determinant of the outcome is the status of the tube at the time of surgery. The following factors influence the outcome:

1. distal ampullary diameter;
2. tubal wall thickness;
3. nature of the tubal endothelium at the neostomy site;
4. extent of adhesions; and
5. type of adhesions.

These factors have been quantified in a scoring system which permits estimation of the likely surgical outcome (Gomel, 1988). Considering that improvements in the results of salpingostomy with the use of microsurgical techniques have been much less impressive than for other tubal reconstructive procedures, considering further that IVF offers a credible alternative therapeutic option, there is a greater place today for laparoscopic salpingostomy in appropriately selected cases, especially since this procedure can be performed during the initial diagnostic laparoscopy.

References

Bruhat MA, Mage G, Manhes H *et al.* (1983) Laparoscopy procedures to promote fertility: ovariolysis and salpingolysis results of 93 selected cases. *Acta Europaea Fertilitatis* **14**: 476–479.

Bruhat MA, Dubuisson JB, Pouly JL *et al.* (1989) La Coeliochirurgie. In *Encycl Med Chir, Techniques Chirurgicales, Urologie-Gynecologie* 6: 38. Paris: Editions Techniques Ed.

Daniell JF & Herbert CM (1984) Laparoscopic salpingostomy utilizing the CO_2 laser. *Fertility and Sterility* **41**: 558–563.

Dubuisson JB, Bouquet de Jolinière J *et al.* (1990) Terminal tuboplasties by laparoscopy: 65 consecutive cases. *Fertility and Sterility* **54**: 401–403.

Fayez JA (1983) An assessment of the role of operative laparoscopy in tuboplasty. *Fertility and Sterility* **39**: 476–479.

Gomel V (1975) Laparoscopic tubal surgery in infertility. *Obstetrics and Gynecology* **46**: 47–48.

Gomel V (1977) Salpingostomy by laparoscopy. *Journal of Reproductive Medicine* **18**: 265–268.

Gomel V (1978) Salpingostomy by microsurgery. *Fertility and Sterility* **29**: 380–387.

Gomel V (1983a) *Microsurgery in Female Infertility*, pp 147–149. Boston: Little, Brown and Co.

Gomel V (1983b) Salpingo-ovariolysis by laparoscopy in infertility. *Fertility and Sterility* **340**: 607–610.

Gomel V (1983c) *Microsurgery in Female Infertility*, pp 143–144. Boston: Little Brown and Co.

Gomel V (1988) Distal tubal occlusion. *Fertility and Sterility* **49**: 946–948.

Gomel V (1989) Operative laparoscopy: time for acceptance. *Fertility and Sterility* **52**: 1–11.

Gomel V, Taylor PJ, Yuzpe AA & Rioux JJ (1986) *Laparoscopy and Hysteroscopy in Gynecologic Practice* pp 77–79. Chicago: Year Book Medical Publishers.

McComb P & Paleologou A (1991) The intussusception salpingostomy technique for the therapy of distal ovoductal occlusion at laparoscopy. *Obstetrics and Gynecology* **78**: 443–447.

Mettler L, Giesel H & Semm K (1979) Treatment of female infertility due to tubal obstruction by operative laparoscopy. *Fertility and Sterility* **32**: 384–388.

13

Ectopic Pregnancy

JEAN LUC POULY, CHARLES CHAPRON AND ARNAUD WATTIEZ

Polyclinique Gynécologie-Obstétrique, Médecine de la Reproduction, Université de Clermont-Ferrand, France

Conservative laparoscopic treatment of ectopic pregnancy (EP) was first described by Manhes and Bruhat. Their first series was published in 1977 (Bruhat et al., 1977). Later on, some others (Semm, 1979; Dubuisson et al., 1987) described the technique of laparoscopic salpingectomy for EP. During the last 5 years operative laparoscopy has become the gold standard in the management of EP.

Today, the aspects of the management as yet unclear are: the respective indications of conservative and radical treatment, the contraindications and the role of ultrasound.

Techniques (Bruhat et al., 1991b)

Conservative Laparoscopic Treatment
(Bruhat et al., 1980; Manhes et al., 1983; Pouly et al., 1986)

The patient must be placed in a dorsal position (and not in lithotomy position) as for any operative laparoscopy. After the diagnosis has been confirmed, laparoscopic treatment is performed providing there are no contraindications. Two suprapubic trocars are introduced, one at each end of an imaginary Pfannenstiel incision. On the side of the EP a 5 mm trocar is introduced through which an atraumatic grasping forceps is inserted and on the opposite side an 8 mm one for the insertion of the Triton. The Triton is a multipurpose 7 mm diameter instrument specially designed for this procedure. Within the main central channel of this instrument, there is a smaller irrigation channel, 0.8 mm in diameter, which permits lavage under pressure. An insulated and retractable monopolar needle is located opposite the irrigation channel. The 5 mm aspiration channel forms the remaining portion of the instrument.

The conservative laparoscopic treatment of EP should be carried out systematically. First of all, the fallopian tube bearing the EP should be well exposed. If a haemoperitoneum is present, repeated lavage of the peritoneal cavity is carried out. The tube is held by a grasping forceps, just proximal to the ectopic sac.

Prophylactic haemostasis is performed before the surgical procedure is begun. 5 IU of ornithine vasopressin is diluted in 20 ml of saline. A 19 gauge spinal needle is pushed under laparoscopic control through the abdominal wall. The solution is injected into the mesosalpinx. The most certain method is to perform two injections, the first, close to the uterine end of the tube and the other along the infundibulopelvic ligament. Others prefer multiple injections in the mesosalpinx in close proximity to the EP. The injection must be performed under strict visual control to avoid the risk of intravascular injection that could lead to profound hypotension. Immediately following the injection, the tube looks blanched and any bleeding usually stops.

Salpingotomy is then performed. The retractable electrode of the Triton is drawn out and a linear incision is made on the antimesenteric surface at the proximal portion of the EP. The monopolar electrode must be applied lightly onto the tubal surface as incision must be obtained only by electrofulguration. Pressure with the electrode could lead to extensive coagulation and destruction of the tubal wall. The length of the salpingotomy incision should be about 10 mm so as to allow easy insertion of the Triton through it. In order to avoid making a false track with the Triton, all three layers of the tube should be incised.

Extraction of trophoblast is performed as follows. By progressive twisting movements, the Triton is introduced through the tubal incision and by repeated suction and lavage, the trophoblastic tissue and the clots are removed. If the EP is too large to be removed in one step by aspiration, repeated extractions must be performed with the help of a morcellator. Even when the tube appears collapsed, it is necessary to confirm that no trophoblastic tissue is left behind. An atraumatic forceps with long serrated blades is introduced through the incision with the blades closed and, once inside, the blades are opened wide, thereby exposing the interior of the tube. A close view with the laparoscope permits clear visualization of any trophoblastic remnants that would appear as rather pale tissue.

Finally, a thorough peritoneal toilet is performed. The incision is left open and not sutured. An intra-abdominal drain is not left *in situ* unless a large haemoperitoneum is present.

Postoperative hospital stay is usually for 24–48 hours and the serum hCG levels must be monitored until they fall to zero.

Certain operative difficulties may be encountered during the course of this procedure. If EP is in the process of tubal abortion, milking of the tube is a possible alternative. In our experience (Bruhat *et al.*, 1980), we have observed that this is only possible if there is no haematosalpinx as otherwise the trophoblast, which is generally located proximal to the haematosalpinx, will often be left behind. If the EP is very small it is better not to perform a prophylactic haemostasis as this would lead to tubal oedema and hence, difficulty in the visualization of the EP. In cases of large EP, aspiration is often incomplete. Thus, the removal of the residual trophoblastic tissue with the help of a grasping forceps is often required.

Laparoscopic Salpingectomy (Dubuisson *et al.*, 1987)

Laparoscopic salpingectomy is usually performed in a retrograde manner, beginning at the isthmus (Dubuisson *et al.*, 1987). At first, blood clots and trophoblastic fragments are aspirated from the pouch of Douglas. A grasping forceps is then introduced through a suprapubic trocar on the side of the EP. This grasps the tube at the isthmoampullary junction so as to expose the uterine attachment of the tube. Two trocars are introduced suprapubically on the opposite side: one for scissors and the other for bipolar coagulation or thermocoagulation forceps. Coagulation is started on the tubal isthmus flush with the uterus. With successive coagulation and cutting, extending from the isthmus and running along the mesosalpinx close to the tube right up to the infundibulopelvic ligament, the tube can be completely excised. The tube is removed with the help of a pair of long Palmer's polyp forceps which is introduced through one of the two suprapubic incisions or through a posterior culdotomy. The procedure is terminated by a thorough peritoneal toilet. A complementary coagulation of the uterine cornua may be performed, if necessary. Postoperative stay is usually 24–48 hours in hospital and subsequent monitoring of the hCG levels.

This technique is suitable for fimbrial, ampullary and isthmic locations of the EP. Difficulties arise due to the large size of the haematosalpinx that are not easy to remove. In such cases, it is often better to perform a salpingotomy so as to reduce the tubal volume and then to perform the salpingectomy. Another difficulty arises due to the presence of adhesions between the tube and the ovary. If these are very thick and adhesiolysis is impossible, one must choose between conservative treatment and adnexectomy.

Laparoscopic Treatment with Methotrexate (Pansky *et al.*, 1989; Zakut *et al.*, 1989; Kooi and Kock, 1990)

This method can be applied only if there is no haemoperitoneum. The tube is stabilized with a grasping forceps and a spinal needle is introduced through the abdominal wall and inserted into the EP under laparoscopic control. After aspiration, 2–5 cm^3 of a solution containing from 10–40 mg of methotrexate is injected into the EP. Postoperative course includes hospitalization for 24 hours and strict surveillance of the rate of fall of hCG.

Role of Lasers in the Laparoscopic Treatment of EP

The CO_2 (Johns and Hardie, 1986) and the Nd:YAG (Keckstein *et al.*, 1990) lasers have been used frequently for the treatment of EP. The CO_2 laser is mainly used for effecting the salpingotomy incision wherein it replaces the monopolar electrode. It suffers from the disadvantage that CO_2 laser energy is absorbed by fluid and is thus less effective in the presence of haemorrhage.

The non-contact Nd:YAG laser, as it leads to a large zone of coagulation necrosis, is effective in destroying the trophoblast and also in achieving haemostasis in cases of ruptured ectopics.

It should always be remembered that a laser is only an instrument and not a technique.

Operative Results, Indications and Contraindications

The laparoscopic treatment of EP is not infallible. After conservative laparoscopic treatment, the commonest problem encountered has been residual trophoblastic tissue within the tube. The spontaneous evolution in this case is the formation of a haematocoele rather than acute haemorrhage. The clinical diagnosis is generally made only after a delay of 15–20 days at a stage when significant pelvic adhesions are present. This complication occurs in 5% of the cases (Pouly et al., 1986; Donnez and Nisolle, 1989; Chapron et al., 1991a). This does not mean that the laparoscopic treatment is at fault as a similar incidence of 4.8% has been reported by Di Marchi et al. (1987) after conservative treatment by laparotomy. But the failure rate rises to 16% in cases of laparoscopic tubal milking (Pouly et al., 1986; Chapron et al., 1991a). Thus we never perform this procedure, always preferring salpingostomy when a conservative laparoscopic procedure is carried out.

Early detection of failures is possible by surveying the rate of fall of serum hCG. A comparison of the relative hCG rate was made between 69 successful cases and 7 failures (Pouly et al., 1991b). From this study, we could demonstrate that early detection of treatment failures is possible on the second or the third postoperative day if the fall of the hCG rate was not significant. Depending upon the rate of fall of the hCG in relation to the postoperative day, four situations can be clearly defined (Figure 13.1):

Zone A: success is ensured and no further monitoring of hCG is required.

Zone B: the treatment is likely to be successful, but continuous monitoring to demonstrate a downward trend until hCG is undetectable is necessary, especially in cases where the initial hCG level had been high.

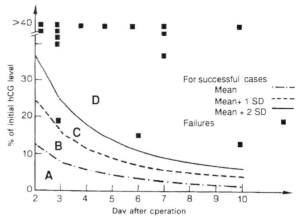

Figure 13.1 Corrected curves of hCG levels given as relative values, according to the postoperative days in successful cases (curves per means values, mean + 1 SD. mean + 2 SD) and in cases of failure (black squares). Diagram indicating the postoperative procedure: zone A, monitoring unnecessary; zone B, likely successful treatment but continuous monitoring until zero, if high initial hCG level (> 200 ng/ml); zone C, strict monitoring until hCG level returns to zero; zone D, very likely failure.

Zone C: there is a moderate risk of failure and the drop of hCG level must be very carefully monitored every 2 days until undetectable.

Zone D: the treatment must be considered as a failure. In these cases of early detection of failure we propose the following alternatives:

- a second laparoscopic salpingotomy or a laparoscopic salpingectomy if there are any clinical indicators of persistent EP (abdominal-pelvic pain; intra-abdominal haemorrhage, etc.).
- medical treatment in the form of methotrexate (i.m.) when the diagnosis of failure is purely based on beta-hCG in the absence of any clinical manifestations.

By studying these failures, we concluded that they mainly occurred in the following situations:

- haematosalpinx larger than 4 cm in diameter; usually greater than 6 cm.
- large haemoperitoneum over 2000 cm^3.
- high initial hCG level over 20 000 IU/l.
- and in cases of transfimbrial extraction (milking) of EP.

On the other hand, conservative treatment is not always easy to perform and may have to be aborted in certain cases such as marked obesity, large haemoperitoneum, extensive adhesions, very large EP.

Interstitial pregnancy is not an indication for

endoscopic treatment even though few cases treated by conservative laparoscopic treatment have been reported (Hill *et al.*, 1989; Reich *et al.*, 1990). In most of these cases, the salpingotomy incision induces considerable and sometimes life-threatening haemorrhage that often requires an emergency laparotomy.

Therefore, we consider the following to be the contraindications for conservative laparoscopic treatment:

1. Absolute contraindications:
   contraindications to anaesthesia for laparoscopy.
   shock.
   haematosalpinx larger than 6 cm.
   hCG titre greater than 20 000 IU/l.
2. Relative contraindications:
   haemoperitoneum greater than 2000 cm³.
   acute and significant haemorrhage.
   marked obesity.
   extensive and dense pelvic adhesions.
   haematosalpinx over 4 cm.
   interstitial pregnancy.

The selection criteria depends, to a large extent, upon the experience of the operating surgeon.

After laparoscopic salpingectomy, failures are rare. Occasionally, peritoneal implantation of trophoblastic tissue occurs and induces haematocoele formation (Dubuisson *et al.*, 1990). This complication is rare, occurring in less than 0.5%. For this reason hCG surveillance must be carried out about 2 or 3 days after the surgical procedure. Contraindications to laparoscopic salpingectomy are the following: shock and interstitial pregnancy are the main ones. Marked obesity and extensive pelvic adhesions are relative contraindications. A large haemoperitoneum, acute haemorrhage and a large haematosalpinx are not contraindications to this treatment.

Methotrexate injection of EP at laparoscopy is associated with a 10% failure rate (Pansky *et al.*, 1989). This occurs when this antifolate is unable to stop the growth of the trophoblastic tissue. After this mode of treatment, hCG levels must be subject to strict surveillance for a prolonged period as the hCG fall is very gradual and detection of failures is possible only after 4–10 days with a large risk of acute haemorrhage during this period. Moreover, methotrexate injection leads to increased intratubal pressure that can culminate in its rupture, this occurring during the injection or in the first 4 postoperative hours. Contraindications to this treatment is a ruptured EP. In all the other cases, this treatment is suitable and is mainly indicated in those cases wherein laparoscopic treatment is contraindicated or difficult, i.e. interstitial pregnancy, high hCG rate, obesity and EP largely involved in pelvic adhesion.

Fertility

Fertility results after conservative or radical laparoscopic treatment are comparable, if not better, with those observed after similar treatment by laparotomy, with or without microsurgical techniques (Tables 13.1 and 13.2). Through a retrospective study of 223 patients, desirous of childbearing, who were treated by laparoscopic salpingostomy, the intrauterine pregnancy (IUP) and recurrence rates were found to be 67% and 12% respectively (Pouly *et al.*, 1991a). These results, similar to those reported by De Cherney and Diamond (1987) and Donnez and Nisolle (1989) demonstrate that conservative laparoscopic treatment of EP preserves subsequent fertility.

The analysis of post-EP fertility after laparoscopic treatment, based on our results (Pouly *et al.*, 1991a), allowed us to draw the following conclusions:

1. The study of fertility results after laparoscopic treatment of EP, based on the operative procedure performed and the status of the contralateral tube, demonstrate that prognosis is better after conservative than after radical treatment (Table 13.3). The IUP rate is superior after conservative treatment and salpingectomy does not decrease the risk of recurrence (Dubuisson *et al.*, 1990; Pouly *et al.*, 1991a).
2. The post-EP fertility appears to be unrelated to the tubal pregnancy characteristics (Pouly *et al.*, 1991a). The site of the EP and whether the tube was ruptured or not had no significant influence on the IUP, recurrence and fertility rates. The practical implications of the afore-mentioned deductions are the following:
   (a) It is not necessary to systematically realize a salpingectomy in cases of tubal rupture only in order to preserve the fertility.
   (b) Isthmic ectopic pregnancy can also be treated by conservative laparoscopic treatment. For these, laparoscopic salpingotomy is reliable and the future fertility is not significantly different from that obtained after conservative treatment by laparotomy (Chapron *et al.*, 1992b).
3. Laparoscopy from only the diagnostic point of view, plays only a very small role in establishing the fertility prognosis after EP. According to our study, from all the information obtained

Table 13.1 Fertility after treatment by laparotomy of ectopic pregnancy

Operative procedure	N	IUP		EP	
		No.	%	No.	%
Radical treatment					
Bender (1956)	232	98	41	18	17
Vehaskari (1960)	219	105	48	18	8
Timonen & Nieminen (1967)	558	273	49	67	12
Franklin et al. (1973)	385	235	61	104	27
Sherman et al. (1982)	104	75	72	6	6
Tuomivaara & Kaupila (1988)	237	164	69	31	13
Total	1741	950	54	244	14
Conservative treatment					
Timonen & Nieminen (1967)	185	98	53	22	12
Sherman et al. (1964)	47	39	83	3	6
Tuomivaara & Kaupila (1988)	86	57	66	12	14
Makiren et al. (1989)	42	29	69	12	29
Langer et al. (1990)	118	83	70	13	11
Total	478	306	64	62	13
Microsurgical treatment					
Janecek (1979)	10	6	60	2	20
DeCherney et al. (1980)	9	5	55	0	0
Oelsner et al. (1987)	51	26	51	13	25
Total	70	37	53	15	21

Adapted from Bruhat et al. (1991a).

Table 13.2 Fertility after laparoscopic treatment of ectopic pregnancy

Authors	Operative procedure	N	IUP		EP	
			No.	%	No.	%
DeCherney et al. (1987)	C	69	36	52	7	16
Donnez & Nisolle (1990)	C	138	70	51	14	10
Pouly et al. (1991a)	C	223	149	67	27	12
Total		430	255	59	48	11
Reich et al. (1988)	C + R	38	19	50	11	29
Mecke et al. (1989)	C + R	74	42	57	10	14
Total		112	61	54	21	18
*Dubuisson et al. (1990)	R	125	30	24	16	13

C, conservative laparoscopic treatment; R, radical laparoscopic treatment.

at diagnostic laparoscopy, only two factors, namely the existence of homolateral adhesions and the controlateral tubal status, had any significant effect on the future fertility prognosis (Pouly et al., 1991a). These results are in agreement with those of others who have reported the deleterious effects of adhesions (Sandvei et al., 1987; Thorburn et al., 1988; Vermesh, 1989) and the influence of the contralateral tubal status (Hallat, 1986; Langer et al., 1987; Oelsner et al., 1987; Tuomivaara and Kaupila, 1988) on future fertility prognosis.

4. Most of the factors that determine the future fertility prognosis are indicated by the past history of the patient (Pouly et al., 1991a). Factors in the history which have significant deleterious effects on the the post-EP fertility are: previous history of EP, salpingitis, solitary tube, tubal microsurgery and laparoscopic adhesiolysis. The fertility rate is significantly

Table 13.3 Fertility results after laparoscopic treatment of ectopic pregnancy according to operative procedure and contralateral tubal status

Authors	Contralateral tube normal					Contralateral tube patent but pathological				
		IUP		EP			IUP		EP	
	N	No.	%	No.	%	N	No.	%	No.	%
Pouly *et al.* (1991a)	145	120[a]	83	11[b]	8	31	13[c]	42	6[d]	19
Dubuisson *et al.* (1990)	32	15[a]	47	6[b]	19	39	10[c]	26	10[d]	26

[a], $P < 0.001$; [b], [c], [d]; $P = $ NS.

higher for patients without any such past history than for patients presenting with one or more of these aforementioned factors. Simple and cumulative IUP rates are significantly lower for patients presenting with one or more of these factors than for patients without any antecedents. Past history also delays the onset of IUP. Finally, these factors increase the risks of recurrence which usually occurs ipsilaterally (Chapron *et al.*, 1992b). Some authors have also reported the negative impact of infertility (Thorburn *et al.*, 1988; Vermesh, 1989) and prior salpingitis (Nagamani *et al.*, 1984; Sandvei *et al.*, 1987; Tuomivaara and Kaupila, 1988) on future fertility.

5. Using a multivariate analysis we evaluated the relative responsibility of each of the factors which significantly decreased the post-EP fertility (Table 13.4). By taking into account these factors and their approximate coefficients we propose a *therapeutic scoring system for ectopic pregnancy* (Table 13.4) (Pouly *et al.*, 1991a). With this score, we propose the following management of EP in order to preserve future fertility:

Table 13.4 Therapeutic scoring system for ectopic pregnancy

Prior history of one ectopic pregnancy	2
For each additional ectopic pregnancy	1
Prior history of laparoscopic adhesiolysis*	1
Prior history of tubal microsurgery*	2
Solitary tube	2
Prior history of salpingitis	1
Homolateral adhesions	1
Contralateral adhesions†	1

* Only one is taken in count.
† If the tube is absent or blocked, count as 'solitary tube'.
+ Score 0–4, conservative laparoscopic treatment; + Score 5, radical laparoscopic treatment; + Score 6 and above, radical laparoscopic treatment and contralateral sterilization followed by IVF.

- Score 0–4: conservative laparoscopic treatment by salpingostomy.
- Score 5: radical laparoscopic treatment, i.e. salpingectomy.
- Score 6 and +: radical laparoscopic treatment and contralateral tubal sterilization followed by IVF-ET.

Conclusion

As with laparotomy, the laparoscopic treatment of ectopic pregnancy can be either conservative or radical. After conservative laparoscopic treatment by salpingotomy the risk of failure can be estimated to range between 4 and 6%. Early detection of these failures due to incomplete removal of the trophoblast is possible from the second or third postoperative day by a postoperative surveillance of the drop in hCG levels. The fertility results after laparoscopic treatment of ectopic pregnancy, whether expressed without correction or in cumulative rate, are comparable if not better than those observed after similar treatment by laparotomy. These fertility results, together with the considerable advantages of endoscopy over laparotomy, mean that today laparoscopic treatment is without question the best surgical treatment for EP. The study of the post-ectopic fertility results after laparoscopic treatment demonstrate that prognosis is better after conservative treatment than after salpingectomy. For us laparoscopic salpingotomy without tubal suturing is the surgical treatment of choice for ectopic pregnancy when it is desired to safeguard future fertility (Chapron *et al.*, 1991b). The post-ectopic fertility is unrelated to the tubal characteristics (location, size, rupture) but mainly depends on the patient's previous history (salpingitis, ectopic pregnancy, solitary tube, tubal infertility). By assessing the various factors significantly affecting future fertility by multivariate analysis we have established a *therapeutic scoring system for ectopic pregnancy*. In practice this therapeutic scoring system allowed us, with the aim of maximizing the patient's future fertility, to choose between one of the three following possibilities: conservative laparoscopic treatment by salpingotomy; radical laparoscopic treatment by salpingectomy; radical laparoscopic treatment and contralateral sterilization.

References

Bender S (1956) Fertility after tubal pregnancy. *Journal of Obstetrics and Gynaecology of the British Commonwealth* 63: 400–403.

Bruhat MA, Manhes H, Choukroun J & Suzanne F (1977) Essai de traitement per coelioscopique de la grossesse extra-utérine. A propos de 26 observations. *Revue Française de Gynécologie et d'Obstétrique* 72: 667–669.

Bruhat MA, Manhes H, Mage G & Pouly JL (1980) Treatment of ectopic pregnancy by means of laparoscopy. *Fertility and Sterility* 33: 411–414.

Bruhat MA, Mage G, Chapron C et al (1991a) Present-day endoscopic surgery in gynecology. *European Journal of Obstetrics, Gynecology and Reproductive Biology* 41: 4–13.

Bruhat MA, Mage G, Pouly JL et al. (1991b) *Operative Laparoscopy*. New York: Medsci/McGraw-Hill. 228pp.

Chapron C, Querleu D & Crepin G (1991a) Laparoscopic treatment of ectopic pregnancies. A one hundred cases study. *European Journal of Obstetrics, Gynecology and Reproductive Biology* (in press).

Chapron C, Pouly JL, Manhes H et al. (1991b) Treatment of tubal pregnancy (letter). *Fertility and Sterility* 56: 374–375.

Chapron C, Pouly JL, Mage G et al. (1992a) Récidives après traitement coelioscopique conservateur d'une première grossesse extra-utérine. *Journal de Gynécologie, Obstétrique et Biologie de la Reproduction* 21: 59–64.

Chapron, C, Pouly JL, Wattiez et al. (1992b) Results of conservative laparoscopic treatment of isthmic ectopic pregnancies: a 26 cases study. *Human Reproduction* 7: 422–424.

DeCherney AH & Diamond MP (1987) Laparoscopic salpingostomy for ectopic pregnancy. *Obstetrics and Gynecology* 70: 948–950.

DeCherney AH, Polan, ML, Kort H & Kase N (1980) Microsurgical technique in the management of tubal ectopic pregnancy. *Fertility and Sterility* 34: 324–327.

Di Marchi JM, Losasa TS & Lobara TY (1987) Persistent ectopic pregnancy. *Obstetrics and Gynecology* 70: 555–558.

Donnez J & Nisolle M (1989) Laparoscopic treatment of ampullary tubal pregnancy. *Journal of Gynecological Surgery* 5: 157–162.

Dubuisson JB & Aubriot FX & Cardone V (1987) Laparoscopic salpingectomy for tubal pregnancy. *Fertility and Sterility* 47: 225–228.

Dubuisson JB, Aubriot FX, Foulot H et al. (1990) Reproductive outcome after laparoscopic salpingectomy for tubal pregnancy. *Fertility and Sterility* 53: 1004–1007.

Franklin EW, Ziederman A & Laemmle P (1973) Tubal ectopic pregnancy: etiology and obstet and gynecologic sequelae. *American Journal of Obstetrics and Gynecology* 117: 220–225.

Hallatt JG (1986) Tubal conservation in ectopic pregnancy: a study of 200 cases. *American Journal of Obstetrics and Gynecology* 154: 1216–1221.

Hill JA, Segars JH & Herbert III CM (1989) Laparoscopic management of interstitial pregnancy. *Journal of Gynecologic Surgery* 5: 209–212.

Janecek J (1979) Résultats de la chirurgie reconstructive dans les grossesses extra-utérines non rompues. *Revue Médicale de la Suisse Romande* 99: 603.

Johns DA & Hardie RP (1986) Management of unruptured ectopic pregnancy with laparoscopic carbon dioxide laser. *Fertility and Sterility* 46: 703–705.

Keckstein J, Hepp, S & Schneider V (1990) A new technique for conservation of the fallopian tube in unruptured ectopic pregnancy. *British Journal of Obstetrics and Gynaecology* 97: 352–354.

Kooi S & Kock HCLV (1990) Treatment of tubal pregnancy by local injection of methotrexate after adrenaline injection into the mesosalpinx: a report of 25 patients. *Fertility and Sterility* 54: 580–584.

Langer R, Bukovsky I, Sherman A et al. (1987) Fertility following conservative surgery for tubal pregnancy. *Acta Obstetrica et Gynecologica Scandinavica* 66: 649–652.

Langer R, Raziel A, Ron-El R, Bukovski I & Caspie E (1990) Reproductive outcome after conservative surgery for unruptured tubal pregnancy. A 15 year experience. *Fertility and Sterility* 53: 227–231.

Makinen JI, Salmi TU, Nikkanen VPJ & Koskinen EYJ (1989) Encouraging rates of fertility after ectopic pregnancy. *International Journal of Fertility* 34: 46–51.

Manhes H, Mage G, Pouly JL, Ropert JF & Bruhat MA (1983) Traitement coelioscopique de la grossesse tubaire: améliorations techniques. *Presse Médicale* 12: 1431.

Mecke H, Semm K & Lehmann-Willenbrocke E (1989) Results of operative pelviscopy in 202 cases of ectopic pregnancy. *International Journal of Fertility* 34: 93–100.

Nagamani M, London S & St Amand P (1984) Factors influencing fertility after ectopic pregnancy. *American Journal of Obstetrics and Gynecology* 149: 533–535.

Oelsner G, Morad J, Carp H, Mashiach S & Serr DM (1987) Reproductive performance following conservative microsurgical management of tubal pregnancy. *British Journal of Obstetrics and Gynaecology* 84: 1078–1083.

Pansky M, Bukovsky I, Golan A et al. (1989) Local methotrexate injection; a non surgical treatment of ectopic pregnancy. *American Journal of Obstetrics and Gynecology* 161: 393–396.

Pouly JL, Manhes H, Mage G, Canis M & Bruhat MA (1986) Conservative laparoscopic treatment of 321 ectopic pregnancies. *Fertility and Sterility* **46**: 1093–1097.

Pouly JL, Chapron C, Manhes H *et al.* (1991a). Multifactorial analysis of fertility following conservative laparoscopic treatment of ectopic pregnancy through a 223 cases series. *Fertility and Sterility* **56**: 453–460.

Pouly JL, Chapron C, Mage G *et al.* (1991b) The drop in the levels of hCG after conservative laparoscopic treatment of ectopic pregnancy. *Journal of Gynecologic Surgery* **7**: 211–217.

Reich H, Johns DA, De Caprio J, McGlynn F & Reich E (1988) Laparoscopic treatment of 109 consecutive ectopic pregnancies. *Journal of Reproductive Medicine* **33**: 885–890.

Reich H, McGlynn F, Budin R, Tsoutsoplides G & De Caprio J (1990) Laparoscopic treatment of ruptured interstitial pregnancy. *Journal of Gynecologic Surgery* **6**: 135–138.

Sandvei R, Ulstein M & Wollen AL (1987) Fertility following ectopic pregnancy with special reference to previous use of an intrauterine contraceptive device (IUCD). *Acta Obstetrica et Gynecologica Scandinavica* **66**: 131–137.

Semm K (1979) New methods of pelviscopy (gynecologic laparoscopy) for myomectomy, ovariectomy, tubectomy and adnexectomy. *Endoscopy* **2**: 85.

Sherman D, Langer R, Sadovski G, Bukovski I & Caspi E (1982) Improved fertility following ectopic pregnancy. *Fertility and Sterility* **37**: 497–502.

Thorburn J, Philipson M & Lindblom B (1988) Fertility after ectopic pregnancy in relation to background factors and surgical treatment. *Fertility and Sterility* **49**: 595–601.

Timonen S & Nieminen U (1967) Tubal pregnancy: choice of operative method of treatment. *Acta Obstetrica et Gynecologica Scandinavica* **46**: 327–339.

Tuomivaara L & Kaupila A (1988) Radical or conservative surgery for ectopic pregnancy? A follow-up study of fertility of 323 patients. *Fertility and Sterility* **50**: 580–583.

Vehaskari A (1960) The operation of choice for ectopic pregnancy with reference to subsequent fertility. *Acta Obstetrica et Gynecologica Scandinavica* **39**: 1–7.

Vermesh M (1989) Conservative management of ectopic gestation. *Fertility and Sterility* **51**: 559–567.

Zakut U, Sadan O, Katz A, Dreval D & Bernstein D (1989) Management of tubal pregnancy with methotrexate. *British Journal of Obstetrics and Gynaecology* **96**: 725–728.

14

Techniques of Mass Sterilization

SHIRISH S. SHETH

Hon. Professor of Obstetrics & Gynaecology, King Edward Memorial Hospital, Bombay, India

Population control is essential in the third world where a high growth rate of population coupled with poverty has a devastating effect. This tremendous increase in population is due to ignorance, illiteracy, religious or cultural beliefs and political apathy. A staggering infant mortality of 100–150 per 1000 is often compensated by having more children. According to the World Development Report (1987), the average number of children per family in 1985 was 5.59 in Bangladesh, 4.5 in India, 4.25 in Mexico, 6.74 in Pakistan and 8 in Yemen.

There is a dire need for a method of permanent contraception or sterilization. Mass voluntary sterilization can be performed on either partner. The demand for female sterilization procedures far surpasses vasectomies. In such a grim scenario, it is immaterial whether sterilization is by vasectomy or tubectomy. Globally, more than 120 million couples use sterilization as their contraceptive method of choice and women at an increasingly younger age are choosing this method (Rioux, 1989). This method protects 46% of couples in Puerto Rico. 34% in the USA, 30% in Panama, 25% in China, 23% in Thailand, 21% in India, 20% in The Netherlands, 16% in England and Wales, 14% in Mexico and 6–33.1% in Brazil. All over India, 4.2 million sterilization operations were carried out between 1985 and 1986 (Umashankar, 1988).

Choice of Method

Endoscopy has revolutionized the practice of gynaecology (Phillips, 1990). In the last decade, the University Department of Obstetrics and Gynaecology at Kiel, Germany has pioneered tremendous technical developments in operative laparoscopy (Semm, 1987).

Female sterilization on a mass scale can be by tubal occlusion by the laparoscopic method or at mini-laparotomy or by the vaginal route through posterior colpotomy. The culdoscopic method is obsolete and the hysteroscopic one still in an experimental stage (see Chapter 13). Whether the tubes are occluded by one method or another depends on the expertise and capabilities of the operator. If the operator has vast experience with mini-laparotomy and is relatively unskilled at laparoscopy, it is obvious that he should use the former method. However, scientific evidence has shown a clear superiority of the laparoscopic method, except in the immediate post-partum period where Bhatt et al. (1983) have shown a clear advantage of mini-laparotomy over other methods.

The laparoscopic method is quick, the abdomen is not opened nor the vagina cut. Consequently, the hospital stay is shorter. Being safe and fast and easy to perform, it is the ideal method for mass sterilization and the most acceptable to patients. In the USA, laparoscopic sterilization is the most common laparoscopic procedure as well as the most favoured method of sterilization of women (Soderstrom, 1977).

The vaginal method of sterilization had its brief period of glory prior to the advent of the laparoscope, particularly amongst advocates of vaginal surgery (Sheth et al., 1973). It needs expertise in opening the pouch of Douglas and gaining access to the fallopian tubes. If it is performed by an inexperienced operator, there can be trauma to the tubes, mesosalpinx and even the ovaries and/or the uterus. In the absence of asepsis, there can be many complications. The worst results are when this method of tubal sterilization by an inexperienced operator is combined with termination of pregnancy in a septic environment. These disadvantages have brought the operation into disrepute. It only has a limited role in tubal sterilization, e.g. when a laparoscope or the expertise in its use is not available.

According to Bhiwandiwala et al. (1982b) the physician should continue to use the method with which he is most familiar and comfortable; differences in techniques usually can be overriden by experience.

Methods of Tubal Occlusion

The tubes may be occluded by:

1. cautery, unipolar or bipolar;
2. clip, Filshie (Filshie, 1983) or Hulka;
3. ring or Yoon band (Yoon, 1990).

The choice will depend upon the operator's experience, the relative advantages and disadvantages and the cost.

Electrocoagulation

Electrocoagulation without transection or resection of the fallopian tube has the largest record of practice of all the methods of sterilization in the United States (Levy and Soderstrom, 1990). The bipolar method was designed to decrease some of the hazards, though burns have occurred even with this. However, Semm (1987) using endocoagulation, which causes protein denaturation by heating the tissue to 100–120°C, then cuts the tube with hook scissors without damaging the adjacent vessels. This destroys only 1 cm of the tubes which can later be re-anastomosed should the need arise.

The disadvantages of the cautery are burns of the abdominal wall and bowel, and problems caused by accidental stepping on the footswitch and erratic power supply in the developing world. Bhathena et al. (1985) reports inadvertent burns of the surrounding tissues in six cases, of which three required laparotomy.

The clip technique is preferred in the young, particularly if the option of reversal is to be considered. However, in the poorer nations, where cost plays a major role, the ring is used. The falope ring technique, presently popular in India, has a low complication rate and a low failure rate of 0.2–0.7 (Motashaw, 1983).

The Sterilization Camp

A 'camp' provides expert medical or surgical assistance to a large number of needy persons in a short time in an orderly organized manner. The patients usually belong to the less privileged or deprived section of society who do not have access to even basic facilities.

In the developing world, such a mass scale approach is used for the diagnosis and treatment of cataract, squints, cardiac disorders, plastic or orthopaedic procedures for the handicapped and for sterilization of males and females.

A large number of people turn out to avail themselves of such a facility. A successful outcome enhances the reputation of such a programme and generates more volunteers.

A number of laparoscopic tubal sterilization camps have been conducted by teams of volunteers travelling around India (Bhathena et al., 1985; Sheth, 1988; Mehta, 1989).

Where to Organize a Mass Sterilization Camp for Women

Mass voluntary sterilization camps should be organized in geographical areas or countries with a very high growth of population. Couples with more than an adequate number of children are approached for the procedure. They will remain unsterilized and continue to add to the size of their family to their own detriment and to that of the nation. These camps can be held under the auspices of government, municipal, district or local authorities, or service organizations, such as Rotary or Lions clubs, or women's community groups.

PREREQUISITES

1. A large number of willing women. Anything less than 25 operations per day may not be an

incentive for the visiting team who come from afar.

2. Surgeons with experience of laparoscopic sterilization. A camp is not the site for juniors to learn or the inexperienced to practise.
3. Trained anaesthesiologist and Boyle's apparatus.
4. Availability of running water to cleanse the instruments.
5. A continuous supply of electricity for the light source.
6. Facilities for laparotomy should the need arise.
7. A doctor to assess the patients preoperatively and a social or health worker to ascertain the number of living children. In some parts of the world with high paediatric mortality, two children are preferred of which at least one should be a son aged more than 4 years. This is for cultural and religious reasons.
8. Local support from the government and/or municipality is essential.

THE TEAM

The team consists of:

1. Experienced surgeons—one to four or more, depending upon the size of the camp
2. Theatre nursing staff—one or two.
3. Theatre assistants—one or two, to look after the equipment.

It is better to have the same individuals in the team rather than new entrants, so as to have a cohesive group, accustomed to working harmoniously. The reputation and experience of the team are the pillars upon which the success of the camp is built. Not many skilled and experienced gynaecologists are willing to take part in these camps. There may not be any financial incentives, so it involves commitment to a cause. Travel can be arduous since the distances covered may be large. One has to sacrifice family life, private practice and take leave of absence from work.

If the local gynaecologist in the region or district where the camp is being held is an experienced surgeon and has the necessary confidence, it is a wise decision to include him in the team. This, besides fostering good public relations, can help in the initiation of future camps, which will then use his expertise. Local nursing and other staff, if included in the programme, can also be an asset.

Preparations for Holding a Camp

It is necessary to have adequate propaganda by means of pamphlets, posters, banners and visits by social workers. Information is provided as to the credentials of the operating team, e.g. stressing the fact that they are from a famous medical institution or a metropolitan city.

Details of the method of sterilization help to motivate the women. Emphasis is laid on the positive aspects of the procedure. They are told that the abdomen is not cut open, there is only one stitch, the vagina is intact, the stay is only for a few hours and does not usually involve an overnight absence from home. These facts assuage the fears of the women and then sterilization becomes acceptable. The women and their family members are also assured that it is a safe and efficient procedure which will not disturb their family life and they can resume their normal routine quickly.

Transport to and from the operation site must be arranged as otherwise, even if motivated, the women will not be able to avail themselves of the procedure. Buses, jeeps, ambulances, vans, cars and even bullock carts have been used to fetch the patients from the surrounding countryside and take them back. They need to be reassured regarding return transport and medical help, should it be required.

Paramedical staff are needed to register the cases, take the consent of both husband and wife and bring in and take out the patients. An operating room with the necessary facilities must be arranged and an adequate number of units to provide light and pneumoperitoneum apparatus. Postoperative lying-in facilities for 4–24 hours are needed. In some countries, incentive money is paid to the patient, the surgeon and the motivator. Arrangements for the hosting of the surgical team must be satisfactory. Well maintained public relations ensure the success of the camp to be held and any future ones in the area.

The medical team at the venue will need to start well before the operating team is due to arrive. Many of the women are uneducated and illiterate. A patient hearing of their apprehensions, queries and doubts is needed and satisfactory answers given. This is where involvement of the local health authorities and organizers pays rich dividends as they will have a better rapport with the people of that area. The failure rate and available alternatives, if the need should arise, should be explained. The physical and social fitness of the woman should be checked.

Women with severe anaemia (Hb less than 7 g/dl), cardiac disease or severe malnutrition are not accepted. A routine urine examination should be done. Tetanus toxoid is given and sensitivity to lignocaine tested. Pregnancy must be excluded as sterilization with termination of pregnancy performed in an unfamiliar set-up can prove risky. Occasionally there are surprises, e.g. conception has occurred during lactational amenorrhoea and laparoscopy reveals a slightly enlarged, congested pregnant uterus. Those that have delivered just 48–72 hours prior to the holding of the camp are not accepted as the uterus will be rather high for the procedure. It is advisable not to hold a mass diagnostic camp for other diseases along with a mass sterilization camp as a mix-up can be disastrous, e.g. tubal occlusion mistakenly performed on an infertile patient.

Naturally an operation theatre is the ideal place to perform this procedure. However, in the camp scenario, the premises used were school halls, classrooms, guest houses or parts of an auditorium which had been converted temporarily into an operating room. The space allotted should be at least 15 × 12 feet. The tables were sometimes regular operation tables but often ordinary tables were used with blocks or bricks at the foot end to achieve the Trendelenburg position.

The number of tables varies from two to six, depending upon the number of surgeons, available space and the number of operations to be performed. A surgeon may choose to have two or three tables at his command. A patient is operated on one table and whilst that patient is being shifted, the surgeon starts a pneumoperitoneum on the second table. In the meantime another patient is being positioned on the third table, so that i.v. premedication, painting, draping and infiltration of local anaesthesia can be attended to by an assistant (Table 14.1, Figure 14.1).

EQUIPMENT

This consists of:

1. single puncture operating laparoscopes or double puncture laparoscopes;
2. falope ring applicators, Veress needles, trocar and cannula;
3. fibreoptic light source or a variant;

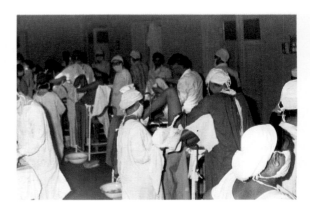

Figure 14.1 Theatre scenario.

4. a pneumoperitoneum apparatus or a variant, e.g. an air pump.

In operative laparoscopy, the single puncture technique is not recommended (Sutton, 1990). However, for mass sterilization by the laparoscopic method, single puncture equipment was preferred to the double puncture for the following reasons:

1. Tubal occlusion is the only operation to be performed.
2. One stitch is preferred by patients instead of two puncture sites.
3. The time for operation is less. When a large number of laparoscopic sterilizations are being performed, every minute counts.
4. The amount of manipulation required is less.
5. A second set of trocar and cannula is not needed and this saves time.

The equipment needed is dependent on the number of tables. One set of pneumoperitoneum apparatus and a light source between two tables can suffice. These can be operated by a single paramedic or a non-medical person. The presence of an overall supervisor streamlines the working of all the tables.

The equipment used needs to be cleansed under running water and kept for at least 10 minutes in sterilizing solution (Cidex or formalin) before its use in the next patient. If this is not possible, a compromise can be made by cleaning the trocar thoroughly in soapy water, preferably containing 1000 p.p.m. of chlorine and then rinsing and boiling in clean water for 5 minutes (Woodford, 1988). The laparoscope should be rinsed in 80% ethanol and dried. At times, unfortunately, undesirable compromises are made. It helps a great deal to have a greater number of Veress needles, trocars and cannulae and clip or ring applicators as these are the instruments which come into direct contact with

Table 14.1 Mass laparoscopic sterilization camps

No. of operation tables	2–6
No. of operations/table/hour	6–15
No. of working hours/day	8–14
Surgical time for each operation	2–10 min
No. of operations/day	100–500
Postoperative stay in hours	6–18

Venue: government hospitals, cottages, school or guest house premises.

body tissues, such as the peritoneum and the fallopian tubes.

LIGHT

A fibreoptic light source is ideal for laparoscopic tubal sterilization but may not be available in isolated areas. It is cumbersome for a visiting team to carry it, besides being unsafe for the equipment. Mini-light sources which are handy and easy to transport may be used (Figure 14.2). The light emitted is sufficient for the purpose though the operator may need to get visually acclimatized to it. The light is insufficient, however, for an inexperienced operator in a difficult case or for a diagnostic laparoscopy. It can either work on the main electrical source or battery, which is an advantage in case of power failure in areas of the developing world with an erratic power supply.

Anaesthesia

In the vast majority of patients, laparoscopic sterilization can be performed under local anaesthesia and premedication. General anaesthesia is not necessary unless:

1. premedication and local anaesthesia prove inadequate;
2. the patient is highly strung and apprehensive;
3. there is extreme obesity;
4. extra manipulation is needed because of adhesions, an enlarged uterus or a non-cooperative patient.

It is mandatory to have a competent anaesthetist and Boyle's apparatus in the operation theatre. The choice of premedication is best left to the anaesthetist. Usually, atropine 0.6 mg subcutane-

ously and 50 mg meperidine and 10–20 mg triflupromazine hydrochloride or 10 mg diazepam i.m. or i.v. are given. Local infiltration with 3–5 ml of 1% lignocaine hydrochloride around the site for surgery supplements the premedication.

Pneumoperitoneum

Creating a pneumoperitoneum is an integral part of laparoscopy and should always precede the insertion of a trocar and cannula. Although a few endoscopists advocate the direct insertion of a trocar and cannula, this is incorrect and can be dangerous. The ideal gas to use is carbon dioxide, but this may not be available in some parts of the world, necessitating the use of alternatives, such as nitrous oxide or oxygen. These may not be easy to procure in quantities sufficient for a large number of patients and are expensive. In such circumstances, atmospheric air is an acceptable compromise. Room air can be freely instilled by using an air pump, similar to the one used in a fish tank to release air bubbles (Figure 14.3). An inexperienced operator should not use air. Even experienced operators must exercise caution as there is a greater chance of embolism and death. The use of a cautery is contraindicated when a combustible gas is used.

The equipment supplying gas should be easy to transport as often the local organizers of the camp may not be able to provide an adequate number of units.

The amount of gas used varies between 1000 and 2000 ml. This can be measured by an air indicator or by clinical judgement of the abdomen as it is distending. In a thin woman, only 500–1000 ml may be required whereas an obese one may need up to 3 litres.

Unlike a diagnostic laparoscopy, the purpose

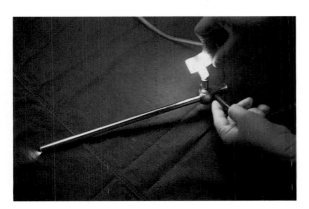

Figure 14.2 Minilight with laparoscope.

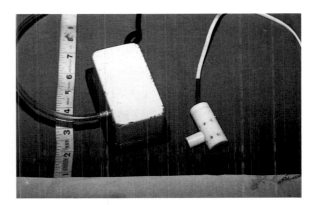

Figure 14.3 Minilight and air pump device.

here is only to visualize the uterine fundus, the medial half of the fallopian tubes, the round ligaments, the utero-ovarian ligaments and part of the ovary.

If one fails to create a pneumoperitoneum the abdominal findings need to be reassessed before the Veress needle is inserted through the pouch of Douglas by colpopuncture. If there is no contraindication, this should pave the way for a successful pneumoperitoneum.

The cul-de-sac method was used in 350 cases of outpatient laparoscopy by Dirk *et al.* (1980) and they suggest this as the method of choice for the creation of a pneumoperitoneum. Sheth (1976) created pneumoperitoneum by this method in 120 cases during laparoscopy without any complications or a failure. He strongly feels that this route should be used in the obese and those who have had previous multiple abdominal operations, so that women are not deprived of tubal sterilization.

Procedure

The tables are placed parallel to each other with one light and gas source in between, so as to service the two tables. Each operator manages one table but the more experienced, particularly the speedier ones, usually manage two. The painting, draping and local infiltration of 3–5 ml of 1% lignocaine hydrochloride is done by an assistant, so that the surgeon is left free to perform the actual laparoscopic sterilization procedure swiftly.

The patient either walks to the table or is carried on a stretcher if premedication has been given earlier. Pneumoperitoneum is created in the usual manner. Single puncture laparoscopes are preferred through which the chosen occluding device is applied at a distance of 3 cm from the cornual ends. An assistant, usually a highly experienced nurse, inserts the uterine manipulator and almost feeds the fallopian tube to the applicator. In areas with a population that is orthodox, conservative and with many cultural taboos, the women and their relatives object to exposure of the genitalia for sterilization procedures. Hence, in this group, some operators have performed all tubal sterilizations without using uterine manipulators. The woman was covered with a sheet covering the genitalia. A steep head low of almost 30–40° helped to keep the abdominal organs away and make the uterus, tube and ovaries accessible. When the tubes have

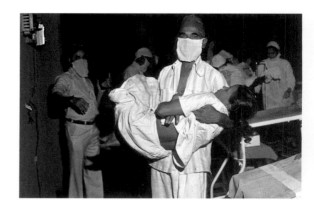

Figure 14.4 Postoperatively, the patient is lifted by one person, due to constraints of space and time.

been occluded, the abdomen is deflated as much as possible and one mattress stitch inserted. The patient is usually lifted bodily by one person (Figure 14.4) and carried to the recovery area. The use of a stretcher or trolley for bringing in and taking out the patient is only feasible if there is plenty of room in the operating area.

Postoperatively the patient is observed for 6–12 hours. There may be an overnight stay if the patient is operated on in the evening, as travel can be difficult in rural areas. At times, due to paucity of facilities, many patients are put on the floor or share a bed (Figures 14.5 and 14.6).

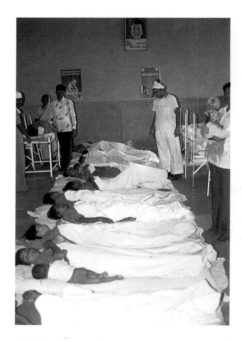

Figure 14.5 Postoperative recovery area in a rural camp.

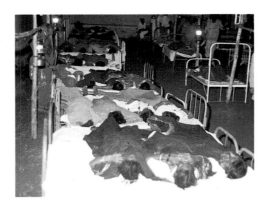

Figure 14.6 Many postoperative patients sharing a bed, at a rural camp.

Table 14.2 Complications in 30 000 laparoscopic sterilizations in rural camps

Complications	Number
Perforation of uterus	268
Transection of tube	56
Mesosalpingeal haematoma	74
Slight bleeding from tube mesosalpinx	194
Extraperitoneal pneumoperitoneum	118
Failed pneumoperitoneum	60
Failure to apply the silicone rubber band	96
Trocar injury	
Intestinal injury (laparotomy required)	3
Abdominal wall haematoma (evacuation required)	1
Wound infection	560
Total	1430

Wound infections were mild, and there were no deaths. (Courtesy *Lancet*, Dec. 17, 1988).

Complications

The complication rate is extremely low if the procedure is done carefully by an experienced surgeon in ideal surroundings. However, even then major catastrophes, such as bowel perforation or laceration or injury to a large vessel, including the aorta, and causing immediate death have occurred. Hence the procedure must be treated with respect and done with the utmost care. Brooks and Marlow (1977) have rightly said: 'While laparoscopy is a relatively safe procedure, there are times when its use can be extremely hazardous.'

Chamberlain and Brown (1978) found a complication rate of 4.1% in 29 661 laparoscopic sterilizations. A WHO multicentre, multinational randomized study (1982) found that the incidence of complications at the time of operation are greater with the laparoscopic approach, 7% of women experiencing major or minor complications. Bhatt *et al.* (1983) analysing 68 visceral injuries at sterilization found the highest incidence of 10.4 per 1000 with the laparoscopic method, whilst with posterior colpotomy it was 1.64 per 1000 and with laparotomy it was 0.98 per 1000. However, in his series, laparoscopy was done in only 7.1% of cases, and a large number of the patients were in the post-partum or post-abortal period. Quilligan and Zuspan (1986) found minor complications occur less frequently with laparoscopic sterilization than with sterilization via colpotomy or at laparotomy.

Haste and inexperience naturally compound the problem, more so in an unfamiliar surrounding like a rural camp. The complication rate is more in the post-partum and post-abortal periods (Hughes, 1977; Mumford and Bhiwandiwala, 1981). However, the patients at a mass voluntary sterilization camp are the so-called interval, non-obstetric or gynaecological cases.

In a mass sterilization programme for 9066 illiterate women, Bhathena *et al.* (1985) had an overall complication rate of 5.3%, uterine perforations accounting for 1.2%. There were no deaths, serious complications occurred in 0.1% and the laparotomy rate was 0.5%. Mehta (1989) had a major complication rate of 3.2 per 100 000. In a series of 30 000 laparoscopic sterilizations (Table 14.2), Sheth (1988) reported complications in 4.7%, with three cases needing laparotomy. Minor wound infections were the commonest complications with perforation coming next, accounting for 268 cases. This could be due to the manipulator being inserted by assistants that keep changing.

There is a risk of transmission of blood-borne viral infections, particularly hepatitis B and C and also the human immunodeficiency virus (HIV).

Mortality

Cardiorespiratory complications during general anaesthesia are the leading cause of death (Peterson *et al.*, 1982).

A sterilization death is one that can be directly attributed to sterilization or one that occurs within 30 days of the procedure and cannot be explained satisfactorily by any other cause.

Chamberlain and Brown (1977) cite a death rate of 10 per 100 000 in the United Kingdom, whilst the American Association of Gynecologists report a death rate of 4 per 100 000 (Phillips *et al.*, 1977).

Table 14.3 Laparoscopic sterilizations and mortality

Report	No. of laparoscopic sterilizations	Failed attempts per 1000	Complication rate (%)	Laparotomy rate per 1000	Death rate per 100 000
AAGL, 1976 (Phillips *et al.*, 1977)	77 103	NR		2.7	4
RCOG, 1976–77 (Chamberlain and Brown, 1978)	29 577	7.50	4.1	12.10	10.2
Bhathena *et al.** (1985)	9 066	5.0	5.3	2.0	0
Mehta* (1989)	250 136	0.2	1.5	0.003	4.8
Sheth* (1988)	30 000	2.1	4.7	0.10	0

* Mass sterilizations report.

Bhatt *et al.* (1983) found a mortality rate of 7.15 per 10 000 sterilizations performed by different methods, although there were none when the laparoscopic method was used. Seven out of 23 deaths in 32 177 sterilizations were due to anaesthetic problems. Mehta (1989) reports 12 deaths in 250 136 operations with a death rate of 4.8 per 100 000.

At mass voluntary sterilization rural camps, where the laparoscopic method was used, Bhathena *et al.* (1985) had no deaths in 9066 cases, and neither did Sheth (1988) in 30 000 cases, though three women had to have a laparotomy (Table 14.3).

In the developing world, maternal mortality is very high, ranging from 100 to 700 per 100 000 in contrast to 4–6 per 100 000 in the developed nations. A significant number of deaths per 10 000 cases can thus be prevented by sterilization as 10 000 sterilizations will prevent at least 10 000 pregnancies (Figure 14.7).

10,000 LS STERILISATIONS

10,000 PREGNANCIES PREVENTED, AT LEAST.

Maternal Mortality 100 to 700 / 100,000 in developing World.

Laparoscopic Sterilisation death rate 1 per 5,000 – 10,000.

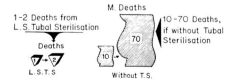

Figure 14.7 Laparoscopic sterilizations and mortality.

Follow-up

Vessey *et al.* (1983) found little evidence of increased gynaecological disorders in those undergoing tubal sterilization when compared with well matched controls.

In the developing world, follow-up of women who have taken part in a mass sterilization programme is poor, and in the rural areas it is worse. The local health officers or organizers are usually in charge, and any major complication would be brought to light or even magnified as compensation may be demanded. Women in the rural areas have remarkable resistance and wound infections are usually mild. They also have a great tolerance for pain and discomfort.

When mass laparoscopic sterilization is performed, one may come across unexpected abnormalities, e.g. a congenital malformation, a mass or pelvic inflammatory disease, particularly abdominal and/or pelvic tuberculosis. In an analysis of the last 10 000 patients in a series of 30 000, Sheth (1988) found that 2.5% had evidence of some abnormality such as a congenital malformation, an ovarian cyst or pelvic inflammatory disease. Since a mass sterilization programme is not the forum for handling such cases, they should be referred for appropriate therapy and follow-up.

Failure

Every sterilization method, including hysterectomy, has failed and pregnancy has occurred. Phillips *et al.* (1977) report that in a substantial proportion of failures, the pregnancy is ectopic. Extensive coagulation and division can give rise to a greater chance of ectopic pregnancy. However, the incidence of ectopic pregnancy is much less, 2–8 per 1000, when the occluding device is a clip, as shown by an international multicentre study (Hulka, 1990).

Bhathena *et al.* (1985) cites a pregnancy rate of 0.1% and Liskin *et al.* (1985) 1.3% with laparoscopic sterilization. Mehta (1989) had a failure rate of 0.1% with the falope ring whilst Rock mentions a pregnancy rate of 0.2–0.5% (Rock *et al.*, 1987). Bhiwandiwala *et al.* (1982a) had luteal phase pregnancy in 0.12%. In a mass sterilization programme, the incidence of luteal phase pregnancy will be higher.

Reversal

Below the age of 30 years, reversal of sterilization is usually requested by women who remarry after divorce or the death of a spouse (Gomel, 1978). In the developing world, a high paediatric mortality may also be the reason for reversal.

Mechanical devices to occlude the fallopian tubes are recommended to eliminate the hazards of techniques using electricity. The clip is good for the young in case reversal is required (Editorial, 1980). Isthmic anastomosis, after clip reversal, leads to 87% intrauterine pregnancies (Hulka *et al.*, 1982).

Couples who may want a child in the future or are doubtful about permanent contraception should not opt for laparoscopic sterilization by any of the currently available techniques. The laparoscopic method of tubal sterilization must be considered as permanent and therefore irreversible, despite its high reversibility rate.

Factors that can Adversely Affect the Camp

The patient and the relatives can be easily displeased if there is a hurried positioning of the patient on the table; the per vaginam examination or speculum insertion is done quickly or the physical act of lifting the patient is done in an undignified manner. Any shouting or screaming by the patient during the operation, or an operated woman in a precarious state, or a complication occurring which necessitates a laparotomy can upset the large apprehensive crowd waiting for the outcome of the operation. If a death occurs, the news will spread like wild fire

and the entire crowd will promptly decide against the procedure and vanish from the scene. A mishap at a camp is disastrous as it can get unduly magnified and bring the procedure into disrepute. Any indifference or non-cooperation on the part of the local authorities towards the holding of a camp in that area can also adversely affect the outcome.

Economic Considerations

The equipment required for laparoscopic sterilization is expensive. However, with mini-laparotomy the cost of hospital stay is considerable. Laparoscopic mass sterilization which requires patients to stay only for a few hours is thus far more economical.

Summary

In the overpopulated countries of the developing world, a large mass of its population living in rural areas is deprived of the facility of gynaecological specialists and good hospital care. Despite social, cultural and religious taboos, there is nevertheless a large number of women now sufficiently aware of the advantages of sterilization. But for the facilities provided by mass sterilization camps, these women would in most cases have gone through life procreating and adding to the population boom. Laparoscopic sterilization on a mass scale is the ideal method for interval cases subject, however, to having skilled surgeons and staff and the appropriate equipment. Although some compromises necessarily have to be made in the developing world, the technique achieves the purpose with very good results, not the least of which is the gratitude of the patients. It is hoped that countries with similar problems will use experienced laparoscopists to control their population.

Acknowledgement

My sincere thanks go to Dr V. Karani MD for her painstaking help in compiling this manuscript.

References

Bhathena RK, Jassawalla MJ & Patel DN (1985) Laparoscopic sterilization in camps in rural India. *British Journal of Family Planning* 10: 121–126.

Bhatt RV, Dawn CS, Gogoi MP *et al.* (1983) Immediate sequelae following tubal sterilisation: a multicentre study of the ICMR Task Force on Female Sterilisation. *Contraception* 28: 369–384.

Bhiwandiwala PP, Mumford SD & Feldblum PJ (1982a) Menstrual pattern changes following laparoscopic sterilisation: a comparative study of electrocoagulation and the tubal ring in 1025 cases. *Journal of Reproductive Medicine* 27: 249–255.

Bhiwandiwala PP, Mumford SD & Feldblum PJ (1982b) A comparison of different laparoscopic sterilisation occlusion techniques in 24,439 procedures. *American Journal of Obstetrics and Gynecology* 144: 329–331.

Brooks PG & Marlow J (1977) Indications and contraindications. In *Laparoscopy*, pp 52–59: Baltimore, USA: Williams & Wilkins.

Chamberlain GVP & Brown JC (eds) (1978) *The Report of the Working Party of the Confidential Enquiry into Gynaecological Laparoscopy*, pp 3, 8, 27, 109, 116, 152. London: Royal College of Obstetricians and Gynaecologists.

Dirk AF, Van Lith KJ, Van Schie W *et al.* (1980) Cul de sac insufflation: an easy alternative route for safely inducing pneumoperitoneum. *International Journal of Gynaecology and Obstetrics* 17: 375–378.

Editorial (1980) Female sterilisation—no more tubal coagulation. *British Medical Journal* 280: 1037.

Filshie GM (1983) The Filshie clip. In Van Lith DAF, Keith LG & Van Kall EV (eds) *New Trends in Female Sterilisation*. Chicago: Year Book Medical Publishers.

Gomel V (1978) Profile of women requesting reversal of sterilisation. *Fertility and Sterility* 30: 30–39.

Hughes GJ (1977) Sterilisation failure. *British Medical Journal* ii: 1337–1339.

Hulka JF, Noble AD, Letchworth AT *et al.* (1982) Reversibility of clip sterilisations. *Lancet* 2: 927.

Hulka JV (1990) *Technique of Sterilisation: Manual of Endoscopy*, pp 63–71. California, USA: American Association of Gynecologic Laparoscopists.

Levy BS & Soderstrom RM (1990) *Electrical Techniques of Sterilisation: Manual of Endoscopy*, pp 57–61. California, USA: American Association of Gynecologic Laparoscopists.

Liskin L, Rinchart W, Blackburn R *et al.* (1985) Minilaparotomy and laparoscopy: safe, effective and widely used: *Population Reports (C)* (9),XIII,2: C125–167, C140–141.

Motashaw ND (1983) *The Falope Ring Technique: New Trends in Female Sterilisation*, pp 97–104: Chicago and London: Year Book Medical Publishers.

Mehta PV (1989) A total of 250,136 laparoscopic sterilisations by a single operator. *British Journal of Obstetrics and Gynaecology* 96: 1024–1034.

Mumford SD & Bhiwandiwala PP (1981) Tubal ring sterilisation experience with 10,086 cases. *Obstetrics and Gynecology* 57: 150–157.

Peterson HB, Greenspan JR & DeStefano F (1982) Death associated with laparoscopic sterilisation in the United States. *Reproductive Medicine* 27: 345–347.

Phillips J, Hulka B, Hulka J *et al.* (1977) Laparoscopic procedures: the American Association of Gynecologic Laparoscopists: membership survey for 1975. *Journal of Reproductive Medicine* 18: 227–232.

Phillips JM (1990) Preface. In *Manual of Endoscopy*. California, USA: American Association of Gynaecologic Laparoscopists.

Quilligan EJ & Zuspan F (1986) *Operative Obstetrics*, pp 795–803. New York: Appleton Crofts.

Rioux JE (1989) *Female Sterilisation and its Reversal*, pp 275–291. London: Butterworths.

Rock JA, Guzick DS, Katz E *et al.* (1987) Tubal anastomosis: Pregnancy success following reversal of falope ring or monopolar cautery sterilisation. *Fertility and Sterility* 48: 13–17.

Semm K (1987) Surgical pelviscopy: review of 12,060 pelviscopies. In *Progress in Obstetrics and Gynecology*, vol 6, pp 333–345. London: Churchill Livingstone.

Sheth SS (1976) Transvaginal induction of pneumoperitoneum prior to laparoscopy. *Asian Journal of Obstetrics and Gynecology* 50–54.

Sheth SS (1988) Round the world: laparoscopic female sterilisation camps. *Lancet* 1415–1416.

Sheth SS, Kothari ML & Munshi V (1973) Postabortal colpotomy and sterilisation. *Journal of Obstetrics & Gynaecology of the British Commonwealth* 80 (3): 274–275.

Soderstrom RM (1977) *Operative Sterilisation: An Overview*, vol 15, pp 159–166. Baltimore, USA: Williams & Wilkins.

Sutton C (1990) The treatment of endometriosis. In *Progress in Obstetrics and Gynaecology*, pp 251–272. London: Churchill Livingstone.

Umashankar PK (1988) *Family Welfare Programme in India 1986–87*, pp 17–19. New Delhi: Ministry of Health & Family Welfare.

Vessey M, Huggins G, Lawless M *et al.* (1983) Tubal sterilisation findings in a large prospective study. *British Journal of Obstetrics and Gynaecology* 90: 203–209.

WHO Task Force on female sterilisation (1982) Minilaparotomy or laparoscopy for sterilisation—a multicentre, multi-national randomised study. *American Journal of Obstetrics and Gynaecology* 143: 645.

Woodford FP (1988) *Decontamination of Instruments and Appliances used in the Vagina*. Department of Health: Ref. EL (88) (MB) 210 plus Annex.

World Bank (1987) *World Development Report 3*. London: Published for the World Bank (Oxford University).

Yoon I (1990) Yoon falope ring technique of sterilisation. In *Manual of Endoscopy*, pp 73–75. California, USA: American Association of Gynecologic Laparoscopists.

15

Laparoscopic Ovarian Surgery: Preoperative Diagnosis and Imaging

LACHLAN de CRESPIGNY

Royal Women's Hospital, Melbourne, Australia

Introduction

The appropriate selection of a patient for laparoscopic ovarian surgery necessitates the availability of reliable information on the aetiology of the pelvic mass. A high quality ultrasound service therefore is essential as it is the imaging modality of choice for the assessment of pelvic pathology. Continuing refinements in technology with resultant improvements in the resolution of ultrasonic equipment has made it an accurate method of assessing a pelvic mass, having the flexibility to allow any suspicious area to be scrutinized from different angles. In relative terms it is a low cost investigation.

A most important advance in the diagnosis of pelvic pathology using ultrasound is the development of the endovaginal transducer. Not only does this avoid the necessity of an uncomfortably distended bladder as a prerequisite to imaging the ovaries, but it also provides improved resolution since the transducer is closer to the area under investigation. More recently colour Doppler has been introduced with its capacity to demonstrate the presence or absence of neovascularization in the wall of a cyst. This feature is proving to be of value in determining whether a cyst is benign or malignant.

Equipment and Technique

Although detailed technique is not relevant to this chapter, several points are worth making.

1. Best results using ultrasound are obtained with 'state of the art' high-resolution equipment. Such equipment, plus the necessary expertise in interpreting the images, is not widely available except at referral centres.
2. A transducer with a small 'footprint' is usually necessary for transabdominal gynaecological scanning—the bones of the pelvis limit access if a large transducer is used. This means that most linear array transducers and many of the curved linear arrays are often inappropriate.
3. An endovaginal scanner is essential. Although a transvaginal ultrasound examination is not necessary in all patients, it is of particular value when transabdominal images are suboptimal, e.g. obesity, and in the evaluation of a pelvic mass (Leibman et al., 1988). These workers showed that transvaginal scanning provides improved images of adnexal masses in 78% of cases and of uterine fibroids in 74%.
4. Viewing of hard copy images will not provide as good results as when the sonologist who is preparing the report does the scanning personally (Benacerraf et al., 1990). Indeed, reporting ultrasound images from hard copy may not provide even as good results as clinical examination (O'Brien et al., 1984). When the sonologist him/herself does the scanning then even transabdominal scanning alone (without transvaginal scanning) is superior to clinical examination (Andolf and Jorgensen, 1988).

Transvaginal ultrasound often provides improved imaging in obstetrical and gynaecological scanning of the pelvis. This has been translated

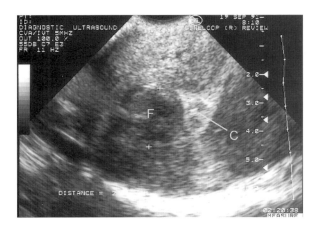

Figure 15.1 A transvaginal section of the uterus which virtually fills the image. The cavity line (C) is demonstrated with a fibroid (F marked with callipers) visible abutting the cavity line.

into earlier diagnosis of pregnancy (de Crespigny *et al.*, 1988), and more accurate assessment of patients with a suspected ectopic pregnancy (de Crespigny, 1988; Kivikoski *et al.*, 1990). The improved resolution of transvaginal scanning provides the ability to diagnose uterine fibroids more accurately, especially if small, and to define their position. In particular, the proximity of the fibroid to the uterine cavity line may be precisely defined (Figure 15.1). Difficulty in distinguishing a solid ovarian tumour from a fibroid is not uncommon using transabdominal scanning but unusual with transvaginal scanning. The ability to move a pelvic mass with the end of the transducer is a further aid to diagnosis.

The exclusion of an ovarian cyst using ultrasound necessitates the clear visualization of each ovary (Figure 15.2). Transvaginal scanning allows the ovaries to be identified more often than transabdominal scanning in the presence of uterine fibroids, especially in peri- and postmeno-

pausal women and in those who have had a hysterectomy (Coleman *et al.*, 1988). In the presence of uterine enlargement the ovaries may be difficult to locate transabdominally. Ovaries situated in the pouch of Douglas are more readily visualized with transvaginal ultrasound, while those high above the uterine fundus may be better seen transabdominally.

Logic dictates that transvaginal scanning should provide improved clinical information (Figure 15.3a, b). Unfortunately the two methods of scanning have not commonly been compared in a study setting. A common approach clinically is to perform transvaginal ultrasound when transabdominal views are suboptimal or the diagnosis uncertain; following this routine Lande *et al.* (1988) found transvaginal ultrasound added diagnostically useful information in 25 of 28 patients with adnexal cysts. Liebman *et al.*

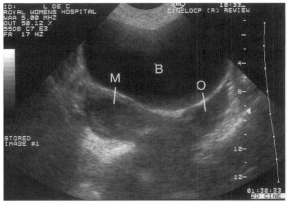

(a)

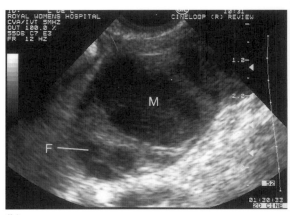

(b)

Figure 15.3 (a) A transverse transabdominal section of the pelvis. Behind the bladder (B) is a normal right ovary (O) and a left mass (M) which is poorly defined and centrally echo poor. (b) On transvaginal ultrasound this same mass (M) is a clearly defined relatively echo free cyst. The adjacent follicles (F) in the cyst wall indicate the cyst is ovarian, the features being those of a benign blood-filled cyst.

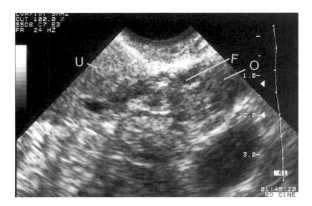

Figure 15.2 A transvaginal image of a normal ovary (O) containing small atretic follicles (F), adjacent to the uterus (U).

(1988) compared transabdominal and transvaginal ultrasound in patients with a palpable mass and found that in 81% transvaginal ultrasound better delineated the internal architecture of the lesion or its relationship to other pelvic structures. Transvaginal ultrasound should therefore be part of the ultrasound examination of a pelvic mass unless declined by the patient.

Indications for Ultrasound

The major indications for gynaecological ultrasound include the following.

Pelvic Pain

While an ovarian cyst is uncommonly found in the absence of a clinically detected mass, ultrasound is particularly valuable when the clinical examination is difficult or impossible such as when the patient is obese or refuses a vaginal examination. In other situations, diagnostic ultrasound may enable the clinician and patient to continue with conservative treatment with confidence when no mass is detected, rather than resort to diagnostic laparoscopy. In this regard it is worth emphasizing that while ultrasound is expected to detect even a small pelvic mass, the examination will be normal if the cause of the pain is not associated with a mass, e.g. pelvic adhesions or small areas of endometriosis. In addition, while the fallopian tube may be seen, especially using a vaginal transducer, a normal tube is not usually visualized with ultrasound.

Pelvic Mass

The major areas in which ultrasound can influence management in patients with a clinical suspicion of a pelvic mass may be summarized as:

1. Confirmation of mass: is there a pelvic mass present? Appropriate use of diagnostic ultrasound in such patients avoids the necessity for surgery where there is uncertainty clinically, e.g. in an obese patient.
2. Site of the mass: is a palpable mass ovarian in origin or does it arise from the uterus or other pelvic organs?
3. Insignificant masses: when a mass is palpable is it significant? This applies in the presence of a small cyst in the premenopausal woman or a palpable postmenopausal ovary.
4. Assessment of possible malignancy: ultrasound cannot provide a pathological diagnosis, but is valuable in helping to determine the likelihood of malignancy. Some benign ovarian cysts have characteristic features, e.g. benign cystic teratoma.
5. Treatment: what is the appropriate management? Treatment may be more rationally planned in light of the findings of (1) to (4) above: is treatment necessary and if so, is cyst aspiration, laparoscopy or laparotomy appropriate? If laparotomy is indicated, the ultrasound findings assist in determining the degree of urgency, whether a gynaecological oncologist should be present, and, depending on the likelihood of malignancy, may help decide which incision is to be used.

Ultrasound Screening for Ovarian Cancer

The major justification for such screening is that less than 30% of primary ovarian cancers are confined to the ovary at the time of diagnosis and the overall 5-year survival rate is less than 25%. Ovarian cancer screening aims to detect lesions at an early stage when the 5-year survival is around 80% (Sigurdsson et al., 1983). The detection rate is low with population screening: Campbell et al. (1989, 1990) identified five patients with primary ovarian cancer in 15 977 screening examinations of women aged 45 and above. To detect those primary tumours (the chance of detecting an ovarian cancer at a single examination was 0.03%), the incidence of false positives was 3.6% at the first ultrasound examination but reduced with subsequent examinations. Such a programme therefore generates a large workload of benign pathology requiring management much of which, with careful patient selection, could be managed using laparoscopy or even cyst aspiration.

On close examination of the cost benefit of ultrasound screening for ovarian cancer Creasman and Di Saia (1991) conclude that it is premature to recommend population screening. It is worth noting the American College of Obstetricians and Gynecologists Committee consider that 'no available techniques are currently suitable for routine screening', a view supported by Westhoff and Randall (1991). Creasman and Di Saia (1991) suggest that only a minority (< 5%) of patients with ovarian cancer have a positive family history, but in this group ultrasound screening may be justified. It should probably be commenced at a young age because in hereditary forms of cancer onset occurs early, usually between the ages of 35 and 45 (Lynch *et al.*, 1982).

A Normal Ovary

The normal ovary is ovoid in outline (Figure 15.2), measures an average of 6.5 ml (5.4–7.6 ml) in premenopausal women (Munn *et al.*, 1986), but is smaller following the menopause (3.6 ± 1.4 ml, Goswamy *et al.*, 1988) and prior to the menarche. Prior to ovulation in spontaneous cycles the ovarian follicle may reach up to 2.5 cm (O'Herlihy *et al.*, 1980) but may be larger in stimulated cycles. In addition, the ovary usually contains several small, mostly peripheral 'cysts' of up to 10 mm which are presumably atretic follicles (Figure 15.2). These are seldom seen following the menopause.

The number of small 'cysts' is increased in polycystic ovarian disease. The ovaries in this condition have been described as having multiple cysts (10 or more) 2–18 mm in diameter, distributed around the ovarian periphery, with an increased amount of stroma (Figure 15.4) or (less commonly) multiple small cysts 2–4 mm in diameter distributed throughout abundant stroma (Adams *et al.*, 1985).

Both ovaries should be able to be visualized using ultrasound in nearly all women. In a series of 321 consecutive patients the author was able to locate both ovaries (when present) in all but one patient—she had had a hysterectomy and there was uncertainty as to whether a single ovary had or had not been removed. Two hundred and forty patients had the ultrasound examination for follicular assessment in either stimulated or non-stimulated cycles. Fifteen patients were postmenopausal. Thirteen of the patients had a transabdominal scan only, eight had transabdominal plus transvaginal, and the remainder transvaginal scans only.

The ovary may be readily differentiated from bowel by watching for peristalsis. Localized collections of tortuous adnexal vessels may occasionally be confused with the ovary but are differentiated easily by examination using colour Doppler. The ovaries may be more difficult to visualize following hysterectomy and after the menopause.

Differential Diagnosis of an Ovarian Mass

The major method of differentiating an ovarian from a non-ovarian pelvic mass is to visualize a normal ovary separate from the mass. If the ovary is moved with the vaginal transducer, an extra-ovarian mass will usually not move with it. A further diagnostic feature is the shape of the ovary—if the ovary is visible adjacent to the mass but is its normal ovoid shape, then the mass is likely to be extra-ovarian, but if the ovary is flattened around the mass then it is usually ovarian (Figure 15.5).

The most frequent differential diagnosis of an ovarian mass on clinical examination is a uterine fibroid, especially if the fibroid is pedunculated. On transvaginal ultrasound the fibroid can be seen as part of the uterus and if pedunculated, the pedicle visualized (Figure 15.6). The fibroid moves with the uterus and the normal ovary is

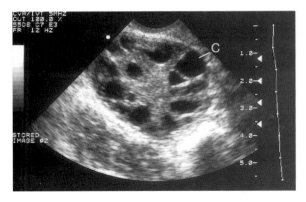

Figure 15.4 A transvaginal section of a polycystic ovary with multiple small, mostly peripheral cysts (C).

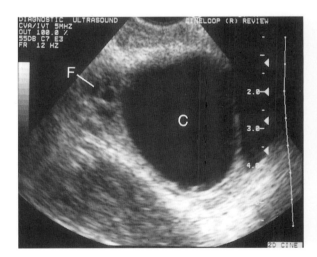

Figure 15.5 A 'simple' ovarian cyst (C) with the ovary containing small atretic follicles (F) in the cyst wall.

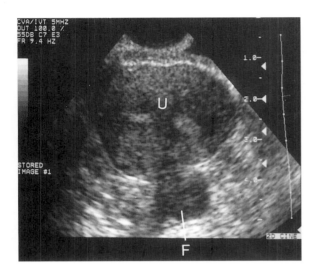

Figure 15.6 A transvaginal image of the uterus (U) with a subserous fibroid (F) posteriorly. The ovaries were visible separately.

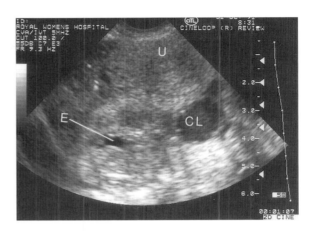

Figure 15.8 Behind the uterus (U) is a 5 mm cystic lesion surrounded by an echo-dense rim of tissue which is the typical appearance of an ectopic pregnancy (E). A small blood-filled cyst, presumably the corpus luteum (CL), is visible adjacent to the ectopic pregnancy.

separately visualized. Other fibroids may also be seen.

A hydrosalpinx may be difficult to distinguish from an ovarian cyst. On ultrasound section both appear to be spherical, thin-walled, fluid-filled structures but by examining sections at different angles then the tortuous shape of the dilated tube is usually identified and its epithelial infolding noted (Figure 15.7). The ovary should be visible separately. This also applies to other non-ovarian masses such as a fimbrial cyst or an ectopic pregnancy (Figure 15.8). It is often difficult to identify the site of origin of an extra-ovarian cyst.

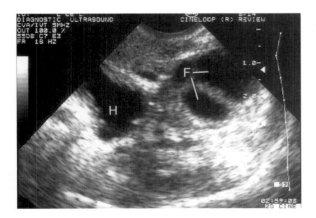

Figure 15.7 The ovary is visible containing several follicles (F). A separate fluid filled lesion with epithelial folds is visible (H) which was subsequently confirmed to be a hydrosalpynx.

Ovarian Cysts

It is worth noting that diagnostic ultrasound frequently offers more information about the nature of a cyst than inspection of its surface at laparoscopy or laparotomy. Using ultrasound, the cyst contents may be carefully scrutinized and magnified, which has been called 'sonomicroscopy' (Goldstein, 1990) and the presence and characteristics of any solid areas noted.

UNILOCULAR SIMPLE CYSTS

In a spontaneously cycling woman, any cyst of greater than 2.5 cm diameter should be considered as being too large to be a follicle (Figure 15.5). The significance of such a 'simple' cyst depends upon its size and the patient's age.

The histological diagnoses include follicular cysts, simple serous cysts, endometriosis, benign mucinous and serous cystadenomas. Few are malignant—of 57 patients with advanced ovarian cancer, in no case was the primary tumour entirely cystic (Paling and Shawker, 1981).

Only some 5% of ovarian cancers are less than 5 cm at the time of diagnosis (Scully, 1982)—larger ovarian cysts are more likely to be malignant even when the cyst is unilocular with no solid element. Herrmann et al. (1987) found no malignancies among 48 'simple' cysts of less than 10 cm diameter but one malignancy in the nine patients with a cyst of greater than 10 cm diameter. Similarly, Meire et al. (1978) found there to be no malignancies among the 23 unilocular cysts of less than 5 cm in diameter but two malignancies in the 19 patients in whom the cyst was greater than 5 cm in diameter.

Even in older women, small 'simple' cysts are rarely malignant. In 1989 two series were published which together totalled 100 patients who had anechoic, unilocular, thin-walled, fluid-filled cysts of less than 5 cm in diameter. The patients in one study were all over 50 years of age (Andolf and Jorgensen, 1989) and in the other were all postmenopausal (Goldstein et al., 1989). On follow-up none was found to be malignant. In an earlier study (1983–85) of 13 postmenopausal patients who had a cyst of less than 10 cm in diameter, one borderline malignancy was found using transabdominal ultrasound (Hall and McCarthy, 1986). It is reasonable to expect that even this tumour would have been more likely to be suspected using the improved equipment now available, especially transvaginal ultrasound and colour Doppler.

The management of a small 'simple' ovarian cyst therefore depends more on its malignant potential than the very small risk of actual malignancy. It has been suggested that serous and mucinous cystadenomas only occasionally undergo malignant change—surface epithelial inclusion glands are thought to be the source of most of the common epithelial carcinomas of the ovary (Scully, 1982). There can therefore be little justification in treating all small 'simple' ovarian cysts as potential cancers.

SIMPLE CYSTS WITH ECHOES IN THE FLUID

The presence of fine echoes throughout the cyst fluid frequently indicates that blood is present either as a result of haemorrhage into the cyst (Reynolds et al., 1986) or to endometriosis.

Endometriotic or other blood-filled cysts may contain dense echoes (Figure 15.9) or fine echoes—there is some relationship between the viscosity of the blood-filled cyst and its echodensity on ultrasound. However, not all blood-filled cysts contain such echoes and not all cysts with uniform echoes contain blood (de Crespigny et al., 1989).

FEATURES OF MALIGNANCY

Multilocular cysts, particularly when the septae are thick, and those with solid areas within the cyst are more likely to be malignant. Even small solid areas are of concern (Moyle et al., 1983). These features have been combined into a scoring system by Sassone et al. (1991) which confirms the empirical results of others—namely that using ultrasound one can effectively select out a group at extremely low risk of malignancy (their classification showed a negative predictive value of 100%), but many benign cysts have some of the adverse features, i.e. benign cysts may be large, multilocular (Figure 15.10) or have solid areas (Figure 15.11) (Sassone et al. found a positive predictive value of 37%). There are, however, undoubtedly a group with many of the adverse features which clearly have a very high chance of malignancy, e.g. complex looking solid and cystic multilocular ovarian tumours (Figure 15.12).

SPECIAL TUMOURS WITH CHARACTERISTIC FEATURES

On first appearances a benign cystic teratoma may be suspicious of malignancy since it is a complex solid and cystic lesion. Dermoid cysts, even when large, may be missed, as their echodense contents may reflect ultrasound and they are mistaken for normal bowel. On closer

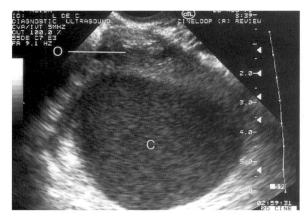

Figure 15.9 An adnexal cyst (C) contains dense echoes. The ovary (O) is in the cyst wall and contains several small cystic lesions of < 5 mm diameter. The cyst was removed surgically and proved to be an endometrioma.

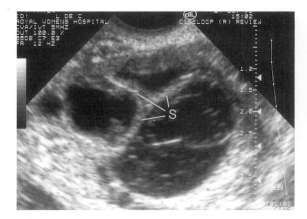

Figure 15.10 This trilocular cyst has thick septa (S). The patient had a past history of endometriosis and this was subsequently confirmed at surgery.

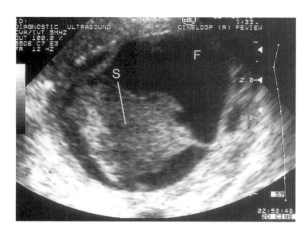

Figure 15.11 This cyst contains a large solid area (S) as well as fluid (F). The solid area wobbled within the cyst when the ovarian cyst was shaken with the vaginal transducer. This represents clot and the cyst subsequently resolved.

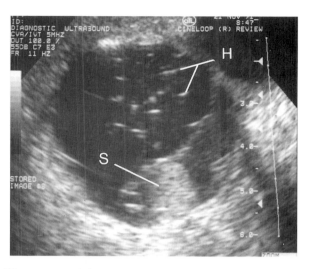

Figure 15.13 A benign cystic teratoma. The dense solid area (S) and the cyst containing fine dense echogenic lines (hair—H) are characteristic.

Colourflow and Duplex Doppler

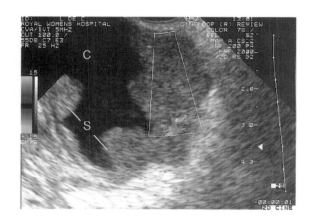

Figure 15.12 A solid (S) and cystic (C) ovarian tumour. The coloured area indicates neovascularization within the solid areas. The RI was low and the pathology later indicated a mucinous cystadenocarcinoma.

inspection the bizarre echo pattern is characteristic. Bronshtein *et al.* (1991) have shown that individual hair fibres seen with transvaginal ultrasound are hyperechoic sparkling dots or delicate white lines. An awareness of this characteristic allowed the group to diagnose 25 dermoid cysts with 100% accuracy (Figure 15.13).

Other cysts with characteristic appearances include thecomas—a hypoechoic mass with acoustic shadowing (Athey and Malone, 1987)—and Krukenberg tumours whose pattern includes irregular hyperechoic areas and moth-eaten cyst formation (Shimizu *et al.*, 1990).

Many high quality vaginal ultrasound transducers now have a colourflow imaging capability. This allows the imaging of small blood vessels which would not be visible without colour and are often too small to be seen even with transabdominal colourflow imaging. Coloured areas within a tumour show the presence of neovascularization (see Figure 15.12)—benign tumours and normal ovarian tissue do not usually show areas of colour. The presence of blood flow within even small ovarian tumours correlates well with laboratory work which shows that angiogenesis occurs in hyperplastic tissue and is important for the conversion of normal epithelium into cancer (Folkman *et al.*, 1989). There is, however, increased vascularity within the ovarian parenchyma in the luteal phase of the cycle, around the time of ovulation and during pregnancy; hence it is suggested that examinations be performed between day 1 and day 8 of the cycle (Bourne *et al.*, 1989).

Duplex Doppler is combined ultrasound imaging with pulsed Doppler. This allows an area of interest to be identified on the B-mode image then examined with pulsed Doppler. Using transvaginal colour Doppler to identify small vessels within a lesion, the blood flow characteristics within that vessel may be examined with duplex Doppler. A number of formulae have been used to relate the systolic and diastolic blood flow within a vessel. The pulsatility index (PI) and resistance index (RI) are two such measures, and these reflect the blood flow impedance distal to the point of sampling. A low PI or RI indicates a low impedance to blood flow in the distal vasculature as seen in neoplasia, a high PI or RI (associated with absent intratumoral neovascularization with colour Doppler) is said to exclude ovarian cancer.

It has become clear that transvaginal colour Doppler (Figure 15.14) is a valuable method of differentiating benign and malignant ovarian tumours (Bourne *et al.*, 1989; Fleischer *et al.*, 1991; Kurjac *et al.*, 1991). Kurjac and his colleagues found colour flow to be present and the RI to be ≤ 0.4 in 54 of 56 malignant adnexal tumours, and no colour flow and an RI > 0.4 in 623 of 624 benign adnexal tumours, although others have been unable to reproduce their results. It has been suggested that utilization of this technology should provide an improved method of selection of those patients suitable to undergo conservative treatment for an ovarian cyst such as cyst aspiration (Editorial, 1990). Perhaps the most important contribution by colour Doppler will prove to be its capacity to demonstrate that a cyst with some adverse feature (such as large size, multilocular or containing solid areas) is likely to be benign.

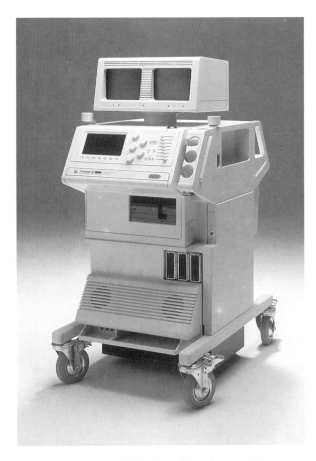

Figure 15.14 ATL colour Doppler machine.

Other Imaging Modalities

Computerized tomography (CT) provides high quality images of the ovaries but does not give more information than ultrasound (Walsh *et al.*, 1978). Both CT and ultrasound are similarly accurate in evaluating pelvic masses but CT is better at detecting abdominal metastatic disease since bowel gas interferes with ultrasound images (Sommer *et al.*, 1982).

Magnetic resonance imaging (MRI) provides clear pictures of pelvic organs and shows the extent of infiltration of ovarian tumours, but normal ovaries are difficult to identify with certainty (Johnson *et al.*, 1984). This modality provides more soft tissue contrast than CT and is biologically safe. It is said to be more sensitive than ultrasound in the diagnosis of endometriosis and more sensitive and specific than either CT or ultrasound in the evaluation of an ovarian mass, and more sensitive but less specific than ultrasound in discriminating malignant from benign conditions (Scoutt and McCarthy, 1991).

The accuracy, convenience, relatively low cost and availability of high-resolution ultrasound equipment has resulted in it remaining the principal and usually sole imaging modality in assessing pelvic pathology despite the undoubted contribution both CT and MRI can offer in some clinical situations.

Management of the Pelvic Mass

An ultrasound examination by an experienced sonographer using state-of-art equipment should be part of the preoperative assessment of patients undergoing laparoscopic surgery for an ovarian cyst. When septations are present it is recommended that a technique is used which avoids rupture of the mass (Levene, 1990). In a report of a survey of ovarian neoplasms which had been treated laparoscopically Maiman *et al.* (1991) suggested that 'strict uniform sonographic criteria must be adhered to in patient selection for the laparoscopic approach to ovarian masses'.

The 'Simple' Cyst

The management of a patient with a unilocular, thin-walled ovarian cyst without any solid areas (and preferably no neovascularization detectable using colour Doppler and a high resistance index) depends on both the size of the cyst and the age of the patient. Spontaneous resolution of a small simple ovarian cyst even in postmenopausal women is common (Andolf and Jorgensen, 1989) and thus expectant management is often appropriate if the cyst is asymptomatic. However, if associated with pain, treatment may become necessary.

Ultrasound guided cyst aspiration in carefully selected patients has been shown to relieve pain with a low incidence of recurrence of the cyst (de Crespigny *et al.*, 1989). It is suggested that aspiration is applicable in a premenopausal woman if the cyst is less than 10 cm as malignancy is then rare. Surgery is commonly the treatment of choice for an ovarian cyst in a postmenopausal woman since functional cysts are not expected, but cyst aspiration may sometimes be a reasonable alternative if the cyst is no greater than 5 cm diameter and appears 'simple' using a high quality transvaginal scanner. Aspirated cyst fluid should be submitted for cytological examination and oestradiol estimation, the latter giving support to a diagnosis of a functional cyst. A follow-up ultrasound examination is advocated to exclude cyst recurrence. More invasive treatment, such as laparoscopic surgery, is indicated in the presence of severe pain (since this is uncommon in an uncomplicated cyst) or for a recurrent or large cyst. Such an approach allows complete removal, or at least a biopsy of the cyst wall to be taken.

Blood-filled Cyst

When fine echoes are visible throughout the cyst, usually indicating a blood-filled cyst, ultrasound guided aspiration may still be performed, but not infrequently some or all of the contents may be too viscous to allow aspiration. Although cyst aspiration does provide pain relief, recurrence is common. Thus surgery may be a more appropriate form of management. Since malignancy is rare, a conservative approach may be used.

Other Apparently Benign Cysts

Benign cystic teratomas and cysts with several thin-walled locules are best treated surgically. A conservative approach, such as laparoscopy, may again be applicable.

Possibly Malignant Cysts

Cysts which show adverse features such as large or multilocular cysts (especially if thick-walled),

those with solid areas, those with neovascularization seen with colour Doppler and a low resistance index on duplex Doppler, require surgery. A laparotomy is usually the approach for such cysts.

Summary

High-resolution ultrasound equipment has allowed the gynaecologist to develop a more rational approach to management of an adnexal mass. This is possible in centres in which 'state of the art' ultrasound equipment is available, including a vaginal transducer and preferably colour Doppler, together with an experienced sonologist. No longer can there be any justification in recommending surgery for all premenopausal women with a palpable ovarian mass which persists for a month, as advocated in the classic textbook of *Bonney's Gynaecological Surgery* (Howkins and Stallworthy, 1974). Similarly, laparotomy and total abdominal hysterectomy and bilateral salpingo-oophorectomy is not necessarily essential for all postmenopausal women with a palpable ovary on clinical examination (Barber and Graber, 1971). An ultrasound examination should now be part of the diagnostic work-up of an ovarian cyst and, depending on the patient's symptoms, her age, the clinical findings and the ultrasound features, a decision may be made between conservative management, cyst aspiration, laparoscopic surgery and laparotomy.

Acknowledgements

The author wishes to acknowledge Dr Hugh Robinson for his comments and advice and Mrs Kerrie Carson who typed this chapter.

References

Adams J, Polson DW, Abdulwahid N *et al.* (1985) Multifollicular ovaries: clinical and endocrine features and response to pulsatile gonatropin releasing hormone. *Lancet* **2**: 1375–1378.

Andolf E & Jorgensen C (1988) The prospective comparison of clinical ultrasound and operative examination of the female pelvis. *Journal of Ultrasound in Medicine* **7**: 617–620.

Andolf E & Jorgensen C (1989) Cystic lesions in elderly women diagnosed by ultrasound. *British Journal of Obstetrics and Gynaecology* **96**: 1076–1079.

Athey PA & Malone RS (1987) Sonography of ovarian fibromas/thecomas. *Journal of Ultrasound in Medicine* **6**: 431–436.

Barber HRK & Graber FA (1971) PMBO Syndrome (postmenopausal palpable ovary syndrome). *Obstetrics and Gynecology* **38**: 921–923.

Benacerraf BR, Finkler NJ, Wojciechowski C & Knapp RC (1990) Sonographic accuracy in the diagnosis of ovarian masses. *Journal of Reproductive Medicine* **35**: 491–495.

Bourne T, Campbell S, Steer C, Whitehead MI & Collins WP (1989) Transvaginal colour flow imaging: a possible new screening technique for ovarian cancer. *British Medical Journal* **299**: 1367–1370.

Bronshtein M, Yoffe N, Brandes JM & Blumenfeld Z (1991) Hair as a sonographic marker of ovarian teratomas: improved identification using transvaginal sonography and simulation model. *Journal of Clinical Ultrasound* **19**: 351–355.

Campbell S, Bhan V, Royston P, Whitehead MI & Collins WP (1989) Transabdominal ultrasound screening for early ovarian cancer. *British Medical Journal* **299**: 1363–1367.

Campbell S, Royston P, Bran V, Whitehead MI & Collins WP (1990) Novel screening strategies for early ovarian cancer by transabdominal ultrasonography. *British Journal of Obstetrics and Gynaecology* **97**: 304–311.

Coleman BG, Arger PH, Grumbach K et al. (1988) Transvaginal and transabdominal sonography: prospective comparison. *Radiology* **168**: 639–643.

Creasman WT & Di Saia PJ (1991) Screening in ovarian cancer. *American Journal of Obstetrics and Gynecology* **165**: 7–10.

de Crespigny L (1988) Demonstration of ectopic pregnancy with transvaginal ultrasound. *British Journal of Obstetrics and Gynaecology* **95**: 1253–1256.

de Crespigny L, Cooper D & McKenna M (1988) Early detection of uterine pregnancy with ultrasound. *Journal of Ultrasound in Medicine* **7**: 7–10.

de Crespigny L, Robinson HP, Davoren RAM & Fortune D (1989) The 'simple' ovarian cyst: aspirate or operate? *British Journal of Obstetrics and Gynaecology* **96**: 1035–1039.

Editorial (1990) First catch your deer. *Lancet* **336**: 147–149.

Fleischer AC, Rogers WH, Rao BK, Kepple DM & Jones HW (1991) Transvaginal color doppler sonography of ovarian masses with pathological correlation. *Ultrasound in Obstetrics and Gynaecology* **1**: 275–278.

Folkman J, Watson K, Ingber D & Hanahan D (1989) Induction of angiogenesis during the transition from hyperplasia to neoplasia. *Nature* **339**: 58–61.

Goldstein SR (1990) Early pregnancy failure—appropriate terminology. *American Journal of Obstetrics and Gynecology* **163**: 1093.

Goldstein SR, Subramanyam B, Snyder JR et al. (1989) The postmenopausal cystic adnexal mass: the potential role of ultrasound in conservative management. *Obstetrics and Gynecology* **73**: 8–10.

Goswamy RK, Campbell S, Royston JP et al. (1988)

Ovarian size in postmenopausal women. *British Journal of Obstetrics and Gynaecology* **95**: 795–801.

Hall DA & McCarthy KA (1986) The significance of the postmenopausal simple adnexal cyst. *Journal of Ultrasound in Medicine* **5**: 503–505.

Herrmann UJ, Locher GW & Goldhirsch AA (1987) Sonographic patterns of ovarian tumours: prediction of malignancy. *Obstetrics and Gynecology* **69**: 777–781.

Howkins J & Stallworthy J (1974) *Bonney's Gynaecological Surgery*, p 586. London: Baillière Tindall.

Johnson IR, Symonds EM, Worthington BS et al. (1984) Imaging ovarian tumours by nuclear magnetic resonance. *British Journal of Obstetrics and Gynaecology* **91**: 260–264.

Kivikoski AI, Martin CM & Smeltzer JS (1990) Transabdominal and transvaginal ultrasonography in the diagnosis of ectopic pregnancy: a comparative study. *American Journal of Obstetrics and Gynecology* **163**: 123–128.

Kurjak A, Zulad I & Alfirevic Z (1991) Evaluation of adnexal masses with transvaginal colour ultrasound. *Journal of Ultrasound in Medicine* **10**: 295–297.

Lande IM, Hill MC, Cosco FE & Kator NN (1988) Adnexal and cul-de-sac abnormalities: transvaginal sonography. *Radiology* **166**: 325–332.

Leibman AJ, Kruse B & McSweeney MB (1988) Transvaginal sonography: comparison with transabdominal sonography in the diagnosis of pelvic masses. *American Journal of Roentgenology* **151**: 89–92.

Levene RL (1990) Pelviscopic surgery in women over forty. *Journal of Reproductive Medicine* **35**: 597–600.

Lynch HT, Albano WA, Lynch JF, Lynch PM & Campbell A (1982) Surveillance and management of patients at high genetic risk for ovarian carcinoma. *Obstetrics and Gynecology* **59**: 589–596.

Maiman M, Seltzer V & Boyce J (1991) Laparoscopic excision of ovarian neoplasms subsequently found to be malignant. *Obstetrics and Gynecology* **77**: 563–565.

Meire HB, Farrant P & Guha T (1978) Distinction of benign from malignant ovarian cysts by ultrasound. *British Journal of Obstetrics and Gynaecology* **85**: 893–899.

Moyle JW, Rochester D, Sider L, Shrock K & Krause P (1983) Sonography of ovarian tumours: predictability of tumour type. *American Journal of Roentgenology* **141**: 985–991.

Munn CS, Kiser LC, Wetzner SM & Baer JE (1986) Ovary volume in young and premenopausal adults: US determination. *Radiology* **159**: 731–732.

O'Brien WF, Buck DR & Nash JD (1984) Evaluation of sonography in the initial assessment of the gynaecologic patient. *American Journal of Obstetrics and Gynecology* **149**: 598–601.

O'Herlihy C, de Crespigny L, Lopata A et al. (1980) Pre-ovulatory follicular size: a comparison of ultrasound and laparoscopic measurements. *Fertility and Sterility* **34**: 24–26.

Paling MR & Shawker JH (1981) Abdominal ultrasound in advanced ovarian carcinoma. *Journal of Clinical Ultrasound* **9**: 435–441.

Reynolds T, Hill MC & Glassman LM (1986) Sonography of haemorrhagic ovarian cysts. *Journal of Clinical Ultrasound* **14**: 449–453.

Sassone AM, Timor-Tritsch IE, Artner A, Westhoff C

& Warren WB (1991) Transvaginal sonographic characterization of ovarian disease: evaluation of a new scoring system to predict ovarian malignancy. *Obstetrics and Gynecology* 78: 70–76.

Scoutt LM & McCarthy SM (1991) Imaging of ovarian masses: magnetic resonance imaging. *Clinical Obstetrics and Gynecology* 34: 443–451.

Scully RE (1982) Minimal cancer of the ovary. *Clinics in Oncology* 1 (2): 379–387.

Shimizu H, Yamasaki M, Ohama K, Nozoki T & Tanaka Y (1990) Characteristic ultrasonographic of the Krukenberg tumour. *Journal of Clinical Ultrasound* 18: 697–703.

Sigurdsson K, Alm P & Gullberg B (1983) Prognostic factors in malignant epithelial ovarian tumours. *Gynecologic Oncology* 15: 370–380.

Sommer FG, Walsh JW, Schwartz PE *et al.* (1982) Evaluation of gynecologic pelvic masses by ultrasound and computed tomography. *Journal of Reproductive Medicine* 27: 45–50.

Walsh JW, Taylor KJW & Wasson JFM (1978) Prospective comparison of ultrasound and computed tomography in the evaluation of gynecologic pelvic masses. *American Journal of Roentgenology* 131: 955–959.

Westhoff C & Randall MC (1991) Ovarian cancer screening: potential effect on mortality. *American Journal of Obstetrics and Gynecology* 165: 502–505.

16

Laparoscopic Ovarian Surgery and Ovarian Torsion

ALAIN J.M. AUDEBERT

Institut Robert B. Greenblatt, Bordeaux, France

Ovarian surgery is one of the most frequently performed laparoscopic procedures (Peterson *et al.*, 1990); in routine practice the increased use of pelvic imaging (sonography), in cases of any gynaecological symptom or as a screening exploration in women at risk explains why more and more ovarian masses are encountered. The diagnostic and therapeutic challenge for the clinician has to be solved in order to prov 'e the best immediate and long-term benefits for the patient.

In trying to simplify the situation, the major objective is to identify:

1. the functional ovarian cyst requiring, in most of the cases, no treatment if a strict clinical and sonographic observation can be achieved;
2. the borderline cases and malignant ovarian neoplasms requiring the conventional and adequate surgical approach by laparotomy;
3. the benign ovarian neoplasm offering, under strict conditions, a major role to a therapeutic approach by laparoscopy.

In fact, at any step in the presently available diagnostic strategy one cannot be sure of the real nature of the ovarian lesion to be treated in the absence of a complete pathological report; this means that, at any moment, one has to be prepared and able to change the planned therapeutic approach in order to give the patient the best chances according to the new situation.

Ovarian torsion requires an early diagnosis in order to perform a conservative treatment and is easily achieved by laparoscopy.

Oncological Considerations

Careful selection of cases appropriate for laparoscopic surgery is mandatory because the risk of treating an unsuspected ovarian malignancy by laparoscopy is a real one. In a recent survey, 42 such cases were reported (Maiman *et al.*, 1991). The main difficulty is the identification of early ovarian cancer especially in young women. With an advanced lesion the diagnosis is usually suspected before laparoscopy or when the ovarian neoplasm is ultrasonically visualized before any additional procedure is undertaken. The risk of spreading the cancer in the event of rupturing an ovarian malignancy may compromise the patient's survival unless additional cytotoxic therapy is administered (Schwartz, 1991a). However, the literature is controversial; puncture of an ovarian malignancy immediately followed by laparotomy probably bears less risk of dissemination than a spontaneous rupture.

The incidence of malignant epithelial ovarian neoplasms is variable. In northern America and in northern Europe the reported rates are close to 10 per 100 000 women. The incidence is correlated with the age of the patients. For the women aged less than 35 years, with a 'simple' ovarian cyst the incidence of malignancy is 4.5 for 100 000 women. In cases of unilocular cyst less than 10 cm in diameter the risk of malignancy appears very low (Meire *et al.*, 1978).

Borderline ovarian tumours represent 9.2–16.3% of epithelial ovarian neoplasms (Chambers *et al.*, 1988). After ovarian cystectomy the risk of

Table 16.1 Risk factors for ovarian malignancy

Absence of child, low parity, infertility
Middle or upper socioeconomic class
White
Age > 50 years
Family history of ovarian, breast or endometrial
cancer
No OC use

recurrence for stages Ia and Ib is around 10% (Lim-Tan et al., 1988). The reported frequency of microscopic tumours with a grossly normal-appearing contralateral ovary varies from 5% to 10% (McGowan et al., 1985). Immediate formal surgery in the event of puncture of such a lesion does not seem to hamper the prognosis (Tasker and Langley, 1985).

The known risk factors for ovarian malignancy are listed in Table 16.1.

The largest published series of ovarian cysts managed by laparoscopy includes 652 cysts (Canis et al., 1992); six ovarian cancers and six borderline malignant neoplasms were all identified at the time of the diagnostic laparoscopy and treated immediately by laparotomy.

Our own data, evaluated in November 1991, include 308 women (some with bilateral lesions): eight malignant or borderline neoplasms were demonstrated by the pathological report. Only one was managed by laparoscopy in a woman aged 35 years. She is carefully and regularly checked and the second ovary was removed 3 years later; no evidence of malignancy was detected.

These two important series demonstrate that with a careful approach the risk of operating on an undetected malignancy is very low.

Pre-Laparoscopic Assessment of an Ovarian Mass

The pre-laparoscopic assessment of an ovarian mass is more efficient with the newer develop-

Table 16.2 Incidence of malignancy in two large series of laparoscopic surgical removal of ovarian neoplasms

Author	No. of cases	Cancer	Borderline	Operated by laparoscopy
Canis et al. (1992)	652	6	6	0
Audebert	308	4	4	1 borderline

ments in pelvic imaging. Abdominal ultrasound and, more recently, transvaginal ultrasound are the best diagnostic tools presently available. Significant progress has been made in establishing satisfactory guidelines for detecting a suspected malignant ovarian neoplasm in addition to other information (risk factors, age, clinical examination, tumour markers).

The main ultrasound findings suspicious for malignancy are size (more than 5 cm in diameter), the presence of thick septae, solid parts or papillary projections, bilaterality, indefinite margins and the presence of ascites (Hermann et al., 1987; Grandberg et al., 1990). Trained operators, using strict ultrasonic criteria, are able accurately to predict benign masses in 96% of patients studied (Hermann et al., 1987). When a clear unilocular cyst is diagnosed by ultrasound, the predictability for benign neoplasms is in the range of 90–95% (Meire et al., 1978; Hermann et al., 1987). In 152 women aged 50 years or more, no malignancy was detected in pure cystic lesions less than 5 cm in diameter (Andolf and Jorgensen, 1989). In another series of 102 postmenopausal women who had abdominal ultrasonic evaluation of adnexal masses before surgery, a negative predictive value of 94% was established (Luxman et al., 1991), meaning that 6 of 100 postmenopausal women with a 'simple' cyst may have a malignant tumour; 2 of 33 patients with a 'simple' cyst smaller than 5 cm in diameter had malignant ovarian tumours. These controversial results illustrate the limits of the ultrasonic assessment. The diagnostic role of colour Doppler sonography has yet to be evaluated in this situation.

The present serological markers have a variable specificity according to the nature of the ovarian neoplasm; they are relatively specific for ovarian germ cell malignancies but these malignancies are rare (Schwartz, 1991b). CA 125 is the most

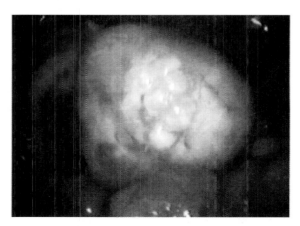

Figure 16.1 External excrescences on the surface of a borderline malignant ovarian neoplasm.

commonly used marker for epithelial ovarian neoplasms. Its poor sensitivity and specificity limit its use except in postmenopausal women. In this group of patients an elevated CA 125 in association with any other positive diagnostic test has a positive predictive value approaching 100%. When used alone, CA 125 has a positive predictive value of 36% for premenopausal women and 87% for postmenopausal women with pelvic masses (Finkler *et al.*, 1988).

In fact, if the role of ultrasonography in diagnosing suspicious malignancy is important, a common practical question to be answered in the case of a unilocular cyst identified in a young woman by ultrasonography is: 'Is it a functional ovarian cyst?' When uncomplicated, these cysts frequently undergo spontaneous resolution and do not need any form of treatment. In women with a persisting ovarian cyst submitted to laparoscopy the incidence of functional cysts varies from 16% to 43.5%. Every effort should be made to reduce this incidence. On some occasions the cyst may be aspirated under ultrasound control in order to obtain a cytological confirmation; this procedure has to be performed with caution because cytological examination of cystic fluid may frequently be unreliable. In a series of 59 ovarian cysts the sensitivity and the specificity of cytology alone was respectively of 67% and 91% (Diernaes *et al.*, 1987). The cytological examination of the fluid of 35 functional cysts was concordant with pathological examination in only 22 cases (Abeille *et al.*, 1988); the risks of failing to identify an ovarian malignancy and implantation of malignant cells along the needle track have to be further evaluated. Determination of steroids and tumour markers can be made in the fluid of the cyst: in functional cysts steroid concentrations are elevated and CA 125 concentrations are usually low (Abeille *et al.*, 1988). Combination of these various tests with the gross

appearance of the fluid allows a correct diagnosis to be established in most cases. Ultrasound guided cystoscopy with 0.5 mm scope is presently being evaluated.

Laparoscopic Assessment of an Ovarian Neoplasm

Preliminary to any procedure, a careful assessment of the ovarian neoplasm programmed for operative laparoscopy has to be made according to a predefined protocol.

1. The first procedure to be performed is the inspection and aspiration of the fluid collected in the pouch of Douglas for cytology before any contamination.
2. All the surface of the pelvic and abdominal peritoneum is then carefully exposed for proper visualization with a probe; the same procedure is performed for the digestive tract, the omentum and the liver. Some lesions may provide the diagnosis (endometriotic implants) or directly lead to a laparotomy being performed.
3. The ovarian surface of both ovaries is at that time alternatively scrutinized and other masses originating from the tube (hydrosalpinx) or the paraovarian region (vestigial cyst) are eventually identified. External papillary projections are easily detected. The connection of the ovary with surrounding structures is determined; in case of adhesions hiding the ovary partially or totally, a gentle adhesiolysis may first have to be performed. The lengthening of the utero-ovarian ligament is usually an indirect sign of a non-functional ovarian cyst.

   At this stage one has to be able to identify a malignant or borderline malignant ovarian neoplasm indicating immediate laparotomy. If it is not the case, additional diagnostic procedures are then performed.
4. The ovary is gently grasped with a forceps and mobilized in order to select the most appropriate site for puncture preferentially at

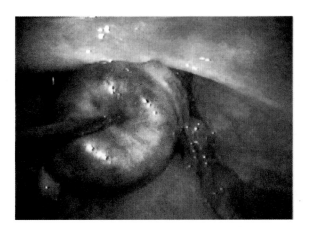

Figure 16.2 Puncture of a benign ovarian cyst.

Table 16.3 Laparoscopic assessment of ovarian neoplasms: procedures performed systematically (benign neoplasm)

Aspiration of peritoneal fluid for cytology
Inspection of the abdominal cavity, omentum, liver
Inspection of ovarian surface and ovarian ligaments
Puncture of the ovarian cyst
Cystoscopy
Frozen sections

the apex of the cyst and at a distance from the ovarian blood supply. If internal papillary projections have been eliminated by the ultrasonic examination, a fine needle can be used for aspiration of the fluid content, avoiding any spillage, and identification according to its characteristics frequently orienting the diagnostic when typical. In a series of 144 cases the macroscopic appearance of the cystic fluid was properly correlated with the pathological report in 82% of the cases (Abeille *et al.*, 1988).

5. If a 'cystoscopy' is planned it is better to introduce an appropriate trocar directly into the cyst for aspiration and lavage with a cannula, then replace by the small endoscope in order to visualize all the internal surface of the cystic wall and look for any excrescence. Another possibility is to enlarge with scissors the site of puncture and expose the interior of the cyst with two grasping forceps. Any suspicious lesion may stop any further laparoscopic procedure except lavage of the pouch of Douglas which contains 20–60 ml and a laparotomy is immediately performed.

In some cases, if it is preferred to remove an intact cyst or the whole ovary, no puncture is performed before the excision procedure. In other cases an absolute identification of the nature of the ovarian neoplasm is impossible.

6. It is then recommended that frozen sections be taken for proper diagnosis.

At the end of this diagnostic stage any evident or suspicious malignancy of the ovarian neoplasm must be excluded in order to proceed to a laparoscopic treatment. In our series of 308 patients, the eight malignant or borderline malignant ovarian neoplasms were correctly identified; three other patients operated on by laparotomy because of high suspicion of malignancy were found afterwards, after the pathological examination, to have, in fact, a benign lesion. In another

report of 652 ovarian cysts 12 malignant lesions were recorded and immediately treated by laparotomy; in 12 other cases a laparotomy was performed for benign neoplasm thought to be malignant at the time of the laparoscopic assessment (Canis *et al.*, 1992). In a previous series of the same authors the positive predictive diagnosis of benignity was accurate in all the cases (100% specificity); the sensitivity for diagnosing a malignant lesion was also 100% (Mage *et al.*, 1987). The correlation between laparoscopic presumptive diagnosis and pathological examination is not as good, with a correct identification in only 80% of the cases.

Only macroscopic benign appearing neoplasm will be treated by laparoscopy (unilocular lesions, cysts with smooth wall). Severe dense adhesions may also oblige the surgeon to perform a laparotomy on some occasions, but this is not specific for ovarian surgery. This indicates that all patients have initially to give their consent in case a laparotomy is required. All benign ovarian neoplasms can be treated by laparoscopy, including ovarian endometriomas and teratomas (Nezhat *et al.*, 1989) depending upon the experience of the operator and the use of a proper technique. During the past 3 years we, as others, have been able to remove by laparoscopy all the ovarian endometriomas (more than 100) and teratomas (25 cases).

Laparoscopic Ovarian Surgery

With this terminology we include only major procedures, with complete intraperitoneal removal or destruction of the ovarian neoplasm, excluding simple ovarian puncture and biopsy or excision of a part of the cyst wall (fenestration); we consider that these procedures have more of a diagnostic than a therapeutic role.

General Principles

All the general principles described for laparoscopic surgery are applied for ovarian surgery:

1. proper selection and preoperative counselling of patients;
2. general endotracheal anaesthesia;
3. urinary drainage with a foley catheter;
4. capacity to perform immediate laparotomy if necessary;

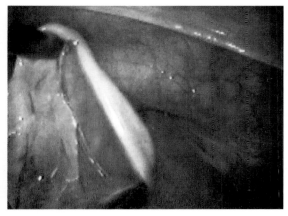

Figure 16.3 Inspection of the internal lining of a cyst.

5. uterine manipulator placed inside the uterus;
6. experience in operative laparoscopy.

Equipment

Mandatory equipment for laparoscopic ovarian surgery includes:

1. a video camera and monitor system;
2. a high-flow controlled insufflator;
3. bipolar cautery forceps and generator;
4. a suction and irrigating system;
5. a needle for suction, laparoscopic scissors and grasping forceps;
6. an 11 mm grasping forceps for extraction of excised tissues;
7. endoscopic sutures and endoscopic stapling device;
8. a monopolar instrument for cutting, or laser;
9. a small endoscope for 'ovarian cytoscopy';
10. biological tissue glue.

These last two are still undergoing further development and evaluation.

Technique of Ovarian Cystectomy

The technique of ovarian cystectomy has been previously described in detail (Bruhat *et al.*, 1989; Johns, 1991); so we will only focus on certain aspects. With possible malignancy having been certainly ruled out, the ovary is gently mobilized with grasping forceps, on some occasions after preliminary adhesiolysis. The size and the intra-ovarian location of the cyst are determined in order to select the proper site for the incision of the ovarian albuginea. The ideal site is the antimesenteric portion of the ovary, away from the blood vessels of the hilus. Two different approaches can be used depending on whether a previous puncture and cystoscopy have been performed: in the case of puncture, the opening is enlarged with scissors, unipolar electrode or laser and the cyst wall grasped, the ovary being stabilized by another pair of grasping forceps. The length of the incision is adapted to the size of the cyst. The cystic wall is then progressively and gently stripped from the ovary. This procedure is more or less easy to perform depending on the strength of the wall (the functional cysts are usually very smooth) and its adherence to the adjacent ovarian cortex. On some occasions, excision of the adjacent ovarian cortex is necessary. Haemostasis is attained when necessary with fine bipolar forceps.

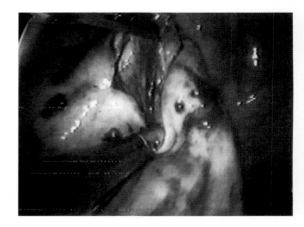

Figure 16.4 The cyst wall is grasped through the ovarian incision.

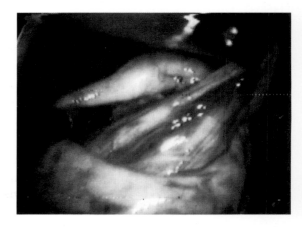

Figure 16.5 The cyst wall is stripped out of the ovary.

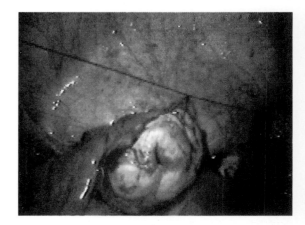

Figure 16.6 Suture of the ovary after cystectomy.

The dissection can also be achieved with a laser or facilitated by aquadissection with an irrigating probe. The ovarian wound is irrigated and haemostasis completed when necessary. The ovarian incision can be left open or approximated by three techniques: fine monofilament suture of the edges, tissue glue or by coagulation of the ovarian cortex adjacent to the surface which will

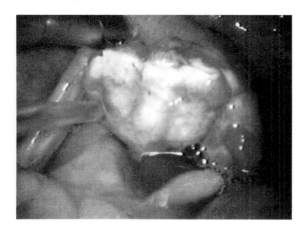

Figure 16.7 End result after suture of the ovary.

in some instances evert the opening. The excised tissue is removed from the abdominal cavity through an adapted trocar (11 mm sleeve in most of the cases) with strong grasping forceps. Fragmentation with scissors or a tissue morcellator is performed if the amount of tissue is excessive. Lavage of the pelvis and aspiration of all debris with warmed Ringer's lactate completes the procedure, as haemostasis is re-checked by underwater inspection. A large volume of warmed Ringer's lactate is left *in situ* in order to reduce the risk of postoperative adhesion formation. The solution should stay clear, otherwise the pelvis should be again irrigated.

When the ovarian cyst has not been punctured, the same procedures can be applied with great care to avoid rupture of the cyst wall. The ovarian incision is larger in this case. The technique is preferred if leakage of the cystic fluid is not advisable as with a teratoma or mucinous cyst. The removal of the cyst from the abdominal cavity can be achieved, although not always easily, through an enlarged abdominal incision used to introduce one of the trocars or through a colpotomy incision. Another possibility is to aspirate the cyst contents and to fragment the cyst, previously placed in a plastic bag held by two grasping forceps. Properly done this procedure avoids any spillage and may be safer than the other techniques where unexpected rupture of the cyst can occur at the time of removal if the incision is not large enough.

In all the cases the removed tissues are submitted for pathological evaluation.

Destruction of the Ovarian Cyst Lining
in situ

This method is usually done when stripping out the wall cyst is difficult and when it is sure

that no malignancy is suspected (endometrioma, functional cyst); contrary to some authors (Donnez, 1989; Fayez and Vogel, 1991), we try to avoid this procedure because only a part of the cyst wall can be evaluated by the pathologist.

The top of the cyst is removed; the content of the cyst is aspirated and irrigated; the whole surface of the lining is carefully inspected. Ablation is then attained with any type of laser or by bipolar coagulation; for the large cysts it is not always easy to expose properly the whole surface which is mandatory to reduce the risk of recurrence (especially in the case of endometrioma). One has to be very careful when the cyst is adherent to the pelvic wall in order to avoid the risk of damaging underlying structure. The depth of destruction must previously be accurately determined for the selected method. It is important then to check if haemostasis is correct and that ablation of the wall cyst is fully attained.

Laparoscopic Oophorectomy

Laparoscopic oophorectomy or salpingo-oophorectomy are preferred when the cyst fills all the ovary or in postmenopausal women. The first report was published in 1979 (Semm, 1979). The availability of endoscopic sutures and stapling devices has facilitated this type of laparoscopic surgery.

It is important to mobilize the ovary or the adnexa in order to evaluate whether the vessels are easily exposed and skeletonized at a sufficient distance from the pelvic wall and to facilitate identification of important structures such as the ureter through the peritoneum. If the ovary cannot be mobilized sufficiently, an irrigating probe is passed into the retroperitoneal space through a small incision in an avascular area of the anterior leaf of the broad ligament; the peritoneum is dissected away from the side wall by Ringer's lactate.

The skeletonized infundibulopelvic vessels and utero-ovarian ligaments are ligated with Endoknot suture or application of clips and trans-sected. The pedicles have to be checked; it is safer in addition to apply an Endoloop suture. An alternative method is the use of bipolar coagulation or thermocoagulation. The forceps are carefully applied on the pedicles, at a safe distance from the side wall. When proper desiccation is obtained the pedicles are trans-sected; we use this technique preferentially.

If the fallopian tube is to be removed the same approach is applied. Haemostasis is inspected and

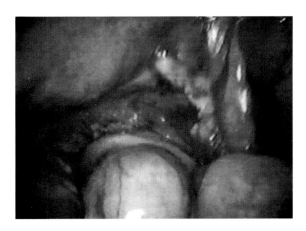

Figure 16.8 Laparoscopic oophorectomy with bipolar coagulation technique.

eventually completed. The removal is performed as previously described. Irrigation and lavage of the pelvic cavity finish the procedure.

Complications

As in other surgical laparoscopic procedures various complications may occur. Complications are unfortunately rarely reported in the literature.

During the operation uncontrolled bleeding, injury to other structures, or unsuccessful removal will require adequate treatment by laparotomy. In our experience and in another series (Mage *et al.*, 1987), with a combined number of cases close to 1000, no such complication was encountered. In a prospective study comparing different methods for treating 124 ovarian endometriomas, no intraoperative complication was recorded (Fayez and Vogel, 1991). Laparotomy was performed only in case of unsuspected malignant neoplasm identified at the time of the laparoscopy. Rupture of the cyst with spillage of its fluid content may be deleterious with mucinous lesions, teratomas or endometriomas. In order to avoid postoperative adhesion formation or peritonitis, a long and meticulous lavage is required until the irrigation solution is completely clear. Subsequent abdominal pain and ovarian abscess have been reported (Mage *et al.*, 1987). The occlusive syndrome and postoperative haemorrhagia may also occur.

The incidence of postoperative adhesion has been properly evaluated only for endometriomas. Adhesions are statistically more frequent with excision techniques (100%) in comparison with stripping of the lining (37%), laser ablation (30%) or drainage (27%) (Fayez and Vogel, 1991). For the other types of ovarian neoplasms it is difficult to gather a sufficient number of second-look laparoscopies. Excluding endometriomas, the fertility after laparoscopic management of ovarian cysts is satisfactory: 34 (89.5%) of 38 patients wishing conception had a subsequent pregnancy (Canis *et al.*, 1992). Recurrence of the cyst is also more frequent for endometriomas; it has not been proved that complementary medical treatment following the laparoscopy reduces the risk.

Laparoscopic Treatment of Ovarian Torsion

Acute abdominal pain originating from the ovary is due in most of the cases to an ovarian abscess, intracystic haemorrhage, with or without rupture, or ovarian torsion. The latest cause is rare and may also be associated with subacute or chronic pain. Ultrasonography may help the diagnosis with a predictive value of 88% (Graif and Itzchak, 1988); laparoscopy is promptly indicated for early diagnosis and treatment and possibly salvage of the ovary (Manhès *et al.*, 1984).

Usually ovarian torsion is due to an abnormality of the adnexa (ovarian cyst, ectopic pregnancy, paraovarian cyst, or long utero-ovarian ligament).

Untwisting the ovary or the adnexa is simply attained with a blunt probe or grasping forceps. Conservative treatment is preferred when the condition of the tissues appears favourable but tissue necrosis indicates the need for complete removal.

Causal factors must be adequately treated also as previously described. It is not always easy to identify the causal abnormality when ischaemia is present. Shortening of the utero-ovarian ligament, if indicated, can be done by laparoscopy using the same techniques used by laparotomy; ovarian fixation can be achieved by adequate suturing with two endoscopic needleholders and fine monofilament suture.

Second-look laparoscopy a few weeks later is mandatory when conservative treatment has been applied to severe lesions (Bruhat *et al.*, 1989).

Conclusion

Laparoscopic treatment of benign ovarian neoplasms can be properly achieved in the great majority of the cases. The advantages of laparoscopic surgery is nowadays well established but such surgery requires adequate instrumentation and training.

Laparoscopic operative techniques for ovarian neoplasms are now correctly standardized; results compare favourably with surgery by laparotomy.

A strict selection of patients is necessary to exclude malignant neoplasms requiring conventional treatment by laparotomy. Fear of missing the diagnosis of malignancy dictates a policy of meticulous evaluation until laparoscopic treatment is indicated. However, proper guidelines have still to be established and validated.

References

Abeille JP, Mintz M & Pez JP (1988) Intérêt de certains dosages dans les liquides des kystes annexiels: à propos de 144 cas. *Contr. Fertil. Sexual.* **16**: 3315–3320.

Andolf E & Jorgensen C (1989) Cystic lesions in elderly women, diagnosed by ultrasound. *British Journal of Obstetrics and Gynaecology* **96**: 1076–1079.

Bruhat MA, Mage G, Pouly JL et al. (1989) Coélioscopie opératoire vol. 1. Paris: Medsci/McGraw-Hill.

Canis M, Mage G, Wattiez A et al. (1992) Résultats à court terme et long terme après traitement coélioscopique des kystes de l'ovaire. *Fertil. Contr. Sexual.* 1992 (in press).

Chambers JT, Merino MJ, Kohorn EI & Schwartz PE (1988) Borderline ovarian tumors. *American Journal of Obstetrics and Gynecology* **159**: 1088–1094.

Diernaes E, Rasmussen J, Soerensen T & Hasch E (1987) Ovarian cyst management by puncture. *Lancet* **1**: 1084.

Donnez J (1989) *Laser Operative Laparoscopy and Hysteroscopy*, vol. 1. Leuven, Belgium: Nauwelaerts Printing.

Fayez JA & Vogel MF (1991) Comparison of different treatment methods of endometriomas by laparoscopy. *Obstetrics and Gynecology* **78**: 661–665.

Finkler NJ, Benacererraf B, Lavin PT, Wojciechowski C & Knapp RC (1988) Comparison of serum CA 125, clinical impression and ultrasound in the preoperative evaluation of ovarian masses. *Obstetrics and Gynecology* **72**: 659–664.

Gabriel R, Quereux C & Wahl P (1989) Kystes fonctionnels de l'ovaire. *Encycl. Méd. Chir (Paris-France), Gynécologie* **158**: A10,7-1989, 4 p.

Graif M & Itzchak Y (1988) Sonographic evaluation of ovarian torsion in childhood and adolescence. *American Journal of Roentgenology* **150**: 647–649.

Grandberg S, Norstrom A & Wikland A (1990) Tumors in the pelvis as imaged by vaginal sonography. *Gynecologic Oncology* **37**: 224.

Herrmann UJ, Locher GW & Goldhirsch A (1987) Sonographic patterns of malignancy: prediction of malignancy. *Obstetrics and Gynecology* **69**: 777–781.

Johns A (1991) Laparoscopic oophorectomy/oophorocystectomy. *Clinical Obstetrics and Gynecology* **34**: 460–466.

Lim-Tan SK, Cajigas HE & Scully RE (1988) Ovarian cystectomy for serous borderline tumors: a follow-up study of 35 cases. *Obstetrics and Gynecology* **72**: 775–780.

Luxman D, Bergman A, Sagi J & David MP (1991) The postmenopausal adnexal mass: correlation between ultrasonic and pathologic findings. *Obstetrics and Gynecology* **77**: 726–728.

Mage G, Canis M, Manhes H, Pouly JL & Bruhat MA (1987) Kystes ovariens et coélioscopie—A propos de 226 observations. *Journal de Gynécologie, Obstétrique et Biologie de la Reproduction* **16**: 1053–1061.

Maiman M, Seltzer V & Boyce J (1991) Laparoscopic excision of ovarian neoplasms subsequently found to be malignant. *Obstetrics and Gynecology* **77**: 563–565.

Manhès H, Canis M, Mage G, Pouly JL & Bruhat MA (1984) Place de la coélioscopie dans le diagnostic et le traitement des torsions d'annexes. *Journal de Gynécologie, Obstétrique et Biologie de la Reproduction* **13**: 825–829.

McGowan L, Lesher LP, Norris HJ et al. (1985) Misstaging of ovarian cancer. *Obstetrics and Gynecology* **65**: 568–572.

Meire HB, Farrant P & Gutha T (1978) Distinction of benign from malignant ovarian cysts by ultrasound. *British Journal of Obstetrics and Gynaecology* **85**: 893.

Nezhat C, Winer WK & Nezhat F (1989) Laparoscopic removal of dermoid cysts. *Obstetrics and Gynecology* **73**: 278–280.

Peterson H, Hulka J & Phillips J (1990) American Association of Gynecologic Laparoscopists 1988 membership survey on operative laparoscopy. *Journal of Reproductive Medicine* **35**: 587–589.

Schwartz PE (1991a) An oncologic view of when to do endoscopic surgery. *Clinical Obstetrics and Gynecology* **34**: 467–472.

Schwartz PE (1991b) Ovarian masses: serologic markers. *Clinical Obstetrics and Gynecology* **34**: 423–432.

Semm K (1979) Changes in the classic gynecologic surgery: review of 3,300 pelviscopies in 1971–1976. *International Journal of Fertility* **24**: 13–18.

Tasker M & Langley FA (1985) The outlook for women with borderline epithelial tumours of the ovary. *British Journal of Obstetrics and Gynaecology* **92**: 969–976.

17

Endo-ovarian Surgery for Ovarian Endometriomas

IVO BROSENS

University Hospital Gasthuisberg, Leuven, Belgium

The Structure of the Ovarian Endometrioma

The first case of an ovarian endometrioma published by W.W. Russel in 1899 gave a detailed description of the ovary 'enveloped in adhesions to the posterior face of the broad ligament' and 'the presence of areas which were an exact prototype of the uterine glands and interglandular connective tissue'. However, it took more than two decades before the relationship between the haemorrhagic cyst of the ovary and the ectopic endometrium was established. In 1920 Cullen suggested that active endometrium was involved in the pathogenesis of the 'ovarian haematoma', and he postulated that the uterine mucosa on the surface of the ovary was due to an overflow of the adenomyoma of the rectovaginal septum. It has been the merit of Sampson (1927) to introduce the idea that the small blood-spots on the surface are the first commonly visible sign of ovarian endometriomas. Several authors have subsequently held the view that ectopic endometrium eats its way into the ovary like insects eating into an apple or that chocolate cysts are situated in ovarian follicles or lying wholly in the medulla of the ovary. In 1957 the role of the adhesions in endometrioma formation was clarified by Hughesdon. His work was based on serial sections of ovarian endometriomas and confirmed that 'even in the most advanced lesions the ectopic endometrium never in fact leaves the surface: it remains on, and is never in the ovary'. In 90% of the cases the inner cystic wall could be identified as ovarian cortex (Figure 17.1). Owing

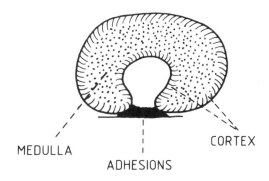

Figure 17.1 Diagram of a small endometrioma sealed by adhesions.

to stretching the inner cortex is not always uniform and recognizable as is the case in large endometriomas. In many cases the ovary does not invaginate centrally but remains on one side as a more or less definite mass and the cavity is surrounded on the other side by a relatively flat wall (Figure 17.2).

Gross Appearance

The term 'chocolate cyst' was coined to describe the endometrial cysts of the ovary, but is purely descriptive and may be misleading if one only notices the chocolate content of a cyst. Aspiration of a cyst is therefore not a reliable diagnostic tool

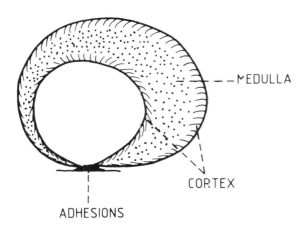

Figure 17.2 Diagram of a large endometrioma with flattening of the ovarian cortex on one side.

as a similar content can be found in haemorrhagic functional cysts and even in some neoplastic tumours.

The gross features of the endometrial cyst are very familiar to the gynaecological surgeon (Figure 17.3a). Several of these characterics are explained by its particular structure. First, the adhesions are an essential feature. The inversed ovarian cavity is sealed by adhesions to form a cystic structure (Figure 17.3b). In many cases the ovary is adherent to an adjacent structure which can extend from the lateral pelvic wall to the back of the uterus. This explains the difficulty of mobilizing the cyst without opening or rupturing it and spilling its content. In some cases the ovary can be free but adhesions and scarification are present and are usually located on the lateral side of the ovary. Second, the cysts of modest size have a thick wall as the wall is the ovary itself. Enlargement of the cyst tends not to produce a general expansion as with other benign, truly intraovarian cysts. As the flattening of the wall usually occurs on the medial side, the remaining ovarian structure is usually found on the lateral side.

Ovarian Cystoscopy

Ovarian cystoscopy was described by Brosens and Puttemans (1989) as a tool to investigate the ovarian cysts which are not suspected of malignancy at the time of laparoscopy and to avoid unnecessary ovarian surgery. The haemorrhagic functional cyst can be simply aspirated. The technique is based on inspection and exploration of the cystic wall using a second endoscopical

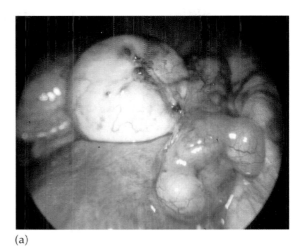

(a)

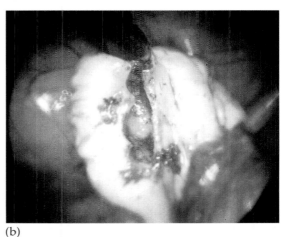

(b)

Figure 17.3 (a) A typical small endometrioma with the scar closing the invagination of the ovarian cortex on the lateral side of the ovary. (b) The inside of the endometrioma is the invaginated ovarian cortex with adhesion on the edge of the invagination.

system (Figure 17.4). After aspiration and flushing, the cyst is entered by the cystoscope, which has a 5 mm diameter. A saline drip connected with the operating channel of the cystoscope is used to expand the wall of the cyst which would otherwise collapse when a large incision is made. A biopsy forceps can then be introduced through the operating channel of the cystoscope and biopsies are obtained from selected areas. Using this technique the benign characteristics can be confirmed and functional cysts such as an haemorrhagic follicular cyst or a cystic corpus luteum can be discerned from an endometrial cyst (Figures 17.5 and 17.6). This technique has been proved to be particularly useful in ovarian adhesive disease, when the outside characteristics are absent or masked.

Inspection of the *endometrial cyst* shows a great variation in the degree of vascularization and the presence of endometrial implants. In some cysts large parts of the wall consist of a uniformly

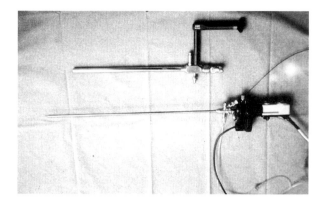

Figure 17.4 The endoscope for endo-ovarian surgery consists of a 2.6 mm rigid endoscope located in a 5 mm sheath which has a 1 mm channel allowing passage of the laser fibre, and small flexible instruments and also has connections for an infusion. The shutter is placed on the eyepiece to protect the camera.

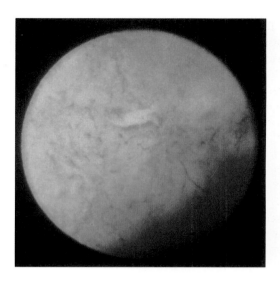

Figure 17.6 Ovarian cystoscopy: the yellow wall of a cystic corpus luteum with a fine capillary vascularization.

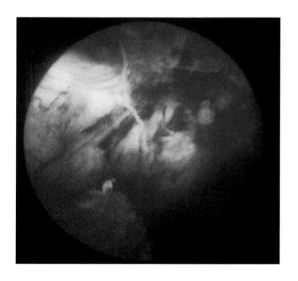

Figure 17.5 Ovarian cystoscopy: detail of the wall of an haemorrhagic corpus luteum cyst.

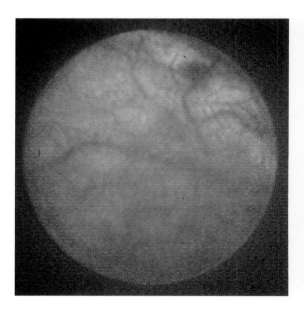

Figure 17.7 Ovarian cystoscopy: mucosa-like implant of endometriosis.

dark, non-vascularized tissue which represents pigmented fibroreactive tissue. In some, probably young, endometriomas the pearl-like surface of the ovarian cortex can still be identified. Endometrial tissue can be identified by its vascularization and sometimes mucosal appearance (Figure 17.7). Again, young or very active endometriomas consist of free, mucosa-like implants covering ovarian cortex from which they can be easily separated, while in older endometriomas much of the wall is fibroreactive tissue with interspersed vascularized implants. Irregular congested vessels are frequently noted close to the ovarian hilus.

Endo-ovarian Laser Surgery

The rationale for endo-ovarian laser surgery is that the lesion causing the endometrioma is located superficially and can be identified using the described technique of ovarian cystoscopy. This technique is minimally invasive and allows localization of the implants. This is proven by the high rate of positive biopsies, while in up to one-third of resected endometriomas only tissue compatible with endometrioma, i.e. fibroreactive tissue with pigmentation, is found.

Endo-ovarian laser surgery of endometrial cysts has been performed with the use of the argon laser (HGM Medical Laser Systems, Inc., Salt Lake City, Utah, USA). This laser uses argon gas as the laser medium and produces a blue-green light representing a composite of approximately 10 different wavelengths, the most pronounced being at 488 and 515 nm. This laser light is colour-dependent which means it is preferentially absorbed by pigments of its complementary colour, red (e.g. haemoglobin), or by black pigments, which contains all colours (e.g. melanin). Unlike the carbon dioxide laser, argon laser light is not absorbed by water, explaining its use both in ophthalmology and inside the ovarian cyst, where saline is used as a distension medium. In unpigmented tissue scattering of laser light is the primary form of heat production. Since absorption and scatter both contribute to the energy conversion of light into heat in either pigmented or unpigmented tissue, higher power densities are usually required for argon lasers to coagulate and/or vaporize human tissue. In gynaecology, therefore, the use of a 20 W model is recommended. Depth of penetration ranges between 0.4 and 0.8 mm, so the potential for damage to adjacent tissue is far less a problem than for instance with a Nd:YAG laser (depth of penetration up to 4.2 mm). Carried through optical fibres that are available in different sizes, the argon laser beam is guided to the target site (Table 17.1). Set-up of this laser through the operative channel of an endoscope is therefore very easy. Since the beam from a fibre is divergent (7°), no backstops are needed and power density is at its maximum at the tip of the fibre. This explains that incisional power can be obtained by touching the target with the fibre tip. In the non-contact mode the distance between the target and the fibre tip determines the tissue effect—rapid or slow vaporization, coagulation (protein denaturation without ablation), or just surface heating. In this mode carbonization and smoke production are negligible. To avoid retinal or camera damage, a special shutter of a precise wavelength is used, covering the endoscope's optical channel only when the laser is activated. This changes the colour but not the visibility of the operating field. For endo-ovarian surgery with the argon laser, a 300 or 600 μm fibre is introduced through the channel of the sheath into the cystic cavity. As mentioned above, the absorption spectrum of the argon laser makes it an efficient instrument for coagulation of the superficial vessels and haemorrhagic foci. The depth of coagulation is easily controlled by adjusting the power density (power output between 8 and 10 W) and the duration of coagulation (mostly in the continuous mode). While the cyst is distended under the continuous flow of a saline infusion the vascularized implants and the superficial haemorrhagic vessels are coagulated. The wall can also be coagulated to a depth of 1–2 mm (Figure 17.8). The KTP (potassium–titanyl–phosphate) laser can also be used for endo-ovarian surgery since it has similar laser-tissue effects and with a wavelength of 532 nm is close to that of the argon laser but produces emerald-green light.

Disadvantages are the relatively small spot size of 600 μm at the tip of the optical fibre. With a diversion of 7° this can be increased when coagulation is performed from a distance of a few millimetres. The visibility is reduced not only by the small size of the optical system (2.6 mm) but also by the absorption of light by the dark surface

Table 17.1 Presentation of the physical characteristics of CO_2, argon, KTP/532 and Nd:YAG lasers

Physical laser characteristics	CO_2	Argon	KTP	Nd:YAG
Wavelength	10 600 nm	488/515 nm	532 nm	1064/1318 nm
Colour dependence	None	Yes	Yes	Yes
Main tissue effect	Vaporization	Coagulation	Coagulation	Coagulation
Penetration depth	0.1 mm	0.4–0.8 mm	0.4–0.8 mm	0.6–4 2 mm
Forward scatter	None	Slight	Slight	Moderate
Absorption in water	Total	None	None	None
Carbonization	+++	+	+	±
Smoke production	+++	+	+	±
Passed through	Mirrors	Fibres	Fibres	Fibres
Beam alignment	+++	–	–	–
Surgical technique	No-touch	No-touch and direct contact	No-touch and direct contact	No-touch and direct contact (sapphire tips or sculpted fibres)

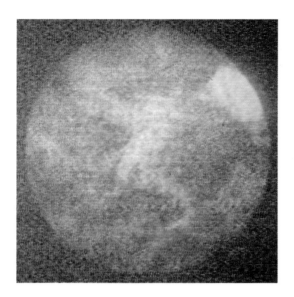

Figure 17.8 Endo-ovarian laser coagulation of an endo-metrioma.

and by the shutter mechanism that is interposed each time the laser is activated to protect the eyes of the surgeon.

A 1-year follow-up study of a first series of 20 patients treated by this technique showed no recurrence of the ovarian endometrioma.

Summary

Ovarian cystoscopy can be applied for accurate diagnosis of non-malignant ovarian cysts at the time of laparoscopy. The wall of the cyst is inspected in detail and selective biopsies are obtained. Unnecessary surgery for non-neoplastic tumours can be avoided and endometrial and cystic tumours can be treated *in situ* using an argon or KTP laser with minimal surgical damage to the ovarian capsule. This laser technique is under further investigation to evaluate its place in the diagnosis and conservative surgical treatment of benign ovarian cysts occurring frequently during reproductive life.

References

Brosens I (1991) Endometriosis related to infertility. *Current Opinion in Obstetrics and Gynecology* **3**: 205–210.

Brosens I & Puttemans P (1989) Double-optic laparoscopy. Salpingoscopy, ovarian cystoscopy and endo-ovarian surgery with argon laser. In Sutton CJG (ed) *Baillière's Clinical Obstetrics and Gynaecology. Laparoscopic Surgery* **3.3**: 595–608.

Cullen TS (1920) The distribution of adenomyomata containing uterine mucosa. *American Journal of Obstetrics and Gynecology* **80**: 130–138.

Hughesdon PE (1957) The structure of endometrial cysts of the ovary. *Journal of Obstetrics and Gynaecology of the British Empire* **64**: 481–487.

Russel WW (1899) Aberrant portions of the Müllerian duct found in an ovary. *Johns Hopkins Hospital Bulletin* **10**: 8–10.

Sampson JA (1927) Peritoneal endometriosis due to menstrual dissemination of endometrial tissue into the peritoneal cavity. *American Journal of Obstetrics and Gynecology* **14**: 422–469.

18

Endoscopic Surgical Approach to the Treatment of Anovulation due to Polycystic Ovary Syndrome— Ovarian Drilling

GABOR T. KOVACS

Box Hill Hospital, Monash University, Victoria, Australia

The surgical treatment of polycystic ovaries to restore regular menstruation and subsequent pregnancy was first reported by Stein and Leventhal in 1935. They described seven amenorrhoeic women who underwent wedge resection, with menstruation returning in all and pregnancy in two. By 1964, Stein was able to report on a series of 108 women who were treated by bilateral ovarian wedge resection (BOWR) during a period of 34 years (Stein, 1964). He reported the return of cyclic menstruation in 95% of patients, and 71 of the 83 who wished to conceive succeeded. Confirmatory evidence for the efficacy of this treatment came from a large study at the Johns Hopkins Hospital, Baltimore (Adashi et al., 1981) which found that ovulation was restored in 91.1% of women after BOWR with an overall crude conception rate of 47.8%. This study also raised the possibility of tubal infertility subsequent to BOWR, where seven out of seven women who were re-investigated because of persistent infertility were found to have significant pelvic adhesions, whereas none of these women had previously been noted to have pelvic abnormalities.

Toaff et al. (1976) also reported on seven women who were investigated by laparoscopy after BOWR but had persistent infertility. They found extensive peritubal/pelvic adhesions in all cases and agreed with Kistner (1968) 'to relegate the surgical approach to a minor position in patients with Stein–Leventhal syndrome'.

The relegation of surgical treatment became a realistic option with the availability of hormonal therapy in the form of clomiphene citrate (Greenblatt et al., 1961) and the purification of human gonadotrophins (Gemzell et al., 1960). Although clomiphene citrate is easy to administer and is relatively inexpensive, in patients with polycystic ovary syndrome (PCOS), ovulation rates of 70–80% with pregnancy rates of 31–94% have been reported (Gindoff and Jewelewicz, 1987). Therefore a significant number of women who do not respond to clomiphene citrate require other treatments. Also, the ovary with PCOS may be more sensitive to clomiphene citrate and multiple pregnancies are more common (Goldfarb and Crawford, 1969).

The first use of human gonadotrophin to induce ovulation was reported by Gemzell et al. in 1960. With the development of commercial preparations, gonadotrophin therapy became a widespread alternative. However, this requires strict monitoring to prevent hyperstimulation (Schenker and Polishuk, 1975) with serious complications, and even when strictly monitored has a multiple pregnancy rate of about 20% (Kovacs et al., 1989a). Furthermore, those women who had elevated baseline levels of luteinizing hormone (LH) and presumably had PCOS, did significantly worse with respect to ovulation and pregnancy with a conception rate of about 40% (Kovacs et al., 1989a).

The use of gonadotrophins also has the disadvantage that it is extremely time intensive for both the women and the medical staff, with several hormone estimations each week necessitating frequent attendances. Also, usually several cycles of ovulation induction are required to achieve pregnancy with a cumulative percentage pregnant of 75% after six cycles of treatment (Kovacs *et al.*, 1984). Recent analysis of our data shows that women with PCOS do no worse but no better than women with hypogonadotrophic amenorrhoea when the outcome of gonadotrophin ovulation induction is analysed by life table analysis (Burger *et al.*, 1991).

The treatment of clomiphene-resistant anovulation was somewhat simplified by the introduction of gonadotrophin releasing hormone (GnRH) infusion, but our experience suggests that this method is most unrewarding for patients with PCOS (Kovacs *et al.*, 1989b).

So after two decades of preference for a hormonal approach to ovulation induction for PCOS, it was of interest when the surgical approach for the treatment was revisited by using a laparoscopic approach by Gjönnaess in 1984. In this initial report he described how 92% of 62 women treated by electrocautery ovulated within 3 months, with a conception rate of 80%, a figure which was better than that for the hormonal approach.

Campo and colleagues (1983) had previously reported the laparoscopic resection of small ovarian fragments in 12 women with less impressive results with an ovulation rate of 45% and conception rate of 42%.

Confirmatory evidence was published from the United States from a small series by Greenblatt and Casper (1987) who managed to get five out of six women with PCOS to ovulate after ovarian electrocautery; from Holland (van der Weiden and Alberda, 1987) with nine out of eleven patients responding, and from Australia in our unit where nine out of ten women ovulated postoperatively (Kovacs *et al.*, 1991). The advantage of laparoscopic electrocautery is that major surgery is avoided, and that this method does not appear to result in the frequent adhesion formation which follows wedge resection of the ovaries. In our own series five of the patients have now been inspected by laparoscopy without any evidence of adhesions. Dabirashrafi (1989) reported adhesions in only one out of nine women who had a second look laparoscopy after electrocautery.

With the endoscopic use of laser, CO_2, argon, YAG and potassium–titanyl–phosphate (KTP) lasers have all been used in the surgical treatment of clomiphene-resistant PCOS (Feste 1990a). It is postulated that lasers have the advantage over electrocautery because the area of damage is limited, there is better haemostasis during laser dissection and tissue regeneration is greater (Huber *et al.*, 1988). Huber and colleagues (1988) reported on their initial experience in a controlled

trial of Nd:YAG laser with a flexible fibre to incise the ovarian capsule in eight women, of whom five ovulated spontaneously. They compared this group to controls who also had PCOS but had undergone only a diagnostic laparoscopy, none of whom had ovulated. They suggested that the incision of polycystic ovaries was a new application for this kind of laser.

The largest published series of laparoscopic laser vaporization is by Daniell and Miller (1989). They reported on their series of 85 women with clomiphene-resistant PCOS treated by either CO_2 or KTP laser vaporization with a postoperative ovulation rate of 71%, with a conception rate of 56%. They concluded that this treatment was effective, safe and without the risk of postoperative adhesions because of the precise destructive characteristic, with little lateral tissue damage.

Mechanism of action

The mechanism of action for the restoration of cyclical ovulation is not understood for any of these methods of wedge resection, cautery or laser vaporization. Stein and Leventhal (1935) postulated that BOWR decreased the mechanical crowding of the cortex by cysts, which again enabled the progress of normal graafian follicles to the surface of the ovary. Gjönnaess (1984) postulated that ovulation was elicited by either non-specific ovarian stromal destruction, or extensive capsular destruction with discharge of the contents of a number of subcapsular follicle cysts, or the local capsular cautery of one specific but unidentified follicle. Daniell and Miller (1989) suggested that by physically opening the subcapsular cysts with the laser, the follicular fluid that contains androgens is removed from the ovarian environment, thus lowering the androgen content of ovaries, resolving the block to ovulation. Other postulated mechanisms of action include decrease in atretic follicles and androgen production, with subsequently less circulating androgen and less peripheral androgen conversion to oestrogen with decreased negative feedback, or that the destruction of follicles results in a reduction of ovarian inhibin with a resultant rise in FSH (Keckstein, 1989).

Hormonal Changes

The hormonal changes associated with BOWR or ovarian drilling (by electrocoagulator or laser vaporization) are just as poorly understood as the mechanism of action. There is consensus that there is a temporary reduction of ovarian steroid production with persistent decrease in testosterone (Judd et al., 1976; Gjönnaess and Norman, 1987; Kovacs et al., 1991). The only reported study on inhibin levels (Kovacs et al., 1991) showed a transient fall in levels, followed by a rise and return to normal within 6 weeks.

Methodology of Ovarian Drilling

In order to carry out endoscopic surgery on the ovary the principles of operative laparoscopy apply. The patient should be under general anaesthesia, and pneumoperitoneum should be induced. It is best to use a high-flow insufflator which enables the rapid replacement of gas when contaminated by smoke or laser plume. At least a triple puncture should be used, with the laparoscope being introduced sub-umbilically, a grasping forceps suprapubically, with the diathermy forceps or CO_2 laser delivery channel through the third cannula. It is also advisable, but not essential for ovarian drilling that a suction irrigator be inserted through a fourth puncture site.

After adequate visualization with the patient in Trendelenburg position and the bowel scooped out of the pelvis, the ovary is grasped by its ligament so that it can be manipulated and steadied. The use of video laparoscopy is the method of choice as this enables the assistant to see what is going on and therefore be of greater assistance. It is also more convenient for the surgeon to operate watching the video screen rather than peering down the laparoscope (Nezhat et al., 1989).

The ovarian surface can then be drilled using either diathermy or laser energy.

The Use of Ovarian Electrocautery with Unipolar Diathermy

This method will be discussed in detail, as all the equipment and skill required are part of the everyday armoury of the operating gynaecologist. Our initial series of ovarian cautery were carried out using this methodology (Kovacs et al., 1991).

Once the ovary has been visualized, grasped and isolated from other tissues, a Semm unipolar diathermy forceps is introduced into the peritoneal cavity through a 5.5 mm cannula. The ovarian

capsule is then grasped with the Semm forceps (Figure 18.2). This is somewhat difficult with the enlarged shiny white ovaries, and we have previously described this as trying to grasp a football with ice-tongs. To help penetration of the capsule, it was found useful to open the forceps wide, touch the ovarian surface at two points, and then pass a current down the forceps. This then enabled one of the jaws of the forceps to be pushed through the capsule and a better grasp of the capsule thus obtained. A pulse of unipolar current of 25–30 W was then passed down the forceps so that the capsule was extensively burnt adjoining the jaws of the forceps. Great care was taken that there should be no other tissue, especially bowel, within close proximity of the ovary. Furthermore, the ovarian tissue was not released so that it should not come in contact with other tissues until it cooled. It is possible to accelerate this cooling by using the irrigator.

It is important that the diathermy source is turned off at all times except when burning is actually being carried out. The forceps needs to be moved several times around the ovarian surface until at least ten burns per ovary have been carried out.

Although this method requires no special equipment, unipolar diathermy is potentially the most dangerous method of ovarian drilling. This is because the current travels through the patient from the active electrode of the forceps to the return plate usually fixed to the buttocks or thigh. If the current takes a short-cut through other tissues, then that tissue, most often bowel, may be burnt. Nevertheless unipolar diathermy is widely and usually safely used in many procedures at laparoscopy and laparotomy. A recent development for unipolar diathermy in ovarian drilling is the development of the Corson needle (Figures 18.3, 18.4). This is an insulated needle introduced through a sheath which is passed down a 5.5 ml cannula. The ovarian ligament can then be grasped with a Semm's forceps and the ovary can be penetrated by the needle under vision. As most of the uninsulated part of the needle is within the ovarian tissue, the risk of flash burns is minimized.

With the availability of the Corson needle, this is my preferred option for ovarian drilling.

Ovarian Cautery with Bipolar Diathermy

In principle the bipolar approach to electrocoagulation is safer than the unipolar, as the current passes only between the two electrodes of

Figure 18.1 Monash Day
Surgery Centre equipped for
endoscopic surgery on an
outpatient day-stay basis.

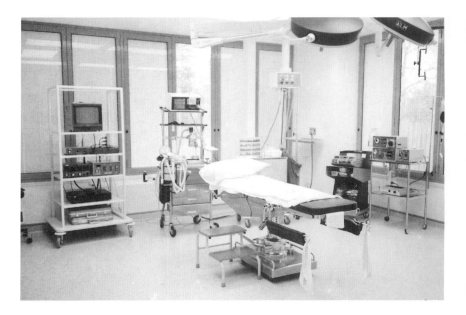

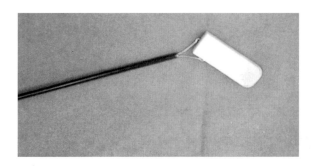

Figure 18.2 The difficulty of grasping the ovary with
unipolar Semm's forceps.

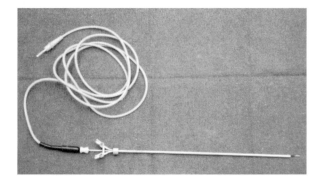

Figure 18.3 The unipolar Corson needle—the instrument of choice for ovarian cautery.

the bipolar forceps and possible damage to surrounding tissues is limited to heating, with electrical burns being eliminated. The disadvantage of bipolar diathermy is the limited instrumentation which is available. Bipolar forceps are limited to paddle-type or button-type coagulators, and do not have the ability to adequately grasp

the ovary, and therefore are not suitable for ovarian drilling.

Unless a better instrument is developed, bipolar coagulation is not a suitable method for ovarian drilling.

The Use of Carbon Dioxide Laser for Ovarian Drilling

The technique of CO_2 laser drilling is described in detail by Daniell and Miller (1989). They recommend introducing the laser through an operating laparoscope with a two-puncture technique, grasping the ovary with forceps inserted suprapubically. I personally prefer to introduce the laser through an infraguide coupled to the laser through a third puncture. They use continuous mode at 25 W to vaporize and drain all the visible subcapsular follicles, and drill randomly placed craters in each ovary. Each crater takes 5–10 seconds of firing to develop. About 25–40 vaporization sites are formed in each ovary. The ovaries are irrigated with heparinized Ringer's lactate, and any excessive bleeding stopped using unipolar electrocautery. The laser plume is vented off regularly.

The Use of Other Lasers

When using a KTP or argon laser, the flexible fibre is introduced 2 inches below the telescope, through a third, 5.5 mm trocar which has a dual channel, enabling the smoke to be evacuated close to its source. (Figures 18.5–18.7 show the KTP/532 laser used to drill polycystic ovaries.)

Figure 18.4 Videolaparoscopic ovarian cautery using the unipolar Corson needle. The video screen.

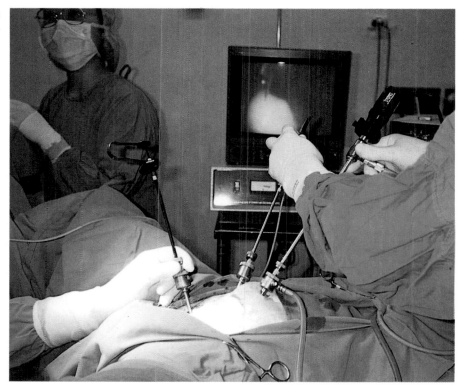

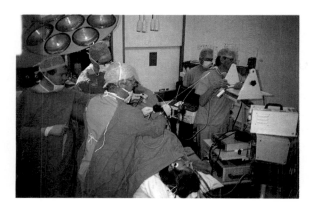

Figure 18.5 KTP/532 Laser Emerald Green Laser light passing down flexible fibres. (Photograph courtesy of Chris Sutton.)

Feste (1990b) recommends a YAG laser with a sapphire tip, with 25 W of power, with a minimum of 15 holes that penetrate the stroma into each ovary.

Yanagibori and colleagues (1989) used the YAG laser with a 0.4 mm diameter contact probe at 100 mm/s incision speed to perform bilateral wedge resection of the ovaries in six women with PCOS. Three of these women achieved pregnancy.

Dangers of Ovarian Drilling

Apart from the usual dangers of laparoscopic procedures performed under general anaesthesia,

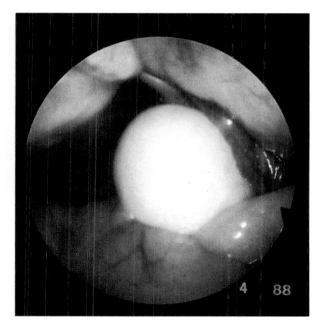

Figure 18.6 Polycystic ovary before treatment. (Photograph courtesy of Chris Sutton.)

ovarian drilling also has the inherent danger that the energy used may damage adjoining organs or structures. Furthermore, there is also the danger that excessive drilling may cause ovarian atrophy (Dabirashrafi, 1989). It is therefore advised that the hilus of the ovary is not cauterized/vaporized, and that the number of holes be individualized depending on ovarian size (Daniell, 1989).

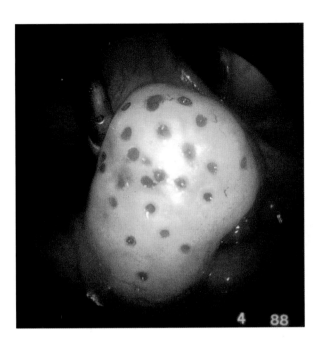

Figure 18.7 Polycystic ovary after laser drills with KTP laser. (Photograph courtesy of Chris Sutton.)

As far as ovarian adhesions are concerned, these are probably minimal, and a study in sheep suggests that CO_2 laser drilling causes no adhesions (Petrucco, 1988).

Conclusions

The treatment of PCOS has now gone around a whole circle. Although surgical treatment preceded hormonal treatment by 30 years, BOWR was abandoned in the 1960s when it became apparent that it not infrequently caused pelvic adhesions. Clomiphene citrate became the first line of treatment of this disorder, and there is no doubt that this still applies, but there are many women who do not respond to this medication.

Whether treatment should then proceed to gonadotrophins or ovarian drilling is still debatable. A randomized comparison of gonadotrophin therapy with electrocautery in clomiphene citrate-resistant anovulatory women was reported by Abdel Gadir and colleagues in 1990. They found that in their three-way trial of 89 women treated by cautery, HMG or pure FSH resulted in similar ovulation and conception rates. The rate of pregnancy loss, however, was significantly lower ($P = 0.2$) in the electrocautery group. This is the first study of its type that has been reported and suggests that ovarian drilling is as good as, if not

better than gonadotrophin therapy. It has been suggested that elevated LH levels result in a higher rate of early pregnancy loss in women with PCOS (Abdulwahid et al., 1985). If ovarian drilling does, in fact, result in a decreased pregnancy loss when compared to hormonal treatment, it will become the preferred method. Furthermore, therapy by ovarian drilling may often be combined with a diagnostic laparoscopy, therefore providing a method of treatment with little extra effort, discomfort or risk. In a recent review of the regimens for ovulation induction for PCOS (Kelly and Jewelewicz, 1990), the possibility of ovarian drilling has been completely omitted. This is no longer acceptable in the 1990s. Although the use of clomiphene citrate is undoubtedly the first line of treatment, the use of ovarian drilling should at least be considered before embarking on gonadotrophin therapy.

Whether electrocautery or a particular laser is used will depend on the training and facilities available to the surgeon. If controlled studies in the future show any of the methods to be significantly better or safer, then of course this method should be used preferentially, but now there appears to be little to choose between them.

References

Abdel Gadir A, Mowafi RS, Alnaser HM et al. (1990) Ovarian electrocautery, human menopausal gonadotrophins and pure follicle stimulating hormone therapy in the treatment of patients with polycystic ovarian disease. *Clinical Endocrinology (Oxford)* **33**: 585–592.

Abdulwahid NA, Adams J, Van Der Spuy ZM & Jacobs HS (1985) Gonadotrophin control of follicular development. *Clinical Endocrinology* **23**: 613–626.

Adashi EY, Rock JA, Guzick D et al. (1981) Fertility following bilateral ovarian wedge resection: a critical analysis of 90 consecutive cases of the polycystic ovary syndrome. *Fertility and Sterility* **36**: 320–325.

Burger HG, Healy DL, Kovacs GT et al. (1991) Ovulation induction in Polycystic Ovarian Disease. *Proceedings of the XIII World Congress of Gynaecology and Obstetrics, Singapore*, September 1991, Vol. 1. Singapore: FIGO.

Campo S, Garcea N, Caruso A & Siccardi P (1983) Effect of coelioscopic ovarian resection in patients with polycystic ovaries. *Gynecological and Obstetrical Investigation* **15**: 213.

Dabirashrafi H (1989) Complications of laparoscopic ovarian cauterization. *Fertility and Sterility* **52**: 878.

Daniell JF (1989) Complications of laparoscopic ovarian cauterization. *Fertility and Sterility* **52**: 879.

Daniell JF & Miller W (1989) Polycystic ovaries treated by laparoscopic laser vaporization. *Fertility and Sterility* **51**: 232–236.

Feste JR (1990a) General aspects of CO_2 laser laparoscopy. In Baggish MS (ed) *Endoscopic Laser Surgery*, pp 67–68. New York: Elsevier.

Feste J (1990b) Laser laparoscopy: CO_2. In Keye WR (ed) *Laser Surgery in Gynecology and Obstetrics*, pp 187–206. Chicago: Year Book Medical Publishers.

Gemzell CA, Diczfalusy E & Tilliger KG (1960) Human pituitary follicle stimulating hormone. Clinical effect of a partially purified preparation. Ciba Foundation Colloquia. *Endocrinology* 13: 191–208.

Gindoff PR & Jewelewicz R (1987) Polycystic ovarian disease. *Obstetrics and Gynecology Clinics of North America* 14: 931–953.

Gjönnaess H (1984) Polycystic ovarian syndrome treated by ovarian electrocautery through the laparoscope. *Fertility and Sterility* 41: 20–25.

Gjönnaess H & Norman N (1987) Endocrine effects of ovarian electrocautery in patients with polycystic ovarian disease. *British Journal of Obstetrics and Gynaecology* 94: 779–783.

Goldfarb AF & Crawford R (1969) Polycystic ovarian disease, clomiphene and multiple pregnancies. *Obstetrics and Gynecology* 34: 307–309.

Greenblatt E & Casper RF (1987) Endocrine changes after laparoscopic ovarian cautery in polycystic ovarian syndrome. *American Journal of Obstetrics and Gynecology* 156: 279–285.

Greenblatt RB, William MD, Barfield WE, Jungck EC & Ray AW (1961) Induction of ovulation with MRL/41. *Journal of the American Medical Association* 178: 101–104.

Huber J, Hosmann J & Spona J (1988) Polycystic ovarian syndrome treated by laser through the laparoscope. *Lancet* 2: 215.

Judd HL, Rigg LA, Anderson DC & Yen SC (1976) The effects of ovarian wedge resection on circulating gonadotropin and ovarian steroid levels in patients with polycystic ovary syndrome. *Journal of Clinical Endocrinology and Metabolism* 43: 347–355.

Keckstein J (1989) Laparoscopic treatment of polycystic ovarian syndrome. In Sutton CJG (ed) *Baillière's Clinical Obstetrics and Gynaecology. Laparoscopic Surgery* 3.3: 563–581.

Kelly AC & Jewelewicz R (1990) Alternate regimens for ovulation induction in polycystic ovarian disease. *Fertility and Sterility* 54 195–205.

Kistner RW (1968) Induction of ovulation with clomiphene citrate. In Behrman SH & Kistner RW (eds) *Progress in Infertility*, p 407. Boston: Little, Brown & Co.

Kovacs GT, Dennis PM, Shelton RJ et al. (1984) Induction of ovulation with human pituitary gonadotrophin. Twelve years' experience. *Medical Journal of Australia* 140: 575–579.

Kovacs GT, Pepperell RJ & Evans JH (1989a) Induction of ovulation with human pituitary gonadotrophin (HPG): the Australian experience. *Australian and New Zealand Journal of Obstetrics and Gynaecology* 29: 315–318.

Kovacs GT, Phillips S, Burger HG & Healy DL (1989b) Induction of ovulation with gonadotrophin releasing hormone—life table analysis of 50 courses of treatment. *Medical Journal of Australia* 151: 21–26.

Kovacs G, Buckler H, Bangah M et al. (1991) Treatment of anovulation due to polycystic ovarian syndrome by laparoscopic ovarian electrocautery. *British Journal of Obstetrics and Gynaecology* 98: 30–35.

Nezhat C, Crowgey S & Nezhat F (1989) Videolaparoscopy for the treatment of endometriosis associated with infertility. *Fertility and Sterility* 51: 237–240.

Petrucco OM (1988) Laparoscopic CO_2 laser drilling of sheep ovaries—interval assessment of histological changes and adhesion formation. *Abstracts of the Seventh Scientific Meeting of The Fertility Society of Australia, Newcastle* p 21.

Schenker JG & Polishuk WZ (1975) Ovarian hyperstimulation syndrome. *Obstetrics and Gynecology* 46: 23–28.

Stein FI & Leventhal ML (1935) Amenorrhea associated with bilateral polycystic ovaries. *American Journal of Obstetrics and Gynecology* 29: 181–191.

Stein FI (1964) Duration of fertility following ovarian wedge resection–Stein–Leventhal syndrome. *Western Journal of Surgery, Obstetrics and Gynecology* 78: 237.

Toaff R, Toaff ME & Peyser MR (1976) Infertility following wedge resection of the ovaries. *American Journal of Obstetrics and Gynecology* 124: 92–96.

van der Weiden RM & Alberda AT (1987) Laparoscopic ovarian electrocautery in patients with polycystic ovarian disease resistant to clomiphene citrate. *Surgical Endoscopy* 1: 217–219.

Yanagibori A, Kojima E, Ohtaka K, Morita M & Hirakawa S (1989) Nd:YAG laser therapy for infertility with a contact type probe. *Journal of Reproductive Medicine* 34: 456–460.

19

Laparoscopic Treatment of Tubo-ovarian Abscess

D. ALAN JOHNS

Richland Medical Center, Fort Worth, Texas, USA

The accepted treatment for pelvic inflammatory disease and tubo-ovarian abscess has changed very little in the last 15 years. Newer, more potent antibiotic regimens have been used, but the mainstay of treatment remains laparotomy with drainage of the abscess and excision of the affected organs (in those patients unresponsive to antibiotic therapy). Most recently, the trend has been toward treating suspected unruptured tubo-ovarian abscesses solely with aggressive antibiotic therapy (Kaplan *et al.*, 1967; Landers and Sweet, 1985). The common result of this approach is extensive, dense pelvic adhesive disease with resultant pain and infertility. The alternative course of therapy (intervention by laparotomy) often results in sterility from hysterectomy or adhesive disease from both the infectious process and the laparotomy. Complications of laparotomy in these patients include wound infection and dehiscence, bowel injury, embolus, sepsis, and recurrence of the pelvic abscess (Pedowitz and Bloomfield, 1964). Thus, the treatment of pelvic abscess remains a challenge.

Pelvic abscesses most commonly occur as a result of infection within the fallopian tube with resultant drainage of pus and bacteria into the abdominal cavity. The most common organisms involved are *Neisseria gonorrhoeae*, *Chlamydia trachomatis*, and the facultative and obligate anaerobes (Faro, 1991). Most often, an intense inflammatory response involving the surrounding tissues (usually bowel, peritoneal surfaces, and omentum) occurs. These adhesions are initially very friable and avascular, but become more dense and vascular with time.

Other causes of pelvic abscesses include ruptured appendix, diverticulitis, postoperative pelvic infection related to pelvic surgery, traumatic injury to the bowel or pelvis, and iatrogenic surgical injuries.

Diagnosis

The diagnosis of tubo-ovarian abscess should be considered in any female presenting with significant pelvic pain (with or without a palpable mass), fever and/or leucocytosis. Ultrasound, X-ray, CT scans, and NMRI (nuclear magnetic resonance imaging) scans may also be helpful in the diagnosis. Laboratory evaluations including CBC and erythrocyte sedimentation rates may also be useful.

Using the most advanced and sophisticated assays and scans coupled with a thorough physical examination, 35% of those patients diagnosed with acute pelvic inflammatory disease are found to have *other* conditions when laparoscopy is used to confirm the diagnosis (Binstock *et al.*, 1986). Because of this, many authors advocate routine use of laparoscopy to confirm the diagnosis when pelvic inflammatory disease is suspected (Jacobson and Westrom, 1969; Chaparro *et al.*, 1978). The most common diagnoses confused with pelvic inflammatory disease and tubo-ovarian abscess include endometriomas (both ruptured and intact), bleeding corpus luteum cysts, mesenteric adenitis, and ectopic pregnancy.

Treatment (Traditional Approach)

When a tubo-ovarian abscess is suspected, the patient should be admitted to hospital immediately and appropriate laboratory evaluation initiated and specimens taken. After hospital admission but prior to laparoscopy, baseline laboratory evaluation includes a complete blood count, including white cell count and differential, liver function studies and clotting studies. Cervical cultures for *Neisseria gonorrhoeae* and *Chlamydia trachomatis* are obtained.

At the time of laparoscopy, fluid from the abscess cavity is sent for both aerobic and anaerobic culture and sensitivity assays. Intravenous antibiotic therapy should be started at the time of admission. After laboratory evaluation has been obtained and antibiotics started, laparoscopy should be performed to confirm the diagnosis and document the extent of the infectious process. At this point, 35–40% of these patients will be found to have conditions other than pelvic infection producing their symptoms (Binstock *et al.*, 1986; Levine and Sanfilippo, 1989).

It was traditionally believed that surgical treatment of an acute pelvic infection often resulted in greater risk of injury to the bowel and reproductive tract than conservative therapy (antibiotics and observation). This was based on literature dating back 20–25 years (Pedowitz and Bloomfield, 1964; Kaplan *et al.*, 1967). Although antibiotic therapy has progressed dramatically in the past 10–20 years and surgical risks have decreased dramatically, this concept remains firmly entrenched.

Initial therapy includes high-dose intravenous antibiotics which are continued until the patient remains afebrile for 48–72 hours. Some authors have recommended continued antibiotic therapy (after the patient has become afebrile) until the pelvic mass has diminished significantly in size by ultrasound examination or CT scan.

If the abscess is visible with ultrasound or palpable in the cul-de-sac, drainage through the cul-de-sac has been advocated (Franklin *et al.*, 1973). Abscesses higher in the pelvis may be drained transabdominally with ultrasound guidance (Gerzoff *et al.*, 1981). The abscess cavity should be thoroughly irrigated until the effluent is clear, and a drain placed within the abscess cavity. Treatment by these methods is occasionally associated with recurrence of the abscess or significant morbidity.

Surgical intervention is recommended in those patients with multiloculated abscesses since multiple abscess cavities are difficult to drain vaginally. Those patients unresponsive to intravenous antibiotic therapy and those with multiloculated abscesses are also subjected to laparotomy with excision of the affected organs, often including hysterectomy and salpingo-oophorectomy. This regimen results in excellent cure rates, but significant morbidity, infertility from pelvic adhesive disease or extirpative pelvic surgery, and long-term hypo-oestrogenic problems. In addition, the cost of long-term, in-hospital intravenous therapy with or without laparotomy is significant.

Laparoscopic Treatment: Modern Approach

In an effort to avoid the cost, morbidity and subsequent infertility problems associated with traditional treatment of tubo-ovarian abscesses, a regimen of laparoscopic treatment of pelvic abscesses (regardless of cause) and the associated acute fibrinous adhesions has evolved (Henry-Suchet *et al.*, 1984). When the laparoscopic approach is used it can be extremely cost effective and advantageous to the patient.

Preoperative Evaluation and Treatment

The patient with a presumptive diagnosis of pelvic abscess is admitted to hospital immediately, appropriate laboratory evaluation is obtained, and intravenous antibiotics initiated. The choice of antibiotics should take into consideration the most common organisms producing pelvic abscesses. In the first instance, I recommend the use of simple, broad spectrum intravenous antibiotics (cefoxitin 2 g I.V. every 4 h until the patient becomes afebrile). Oral doxycycline is used as soon as the patient is taking fluids orally (doxycycline 100 mg every 12 h) for a total of 10 days. Other single agents which could be used include ticarcillin/clavulanate (Timentin), ampicillin/sulbactam (Unasyn), or imipenem/cilastatin (Primaxin). In the rare patient who fails to respond to the combination of laparoscopic surgery and single dose agents, combination therapy (clindamycin and metronidazole) may be used. Once an adequate level of intravenous antibiotics has been attained, laparoscopy is performed for confirmation of the diagnosis and therapy.

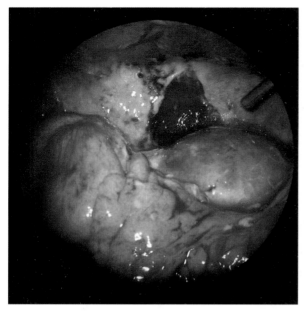

(a)

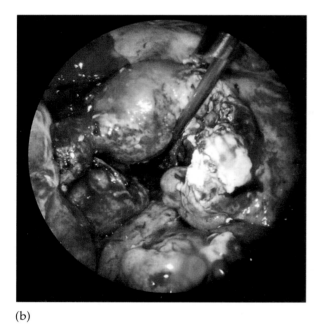

(b)

Figure 19.1 (a) Tubo-ovarian abscess pretreatment; (b) tubo-ovarian abscess post-treatment.

Equipment

The laparoscopic treatment of pelvic inflammatory disease and tubo-ovarian abscess requires a minimum of laparoscopic equipment but extraordinary patience.

A high-flow insufflator is mandatory to maintain an adequate pneumoperitoneum. A uterine manipulator is placed. Occasionally, electrocautery will be necessary for haemostasis, but bleeding is rarely a problem.

The single most important instrument used in the procedure is a hollow, blunt dissecting probe (through which irrigation fluid can be forced). This probe is invaluable for careful, blunt dissection of adhesions involving bowel and pelvic structures. Coupled with 'aquadissection' (dissection of tissue planes with fluid under minimal pressure), the manipulation/dissection probe eliminates the need for scissors, lasers, or other more traumatic (and expensive) instruments.

Any intravenous fluid may be used for aquadissection, but the surgeon should know if this irrigating fluid encourages, supports or retards bacterial growth. Ringer's lactate is the most common fluid used for this dissection. It does not facilitate the growth of most bacteria in pelvic abscesses.

Technique

Under general anaesthesia, the 10 mm diagnostic laparoscope is inserted through an intra-umbilical incision. Two suprapubic incisions (5 mm) are made on either side of the midline, medial to the inferior epigastric vessels.

The patient is placed in the Trendelenburg position and the pelvis and upper abdomen are visually examined. Should the diagnosis of pelvic abscess be confirmed, cultures are obtained. The entire abdominal cavity is then thoroughly rinsed with irrigating fluid to remove blood, pus and debris. The pelvis is carefully inspected and evaluated. The most appropriate course of dissection is then planned.

Using the blunt dissection probe, omentum, small bowel and large bowel are carefully dissected away from pelvic structures. Irrigating fluid forced through the irrigation–dissection probe will often allow dissection planes between bowel and pelvic structures to be identified more easily. This plane may then be opened and extended bluntly or with aquadissection. Most often the abscess cavity will be entered during this initial dissection.

Once the abscess cavity has been entered, the patient should immediately be placed in the reverse Trendelenburg position and cultures obtained. The abscess cavity is then thoroughly irrigated and aspirated until all pus is totally removed. Copious amounts of irrigating fluid are used to cleanse the entire abdominal cavity of pus and debris. In the reverse Trendelenburg position, there is minimal contamination of the upper abdomen.

The adnexal structures are then carefully dissected free. Since these adhesions are filmy and avascular, scissors dissection, laser dissection, and electrosurgery are rarely necessary. Very minimal bleeding will be encountered when careful, blunt 'aquadissection' is used. Once all structures have been identified and dissected, the inflammatory exudate lining the abscess cavity should be removed as much as possible. This is accomplished with aquadissection and tissue grasping forceps. Aquadissection is most helpful in separating the necrotic abscess cavity from pelvic structures and bowel wall.

After dissection of all pelvic structures and removal of inflammatory exudate, the entire abdominal cavity is irrigated with copious amounts of warmed irrigation fluid. After each irrigation, the patient is placed in the reverse Trendelenburg position and the irrigating fluid is aspirated. The process of irrigation and aspiration is continued until the aspirated fluid is clear.

When careful aquadissection is used (and scissors are avoided), very little bleeding will be encountered at the end of the dissection/irrigation process. Any residual bleeding can be controlled easily with microbipolar cautery. At the completion of the procedure, 1–2 litres of irrigation fluid is left in the abdomen in an attempt to 'float' pelvic structures and minimize subsequent adhesive disease. The intra-abdominal fluid also dilutes any remaining bacteria.

The umbilical incision is closed with absorbable sutures. The lower incisions are approximated with collodion. This allows fluid to escape from the lower incisions should abdominal distension occur. Abdominal and vaginal drains are not used.

Postoperative Care

Intravenous antibiotics are continued for 24 hours or until the patient is afebrile. Oral antibiotics are then continued for 5 days. No postoperative dietary restrictions are used and the patient's activity is not limited. Those patients desiring pregnancy are encouraged to undergo a second look laparoscopy within 2 months of their initial procedure for treatment of any residual adhesive disease.

Conclusions

Laparoscopic treatment of pelvic abscess offers many potential advantages:

1. More precise dissection of pelvic structures using the magnification capability of the laparoscope.

2. More thorough removal of pus and necrotic material from the pelvic cavity than would be possible at laparotomy.
3. More thorough and precise irrigation of the upper abdomen by direction of fluid through the dissection–irrigation probe.
4. Minimal intraoperative bleeding due to use of magnification and aquadissection (as opposed to gross scissors and blunt dissection used at laparotomy).
5. Decreased risk of bowel perforation due to more precise dissection of tissue planes utilizing the magnification capabilities of the laparoscope.
6. Elimination of the risk of wound infection and possible evisceration.
7. A shortened patient recovery period (the patient recovers from the abscess, infectious process, and adhesiolysis, *not* from laparotomy).
8. Decreased pelvic pain and infertility from a decrease in pelvic adhesions as a result of laparoscopic treatment.

Our goal in treating pelvic abscess should include prevention of infertility and pelvic pain from resultant adhesive disease. The combination of laparoscopic treatment of pelvic abscesses and intravenous antibiotics offers an effective alternative to traditional long-term antibiotics or laparotomy with radical extirpative pelvic surgery.

Both anecdotal and published data imply significant advantages of the laparoscopic approach to pelvic abscess with few of the hazards of laparotomy in the acutely infected patient (Henry-Suchet *et al.*, 1984; Reich and McGlynn, 1987; Reich, 1989). Large, controlled, randomized studies comparing laparotomy and laparoscopy for treatment of pelvic abscesses with second look data are sorely needed to confirm this perceived advantage.

References

Binstock M, Muzsnai D, Apodaca L, Goldman L & Keith L (1986) Laparoscopy in the diagnosis and treatment of pelvic inflammatory disease. A review and discussion. *International Journal on Fertility* 31:341.

Chaparro MV, Ghosh S, Nashed A *et al.* (1978) Laparoscopy for the confirmation and prognostic evaluation of pelvic inflammatory disease. *International Journal of Gynecology and Obstetrics* 15:307.

Faro S (1991) Why pelvic abscesses form. *Contemporary OB/GYN* 36:69.

Franklin EW, Hevron JE & Thompson JD (1973) Management of the pelvic abscess. *Clinical Obstetrics and Gynecology* 16:66.

Gerzoff SG, Robbins AG, Johnson WC *et al.* (1981) Percutaneous catheter drainage of abdominal abscesses. *New England Journal of Medicine* **305**:653.

Henry-Suchet J, Soler A & Loffredo V (1984) Laparoscopic treatment of tuboovarian abscesses. *Journal of Reproductive Medicine* **29**:579.

Jacobson L & Westrom L (1969) Objectivized diagnosis of acute pelvic inflammatory disease: Diagnostic and prognostic value of routine laparoscopy. *American Journal of Obstetrics and Gynecology* **105**:1088.

Kaplan AL, Jacobs WM & Ehresman JB (1967) Aggressive management of pelvic abscess. *American Journal of Obstetrics and Gynecology* **98**:482.

Landers DV & Sweet RL (1985) Current trends in the diagnosis and treatment of tuboovarian abscess. *American Journal of Obstetrics and Gynecology* **151**:1098.

Levine R & Sanfilippo J (1989) Endoscopic management of tubo ovarian abscess and pelvic inflammatory disease. In Sanfilippo J & Levine R (eds) *Operative Gynecologic Endoscopy*, pp 118–132. Berlin: Springer-Verlag.

Pedowitz P & Bloomfield RD (1964) Ruptures adnexal abscess (tuboovarian) with generalized peritonitis. *American Journal of Obstetrics and Gynecology* **88**:721.

Reich H (1989) Role of laparoscopy in treating TOA and pelvic abscess. *Contemporary OB/GYN* **34**:91.

Reich H & McGlynn F (1987) Laparoscopic treatment of tuboovarian and pelvic abscess. *Journal of Reproductive Medicine* **32**:747.

20

Laparoscopic Uterine Nerve Ablation for Intractable Dysmenorrhoea

CHRIS SUTTON AND NAOMI WHITELAW

Royal Surrey County Hospital, Guildford, Surrey, UK

Dysmenorrhoea continues to be a problem in modern society and some 14% of all visits to the general practitioner of women between the ages of 15 and 50 years is related to this as the primary complaint (Richards, 1979). It is a major cause of periodic absenteeism from the workplace (Sundell et al., 1990) and in the United States of America it has been estimated that 600 million hours are lost annually because of dysmenorrhoea (Ylikorkala and Dawood, 1978). Those women who continue to work despite significant menstrual pain have a reduced productivity, increased accident rate and produce work of diminished quality (Lumsden, 1985; Dawood, 1990). In the United Kingdom around 6.8 million women are thought to be afflicted with this problem and, of these, 2.6 million suffer such unpleasant symptoms that they have to discontinue their normal activities and retire to bed with strong analgesics (Anderson, 1981).

The actual incidence of dysmenorrhoea in different populations is difficult to assess and depends on many complex and variable factors including prevailing social and sexual attitudes in different societies. Prevalence rates vary in different studies from 3% to 90% but probably the best population study comes from Sweden where all 19-year-old girls from the town of Gothenburg were questioned with a 90% response rate (Andersch and Milsom, 1982). Seventy-three per cent of the girls suffered from primary dysmenorrhoa and 15% had severe dysmenorrhoea which affected their working ability and could not be controlled adequately by analgesics or ovulation suppression. It is for this

group of patients that surgery is recommended either by presacral neurectomy, the uterosacral ligament division technique of Doyle (Doyle, 1955) or, more simply, by laparoscopic uterine nerve ablation (LUNA). Before describing this technique it is worth considering the relevant anatomy and to describe in some detail Doyle's procedure which we are trying to imitate with the laser or electrodiathermy at laparoscopy rather than the scalpel at laparotomy.

Anatomy of the Uterine Nerve Supply

The sensory parasympathetic fibres to the cervix and the sensory sympathetic fibres to the corpus traverse the cervical division of the Lee–Frankenhauser plexus (Frankenhauser, 1864) which lies in, under and around the attachments of the uterosacral ligament to the posterior aspect of the cervix. Sympathetic fibres can also be found in this area which have reached the cervix by accompanying the uterine and other arteries.

The parasympathetic components originate from the first to the third and fourth sacral nerves, reaching the plexus by the pelvic nerves (nervi erigentes). In a study of 33 cadavers Campbell (1950) confirmed the finding of earlier workers (Latarjet and Roget, 1922; Davis, 1936) by identifying parasympathetic fibres in the anterior two-thirds of the uterosacral ligaments and demonstrated the presence of small ganglia around the area where the ligaments attach to the cervix.

Theoretically, therefore, division of the uterosacral ligaments at the point of their attachment to the cervix should lead to interruption of most, but not all, of the cervical sensory fibres and some of the corporal sensory fibres and lead to a diminution in uterine pain at the time of menstruation. It is important at the outset for the surgeon and the patient to realize that division of the uterosacral ligaments will not obliterate all the afferent sensory nerve supply and therefore cannot realistically be expected to provide completely painless periods or, indeed, painless childbirth.

Doyle's Procedure

In 1963 Joseph Doyle described the procedure of paracervical uterine denervation which bears his name (Doyle and Des Rosiers, 1963). The procedure could be performed vaginally or abdominally and Doyle suggested that gynaecologists may be more comfortable with the former approach whilst general surgeons would prefer the latter. Employing the vaginal approach a suture was placed through the posterior lip of the cervix at the apex of the vagina and traction on this suture increased the distance of the cervix from the ureter which is clearly demonstrated in his article by a very convincing radiograph of a cervicoureteterogram. The attachments of the uterosacral ligaments to the cervix were then divided between two Heaney clamps and to prevent regrowth of the bisected nerve trunks the posterior leaf of the peritoneal incision was interposed between them. The abdominal approach was recommended if endometriosis was suspected or any gross pathology, such as fibroids, were felt. The pathological tissue was then excised (which may, of course, have had a significant effect on the results) and then traction applied to the uterosacral ligaments by means of a suture placed in the cervix just above the point of their insertion. He carefully scrutinized the course of the ureters and found them rarely to lie close to the ligaments, usually running 1–2 cm laterally. As before, the ligaments were divided between two clamps and in a further refinement of the technique he sutured the ligaments together with stainless steel sutures to the isthmus of the cervix in the midline about 1 cm higher than their original attachment.

Doyle's results were extremely impressive with complete pain relief in 63 out of 73 cases (86%); 35 had primary dysmenorrhoea (85.7% success) and 33 had secondary dysmenorrhoea (86.8% success). Relief was partial in six cases and there were four failures (Doyle, 1954, 1955). With such a satisfactory outcome it is difficult to see why the operation sank into obscurity. Possibly the advent of powerful prostaglandin synthetase inhibitors reduced the demand for relatively drastic forms of intervention. Interest in Doyle's work has recently revived with the development of surgical lasers which can be used endoscopically to perform much the same tissue effect without the need for major surgery.

Counselling and Consenting the Patient

It is important to apprise women of the likely success of the procedure and to make it clear that pain relief cannot be guaranteed and also that we are attempting to ameliorate the discomfort of dysmenorrhoea rather than alleviate it altogether. It certainly cannot be guaranteed to work in all cases and although we have no instances of patients being made worse by the procedure in our own series, Daniell (1989) has reported this and patients should probably be advised accordingly.

As with all laparoscopic procedures there is a definite, albeit small, risk of unexpected complications and patients should be consented for a laparotomy should the need arise.

Initial Pelvic Inspection

Before embarking on operative laparoscopy the surgeon should perform an anatomical tour of the pelvis to identify any structures that could be harmed if inadvertently hit with the laser beam or electrodiathermy. This first step is vital to ensure the safety of operative laparoscopy and should never be omitted since no two pelvises are identical and anatomical variations, particularly concerning the course of the ureter, are not unusual.

The posterior leaves of the broad ligaments are carefully inspected to try to identify the course of the ureters which can rarely lie close to the uterosacral ligaments but usually run 1–2 cm laterally. They can usually be 'palpated' via a probe and often the characteristic peristaltic movements can be recognized beneath the peritoneal surface. The operator should also take note of some thin-walled veins which often lie just lateral to the uterosacral ligaments because if they are accidentally punctured they can cause troublesome bleeding which can be very difficult to stop with the carbon dioxide laser. Haemostatic clips, bipolar diathermy or an endocoagulator should be immediately available if required.

Operative Procedure

Since laparoscopic surgery developed independently in several different centres it is not surprising that there are many different approaches to essentially the same operation. The description given here (Sutton, 1989a) is the method that I have developed and adapted over the past 10 years using the double-puncture technique employing lasers for precise surgical destruction of tissue. The reasons for this preference are given but alternative methods are described for those who do not have access to laser technology.

Laser Uterine Nerve Ablation (LUNA)

The uterosacral ligaments are encouraged to 'stand-out' by the assistant manipulating the uterus to one or other side with an 8 mm Hegar dilator or preferably with a Valtchev uterine mobilizer (Conkin Surgical Instruments, Toronto, Canada). If this fails to delineate them clearly a rigid metal probe is inserted through the suprapubic trocar and pressed on the posterior aspect of the cervix. The position of the ureters should be checked again and any large vessels in the vicinity of the ligaments noted.

The most precise way to ablate the uterosacral ligaments is to vaporize them with a CO_2 laser transmitted down the central channel of the laparoscope (Donnez and Nisolle, 1989) or via the iliac fossa trocar (Sutton, 1986; Figure 20.1). The disadvantage of the single-puncture approach is that a considerable amount of the cross-sectional diameter has to be sacrificed to the laser channel, inevitably resulting in reduced visibility. Furthermore, the actual view is not exactly the same as the path of the laser beam and there have been reports of accidental injury due to unrecognized interposition of a loop of bowel (Borten and Friedman, 1986).

The laser is set at a relatively high power density setting of 10 000–15 000 W/cm² and the uterosacral ligaments are vaporized near the point of their attachment to the posterior aspect of the cervix. The idea of the procedure is to destroy the sensory nerve fibres and their secondary ganglia as they leave the uterus and because of the divergence of these fibres in the uterosacral ligament they should be vaporized as close to the cervix as possible (Figure 20.2). A crater about 1 cm in diameter and 5 mm deep is formed and great care must be taken to vaporize medially rather than laterally to avoid damage to the vessels already identified coursing alongside the uterosacral ligaments (Figure 20.3). A further refinement is to superficially laser the posterior aspect of the cervix between the insertion of the ligaments to interrupt fibres crossing to the contralateral side (Daniell, 1989).

Vaporization continues until the nerve fibres stop splitting but care should be taken not to go too deep since a relatively large artery often lurks in the depth of the ligament and if transected it can bleed copiously. It is relatively easy to vaporize to the correct depth when the uterosacral ligaments are well formed but sometimes their limits are poorly defined and the procedure is

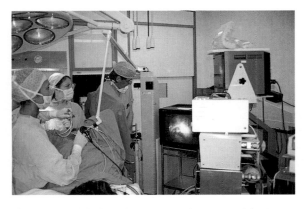

Figure 20.1 CO_2 laser laparoscopy being used for LUNA with double-puncture technique.

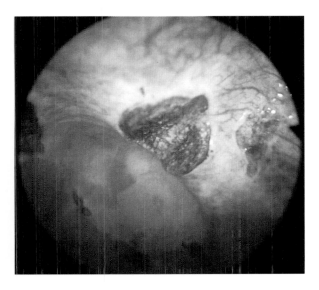

Figure 20.2 LUNA. Vaporization of the right uterosacral ligament showing depth of vaporization until nerve fibres stop splitting.

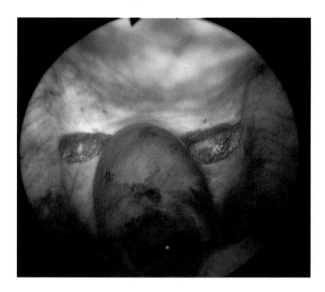

Figure 20.3 LUNA on well developed uterosacral ligaments. Note that a large artery is just visible at the base of the crater on the left.

less than satisfactory simply because it is difficult to be sure that the area vaporized is in the same place as the uterine nerve fibres.

FLEXIBLE FIBRE LASERS

We are increasingly using the KTP/532 laser (Laserscope, San Jose, California, USA) for uterosacral ligament transection because it is very quick, effective and is associated with less bleeding. This laser is a frequency doubled Nd:YAG laser and is transmitted down flexible reusable silicone quartz optical fibres as a visible emerald green light. When dragged across stretched tissue the end of the fibre will vaporize tissue—probably a thermal effect (Keckstein, 1989)—and provides effective cutting but if bleeding occurs the fibre can be held a few millimetres away from the bleeding point and fired to photocoagulate the vessel and seal it. Sometimes it is necessary to flush away the blood with irrigant solution that passes down the same introducer as the laser fibre to achieve haemostasis. If large vessel haemorrhage is encountered it is possible at a flick of a switch to interpose a mirror and seal the artery with the deeper penetrating Nd:YAG laser energy which is produced in the same laser generator.

The argon laser can also be employed but in my experience, although of similar wavelength to the KTP, is not so effective at cutting and produces a blanched zone of coagulation which makes it difficult to assess the depth of penetration. The Nd:YAG laser used on its own should be employed with considerable caution because of

its deep penetration but in skilled hands has been associated with good results (Corson, 1992). Nevertheless I have seen video recordings from other institutions showing catastrophic bleeding from the use of the Nd:YAG laser over the internal iliac artery—a sobering example of the effect this laser has deep below the surface. In order to get round these problems manufacturers have devised artificial sapphire tips and sculpted quartz fibres to focus the energy but such devices only work when contaminated with blood and tissue debris and then heat to 600°C so the effect is purely a thermal one and could be achieved much more cheaply with an electrodiathermy needle or probe (Keckstein et al., 1988). Indeed, laser manufacturers seem to have realized that they have produced a sophisticated 'hot wire' with the introduction of the fibretom (Medilas, MBB, Germany) which incorporates an optoelectronic control system to regulate the heat applied to the tissue. A sensor in the laser measures the temperature of the fibre tip during cutting and a servomechanism automatically controls the laser power to keep the temperature of the tip below the meltdown threshold (Sutton and Hodgson, 1992).

ELECTRODIATHERMY AND
ENDOCOAGULATION

If laser technology is not available these two modalities can be employed but the depth of tissue destruction is difficult to assess and studies in experimental animals and humans show that healing is less efficient than after laser surgery (Bellina et al., 1984). Of the two, endocoagulation (Semm, 1966; Semm and O'Neill-Freys, 1989) is undoubtedly safer (Semm and Mettler, 1980) but much slower. Tissue is heated to about 100°C and when this temperature is reached the acoustic signal changes frequency and is present until the tissue cools to 60°C. This can be rather tedious although the process can be accelerated by flushing the tip with cool saline solution. Removal of the crocodile forceps before this temperature is reached results in the instrument sticking to tissue with resultant bleeding when the jaws are opened.

Although electrosurgical equipment is getting safer, there have been many reports of accidents occurring when the hot tip of the electrode, at about 600°C, inadvertently touches bowel or where radiofrequency current follows the path of least resistance and damages bowel distant to the site of application (Di Novo, 1983), due to its high electrolyte content. Ureteric injuries have also occurred when electrocautery was used for laparoscopic sterilization (Irvin *et al.*, 1975), during electrosurgical resection of endometriosis (Gomel and James, 1991) and, more pertinently, during electrofulguration of an endometriotic implant on the uterosacral ligament (Cheng, 1976). Lichten and Bombard (1987) used electrosurgery to perform LUNA and 81% of a small group of 11 patients reported relief from dysmenorrhoea.

COMPLICATIONS

Apart from the risks of electrosurgery alluded to above, the main problem is haemorrhage either from the thin-walled veins just lateral to the uterosacral ligaments or from arterial bleeding from large vessels lying deep in the uterosacral ligaments. If bleeding does occur attempts should be made to stem the flow by the usual techniques of pressure with a blunt probe and then firing the laser in a rosette fashion around the bleeding point using a defocused beam and a lower power density. If this is unsuccessful other endoscopic techniques of haemostasis should be instantly available, either endocoagulation (Semm, 1966), bipolar desiccation (Reich, 1989) or laparoscopic endoclips (Semm and O'Neill-Freys, 1989). If there is any uncertainty about the effectiveness of haemostasis a redivac drain should be inserted through the suprapubic cannula prior to withdrawing it to lessen the chance of haematoma formation and to monitor any ongoing blood loss. If haemorrhage continues it is safer to resort to laparotomy to stop the bleeding. Two patients have died as a result of postoperative haemorrhage following this procedure in the United States (Daniell, 1989) and patients should never be discharged from a day-care facility if there is a possibility of ongoing intraperitoneal bleeding.

RESULTS

The first laser laparoscopy in the United Kingdom was performed in Guildford, Surrey, in October 1982 using a Sharplan CO_2 laser (Litechnica, Manchester, UK). Since then we have treated more than 1600 women with CO_2 laser laparoscopy and during the past 3 years we have also used a combined KTP and Nd:YAG laser (Laserscope, San Jose, California, USA). Most of the patients treated have suffered from endometriosis and about one-fifth of the women have had laser laparoscopic uterine nerve ablation performed for secondary dysmenorrhoea associated with endometriosis or for primary dysmenorrhoea unresponsive to medical treatment. During the first 5 years we conducted a careful longitudinal study of the patients with endometriosis (Sutton

and Hill, 1990) and as an off-shoot of this enquiry we also followed a group of patients who had severe dysmenorrhoea without pelvic pathology. These patients with primary dysmenorrhoea were asked to record the intensity of their pain on a linear analogue scale, marked from 0 to 10, before the operation and at the follow-up visit 4 months later. All patients were warned that the first period might be slightly more uncomfortable, possibly due to oedema around the nerve fibres during the healing process after laser surgery. The follow-up interview was conducted by one of the vocational trainees from general practice in order to minimize subjective bias that might have been introduced had the surgeon himself seen the patient at the follow-up visit. Patients with secondary (congestive) dysmenorrhoea were informed that if endometriosis was discovered at diagnostic laparoscopy all visible implants would be vaporized and the uterosacral ligaments also vaporized if this was technically feasible. Sometimes only one of the ligaments was anatomically obvious and in that case the procedure was recorded as a partial LUNA only.

In the course of this longitudinal study we followed 100 consecutive patients with dysmenorrhoea associated with endometriosis and 26 patients with no obvious pelvic pathology. We deliberately did not include patients with secondary dysmenorrhoea due to other causes such as fibroids or pelvic congestion.

In patients with primary dysmenorrhoea we used a linear analogue scale to judge the response to treatment. The initial score on average was 9.2 and in 16 patients (73%) the symptoms were improved with an average score among the successful patients of 3.4. Of these, 15 had a complete neurectomy and one had a partial neurectomy due to poor formation of the uterosacral ligament on one side.

No patients were made worse by the procedure but six patients failed to show any improvement and in three of these a partial neurectomy was performed, suggesting an element of technical failure. Of the three patients who failed to show any improvement one subsequently had a hysterectomy and the pathologist noted marked adenomyosis in the myometrium (endometriosis interna), explaining her lack of response to nerve severance. Four patients were lost to follow-up.

Of the 100 women with dysmenorrhoea associated with endometriosis six were lost to follow-up. Eighty-one (85%) reported an improvement in symptoms even though 26 (32%) of them had a partial (unilateral) neurectomy. In three patients the symptoms returned at 6 months to 1 year following the procedure. No patients were made worse but 13 reported no improvement and, interestingly, nine of these had incomplete or partial neurectomies (Sutton, 1989b).

There were no serious complications in this group of patients and all were treated on a day-case or overnight stay basis. In two patients troublesome bleeding was encountered, requiring endocoagulation or haemostatic clips and the insertion of a redivac drain in the pelvis for 12 hours.

Division of the autonomic nerves and ganglia in the Lee–Frankenhauser plexus does not appear to have any adverse effect on bowel or bladder function and no patients have reported any reduction in the ability to enjoy sexual intercourse or achieve orgasm (Daniell, 1992).

Discussion

Although many women are able to cope with the symptoms of dysmenorrhoea, there remains a sizeable proportion of the female population who have to take to their bed for a few days each month and use potent analgesics to obtain pain relief.

Before 1960 many patients were treated surgically with interruption of the inferior hypogastric nerve plexus as it ramifies over the sacral promontory (Black, 1964; Counseller, 1934) or simple division of the uterosacral ligaments, performed either abdominally or vaginally (Doyle, 1955). Early reports of presacral neurectomy yielded disappointing results with failure rates around 11–15% in primary dysmenorrhoea and 25–40% in secondary dysmenorrhoea (Tucker, 1947; Ingersoll and Meigs, 1948). In 1952 White pointed out that the nerve supply to the cervix is not usually interrupted by the presacral neurectomy procedure (White, 1952) and for this reason, and the development of powerful prostaglandin synthetase inhibitors and new steroids to inhibit ovulation, the procedure was all but abandoned by most gynaecologists.

With the advent of the combined oral contraceptive pill a significant reduction in the prevalence of dysmenorrhoea was noted (Royal College of General Practitioners, 1974), a greater influence being exhibited by those preparations which had a progestogen dominant activity (Dygdeman et al., 1979). The discovery that prostaglandins are raised in women with dysmenorrhoea (Chan et al., 1981; Lumsden et al., 1983; Milsom and Andersch, 1984) led to the widespread use of non-steroidal anti-inflammatory drugs to treat this condition

and surgical procedures virtually shrank into obscurity.

Nevertheless there remains a significant proportion of sufferers, as many as 20%, who fail to respond to such pharmacological manipulation (Anderson, 1981; Dawood, 1985; Henzl, 1985) and for these women some form of surgical intervention remains an option. Several recent reports of presacral neurectomy from specialist centres have given excellent results but have involved a large midline incision and all the disadvantages of major surgery (Lee et al., 1986; Tjaden et al., 1990; Fliegner and Umstead, 1991) although with ancillary instruments like the argon beam coagulator it is possible to perform this procedure laparoscopically (Daniell, 1992).

With the increasing popularity of operative laparoscopy in recent years there has been a revival of interest in Doyle's procedure because it is possible to perform the transection or destruction of the uterosacral ligaments either with diathermy coagulation and laparoscopic scissors (Lichten and Bombard, 1987) or the carbon dioxide laser (Daniell and Feste, 1985; Feste, 1985; Donnez and Nisolle, 1989; Sutton, 1989a) or the KTP/532 laser (Daniell, 1989).

The study of Lichten and Bombard (1987) is particularly interesting because it is one of the few, or indeed the only, randomized prospective double-blind study performed in this rapidly developing branch of operative gynaecology. A relatively homogeneous group of women were selected who had severe or incapacitating dysmenorrhoea, who had no demonstrable pelvic pathology at laparascopy and who were unresponsive to NSAIDs and oral contraceptives prescribed concurrently. Coexisting psychiatric illness was evaluated with the Minnesota Multiphasic Personality Inventory and those with an abnormal psychological profile were excluded from the study. The remaining 21 patients were randomized to uterine nerve ablation or control group at the time of diagnostic laparoscopy. Neither the patient nor the clinical psychologist who conducted the interview and the follow-up was aware of the group to which the patient had been randomized. No patient in the control group reported relief from dysmenorrhoea whereas nine of the 11 patients (81%) who had LUNA reported almost complete relief at 3 months and five of them had continued relief from dysmenorrhoea 1 year after surgery. Interestingly, those that reported surgical success also reported relief from associated symptoms of nausea, vomiting, diarrhoea and headaches. Although there were no reported complications in the above study the numbers involved were small and the use of thermocautery in this area is potentially hazardous because of the proximity of the ureter.

We originally chose the carbon dioxide laser because of its ability to vaporize tissue precisely, causing a zone of thermal necrosis only 100 μm beyond the impact site (Wilson, 1988) and, employing the new ultrapulse lasers (Coherent Lasers, Cambridge, UK) the zone of irreversible tissue damage is less than 50 μm. The laser craters in the uterosacral ligaments produce very little postoperative pain, no more than that associated with a diagnostic laparoscopy, because all tissue debris is removed in the laser smoke plume and residual carbon is flushed away by a jet of irrigant solution. There is very little inflammatory reaction, no oedema and healing occurs with virtually no fibrosis, contracture or adhesion formation (Figures 20.4 and 20.5). The main disadvantage of the CO_2 laser is the almost total absorption by water, rendering it ineffective in the presence of anything more than capillary bleeding. Any gynaecologist attempting the procedure of laser uterine nerve ablation should be able to employ endoscopic operative skills to deal with haemorrhage by suture, endocoagulation, clips or diathermy or be prepared to perform a laparotomy to stop the bleeding and the patient should be forewarned of this possible complication.

Because of its ease of use, limited penetration and ability to deal with bleeding we have recently favoured the KTP/532 laser (Figure 20.6) which was initially pioneered in gynaecology by James Daniell in Nashville, Tennessee (Daniell, 1986, 1989). His initial results for LUNA employing the KTP laser are shown in Table 20.1. To anyone who has visited his surgical facility in Nashville

it is abundantly clear that his patients are very well informed and he carefully counsels his patients and tells them that the first period might still be painful and he also tells them that some

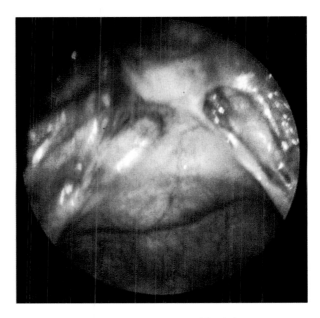

Figure 20.5 LUNA crater at second look laparoscopy— 3 months after KTP/532 laser treatment. (Photograph courtesy of Jim Daniell.)

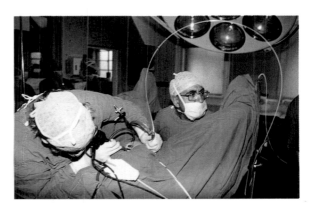

Figure 20.6 KTP/532 emerald green flexible fibre laser.

Table 20.1 LUNA results with KTP laser

	Improved	Same	Worse
Endometriosis			
80 patients	60 (75%)	17 (21%)	3 (4%)
Primary			
dysmenorrhoea			
20 patients	12 (60%)	6 (30%)	2 (10%)
Total			
100 patients	72 (72%)	23 (23%)	5 (5%)

Data from Daniell, 1989.

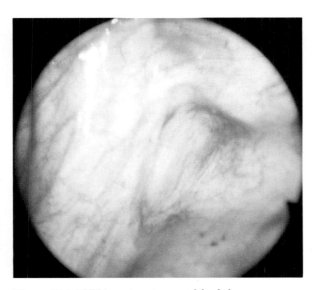

Figure 20.4 LUNA crater at second look laparoscopy— 3 months after CO_2 laser vaporization.

of them may be made worse by the procedure and with 4% of the endometriosis patients and 10% of primary dysmenorrhoea patients this does appear to be the case. The relatively high number in this latter group without pelvic pathology suggests that considerable psychological overlay must be operating here. We do not tell patients that the procedure may make their periods worse and so far no patients have complained of a deterioration in dysmenorrhoea.

Although this technique is frequently used by laser laparoscopists during the investigation of dysmenorrhoea and dyspareunia there are only a few reported series in the literature. Feste (1985) reported his results with 12 patients in a review of 202 patients treated by laser laparoscopy. In a review article Daniell and Feste (1985) reported on their combined results with carbon dioxide laser laparoscopy in a series of 50 patients: 64% with endometriosis and 50% with primary dysmenorrhoea were cured. Feste (1989) presented an update of his work at the World Endometriosis Congress in Houston. He performed laser neurectomy on 196 patients with intractable dysmenorrhoea associated with endometriosis (Figure 20.7) and in the 124 patients that he managed to follow up the success rate was 87%— almost exactly the same as our result even though, at the time, neither surgeon was aware of the technique or laser power used by the other (Table 20.2). It is also interesting that the result is almost exactly the same as that obtained by Doyle in 1963 by laparotomy (Doyle and Des Rosiers, 1963).

Donnez has reported a series of 100 patients who have been followed for more than one year (Donnez and Nisolle, 1989). There was complete relief of symptoms in 50% of the patients whilst

Table 20.2 LUNA results with carbon dioxide laser

	LFU	Improved	Same	Worse
Endometriosis 100 patients	6	81 (86%)	13	—
Primary dysmenorrhoea 26 patients	4	16 (73%)	6	—
Total 126 patients	10	97 (84%)	19	—

41% reported mild to moderate relief. There was no change in the symptoms in 9% but no patients said that their dysmenorrhoea was worse following the procedure.

In this study they also found that many patients complaining of dyspareunia also experienced relief from this symptom and we have also noticed this in the absence of endometriosis, especially in patients with very taut and well demarcated uterosacral ligaments. Donnez's group may, however, have another explanation for this finding since they have found histological evidence of endometriosis in biopsies of the uterosacral ligaments in 52% of patients with pelvic pain when there was no laparoscopic evidence of the disease (Nisolle et al., 1990). There is considerable controversy in the literature about the significance of random peritoneal biopsies but if it is eventually shown that endometriosis exists without its usual outward appearances it calls into question the whole philosophy of vaporizing the deposits with lasers or electrocautery and certainly explains some of our treatment failures.

Summary

The use of the carbon dioxide or fibreoptic lasers at laparoscopy offers a simple and relatively safe approach to the treatment of dysmenorrhoea, both primary and secondary. The procedure takes about 5 minutes to perform and generates a large amount of smoke with the CO_2 laser (less so with the fibreoptic lasers) which has to be efficiently removed but as long as care is taken in recognizing the pelvic anatomy before the laser is fired there should be little possibility of damage to the ureters or the thin-walled veins coursing just medial to the uterosacral ligaments.

Prospective double-blind randomized controlled studies have shown that laparoscopic transection of the uterosacral ligaments close to their insertion in the posterior aspect of the cervix

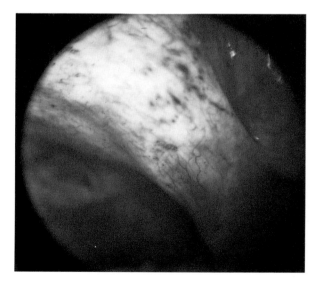

Figure 20.7 Telangiectases in uterosacral ligaments— atypical appearance of endometriosis.

is an effective treatment for dysmenorrhoea that has been unresponsive to drug therapy. Further trials are needed on larger numbers of patients to establish the long-term results but available evidence suggests that this relatively simple procedure is a useful technique in laparoscopic surgery and confers considerable benefit on patients with recalcitrant dysmenorrhoea.

References

Andersch B & Milsom I (1982) An epidemiologic study of young women with dysmenorrhoea. *American Journal of Obstetrics and Gynecology* **144**:655.

Anderson A (1981) The role of prostaglandin synthetase inhibitors in gynaecology. *The Practitioner* **225**:1460–1470.

Bellina JH, Hemmings R, Voros IJ & Ross LF (1984) Carbon dioxide laser and electrosurgical wound study with an animal model. A comparison of tissue damage and healing patterns in peritoneal tissue. *American Journal of Obstetrics and Gynecology* **148**:327.

Black WT Jr (1964) Use of pre-sacral sympathectomy in the treatment of dysmenorrhoea: a second look after 25 years. *American Journal of Obstetrics and Gynecology* **89**:17.

Borten M & Friedman EA (1986) Visual field obstruction in single puncture operative laparoscopy. *Journal of Reproductive Medicine* **31(12)**:1102–1105.

Campbell RM (1950) Anatomy and physiology of sacro-uterine ligaments. *American Journal of Obstetrics and Gynecology* **59**:1.

Chan WY, Dawood MY & Fuchs F (1981) Prostaglandins in primary dysmenorrhoea. *American Journal of Medicine* **70**:535–540.

Cheng YS (1976) Ureteral injury resulting from laparoscopic fulguration of endometriotic implant. *American Journal of Obstetrics and Gynecology* **126**:1045–1046.

Corson SL (1992) Neodymium-YAG laser laparoscopy. In Sutton CJG (ed) *Lasers in Gynaecology*, pp 141–154. London: Chapman and Hall.

Counsellor V (1934) Resection of the pre-sacral nerves: evaluation of end results. *American Journal of Obstetrics and Gynecology* **28**:161.

Daniell JF (1986) Laparoscopic evaluation of the KTP/532 laser for treating endometriosis—initial report. *Fertility and Sterility* **46**:373.

Daniell JF (1989) Fibreoptic laser laparoscopy. In Sutton C (ed) *Baillière's Clinical Obstetrics and Gynaecology. Laparoscopic Surgery* **3(3)**:545–562.

Daniell JF (1992) Advanced operative laser laparoscopy. In Sutton CJG (ed) *Lasers in Gynaecology*, pp 119–139. London: Chapman and Hall.

Daniell JF & Feste J (1985) Laser laparoscopy. In Keye WR (ed) *Laser Surgery in Gynecology and Obstetrics*, Chapter 11, pp 147–165. Boston MA: GK Hall.

Davis A (1936) Intrinsic dysmenorrhoea. *Proceedings of the Royal Society of Medicine* **29**:931.

Dawood YM (1985) Dysmenorrhoea. *Pain and Analgesia* **1**:20.

Dawood YM (1990) Dysmenorrhoea. In Reiter RC (ed) *Chronic Pelvic Pain. Clinical Obstetrics and Gynaecology* **33(1)**: 168–178.

Di Novo JA (1983) Radiofrequency leakage current from unipolar laparoscopic electrocoagulators. *Journal of Reproductive Medicine* **28(9)**:565–575.

Donnez J & Nisolle M (1989) Carbon-dioxide laser laparoscopy in pelvic pain and infertility. In Sutton CJG (ed) *Baillière's Clinical Obstetrics and Gynaecology. Laparoscopic Surgery* **3(3)**:525–544.

Doyle JB (1954) Paracervical uterine denervation for dysmenorrhoea. *Transactions of the New England Obstetrical and Gynecological Society* **8**:143.

Doyle JB (1955) Paracervical uterine denervation by transection of the cervical plexus for the relief of dysmenorrhoea. *American Journal of Obstetrics and Gynecology* **70**:1.

Doyle JB & Des Rosiers JJ (1963) Paracervical uterine denervation for relief of pelvic pain. *Clinical Obstetrics and Gynecology* **6**:742–753.

Dygdeman M, Bremme K, Gillespie A & Lundstrom V (1979) Effects of prostaglandins on the uterus. *Acta Obstetrica et Gynecologica Scandinavica Supplement* **87**:33–38.

Feste JR (1985) Laser laparoscopy. *Journal of Reproductive Medicine* **30**:414.

Feste JR (1989) *Proceedings of the 2nd World Congress of Gynaecological Endoscopy*, p 35. Basel: Karger.

Fliegner JRH & Umstead MP (1991) Presacral neurectomy—a reappraisal. *Australian and New Zealand Journal of Obstetrics and Gynaecology* **31**:76–79.

Frankenhauser G (1864) Die Bewegungenerven der Gebarmutter. *Z. Med. Nat. Wiss.* **1**:35.

Gomel V & James C (1991) Intraoperative management of ureteral injury during laparoscopic surgery. *Fertility and Sterility* **55**:416–419.

Henzl MR (1985) Dysmenorrhoea: achievements and challenges. *Sex Medicine Today* **9**:8.

Ingersoll F & Meigs JV (1943) Presacral neurectomy for dysmenorrhoea. *New England Journal of Medicine* **238**:357.

Irvin TT, Goligher JC & Scott JS (1975) Injury to the ureter during laparoscopic tubal sterilization. *Archives of Surgery* **110**:1501.

Keckstein J (1989) Laparoscopic treatment of polycystic ovarian syndrome. In Sutton CJG (ed) *Baillière's Clinical Obstetrics and Gynaecology. Laparoscopic Surgery*. **3(3)**: 563–582.

Keckstein J, Finger A & Steiner R (1988) Laser application in contact and non-contact procedures: sapphire tips in comparison to 'bare-fibre', argon laser in comparison to Nd:YAG laser. *Lasers in Medicine and Surgery* **4**:158–162.

Latarjet A & Roget P (1922) Le plexus hypogastrique chez la femme. *Gynécologie et Obstétrique* **6**:225.

Lee RB, Stone K, Magelssen D, Belts RP & Benson WL (1986) Presacral neurectomy for chronic pelvic pain. *Obstetrics and Gynecology* **69**:517–521.

Lichten EM & Bombard J (1987) Surgical treatment of dysmenorrhoea with laparoscopic uterine nerve ablation. *Journal of Reproductive Medicine* **32(1)**:37–42.

Lumsden MA (1985) Dysmenorrhoea. In Studd JWW (ed) *Progress in Obstetrics and Gynaecology*, Vol 5, pp 276–292. Edinburgh: Churchill Livingstone.

Lumsden MA, Kelly RW & Baird DT (1983) Primary

dysmenorrhoea: the importance of both prostaglandins C2 and F2 alpha. *British Journal of Obstetrics and Gynaecology* **90**:1135–1140.

Milsom I & Andersch B (1984) Effect of various oral contraceptive combinations on dysmenorrhoea. *Gynecologic and Obstetric Investigation* **17**:284–292.

Nisolle M, Paindeveine B, Bourdon A *et al.* (1990). Histological study of peritoneal endometriosis in infertile women. *Fertility and Sterility* **53**:984–988.

Reich H (1987) Laparoscopic oophorectomy and salpingo-oophorectomy in the treatment of benign tubo-ovarian disease. *International Journal of Fertility* **32**:233.

Reich H (1989) Advanced operative laparoscopy. In Sutton CJG (ed) *Baillière's Clinical Obstetrics and Gynaecology. Laparoscopic Surgery* **3.3**:655–682.

Richards DH (1979) A general practice view of functional disorders associated with menstruation. *Research Clinical Forums* **1**:39–45.

Royal College of General Practitioners (1974) *Oral Contraceptives and Health*. London: Pitman Medical.

Semm K (1966) New apparatus for 'cold-coagulation' of benign cervical lesions. *American Journal of Obstetrics and Gynecology* **95**:963–967.

Semm K & Mettler L (1980) Technical progress in pelvic surgery via operative laparoscopy. *American Journal of Obstetrics and Gynecology* **138**:121–127.

Semm K & O'Neill-Freys I (1989) Conventional operative laparoscopy. In Sutton CJG (ed) *Baillière's Clinical Obstetrics and Gynaecology. Laparoscopic Surgery* **3.3**:451–486.

Sundell G, Milsom I & Andersch B (1990) Factors influencing the prevalence and severity of dys-

menorrhoea in young women. *British Journal of Obstetrics and Gynaecology* **97**:588–594.

Sutton CJG (1986) Initial experience with CO_2 laser laparoscopy. *Lasers in Medical Science* **1**:25–31.

Sutton CJG (1989a) Carbon dioxide laser laparoscopy in the treatment of endometriosis. In Sutton CJG (ed) *Baillière's Clinical Obstetrics and Gynaecology. Laparoscopic Surgery* **3.3**:499–523.

Sutton CJG (1989b) Laser laparoscopic uterine nerve ablation. In Donnez J (ed) *Operative Laser Laparoscopy and Hysteroscopy*, pp 43–52. Louvain, Belgium: Nauwelaerts Publishers.

Sutton CJG & Hill D (1990) Laser laparoscopy in endometriosis: a 5-year study. *British Journal of Obstetrics and Gynaecology* **97**:901–905.

Sutton CJG & Hodgson R (1992) Endoscopic cutting with lasers: a review article. *Journal of Minimally Invasive Therapy* **1**:197–205.

Tjaden B, Schlaff WD, Kimball A & Rock JA (1990) The efficacy of pre-sacral neurectomy for the relief of mid-line dysmenorrhoea. *Obstetrics and Gynecology* **76**:89–91.

Tucker AW (1947) Evaluation of pre-sacral neurectomy in the treatment of dysmenorrhoea. *American Journal of Obstetrics and Gynecology* **53**:226.

White JC (1952) Conduction of visceral pain. *New England Journal of Medicine* **246**:686–688.

Wilson EA (1988) Surgical therapy for endometriosis. *Clinical Obstetrics and Gynecology* **31(4)**:857–865.

Ylikorkala O & Dawood YM (1978) New concepts in dysmenorrhoea. *American Journal of Obstetrics and Gynecology* **130**:833.

21

Laparoscopic Myomectomy

JEAN B. DUBUISSON, FABRICE LECURU AND HERVÉ FOULOT

Clinique Universitaire Port Royal, Paris, France

The indications for laparoscopic surgery have expanded greatly over the past decades as its many advantages over laparotomy have been recognized (Bruhat *et al.*, 1977; Murphy, 1987; Reich, 1989). Myomectomies may also be performed by laparoscopy in selected cases, particularly in subserous and interstitial myomas as published by Semm and Mettler (1980) and by Dubuisson *et al.* (1991). We report our technique and results with laparoscopic myomectomy.

Technique

Laparoscopy is performed transumbilically using a 10 mm endoscope adapted to a video camera. The following instrumentation is used: atraumatic grasping forceps, Semm's myoma enucleator for thermocoagulation, monopolar hook, Semm's needle holder and suture forceps, pelvicleaner (Storz-France). Myomectomy is performed according to the principles of atraumatic infertility surgery in all cases: magnification, meticulous haemostasis, and irrigation with saline solution. Prophylactic antibiotics are administered systematically for 1 week following laparoscopy but vasoconstrictive agents are not used. The simplest technique consists of coagulation and section of subserous myomas when the implantation surface is small (≤ 1 cm^2). For subserous myomas with a large implantation surface and interstitial myomas, the uterus is incised at the site of the myomas without opening the uterine cavity. For the incision, we use thermocoagulation with the Semm enucleator or monopolar coagulation with the hook. It is important to ensure complete haemostasis. Uterine incisions are closed by laparoscopy with sutures to prevent dehiscence of the myometrium after interstitial or submucous myomectomy and to reduce the risk of adhesion formation on a large raw surface (>1 cm^2) after subserous myomectomy. We close the uterus in one or two layers according to the depth of the incision with interrupted or running 3-0 Vicryl (Polyglactine 910, 20 mm needle; Ethicon, Neuilly-France) sutures. Myomas are mostly removed through the suprapubic puncture site after enlargement of the incision (20 mm) with a single tooth tenaculum. Myomas >20 mm are brought to the suprapubic incision and pressed on the peritoneum to prevent loss of CO$_2$: they are then fragmented under laparoscopic control by using a small blade passed through the incision. We are now evaluating the technique of extraction through a posterior colpotomy incision in the same way that we perform the extraction of a distended tube after salpingectomy for ectopic pregnancy (Dubuisson *et al.*, 1987). In cases of large myomas (>80 mm in diameter), a transverse suprapubic incision of 40 mm may be performed for the extraction of myomas after fragmentation. In these rare cases, the uterine incision is closed transparietally, using a classical needle holder placed through the suprapubic incision under laparoscopic control. In all cases, at the end of the procedure, the peritoneal cavity is irrigated with saline solution.

Results

Our experience consists of 147 intraperitoneal myomectomies performed on 70 patients between January 1, 1990 and October 1, 1991. During the same period, 64 myomas were removed by laparotomy in seven patients; thus 91% of myomectomies were performed by laparoscopy. Laparotomy was indicated because of contraindications to laparoscopic surgery, i.e. multiple or huge myomas. Myomas were diagnosed by pelvic examination, ultrasonography or by previous laparoscopy. Hysteroscopy was performed in 30 cases. Hysterosalpingography was performed in all cases of infertility. The main indication for laparoscopy was a pelvic mass in 41 cases (associated with pelvic pain in 15 cases and with infertility in nine cases), infertility in 22 cases, bleeding in six cases and severe endometriosis in one case. Forty-six patients out of 70 (65.7%) were treated preoperatively with a depot gonadotropin-releasing hormone agonist (GnRH, leuproreline 3.75 mg, Enantone, Takeda, Puteaux, France or Triptoreline 3.75 mg, decapeptyl, Ipsen-Biotech, Paris, France) for 2 or 3 months.

One hundred and forty-seven myomas were removed in 70 patients. Fifty-five had a mean diameter between 40 and 110 mm (37.4%). Sixty-eight myomas were subserous, 76 interstitial and 3 submucous. In 46 cases, myomectomy was the only procedure performed. In the 24 other cases, another procedure was associated (tuboplasty, vaporization of endometriosis, ovarian cystectomy, tubal sterilization, removal of a submucous myoma by hysteroscopy). Concerning the operative techniques, the uterine incision was performed with the knife in the 29 first cases. Subsequently, we used the monopolar hook in all 41 cases. Myometrium and serosa were closed with sutures in 43 out of 69 cases. An extension of the suprapubic incision to 40 mm was required for extraction of large myomas in seven cases and we elected to use a posterior colpotomy in eight cases.

We observed no complications and none of the patients required laparotomy or blood transfusion. Follow-up laparoscopy was performed 6 weeks after the initial laparoscopic myomectomy in seven cases. In six cases, no adhesions were noted. In one case, there were severe bowel adhesions to the myomectomy scar adherent to the posterior wall of the uterus (Dubuisson *et al.*, 1992).

Discussion

Preoperative evaluation is crucial in determining operative strategy, according to the number, the size, and the localization of myomas. Lesions within the uterus should be diagnosed by hysterosalpingography or hysteroscopy. In our experience, hysteroscopy should be systematically performed before laparoscopy because it allows the surgeon to differentiate between deep interstitial myomas which should be treated by laparoscopy from submucous myomas that can be treated by hysteroscopy. It may also diagnose submucous myomas associated with subserous or interstitial myomas. In these cases, ablation of the submucous myoma has to be performed during the same operation whether by operative hysteroscopy or laparoscopy. Small interstitial myomas, which may be palpated during laparotomy, can be overlooked during laparoscopy and should therefore be detected by preoperative ultrasound before instituting medical treatment (Fedele *et al.*, 1990). Precise preoperative diagnosis indicates whether laparoscopic myomectomy is possible or whether laparotomy should be performed for large or multiple myomas. Myomectomy should be an atraumatic procedure, minimizing blood loss, preventing disruption of the uterus and reducing the incidence of postoperative pelvic adhesions. Advances in operative endoscopy have allowed myomectomy to be safely performed by laparoscopy. In our experience, the mean operating time is less than 2 hours. The average length of stay in hospital was in the beginning of our series 2–3 days but now the length is usually 1 or 2 days. Operative laparoscopy has several advantages over laparotomy. The postoperative recovery time is much shorter and more comfortable and postoperative pain is reduced. Feeding can usually be resumed the same day and women can ambulate normally by the following day. Large and multiple myomas should not be removed by laparoscopic surgery because of the risk of bleeding, together with difficulty in the extraction of myomas and a prolonged operating time. In our experience, the upper limits are a diameter of more than 100 mm and a number greater than 4. After interstitial or submucous myomectomy, closure of the myometrium by suture is recommended to prevent postoperative bleeding and fragmentation of the uterus using the same techniques as employed at laparotomy. The risk of adhesion formation after laparoscopic myomectomy seems to be low.

Preoperative treatment with GnRH agonists in patients undergoing myomectomy may be beneficial. Gonadotropin-releasing hormone agonist probably causes myoma shrinkage by reducing circulating oestrogen levels. In a randomized, placebo-controlled, double-blind study evaluating the efficacy of leuprolide acetate depot in the treatment of uterine myoma, Friedman et al. (1989a,b) observed a mean reduction in uterine volume of 40%. Maximal reduction was achieved by 12 weeks of therapy with no further change observed after 24 weeks of treatment. Preoperative treatment with these agents facilitates surgery. Matta et al. (1988) observed that gonadotropin-releasing hormone agonist reduces uterine blood flow. A marked reduction in blood loss at surgery has been demonstrated for myomectomy by Shaw (1989) and for hysterectomy by Lumsden et al. (1987). However, Friedman et al. (1989a, b) observed a significant reduction in total intraoperative blood loss only in patients treated with leuprolide acetate with uterine volumes of $\geq 600 \, \text{cm}^3$ before treatment. In our experience, GnRH has the advantage of reducing bleeding during operative laparoscopy. The prevention of uterine bleeding during myomectomy seems particularly important in myomas larger than 40 mm. We used no other drugs because the use of vasopressin, a vasoconstrictive agent, is not allowed in France.

Conclusion

Advances in operative endoscopy have allowed the development of improved techniques for myomectomy by hysteroscopy or laparoscopy. In our experience operative laparoscopy has several advantages over laparotomy and the risks of complications is low in selected cases.

References

Bruhat MA, Manhes H, Choukroun J & Suzanne F (1977) Essai de traitement per coelioscopique de la grossesse extra-utérine. A propos de 26 observations. *Revue Française de Gynécologie et d'Obstétrique* 72:667.

Dubuisson JB, Aubriot FX & Cardone V (1987) Laparoscopic salpingectomy for tubal pregnancy. *Fertility and Sterility* 47:225.

Dubuisson JB, Lecuru F, Foulot H et al. (1992) Myomectomy by laparoscopy: a preliminary report of 43 cases. *Fertility and Sterility* 56:827–830.

Fedele L, Vercellin P, Bianchi S, Brioschi D & Dorta M (1990) Treatment with GnRH agonists before myomectomy and the risk of short-term myoma recurrence. *British Journal of Obstetrics and Gynaecology* 97:393.

Friedman AJ, Harrison-Atlas D, Barbieri RL et al. (1989a) A randomized, placebo-controlled, double-blind study evaluating the efficacy of leuprolide acetate depot in the treatment of uterine leiomyomata. *Fertility and Sterility* 51:251.

Friedman AJ, Rein MS, Harrison-Atlas D, Garfield JM & Doubilet PM (1989b) A randomized placebo-controlled, double-blind study evaluating leuprolide acetate depot treatment before myomectomy. *Fertility and Sterility* 52:728.

Lumsden MA, West CP & Baird DT (1987) Goserelin therapy before surgery for uterine fibroids. *Lancet* 1:36.

Matta WHM, Stabile I, Shaw RW & Campbell S (1988) Doppler assessment of uterine blood flow changes in patients with fibroids receiving the gonadotropin-releasing hormone agonist Buserelin*. *Fertility and Sterility* 49:1083.

Murphy AA (1987) Operative laparoscopy. *Fertility and Sterility* 47:1.

Reich H (1989) New techniques in advanced laparoscopic surgery. In Sutton CJG (ed) *Baillière's Clinical Obstetrics and Gynaecology. Laparoscopic Surgery* 3(3):655–682.

Semm K & Mettler L (1980) Technical progress in pelvic surgery via operative laparoscopy. *American Journal of Obstetrics and Gynecology* 138:121.

Shaw RW (1989) Mechanism of LHRH analogue action in uterine fibroids. *Hormone Research* 32:150.

22

Laparoscopic Pelvic Lymphadenectomy

DENIS QUERLEU* AND ERIC LEBLANC†

*Pavillon Paul Gellé, Roubaix, France
†Centre Oscar Lambret, Lille, France

Current clinical methods of staging pelvic carcinomas are highly inaccurate in detecting metastases to the pelvic lymph nodes (Feigen et al., 1987). The sensitivity of lymphangiography is less than 30%. This technique is unable to visualize internal iliac and other medial node groups. CT scan, as well as magnetic resonance imaging, with sensitivity ranging from 33 to 70% is insensitive if the nodes are not macroscopically enlarged. Lymphoscintigraphy is too unreliable for routine use.

As a consequence, lymph node biopsy remains the only reliable method for appraising the status of pelvic lymph nodes. However, the pathological specimens are taken either during a presurgical staging laparotomy, adding a significant morbidity, or during the surgical step of treatment, at a time when primary treatment decisions have already been taken.

Apart from tumour volume and stage, the presence of lymph node metastasis is the most relevant prognostic factor in most pelvic malignancies, particularly prostatic cancers in the male and carcinoma of the cervix in the female patients, and may influence treatment choice particularly in those patients with early-stage tumours.

Pelvic lymph node picking by a retroperitoneal endoscopic approach has been described (Wurtz et al., 1987). Progress in laparoscopic surgery gives the opportunity to perform a surgically satisfactory pelvic lymphadenectomy, removing the obturator, external iliac and hypogastric lymph nodes. Dargent and Salvat (1989) have described a panoramic retroperitoneal approach. We have described the technique of pelvic lymphadenec-tomy by laparoscopy (Querleu, 1989; Querleu et al., 1991). An investigational programme of laparoscopic para-aortic lymphadenectomy is under way (Querleu, 1992).

Surgical Technique

The technique is carried out on both sides. The patient is placed in the supine position without any flexion of the hips. No cervical tenaculae nor uterine cannulation is necessary. This point is particularly important in cases of carcinoma of the cervix, where trauma to the tumour is unwanted. Under general anaesthesia with tracheal intubation, a pneumoperitoneum is created and an 11 mm laparoscope (Karl Storz, Germany) is placed through a minimal umbilical incision. A video camera is attached. After observation of the liver surface, the appendix and the internal pelvic organs, two 5 mm incisions are made in the right and left inguinal areas, and trocars introduced into the abdomen. Ancillary 4.5 mm scissors, atraumatic forceps and irrigation–aspiration devices are required to be available throughout the procedure. An additional incision is made in the midline above the symphysis pubis, and a 9 mm trocar is inserted, so that the surgeon is ready at any time to use endoscopic clips and later to remove lymph nodes out of the abdomen with a three-arm retractable Dargent forceps (Lépine, Lyon, France).

Pelvic lymphadenectomy is performed on each side as follows. The external iliac vessels, ureter,

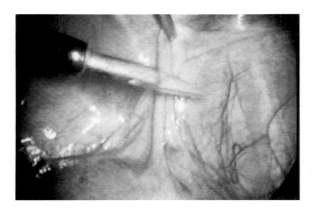

Figure 22.1 Incision of peritoneum between the round and infundibulopelvic ligaments.

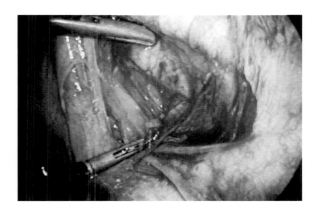

Figure 22.3 Identification and blunt dissection of the external iliac vein.

umbilical artery and, in lean patients, obturator nerve, are identified under the peritoneal surface. The operation begins with an incision with scissors of the pelvic peritoneum between the round and infundibulopelvic ligaments. The round ligament is grasped with the forceps. The peritoneum is cut near the round ligament then easily torn to open the whole area between the round and infundibulopelvic ligaments (Figure 22.1). The incision is made parallel to the axis of the external iliac vessels. The paravesical space is entered, then widened by blunt dissection between the umbilical artery medially and the external iliac vessels laterally. The instrument grasping the round ligament is freed, closed and placed in the paravesical space, pushing medially the umbilical artery. The pelvic floor is easily reached, either medially or laterally to the obturator pedicle, usually without any bleeding. The cellulolymphatic area below the external iliac vein is then clearly visible and safely dissected (Figure 22.2). The inferior aspect of the external iliac vein is separated by blunt dissection with a closed forceps (Figure 22.3). The obturator nerve is

identified and dissected caudally to the point where it leaves the pelvis. The fatty tissue between the obturator nerve and the external iliac vein is then grasped, and thoroughly separated from the pelvic wall. At this point, the pubic bone and the internal obturator muscle are exposed (Figure 22.4). The caudal part of the connective tissue pedicle is then detached by gentle traction from the area of the obturator foramen and of the femoral canal. The tissue flap is then firmly grasped and moved cranially, then carefully dissected from the external iliac vein and artery laterally and the umbilical artery medially (Figure 22.5). At this point, the cellulolymphatic flap is only attached in the inter-iliac bifurcation area. The external iliac artery is freed in the cranial direction, and tissue between the artery and vein may be removed at this time. It is gently separated by traction with a grasping forceps and blunt dissection with the closed tip of another instrument. Additional section of fibrous or lymphatic attachments is sometimes necessary. The tissue sample is thus dissected *en bloc* or in two or three parts, according to the anatomy and firmness of

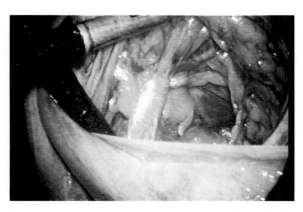

Figure 22.2 Laparoscopic view after opening of the paravesical space.

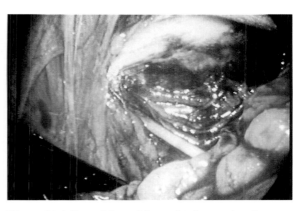

Figure 22.4 Exposition of the pubic bone, the obturator pedicle, the internal obturator muscle.

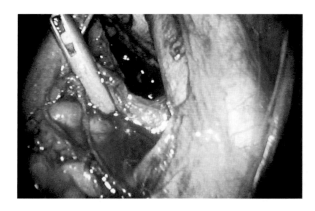

Figure 22.5 Freeing the cellulo lymphatic flap.

the areolar tissue. The sample has then to be extracted from the abdomen by means of the Dargent forceps, avoiding any contamination of the abdominal wall by carcinomatous cells. Haemostasis is checked. A minimal amount of blood may have to be aspirated. At the end of the procedure, the peritoneum is left open to allow drainage of the lymphatic fluid into the abdomen.

In premenopausal patients, a laparoscopic transposition of the ovaries may be added in order to avoid ovarian irradiation. This operation can be completed in the same way as it is done by laparotomy: section of the utero-ovarian pedicles after haemostasis by electrocautery, extra- or intracorporeal knots or, more easily, endo-GIA staplers, section of the peritoneum circumscribing the adnexae, freeing of the ovarian ligament, placement of the adnexae in the paracolic gutters. The ovaries are attached to the lateral peritoneum by endoscopic metallic clips, and are thus ready for later radiological localization.

Results

In our series, 75 patients underwent pretreatment laparoscopic staging between December 1988 and August 1991. Sixty-five of them presented with Fédération Internationale des Gynécologues et Obstétriciens (FIGO) IA2 ($n = 8$), IB ($n = 31$), IIA ($n = 7$), proximal IIB ($n = 19$) carcinoma of the cervix. The other ten patients presented with carcinoma of the endometrium ($n = 3$), borderline tumour of the ovary ($n = 1$), bladder ($n = 3$) and prostate ($n = 3$) cancers. Selection of patients was based upon the potential risks of prolonged pneumoperitoneum and the absence of cytologically positive nodes visible on CT scans. Their age range was 28–69 years (average 48.8). The

primary regional lymph nodes were histologically examined by frozen sections and/or by pathological examination in all but two cases. In these last two observations, metastatic epithelial cells were demonstrated on needle aspirates of unresectable nodes. Ten patients underwent additional ovarian transposition. Duration of the operation was 60–180 minutes (average 115).

One to 15 palpable nodes were removed from each side. Between 3 and 22 nodes were available for pathological examination (mean 9.9, 4.8 on the right side, 4.5 on the left side). In the entire series, 11 patients were node positive, the only patient with carcinoma of the ovary and 10 patients with carcinoma of the cervix (none of the 8 stage IA2 patients, 10 out of the 57 stage IB–IIB patients). Among the 55 node negative patients with carcinoma of the cervix, five underwent Schauta–Amreich radical vaginal hysterectomy. The last 50 patients had Wertheim's abdominal radical hysterectomy with pathological control of occasional remaining primary and of palpable secondary common iliac or para-aortic lymph nodes, 8 of them the same day, 42 of them 1–6 weeks later. No unexpected metastatic node was observed at laparotomy. Finally, if lymph node sampling by laparotomy is used as the gold standard, sensitivity and specificity were 100% in this series.

Observed Complications

Four intraoperative complications were observed. One patient did not tolerate the prolonged pneumoperitoneum, and we had to abandon the procedure after removal of only three nodes. In another case, bleeding from the umbilical artery necessitated bipolar coagulation of the vessel. In a third case, injury to an epigastric artery at a second-puncture entry required elective haemostasis. In one patient venous bleeding in the left paravesical space was controlled by compression with the endoscopic forceps. No emergency laparotomy was necessary during the period of study.

When laparoscopic lymphadenectomy was performed as the only procedure, the postoperative period was uneventful and the patients were discharged from the surgical ward the following day in all but one case. In this case, a pelvic haematoma was observed 5 days after laparoscopic pelvic lymphadenectomy and radium application but it resolved spontaneously. No lymphocyst was observed. No bowel adhesions were noticed

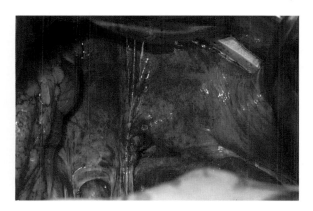

Figure 22.6 Peritoneal healing after pelvic lymphadenectomy.

at further laparotomy, and spontaneous healing of the peritoneum always occurred without intraperitoneal sequelae (Figure 22.6). However, dense fibrosis of the retroperitoneal tissue was noticed in five cases. At the time of submission of the manuscript, we have observed three late recurrences of a cervical tumour in node-negative patients: two recurrences in the vaginal cuff, and one at the pelvic side wall and para-aortic nodes.

Potential Morbidity: Prevention and Management

Selection of patients is based on general contra-indications to prolonged pneumoperitoneum: morbidly obese patients, patients with advanced coronary or respiratory disease. However, these concerns may be overcome by the use of a low abdominal pressure, less than 10 mmHg (1.33 kPa).

Many potential complications may occur during laparoscopic pelvic lymphadenectomy. Although many of them have not yet been observed in our experience, advice concerning their management will be given. Only specific complications will be addressed, and divided into three categories: intraoperative, early and late complications.

Intraoperative Complications

Vascular injury is the major potential risk of laparoscopic pelvic lymphadenectomy, but is much less frequent than one could expect.

Diffuse oozing is comparatively rare, even in moderately obese patients, even when preventive haemostasis by clips is not used. In our experience, haemostasis of capillary vessels is either not necessary, or obtained after irrigation with warm

saline solution. This low incidence of bleeding is likely to be due to the pressure of the pneumoperitoneum.

Injury of large vessels is even rarer, as the magnification provided by the laparoscope allows a precise dissection of the paravesical fossae. Significant bleeding may, however, occur by injury to pelvic arteries or veins. Injury to the branches of the hypogastric artery (particularly uterine artery, superior vesical artery or umbilical artery) is managed by direct haemostasis of the vessel: clips (7 mm clips are preferable) or bipolar haemostasis should be instantly available. In the same way, laceration of pelvic veins (particularly aberrant obturator veins and less commonly obturator, uterine or epigastric veins) may be managed laparoscopically: unless the bleeding stops after 2 minutes of compression of the injured vessel, clips or coagulation should be used.

Injury of the external iliac or hypogastric artery is very unlikely to occur. Experience of the laparotomy approach is that it is usually due to bleeding from an aberrant minor branch, and may be managed by application of a clip. Injury of the external iliac vein or of a main branch of internal iliac veins is the most serious potential risk of pelvic lymphadenectomy. It may occur during node sampling, and is usually due to a lateral laceration of the vessel. Two areas must be dissected with special care: the inferior aspect of the external iliac vein, near the obturator foramen, where inappropriate traction may lead to tearing of aberrant obturator veins at their junction with the external iliac vein, and the area below the hypogastric artery bifurcation. In this respect, operators are strongly advised against attempts at dissection of fixed lymph nodes. When such unresectable nodes are encountered, the diagnosis of metastasis is possible by a cytological examination of fine needle aspirates, preventing the complications of a risky dissection of the node. If bleeding of the external iliac vein occurs, compression may again be successful: a closed forceps may be pushed strongly, thus compressing the vessel against the pelvic sidewall. If haemorrhage persists, the use of clips or coagulation is not advised, as it may worsen the laceration. Introduction of vascular sutures through second-puncture trocars is theoretically possible, but we have never heard about their successful use in external iliac vein injury. As a consequence, external iliac vein laceration may have to be managed by laparotomy.

Bleeding from the ovarian ligament is prevented by gentle handling and retraction of this ligament. If it occurs, management includes placement of clips, staples or bipolar coagulation. If laparoscopic transposition of the ovary is indicated, the surgical technique follows the same principles as that employed at laparotomy: section of the utero-ovarian anastomosis and dissection of the ovarian ligament in order to move the ovary above the pelvic brim. Bleeding may occur predominantly at the level of the uterine cornua, from the uterine artery or veins, and is usually prevented by primary coagulation or application of clips or staples. Coagulation of bleeders is possible in this area.

The risk of *nerve injury* is limited to accidental section of the obturator nerve. This accident is very unlikely to occur, and is prevented by careful dissection of the paravesical fossa, facilitated by the laparoscopic magnification. As section of the obturator nerve has minor motor and sensitive consequences, no repair is warranted.

Ureteral injury is unlikely to occur if only interiliac node sampling has been done. The ureter is not in the operative field, and is usually retracted along with the ovarian ligament, even during dissection of the hypogastric bifurcation. However, the upper area of the dissection must always be managed carefully, avoiding unnecessary grasping of tissues or blind coagulation. If necessary, the ureter may be identified under the peritoneum and dissected free from the pelvic brim to the parameter. Ureteral repair is obviously necessary in case of surgical injury.

Missing lymph nodes is not a complication, but leads to a loss of accuracy of the method, and to inadequate care to unsuspected node-positive patients. The first concern is the risk of missing obturator or external iliac nodes, that may be prevented by careful identification of nerve and vessels, up to the hypogastric bifurcation, and thorough ablation of the cellulolymphatic tissue. In this respect, the learning curve is a problem: beginners are advised to check the quality of node sampling at subsequent laparotomies, by counting the average number of sampled nodes, or by comparing the observed incidence of lymph node metastasis in the cases they manage to that observed in the literature for cervical cancers of the same stage (Averette, 1987).

Missing distant nodes is another problem. Suspect common iliac nodes must be searched and may be sampled during laparoscopy. An incision of the peritoneum above the ureter is made, and identification of the common iliac vessels allows a safe sampling of suspect nodes. In our experience, systematic sampling of nodes in the promontory and common iliac area has been recently introduced. The risk of skip metastasis in the periaortic area must also be addressed. As far

as early cervical cancer is concerned, the incidence of aortic nodes in the absence of pelvic nodes is very low, presumably less than 1%. However, if the technique is applied to cases of advanced cervical carcinoma, periaortic sampling may have to be considered. Our group is involved in a clinical trial assessing the feasibility of periaortic node sampling by laparoscopy. Eight patients have now been operated upon, with no complications.

Early Postoperative Complications

The postoperative period is usually quite uneventful. Many potential complications are possible, but are unspecific: general complications of laparoscopy such as undiagnosed bowel injury, or complications of a radical hysterectomy performed at the same time will not be discussed in this chapter.

Early postoperative haemorrhage has never occurred in our experience. Acute anaemia and clinical signs of haemoperitoneum clearly indicate emergency reoperation. If the patient's condition is relatively stable, it is possible to repeat the laparoscopy. Laparoscopic aspiration of blood and clots is cumbersome but possible and allows a precise localization of the bleeding. The problem can be solved by coagulation or clip application. Otherwise, a laparotomy may be needed.

In cases of moderate bleeding, the patient may develop a pelvic haematoma. Surgical drainage is usually not necessary, as many pelvic haematomas do not require any treatment or may be managed by aspiration under ultrasound monitoring.

Lymphocyst formation is a peculiar complication of lymph node biopsy. Some operators feel that this complication may be prevented by liberal use of surgical clips before division of lymphatic vessels and by closed-suction drainage of the retroperitoneum. This technique may be applied laparoscopically. Although we do not place preventive clips for lymphostasis nor any drain in the dissection area, we have not seen a single case of significant lymphocyst in our experience, probably because we leave the peritoneum opened. Drainage of lymph fluid into the peritoneal cavity is followed by resorption until the leakage of lymph fluid spontaneously stops. If a lymphocyst develops, aspiration under ultrasound monitoring is a safe and efficient management.

Ileus may be caused by the adhesion of the small bowel to the operative field. We advise, when such a complication is suspected, an early second look laparoscopy: recent adhesions are usually quite easy to free laparoscopically.

Late Complications

Leg lymphoedema is rare after pelvic lymphadenectomy, and its incidence should be even lowered by avoiding the removal of the lymphatic area external to the external iliac artery.

Tissue scarring after laparoscopic lymphadenectomy may involve peritoneal or retroperitoneal repair. The peritoneum usually heals with minimal scarring, and no or minimal adhesions. If adhesions develop, there is a risk of late bowel occlusion or of radiation injury. The areolar tissue in the retroperitoneal space heals with a dense fibrosis, making subsequent dissections uneasy and risky. For this reason, it is advisable to perform the radical hysterectomy, if indicated, the same day or not later than 7 days after laparoscopic lymphadenectomy.

Indications

Laparoscopic pelvic lymphadenectomy may become an indispensable tool in gynaecological or urological oncology whenever pathological examination of the pelvic lymph nodes is necessary and adequate in the pretherapeutic staging of pelvic malignancies. In the near future, the perspective of laparoscopic para-aortic lymphadenectomy may extend the indications for laparoscopic staging of pelvic tumours On the other hand, laparoscopic, as well as surgical, staging is useless when the presence of metastatic cells has been documented by fine needle aspiration of suspicious nodes shown by computed tomography scanning.

The first indication in gynaecological oncology is the staging of early, operable, carcinoma of the cervix (Querleu et al., 1991). The risk of 'skip' metastases to the para-aortic nodes without pelvic node involvement is very low (less than 1%) in these cases, and occurs almost only in patients with large tumours (more than 4 cm). As a consequence, stage IB–IIB cases with negative pathological staging may be cured by local therapy (brachytherapy or radical vaginal surgery). On the other hand, radical hysterectomy does not seem justified when metastatic nodes are present (Potter et al., 1990). In addition, some stage IA2 cervical carcinomas without pelvic node metastasis can be treated by cervical conization alone. Laparoscopic staging may thus reduce the cost and effects on fertility of the treatment of early carcinomas of the cervix.

The role of laparoscopic lymphadenectomy may in the future be investigated in the staging of advanced carcinomas of the cervix. However, the poor outcome of patients with para-aortic nodal metastasis, regardless of treatment (Stehman et al., 1991), and the necessity of external irradiation, regardless of pelvic node involvement, limits the role of pathological staging of such tumours to investigational settings.

Laparoscopic pretherapeutic staging of stage I endometrial carcinomas is not very useful for the patient, insofar as surgery is indicated, whatever the node status. Furthermore, the prevalence of lymph node metastasis is low in this condition. However, laparoscopic lymphadenectomy may be included in the surgical step of treatment, in association with vaginal surgery. In the same way, laparoscopic lymphadenectomy and oophorectomy may be an adequate management of unsuspected endometrial adenocarcinomas found in hysterectomy specimens.

Ovarian carcinomas are best treated by laparotomy. However, thanks to progress in laparoscopic surgery, the laparoscopic surgeon may one day meet the criteria for adequate staging and therapy in some cases of early ovarian carcinoma. However, the method cannot be recommended until adequate infra-renal para-aortic node sampling can be routinely completed by laparoscopy.

Laparoscopic staging may become in the near future quite popular among urological oncologists. The prognostic value of lymph node involvement is important enough in cases of bladder or prostate carcinomas to sort out those patients without node metastasis, that may be treated by surgery, from those with metastatic disease, in whom surgery is not indicated.

Conclusion

As far as major laparoscopic surgery is concerned, it should first be stressed that laparoscopic lymphadenectomy is a feasible operation, but only in experienced hands. Thorough knowledge of oncological surgery, including anatomy of the pelvic extraperitoneal spaces and management of vascular injuries, and, of course, of laparoscopic surgery techniques, is mandatory. Complete instrumentation, including a full set of scissors, forceps, irrigation and suction devices, clip applicators, bipolar coagulation, is necessary not only to perform the standard operation, but also to manage potential minor and even major complications. The patient must be informed that an emergency laparotomy may unexpectedly be performed. Therefore, only surgeons experienced in gynecological oncology and operative laparoscopy should undertake this operation. However, potential severe complications are infrequent in clinical practice, and laparoscopic lymphadenectomy may be considered as a safe procedure, and helps to reduce the cost and risks of management of carcinoma of the cervix, as well as other pelvic malignancies.

This technique is the first application of endoscopy in gynaecological or urological oncology, and paves the way to further progress. Laparoscopic radical hysterectomy (Canis *et al.*, 1990) or laparoscopically assisted radical vaginal hysterectomy (Querleu *et al.*, 1991), with full ureter dissection from the iliac area to the bladder, has already been performed and we have introduced in clinical practice para-aortic sampling by laparoscopy. If late results confirm the safety and efficiency of these new techniques, laparoscopy could become a major tool in pelvic oncology.

Summary

Pelvic lymphadenectomy is feasible by laparoscopy. An incision of the peritoneum between the round and infundibulopelvic ligament on each side gives access to the retroperitoneal space. Subsequently, laparoscopic surgery allows precise dissection of external and internal iliac vessels, umbilical artery, and obturator nerve. The peritoneum is left open, and the lymph drains into the peritoneal cavity. The operation was performed in 75 patients, 65 of them with stage I or II cervical carcinoma, between November 1988 and August 1991. An average of 9.9 nodes were removed, and there was no significant morbidity. Sensitivity and specificity were 100% in this experience, but one patient has since recurred with malignancy in the pelvic sidewall and para-aortic area. A laparoscopic staging of gynaecological or urological pelvic malignancies may reduce the incidence of laparotomy in these cases. Node-negative cases may be treated by local irradiation or vaginal surgery alone, whereas node-positive cases are probably not a good indication for surgery at all.

References

Averette HE, Donato DM, Lovecchio JL & Sevin BU (1987) Surgical staging of gynecologic malignancies. *Cancer* **60**:2010–2020.

Canis M, Mage G, Wattiez A *et al.* (1990) La chirurgie endoscopique a-t-elle une place dans la chirurgie radicale du cancer du col utérin? *Journal de Gynécologie, Obstétrique et Biologie de la Reproduction* **19**:921.

Dargent D & Salvat J (1989) *L'Envahissement Ganglionnaire Pelvien.* Paris: Medsci-McGraw-Hill.

Feigen M, Crocker EF, Read J & Crandon AJ (1987) The value of lymphoscintigraphy, lymphangiography and computed tomography scanning in the preoperative assessment of lymph nodes involved by pelvic malignant conditions. *Surgery, Gynecology and Obstetrics* **65**:107–110.

Potter ME, Alvarez RD, Shingleton HM, Soong SJ & Hatch KD (1990) Early invasive cervical cancer with pelvic lymph node involvement: to complete or not to complete radical hysterectomy? *Gynecologic Oncology* **37**:78–81.

Querleu D (1989) Lymphadénectomie pelvienne sous contrôle coelioscopique. *Deuxième Congrés Mondial d'Endoscopie Gynécologique, Clermont-Ferrand, France.*

Querleu D (1991) Hystérectomies de Schauta-Amreich et Schauta-Stoeckel assistées par coelioscopie. *Journal de Gynécologie, Obstétrique et Biologie de la Reproduction* **20**: 747–748.

Querleu D (1992) Laparoscopic paraaortic lymphadenectomy in the staging of advanced carcinoma of the cervix. *International Congress of Gynecologic Endoscopy, AAGL 21st Meeting.* Chicago, 25 September.

Querleu D, Leblanc E & Castelain B (1991) Laparoscopic pelvic lymphadenectomy in the staging of early carcinoma of the cervix. *American Journal of Obstetrics and Gynecology* **164**:579–581.

Stehman FB, Bundy BN, Di Saia P *et al.* (1991) Carcinoma of the cervix treated with radiation therapy I. A multivariate analysis of prognostic variables in the gynecologic oncology group. *Cancer* **67**: 2776–2785.

Wurtz A, Mazeman E, Gosselin B *et al.* (1987) Bilan anatomique des adénopathies rétropéritonéales par endoscopie chirurgicale. *Annales de Chirurgie* **41**:258–263.

23

Laparoscopic Assisted Vaginal Hysterectomy (LAVH)

D. ALAN JOHNS

Richland Medical Center, Fort Worth, Texas, USA

Hysterectomy is the fourth most common inpatient surgical procedure performed in the United States; 656 000 hysterectomies were performed in 1987 alone (Findlay, 1990). Of these hysterectomies, approximately 70% are performed using the abdominal approach and 30% are done vaginally (Kovac et al., 1990). The majority of these procedures are done for benign pelvic conditions such as uterine prolapse, abnormal uterine bleeding, cervical dysplasia, menorrhagia, dysmenorrhoea, stress urinary incontinence, uterine fibroids, and endometriosis.

As instruction in vaginal surgery techniques declines in many residency programmes, the percentage of hysterectomies done by the abdominal approach will almost certainly increase. This trend, unfortunately, is occurring at a time when our health care dollar is stretched beyond its limits.

Traditional contraindications to vaginal hysterectomy are numerous and varied, many contraindications are based more on operator experience than true surgical contraindications (Isaacs, 1990; Smith and Thompson, 1986; Kovac et al., 1990).

These published contraindications include:

1. Previous pelvic surgery.
2. Endometriosis.
3. Previous caesarean section.
4. Significant uterine enlargement.
5. Limited uterine mobility.
6. Pelvic pain.
7. Suspected pathology of the adnexae.
8. Ectopic pregnancy.
9. Acute or chronic pelvic inflammatory disease.
10. Suspected bowel or appendiceal disease.
11. Previous uterine suspension.
12. Invasive cervical or endometrial carcinoma.

Many of these diagnoses are made based on history, pelvic examination, and ultrasound or CT scans of the pelvis. Unfortunately, these parameters are often unreliable when predicting the extent of pelvic pathology (Kovac et al., 1990). The extent and nature of this pathology is a significant factor determining the surgical approach.

In previously published reports, diagnostic laparoscopy carried out prior to planned *abdominal* hysterectomy revealed a large percentage of these patients were candidates for vaginal hysterectomy after visual examination of the pelvis (Kovac et al., 1990). Using diagnostic laparoscopy alone, many abdominal procedures were avoided.

Using operative laparoscopy techniques conceived to treat extensive pelvic endometriosis, myoma, pelvic adhesive disease, ectopic pregnancy, pelvic abscess, and adnexal disease, most patients requiring abdominal hysterectomy for these conditions can enjoy the benefits of vaginal surgery. The vast majority of patients with these benign pelvic conditions can be treated with a combination of operative endoscopy and vaginal surgery. However, the skills required for advanced operative endoscopy and vaginal surgery must both be mastered to combine safely the benefits of both.

Laparoscopy can be utilized in many of these patients with one or more of the contraindications to vaginal surgery.

Previous Pelvic Surgery

Patients who have undergone previous pelvic surgery often have adhesions involving pelvic organs and bowel. Fear of injury to these structures has prevented gynaecological surgeons from using the vaginal approach in these patients.

Diagnostic laparoscopy done prior to hysterectomy allows accurate assessment of the pelvis for adhesive disease. When adhesions are present, scissors or laser dissection frees the uterus and adnexal structures, allowing vaginal surgery to proceed safely. The magnifying capabilities of a laparoscope coupled with precise microsurgical dissection allows safe dissection of bowel, ureter, or adnexal structures.

Endometriosis

When abdominal or vaginal hysterectomy is accomplished by traditional methods, peritoneal and bowel implants of endometriosis often remain untreated. Implants on the pelvic sidewalls or beneath the ovaries may be out of view and missed by the surgeon.

Laparoscopic examination of the pelvis, including peritoneal surfaces, ovaries, and bowel, is an examination under *magnification*. It is therefore less likely endometrial implants will be missed when a careful laparoscopic examination precedes hysterectomy. When endometrial implants are identified, they can be destroyed by electrocautery or laser, or excised (depending on depth of penetration) prior to removal of the uterus or ovaries.

Complete excision of pelvic endometriosis at the time of vaginal hysterectomy may allow preservation of one or both ovaries when they would otherwise be sacrificed to prevent hormonal stimulation of implants left behind. In addition, adhesive disease often accompanying the endometriosis can be treated endoscopically to allow the hysterectomy to be completed vaginally.

Previous Caesarean Section

Patients who have undergone previous caesarean section often have adhesions involving the anterior cul-de-sac, lower uterine segment, and bladder. The possible presence of these adhesions is considered a contraindication to vaginal hysterectomy by some authors. After insertion of the laparoscope, these adhesions can be lysed with scissors or laser. The bladder is then dissected away from the lower uterine segment with the

blunt dissecting probe and aquadissection. This technique is virtually identical to that used during abdominal hysterectomy. Once these adhesions are removed and the bladder dissected from the lower uterine segment, vaginal hysterectomy is feasible.

Pelvic Pain

Patients with unexplained pelvic pain have traditionally been treated by abdominal hysterectomy. It is thought that the cause of the pain may be diagnosed and treated only when the pelvis is evaluated at laparotomy. Vaginal surgery would not allow visual evaluation of the pelvic cavity.

Diagnostic laparoscopy allows evaluation of the pelvis, reproductive tract, and upper abdomen. The source of the pain can often be identified and surgery tailored to those findings. A laparotomy is not necessary for simple diagnosis.

Suspected Adnexal Pathology

Often adnexal pathology is suspected when none exists (Kovac *et al.*, 1990). The presence or absence of adnexal pathology is easily demonstrated at laparoscopy. Should benign adnexal pathology be present, it can be treated with a combination of endoscopic and vaginal surgery or laparotomy as indicated.

Uterine Myoma

Uterine enlargement (most commonly caused by myoma) has been a traditional contraindication to vaginal hysterectomy. Endoscopic freeing of the adnexal structures, round ligaments, uterine arteries, and bladder serosa will allow most myomatous uteri (as large as 20 week size) to be morcellated and removed vaginally.

Once all major vessels have been controlled laparoscopically, simple morcellation and removal of a large fibroid uterus (with no concern for bleeding) becomes a much simpler task.

Ectopic Pregnancy

The patient with a diagnosis of tubal pregnancy who desires hysterectomy may be treated by combining endoscopic removal of the ectopic pregnancy with vaginal hysterectomy. Removal of the affected tube with electrocautery in conjunction with the vaginal hysterectomy is the most common technique used.

Acute or Chronic Pelvic Inflammatory Disease

Pelvic inflammatory disease with associated adhesions or abscess may be successfully treated by laparoscopic techniques. This topic is covered elsewhere in this book.

Should the patient be a candidate for removal of the uterus or adnexae, laparoscopic treatment of pelvic adhesions with freeing of the adnexal structures will most often allow vaginal hysterectomy to be accomplished. Freeing of the adnexae and removal of adhesions or abscess cavity can be accomplished endoscopically prior to vaginal removal.

Minimal Uterine Mobility

When uterine mobility is limited due to shortened or tense pelvic support (uterosacral ligaments), laparoscopy will allow freeing of this support to the point that vaginal hysterectomy can be accomplished. The uterus is freed to (and including) the uterosacral ligaments utilizing endoscopic electrosurgery or staples. Vaginal removal of the uterus can then be easily accomplished.

Pelvic Mass

Most pelvic masses are associated with benign conditions. Introduction of the laparoscope into the peritoneal cavity for diagnosis prior to consideration of the mode of hysterectomy will often save the patient an unnecessary laparotomy.

When benign masses are found, laparoscopic techniques will allow vaginal removal of even the largest of these. When a malignancy is discovered, the appropriate surgical procedure is performed. Laparoscopy performed to make the diagnosis has no deleterious affects on subsequent operative procedures.

Technique

After introduction of the 10 mm diagnostic laparoscope through an intraumbilical incision, two 5 mm suprapubic incisions are made approxi-

mately 4–5 cm on either side of the midline. Care is exercised to avoid the inferior epigastric vessels with these punctures. The pelvis is then thoroughly inspected and pathology evaluated. Adnexal structures to be preserved or removed are closely evaluated. The anterior and posterior cul-de-sacs are inspected for adhesions or endometriosis. The extent of laparoscopic surgery required to allow the procedure to be completed vaginally is then planned (Figure 23.1).

If one or both ovaries are to be removed, the initial step requires entering the retroperitoneal space. This is accomplished by making a nick in the peritoneum between the round ligament and the infundibulopelvic ligament. The retroperitoneal space is then opened with a hollow dissection probe. Irrigating fluid forced through this dissection probe opens the retroperitoneal space and allows easy visualization of retroperitoneal structures. The ureter is identified as it crosses the pelvic brim and dissected (if necessary) to the uterine artery.

The ovarian artery and vein are skeletonized. These two vessels are then controlled with electrosurgery (electrodesiccation), endoscopic sutures, or clips. They can then be safely transected (Figure 23.2).

The anterior and posterior leaves of the broad ligament are opened to the uterine artery. The round ligament is then desiccated with bipolar cautery and transected. Careful blunt aquadissection is used to dissect and identify the uterine artery.

If, in the surgeon's opinion, the artery cannot be adequately controlled vaginally, it is coaptated with bipolar cautery or occluded with laparoscopic staples and transected (see Figure 23.4).

The peritoneum overlying the bladder is then opened with scissors or laser (Figure 23.3). Capillary bleeding will be encountered often during this part of the procedure and can be controlled easily with a microbipolar cautery. The bladder is then bluntly dissected away from the lower uterine segment with the dissecting probe and aquadissection. This step (when accomplished laparoscopically) allows very easy entry into the peritoneal cavity during the vaginal portion of the operation.

If necessary, a laparoscopic colpotomy can then be performed with unipolar cautery, scissors, or laser (Figure 23.5). The uterosacral ligaments can then be desiccated with bipolar cautery and transected (Figure 23.6).

In the rare circumstance where completion of the vaginal portion of the operation is impossible (vaginal stenosis), the anterior cul-de-sac is entered with cautery or laser after the bladder

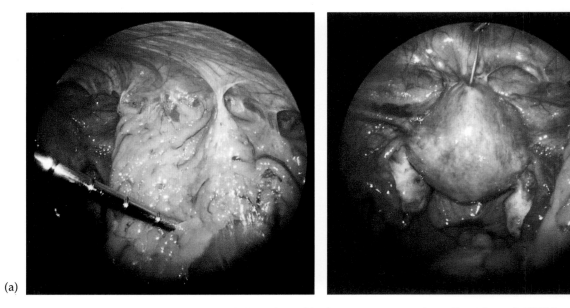

Figure 23.1 (a) Preoperative view of the pelvis. (b) The same patient after adhesiolysis (LAVH Stage 1).

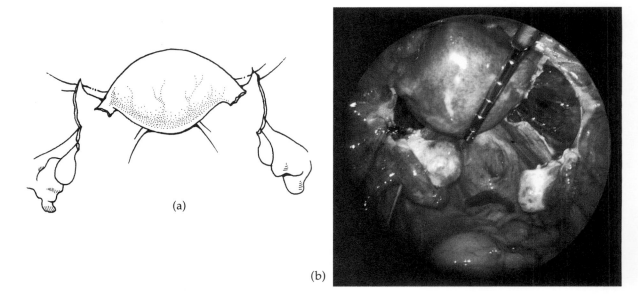

Figure 23.2 Both adnexa have been freed (LAVH Stage 2).

has been blunt dissected away from the lower uterine segment (Figure 23.7). The cervix is then amputated from the apex of the vagina with operating scissors, unipolar cautery, laser, or staple/cutting device.

The uterus can then be removed (after fragmentation) through the vagina with grasping forceps. In rare circumstances, fragmentation and removal through a suprapubic sleeve may be necessary. Semm (1992) has recently described a technique whereby the cervix is left in place and the supracervical portion of the uterus is removed endoscopically. He suggests 'reaming out' the endocervical canal with the Serrated Edged Macro Morcellator (SEMM) after the laparoscopic portion of the hysterectomy has been completed. This

technique is a variation of the supracervical abdominal hysterectomies done many years ago. Its purpose is to retain the cervix and its supporting ligaments while removing as much of the endocervical canal as possible. Any advantages of this procedure await further investigation.

In these circumstances, the vaginal apex can then be closed laparoscopically with interrupted absorbable suture or staples (Figure 23.8) (Reich and DeCaprio, 1989).

When the surgeon is ready to begin the vaginal portion of the procedure, the patient should be repositioned as she would be for vaginal hysterectomy. This repositioning allows better access for removal of the uterus and adnexal structures and closure of the vaginal cuff.

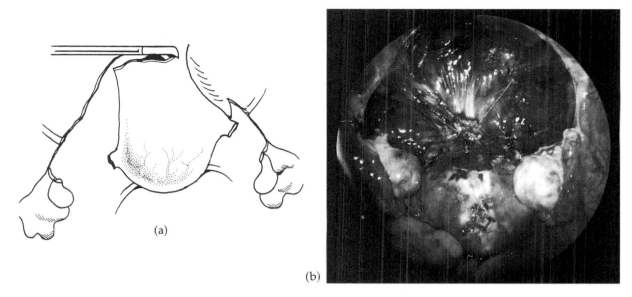

Figure 23.3 (a) Bladder peritoneum entered. (b) The bladder has been dissected from the lower uterine segment (LAVH Stage 3).

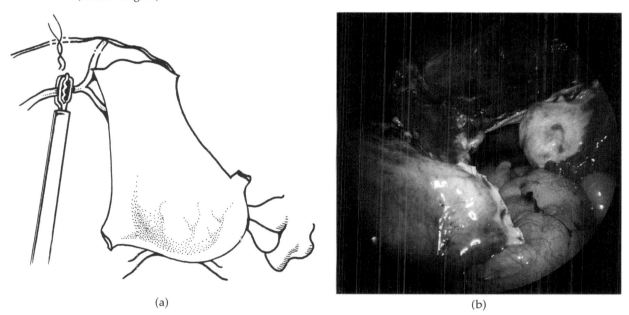

Figure 23.4 (a) Uterine artery coarctated. (b) Uterine artery identified and transected (LAVH Stage 4).

After completion of the procedure, the abdomen is reinflated and the operative field closely inspected with the laparoscope (Figure 23.9). This usually does not require repositioning of the patient. Most often, small areas of capillary bleeding will be identified and are controlled with bipolar cautery. The abdominal cavity is then thoroughly irrigated and all blood and debris removed. Approximately 1000 ml of irrigating fluid is left in the pelvis at the conclusion of the procedure.

The procedure becomes somewhat more difficult when the ovaries are to be preserved. In this case, the round ligament is desiccated and transected. Care must be taken to control

Sampson's artery prior to transection of the round ligament. Acuadissection is then used to identify the posterior leaf of the broad ligament. Large veins course through the entire broad ligament and must be avoided during this dissection. Injury to these vessels will produce considerable bleeding which is very difficult to control.

The ureter is identified as it courses through the retroperitoneal space. The posterior leaf of the broad ligament is then opened above the ureter near the utero-ovarian ligament.

The tube is then desiccated at the urterotubal junction and transected. The remainder of the broad ligament is then desiccated and transected (or stapled and transected). Laparoscopic sutures

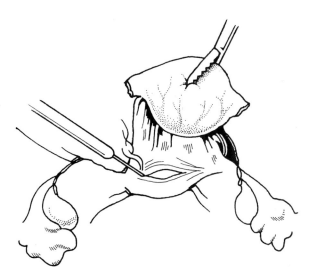

Figure 23.5 Posterior colpotomy.

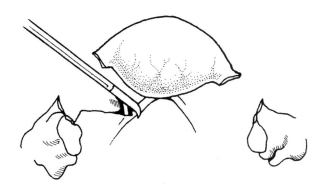

Figure 23.6 Uterosacral ligament transected.

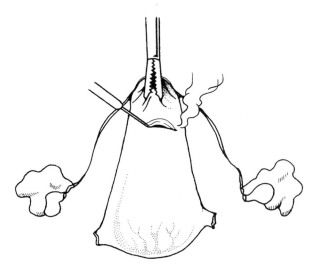

Figure 23.7 Anterior colpotomy.

can also be used during this phase of the procedure. The utero-ovarian ligament is identified, controlled with cautery, staples, or sutures and transected.

The remainder of the laparoscopic portion of

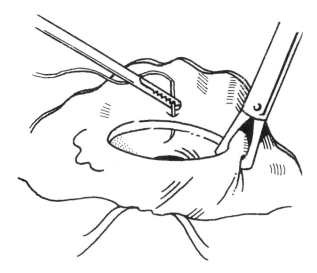

Figure 23.8 Laparoscopic closure of vaginal cuff.

the hysterectomy is then completed as far as necessary to assure vaginal removal of the uterus.

Patients with extensive endometriosis, benign adnexal pathology, or uterine myoma are treated exactly as they would be should laparotomy be used. Laparoscopic techniques are used to free pelvic structures to the point that vaginal hysterectomy can easily be accomplished.

Postoperative Care

A Foley catheter may be used postoperatively, but is removed as soon as possible. Since there is little to no manipulation of the bowel, postoperative ileus is very uncommon. Patients are begun on an unrestricted diet as soon as they desire. Postoperative pain can usually be controlled with oral analgesics within a few hours. Most patients are dismissed from the hospital within 36 hours of their operative procedure.

Conclusions

The combination of laparoscopic techniques with vaginal surgery provides many potential benefits. These include:

1. Providing most patients the benefits of vaginal surgery who would otherwise be committed to abdominal procedures.
2. The decision for laparotomy or vaginal surgery can be made after an accurate laparoscopic evaluation of the pelvis has been made. Minimal guesswork enters into the decision-making process.
3. Those patients with endometriosis benefit from a more complete excision and destruction of

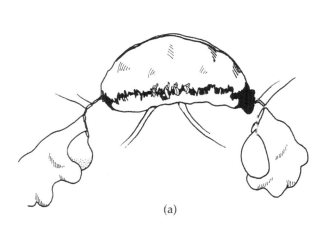

(a)

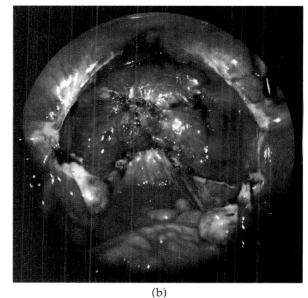

(b)

Figure 23.9 Postoperative view of the pelvis.

their disease. In some, ovaries may be preserved which would otherwise be sacrificed.

4. Since laparoscopic dissection of the bladder from the lower uterine segment is done under direct vision, the incidence of bladder perforation should decrease.

5. The risk of perforation of the rectum during colpotomy should be decreased since the cul-de-sac has been inspected prior to the colpotomy being performed. Any obliteration of the cul-de-sac can be identified and handled accordingly before the colpotomy is performed.

6. When the operative field is inspected laparoscopically after closure of the vaginal cuff, any bleeding can be easily identified and controlled. This bleeding goes unnoticed with traditional vaginal hysterectomy. Control of this bleeding should decrease the risk of postoperative bleeding. This may also decrease the risk of postoperative infection and resultant febrile morbidity.

7. Using electrosurgical laparoscopic techniques, the amount of suturing required to complete the hysterectomy is greatly decreased. Minimal tissue destruction from careful laparoscopic dissection coupled with laparoscopic removal of blood, clots, and debris at the end of the procedure should result in minimal postoperative pain and adhesion formation.

8. When compared to abdominal hysterectomy, vaginal hysterectomy results in a shortened hospital stay (1–2 days versus 3–4 days) and significant savings in hospital cost (Johns, 1991).

9. From morbidity and mortality studies, vaginal

Table 23.1 Laparoscopically assisted vaginal hysterectomy (LAVH) staging

Stage
0	Laparoscopy done—no laparoscopic procedure performed prior to vaginal hysterectomy
1	Procedure included laparoscopic adhesiolysis and/or excision of endometriosis (see Figure 23.1)
2	Either or both adnexa freed laparoscopically (see Figure 23.2)
3	Bladder dissected from uterus (see Figure 23.3)
4	Uterine artery transected laparoscopically (see Figure 23.4)
5	Anterior and/or posterior colpotomy or entire uterus freed

SUBSCRIPT:
0 Neither ovary excised
1 One ovary excised
2 Both ovaries excised

Note: If the extent of the procedure performed laparoscopically varied on the right and left pelvic sidewalls, stage the procedure by the most advanced side.

hysterectomy is safer than abdominal hysterectomy (Bolsen, 1982).

Studies comparing laparoscopic assisted vaginal hysterectomy with conventional vaginal hysterectomy and abdominal hysterectomy are needed at this point to confirm or deny many of these potential advantages. In an attempt to standardize terminology with reference to laparoscopic assisted vaginal hysterectomy, a staging system for LAVH has been devised (Table 23.1) (Johns and Diamond, 1991). Using this staging system, multicentre studies can be undertaken with accurate comparison of techniques used in individual patients.

Combining techniques and skills will hopefully allow more patients to take advantage of the obvious benefits of vaginal surgery. This will require dedication on the part of the gynaecological surgeon of the future. Extensive skills in the techniques of operative laparoscopy and vaginal surgery must be mastered. The health care system and our patients will ultimately benefit.

References

Bolsen B (1982) Study suggests vaginal hysterectomy is safer. *Journal of the American Medical Association* **247**:13.

Findlay S (1990) The health-insurance factor. *US News & World Report* April 30, 1990:57.

Isaacs JH (1990) *Gynecology and Obstetrics. Clinical Gynecology*, Vol. 1, Chap. 50, pp 1–11. Philadelphia: J.B. Lippincott Company.

Johns DA (1991) Medis Groups Frequency Report, Quality Assurance Department, Harris Hospital, Fort Worth. February 27, 1991.

Johns DA & Diamond M (1992) Laparoscopically assisted vaginal hysterectomy (LAVH) staging. Abstract submitted September, 1992.

Kovac SR, Cruikshank SH & Retto HF (1990) Laparoscopy-assisted vaginal hysterectomy. *Journal of Gynecologic Surgery* **6**:185.

Reich H & DeCaprio J (1989) *Laparoscopic Hysterectomy*. Kingston, PA: Nesbitt Memorial Hospital.

Semm K (1992) Pelviscopy. Operative guidelines for minimally invasive surgery. Classical Abdominal Serrated Edged Macro-morcellated Hysterectomy (CASH), pp 7–9. Germany: UFK, Kiel.

Smith HO & Thompson JD (1986) Indications and technique for vaginal hysterectomy. *Contemporary OB/GYN* September 1986, p 125.

24

Laparoscopic Appendicectomy and Colposuspension

RUSSELL MACDONALD

The Hillingdon Hospital, Uxbridge, Middlesex, UK

Laparoscopic Appendicectomy

Why Laparoscopic Appendicectomy?

Prospective clinical research reports that up to 28% of laparotomy appendicectomy specimens are uninflamed and that the diagnosis of acute appendicitis may be falsely positive in 39% of women (Paterson-Brown *et al.*, 1988). Such low diagnostic specificity is acceptable in clinical practice in order to minimize the incidence of ruptured appendicitis. This is particularly so for women, who have a fourfold increased incidence of tubal infertility if appendicectomy is delayed until rupture has occurred (Mueller *et al.*, 1985). However, a reduction in the incidence of normal appendicectomy would seem desirable as even this procedure is associated with significant complications in 17% of cases (Chang *et al.*, 1973).

The value of diagnostic laparoscopy as an adjunct to decision making in cases of acute abdomen, particularly in patients with suspected appendicitis, has not gone unrecognized by general surgeons (Paterson-Brown *et al.*, 1986). There is also documented evidence that it may reduce the 'normal appendicectomy' rate to as little as 1% (Leape and Ramenofsky, 1980). Surgeons, however, have been reluctant to adopt laparoscopy as a diagnostic technique simply because appendicectomy, when required, involves an additional and time-consuming laparotomy. Laparoscopic appendicectomy will, of course, obviate this need. When this operation is accepted into routine surgical practice it is likely that all cases of suspected appendicitis will be confirmed laparoscopically prior to proceeding with laparoscopic appendicectomy.

Operative Technique

Following routine establishment and maintenance of CO_2 pneumoperitoneum with the high-flow and electronically controlled laparoflator, portals are inserted as in Figure 24.1. The operative technique is outlined in Figure 24.2.

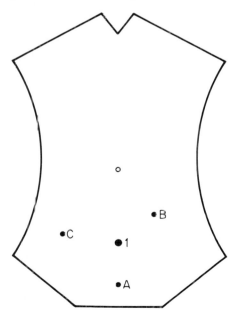

Figure 24.1 Position of laparoscopy portals: 1, 10 mm laparoscope portal; A–C, 5 mm instrument portals.

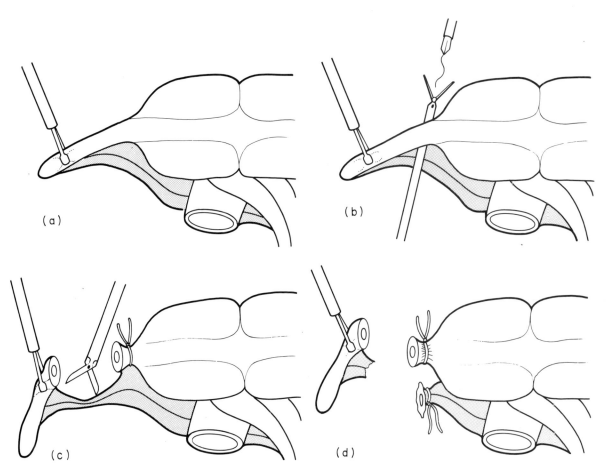

Figure 24.2 Appendicectomy technique. (a) Locate and grasp appendix. (b) With appendix on a stretch pierce mesentery and loop suture round proximal appendix. (c) Tie and divide appendix base with scissors. (d) Tie and divide mesentery. Redrawn from Macdonald *et al.* (1992).

Grasping forceps are inserted through portal A and used to locate the appendix. With gentle traction, the appendix base and mesentery are put on a stretch. Through portal B the mesentery is pierced close to the base of the appendix with pointed grasping forceps. These forceps are then used to crush the appendix base in accordance with standard surgical practice. Suturing is performed through portal C: the suture (1.0 dexon) is passed through this portal, guided around the appendix base by portal B forceps and brought out the abdominal cavity again through portal C. Extracorporeal alternate hitches are then tied and individually slipped into place and secured around the appendix base using a laparoscopic knot-pusher (Figure 24.3). Four hitches are thrown for each knot. The suture and the appendix base are then transected using laparoscopy scissors passed through portal B. The appendix mesentery is then similarly tied and divided.

The 5 mm cannula in portal A is then replaced with a 10 mm cannula and the appendix removed through this portal using 5 mm grasping forceps and a 5 mm reducing sheath. At the end of the procedure the operative field is inspected to

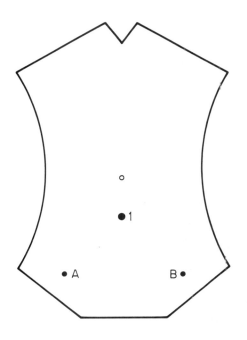

Figure 24.3 Position of laparoscopy portals: 1, 10 mm laparoscope portal; A–B, 5 mm instrument portals.

ensure haemostasis and the abdomen is washed out with normal saline prior to removing the laparoscope.

Postoperatively intravenous antibiotics should be given for 24 hours or until the patient's temperature is normal. The patient may be discharged when independently mobile and tolerating a light diet.

Discussion

The preceding operative technique (Macdonald et al., 1992) differs from the initial description of laparoscopic appendicectomy (Semm and Friedrich, 1987) which closely resembles its laparotomy counterpart (Bailey and Love, 1956). The recommended laparotomy steps are:

1. identification of the appendix base and mesentery;
2. ligation and transection of mesentery;
3. crushing ligation and transection of the stump; and
4. insertion of a purse-string suture.

As the appendix lies anterior to its mesentery it is simpler to ligate and dissect the appendix first. In addition, the insertion of a purse-string is of dubious value and many surgeons have abandoned its routine use (Street et al., 1988). Laparoscopically it is difficult to invert so this suture is not included in our procedure.

Burch Colposuspension

Why Laparoscopic Burch Colposuspension?

Many surgical procedures have been developed for the treatment of stress incontinence. Indeed, a number of these could be classified as minimally invasive and simply involve transvaginal needle bladder neck suspension (Pereyra, 1959; Stamey, 1973; Raz, 1981). However, long-term relief of symptoms seems best when a suprapubic technique is employed (Burch, 1961). The Burch colposuspension is presently favoured as reposition of the bladder neck is more consistent and long lasting.

Continence is maintained only when intraurethral pressure exceeds intravesical pressure (Enhorning, 1961). A sudden increase in intra-abdominal pressure, e.g. during laughing or coughing, is inevitably transmitted to the bladder

and is a potential strain on the continence mechanism. The bladder neck and proximal urethra are normally positioned posterosuperiorly to the pubic symphysis. This location is critical as it allows intra-abdominal pressure changes to be simultaneously directed to the proximal urethra (Stanton, 1985). The net pressure change within the continence mechanism is therefore zero and incontinence does not occur.

Anatomically, stress incontinence usually involves a posterior and inferior displacement of the bladder neck. An increase in intra-abdominal pressure, from whatever cause, will then not simultaneously compress the bladder neck and proximal urethra against the posterosuperior surface of the symphysis pubis. Pressure is only imparted to the bladder and incontinence is likely to occur. Operations for stress incontinence aim to relocate the bladder neck and proximal urethra to their position of function lying on the posterosuperior surface of the pubic symphysis.

All suprapubic colposuspension procedures involve a low Pfannenstiel incision and this has inevitable postoperative morbidity. The anatomy within the space of Retzius can also be seen through this incision. However, little surgical reconstruction is required as the procedure simply involves the insertion of four sutures which attach the vaginal fornices to Cooper's ligament. It would therefore seem ideally suited to a laparoscopic approach. Not only would this obviate the need for a large incision, but the view afforded by retroperitonoscopy is superior to that obtained through a Pfannenstiel and should facilitate suture insertion.

Operative Technique

A retroperitoneal approach is employed. A Veress needle is inserted into the subrectus retroperitoneal space through the lower abdominal wall. The space is opened up pneumatically using carbon dioxide from a high-flow electronically controlled insufflator. The laparoscope and two 5 mm portals are inserted into the space through the points of entry illustrated in Figure 24.3.

The space of Retzius is then opened up using both blunt and aquadissection. Should bleeding occur, this is best arrested with bipolar diathermy. The following landmarks are identified: the superior pubic ramus, the pectineal or Cooper's ligament and the obturator membrane. With the help of an assistant the lateral vaginal fornices are displaced anteriorly and laterally. The bladder is then pushed medially off the vaginal membrane (Figure 24.4b). Following this last step the sutures are inserted.

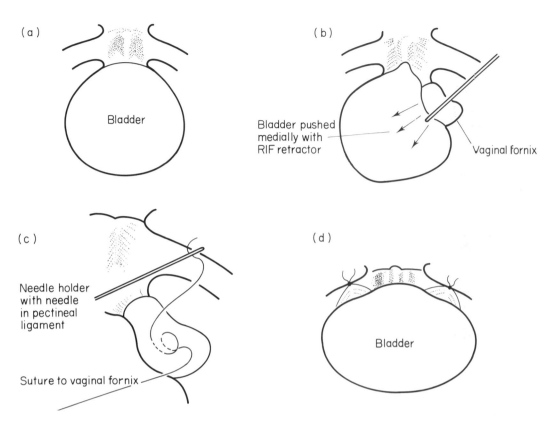

Figure 24.4 Burch colposuspension technique. (a) Open cave of Retzius and identify (1) superior pubic rumus; (2) pectineal ligament; (3) obturator membrane. (b) Assistant digitally displaces right vaginal fornix anterolaterally. Bladder is reflected medially off vaginal fornix. (c) Suture placed through vaginal fornix (figure-of-eight) and pectineal ligament. (d) Both forniceal sutures secured to pectineal ligaments after extracorporeal tieing. RIF, right ilial fossa.

An extracorporeal knot-tying technique is employed. To insert the right forniceal stitch the needle holder and a number 2 Gore-tex suture mounted on a curved needle are inserted through the left iliac fossa portal (Figure 24.4c). The assistant digitally displaces the right vaginal fornix anterolaterally and the bladder is displaced medially using a 5 mm probe inserted through the right iliac fossa portal.

The suture is inserted through the vaginal fornix in the form of a figure-of-eight and then through Cooper's ligament on the superior pubic ramus. As in the laparotomy procedure the vaginal stitch is submucosal and does not pass into the vaginal cavity. The suture and needle are then brought out of the abdominal cavity through the left iliac fossa portal. The left vaginal fornix is then similarly sutured to Cooper's ligament on the left superior pubic ramus by passing the needle holder and suture through the right iliac fossa portal.

The suture is then tied extracorporeally using a knot-pusher. The knot is secured with four to six alternate hitches while the assistant, in turn, pushes each lateral vaginal fornix into a position overlying Cooper's ligament. The bladder is

then filled and a suprapubic catheter inserted. Haemostasis is secured and the laparoscope and cannulae are removed. The catheter is left on free drainage for 5 days after which it is clamped and the patient voids as required. The catheter is removed when two consecutive residuals are less than 150 ml.

Discussion

Laparoscopic Burch colposuspension has not been formally described and few cases have been performed. Pioneering cases were performed by C.Y. Liu of the Chattanooga Women's Laser Centre who initially developed an intraperitoneal version of the above technique (J.J. Wright, 1992, personal communication).

At present the technique is still evolving and it is too early to recommend routine application in clinical practice. Long-term follow-up of a cohort of patients is first required, preferably with pre- and postoperative urodynamic assessment. However, from a practical point of view the procedure is certainly possible and anatomically, colposuspension would seem to be similar to that achieved through a Pfannenstiel incision. Similar clinical results can therefore be expected, but strictly speaking valid long-term comparison requires a properly organized clinical trial.

Summary

The advantages of operative laparoscopy over laparotomy are being recognized and accepted by an increasing proportion of gynaecologists and general surgeons. Such is the present enthusiasm, that the logical approach for the laparoscopist must be to re-examine all laparotomy procedures, reassess their clinical value and if considered efficacious, work out an alternative laparoscopic approach. Reaffirmation of clinical value is, of course, fundamental and essential to genuine progress.

Certain problems are inevitably associated with using laparotomy techniques as a starting block for development. Though the principles are similar, the practice is not. Laparoscopic techniques which mirror laparotomy procedure are therefore unlikely to be of more than transient interest. Real progress in the evolution of surgical laparoscopy must surely depend upon the creation of specialized laparoscopic techniques.

The same comments apply to instrumentation where only an innovative leap will lead to significant development. At present progress is hindered by rigid laparotomy look-alikes. These are difficult to grip, are difficult to manoeuvre, and make far from ideal laparoscopy instruments.

Laparoscopic dissection and incision techniques are rapidly advancing, but deficient technique and instrumentation are clearly apparent during procedures which require reconstruction. At present, laparoscopic reconstruction techniques are restricted to suturing and stapling. Increasingly sophisticated staplers are becoming available, but they are difficult to apply and lack versatility. Until further developments occur surgical laparoscopy will be restricted to procedures which do not require complex reconstruction.

References

Bailey H & Love M (1956) *A Short Practice of Surgery*, Chapter 26, pp 435–455. London: H.K. Lewis and Co. Ltd.

Burch JC (1961) Urethrovaginal fixation to Cooper's ligament for correction of stress incontinence. *American Journal of Obstetrics and Gynecology* **100**:281–290.

Chang F, Hogle H & Welling D (1973) The fate of the negative appendix. *American Journal of Surgery* **126(Dec)**:752–754.

Enhorning G (1961) Simultaneous recording of intravesical and intraurethral pressure. *Acta Chirurgica Scandinavica (Supplement)* **276**:1–68.

Leape L & Ramenofsky M (1980) Laparoscopy for questionable appendicitis. *Annals of Surgery* **191(4)**:410–413.

MacDonald R, Hasan F. Tate J & Lock MR (1992) Laparoscopic appendicectomy. *Minimally Invasive Therapy* **1**:225–229.

Mueller B, Daling J, Moore D *et al.* (1985) Appendectomy and the risk of tubal infertility. *New England Journal of Medicine* **315(24)**:1506–1508.

Paterson-Brown S, Eckersley J, Sim A & Dudley H (1986) Laparoscopy as an adjunct to decision making in the acute abdomen. *British Journal of Surgery* **73(Dec)**:1022–1023.

Paterson-Brown S, Thompson J, Eckersley J, Ponting G & Dudley H (1988) Which patients with suspected appendicitis should undergo laparoscopy? *British Medical Journal* **296**:1363–1364.

Pereyra AJ (1959) A simplified surgical procedure for the correction of stress incontinence in women. *Western Journal of Surgery* **627**:223–230.

Raz S (1981) Modified bladder neck suspension for female stress incontinence. *Urology* **18**:82–90.

Semm K & Friedrich E (1987) *Operative Manual for Endoscopic Abdominal Surgery*, **12.6.3**:98. Chicago: Yearbook Medical Publishers.

Stamey TA (1973) Cystoscopic suspension of the bladder neck for urinary incontinence. *Surgery, Gynecology and Obstetrics* **136**:547–553.

Stanton SL (1985) Stress incontinence: why and how operations work. *Clinics in Obstetrics and Gynecology* **122**:369–377.

Street D, Bodai B, Owens L *et al.* (1988) *Archives of Surgery* **123**:689–690.

25

Pathology and Pathogenesis of Endometriosis

ROBERT P.S. JANSEN

Department of Reproductive Endocrinology and Infertility, Royal Prince Alfred Hospital, Sydney, Australia

Endometriosis is a disease of the pelvic mesenchyme in which tissue with epithelial and stromal characteristics of endometrium develops in situations other than in the uterine mucosa (Sampson, 1940), thus changing the female peritoneal environment. Its pathogenesis, its resultant pathological manifestations and its predisposing factors are thus important to all who wish to understand normal and abnormal appearances of the pelvic peritoneum at laparoscopy. These considerations underlie the principles by which endometriosis can be effectively managed laparoscopically.

Pathogenesis and Predisposition

Environmental Influences

The prevalence of diagnosed endometriosis in women increases through the reproductive years (Ranney, 1975; Mahmood and Templeton, 1990). Epidemiological studies of endometriosis are consistent with the theory that it is the accumulating effect of repeated ovarian and/or menstrual cycles that is the important environmental determinant of endometriosis (or at least for its symptomatic expression). For the development of endometriosis, both ovulation and menstruation may be important.

Follicular growth and ovulation produce transient but very high elevations of oestradiol and progesterone concentrations in the peritoneal fluid (Koninckx et al., 1980), enough to stimulate

the relatively low concentrations of oestradiol and progesterone receptors known to be present in endometriotic tissue compared to receptor concentrations in endometrium (Jänne et al., 1981). The usual histological consequence among general peritoneal lesions is that proliferative and secretory response lags behind histological dating of endometrium sampled simultaneously (Novak and Hoge, 1958; Schweppe et al., 1984), whereas lesions on the ovarian surface, subjected to continuing high exposure from progesterone diffusing from an adjacent corpus luteum, show secretory changes ahead of the endometrium during the luteal phase (Czernobilsky and Morris, 1979; Russell and Bannatyne, 1989). Ovulation and the direct secretion of ovarian steroids into the peritoneal cavity is thus a more potent steroid stimulus to responsive peritoneal tissue than systemic oestrogen administration is.

The evidence that menstruation constitutes a substantial stimulus for the development of endometriosis is striking. Direct implantation of healthy endometrial tissue has been used to produce experimental models of endometriosis in monkeys (DiZerega et al., 1980) and rabbits (Kaplan et al., 1989): functional endometriosis in these circumstances develops almost immediately. The occurrence of endometriosis in abdominal scars after hysterotomy during mid-pregnancy, when healthy decidual tissue may seed the operative wound, is well documented too (Chaterjee, 1980). Indeed, the demonstration of viable endometrium in menstrual fluid (Kruitwagen et al., 1991) and the development of endometriosis in monkeys operated on to divert menstrual fluid into the peritoneal cavity (TeLinde and Scott, 1950; Scott *et al.*, 1953) have been used as evidence that direct implantation of endometrial cells from retrograde menstruation might be the *usual* pathogenetic mechanism for endometriosis. The evidence, however, is against this.

Retrograde menstruation through open fallopian tubes is probably a universal event (Blumenkrantz *et al.*, 1981; Halme *et al.*, 1984), so it is clear that exposure of the peritoneum to menstrual fluid and shed endometrial cells (Kruitwagen *et al.*, 1991) is *not sufficient* for the development of endometriosis. The occurrence of endometriosis in patients with congenital absence of the uterus (El-Mahgoub and Yaseen, 1980; Rosenfeld and Lecher, 1981) and rarely in men (Oliker and Harris, 1971) proves that retrograde menstruation is also *not necessary* for endometriosis to develop. In the menstrual diversion studies in monkeys of the 1940s, endometriosis took up to 55 months to form, which to the authoritative contemporary pathologist Emil Novak implied that induced metaplasia was at least as probable a mechanism as direct endometrial cell implantation (Scott *et al.*, 1953).

Careful and extensive studies by Merill (1966) showed that endometriosis developed at intraperitoneal and subcutaneous sites in 20 of 22 rabbits when they received implants of healthy endometrium enclosed in small diffusion chambers, the walls of which were made of Millipore filter material impenetrable to endometrial cells but permeable to soluble factors released by the usually healthy endometrial tissue. The conclusion was, and is, that there is a soluble factor produced by endometrium that induces endometrioid differentiation in connective tissue. The strength of a menstrual stimulus in producing endometriosis is noticeable among young patients with congenital atresias of the genital tract, in whom endometriosis is very common (Schifrin *et al.*, 1973; Sanfilippo *et al.*, 1986); regression of lesions is said to take place in some of these patients when the outflow obstruction is relieved (Sanfilippo *et al.*, 1986). Patients with congenital abnormalities of the Müllerian system may be predisposed to endometriosis for other reasons, though, because (a) endometriosis is common in women with a bicornuate uterus unaccompanied by outflow obstruction, and (b) endometriosis can occur in the absence of a uterus (El-Mahgoub and Yaseen, 1980; Rosenfeld and Lecher, 1981).

The distribution of endometriosis in areas of the pelvis where menstrual fluid might pool (the pouch of Douglas and uterovesical pouch) has been advanced as evidence for the importance of menstrual fluid in the usual genesis of endometriosis (Jenkins *et al.*, 1986), but this distribution, especially the prevalence of lesions in the ovarian fossas, equally supports an important stimulatory role for ovarian steroids present in the peritoneal fluid at ovulation. Certainly the prevention of retrograde menstruation by tubal ligation for sterilization does not safeguard against either the development or the progression of endometriosis as long as women continue to ovulate (Dodge *et al.*, 1986; Jansen, 1986). Perhaps the only uncontroversial examples of endometrial cell seeding causing endometriosis are those cases in which endometriosis develops in scars after a single operative spill (Chaterjee, 1980; Vermesh *et al.*, 1985), one example of which is hysterotomy for termination of midtrimester pregnancy, when the endometrium is particularly healthy, with a risk of scar endometriosis of about 1% (Chaterjee, 1980).

In summary, there are many examples of endometriosis, clinical and experimental, that cannot be explained by direct endometrial cell implantation, thus leaving epithelial and stromal metaplasia as the critical event. On the other hand there are few situations that cannot be explained by metaplasia, induced in responsive tissue either by soluble factors present in endometrial fluid at the time of commencement of normal endometrial regeneration or by exposure to ovarian steroids, especially when these are present in high concentration in the peritoneal fluid that directly bathes the areas at risk.

This leads to the question, why does endometriosis develop in some women and not in others?

Inherited Influences

Among 123 patients with clinically proven endometriosis studied by Simpson and others (Simpson *et al.*, 1980), 9 of 153 female siblings aged over 18, and 10 of 123 mothers, had also had diagnoses of endometriosis confirmed by similar criteria, giving a prevalence of clinically important endometriosis among first-degree relations of 19/276, or 6.9%; on the other hand, endometriosis had been diagnosed in only one of 104 female siblings of patients' husbands and in only one of 107 husbands' mothers, giving a prevalence among non-genetic relations of 2/211, or 0.9%. This relative risk of 7.3 given a positive family history is consistent with polygenic or multifactorial inheritance of endometriosis. In a case-control study among 43 women with endometriosis, Lamb *et al.* (1986) found a relative risk of 4.9% for endometriosis among first-degree relations and 1.9% among second-degree relations. For a dramatic example of inherited endometriosis, Henriksen in a published discussion (Scott *et al.*, 1953) gave an example of identical triplets who, despite varying reproductive histories, developed virtually identical presentations of endometriosis in their late 20s. The hereditary predisposition for endometriosis is not associated with any particular HLA type (Simpson *et al.*,1984).

Laparoscopic Pathology

Macroscopic Pathology

Chocolate-coloured, blood-pigment-filled cysts and stigmata affecting the pelvic viscera (Figure 25.1) constitute the most characteristic appearance of endometriosis. Parietal peritoneal involvement is more common, however, and the lesions are often small and flat (Figure 25.2). The commonest sites affected by endometriosis are:

1. the pelvic peritoneum of the pouch of Douglas (or cul-de-sac), the uterosacral ligaments and the ovarian fossae;
2. the ovaries;
3. the bladder serosa; and
4. the sigmoid colon (Redwine, 1987a).

Tissues remote from direct contact with the peritoneal fluid can also be involved: the recto-vaginal septum, the vaginal mucosa, the bladder wall, abdominal scars and the pleural cavity and lung parenchyma are progressively rarer locations. Lesions can be restricted in distribution and care must be taken at laparoscopy to displace the

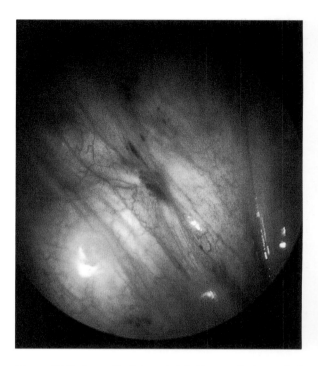

Figure 25.2 A small, flat parietal stigma of pigmented endometriosis. Symptoms may be present out of proportion in severity to the size of the lesion.

intestines from the pelvis and to aspirate all free peritoneal fluid (Figure 25.3), or the diagnosis of endometriosis can be missed.

Non-pigmented and Microscopic Endometriosis

Endometriosis in earlier stages of histogenesis may display only non-pigmented lesions (Jansen

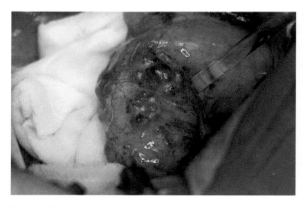

Figure 25.1 Pigmented, cystic visceral lesions of endo-metriosis, involving the serosa of the sigmoid colon, indicative of unquestioned macroscopic endometriosis.

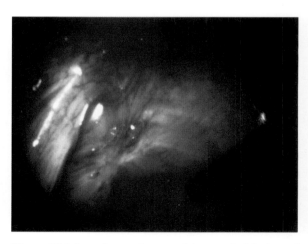

Figure 25.3 Largely unpigmented but typical lesion of endometriosis revealed below the uterosac-ral ligament by aspiration of peritoneal fluid at laparoscopy.

and Russell, 1986; Stripling *et al.*, 1988). Non-pigmented lesions comprise:

1. white opacification of the peritoneum;
2. gland-like excrescences;
3. flame-like vascularized lesions; and
4. otherwise unexplained adhesions between ovary and adjacent peritoneum.

The endometriotic lesion depicted in Figure 25.3 includes both opacified and gland-like areas.

Whether peritoneum that is normal at close laparoscopic inspection can harbour microscopically diagnosable endometriotic elements is controversial (Murphy *et al.*, 1986; Nisolle *et al.*, 1990). A single epithelial gland has a diameter of about 0.5 mm. Opacifications of 1–2 mm are visible laparoscopically with careful inspection and if biopsied may yield enough stroma and glandular elements to allow a diagnosis of endometriosis (Redwine, 1989). Where such care is taken to exclude lesions at laparoscopy, several reports dismiss the notion that normal peritoneum carries a high prevalence of microscopic endometriosis, from patients without endometriosis (Jansen and Russell, 1986) or with it (Redwine, 1988; Redwine and Yocom, 1990).

The histological possibilities among non-pigmented lesions include a variety of peritoneal reactions (Jansen and Russell, 1986), but also a series of apparently related epithelial elements that range in pathological appearance from undifferentiated serosal inclusions and Walthard rests to endometrioid differentiation (endometriosis), fallopian tube-like differentiation (endosalpingiosis) and, rarely, endocervical-like differentiation (endocervicosis). Pigmented lesions may also show these alternative epithelial differentiations. This continuum, especially in adjacent or contiguous lesions (Figure 25.4), lends support to the mechanism of serosal metaplasia over direct epithelial implantation in the usual pathogenesis of endometriosis (Kerner *et al.*, 1981; Russell and Bannatyne, 1989).

Staging

Attempts have been made to classify or 'stage' endometriosis according to its severity. The temptation has been to liken its extent to that of malignancies and to infer a prognosis from such staging. This approach has dangers, because (a) there is little evidence that endometriosis ordinarily spreads in neoplastic fashion from a single focus (Redwine, 1987a); (b) the prevalence of pigmented as opposed to non-pigmented lesions may increase with age, suggesting *in situ* evolution (Redwine, 1987b; Koninckx *et al.*, 1991); (c) the duration of symptoms such as infertility is independent of its extent (Buttram, 1979); and (d) there are paradoxical situations where the chance of obtaining improvement in symptoms from treating endometriosis is inversely related to its extent (Jansen, unpublished observations).

The standard system for categorizing the extent of endometriosis is the modified American Fertility Society classification (American Fertility Society, 1985) into minimal, mild, moderate and severe endometriosis, depending on the sum of points derived from (a) the area of peritoneum involved; (b) the thickness of endometriotic lesions; (c) the presence of endometriotic cysts, especially of the ovary, that contain altered chocolate-like blood products; and (d) the occurrence of adhesions affecting the adnexae or progressively obliterating the pouch of Douglas, or cul-de-sac (Figure 25.5).

Pathophysiological Basis of Treatment

There are two reasons to treat endometriosis:

1. if it causes substantial symptoms, whether pain, excessive uterine bleeding or infertility; or, in the absence of symptoms,
2. if one judges that symptoms are likely to become troublesome before the menopause puts a natural end to the condition's symptomatic progression.

Because symptoms correlate only loosely with anatomical severity (Buttram, 1979), it is better not to make rules for treatment that depend on extent, except that if infertility is present and the

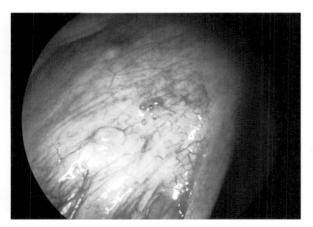

Figure 25.4 Vesicular, non-pigmented peritoneal lesions, consistent with a variety of epithelial metaplasias, including endometriosis.

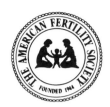

THE AMERICAN FERTILITY SOCIETY
REVISED CLASSIFICATION OF ENDOMETRIOSIS

Patient's Name _____ Date_____

Stage I (Minimal) - 1-5
Stage II (Mild) - 6-15
Stage III (Moderate) - 16-40
Stage IV (Severe) - >40

Laparoscopy_____ Laparotomy_____ Photography_____
Recommended Treatment_____
_____

Total_____

Prognosis_____

PERITONEUM	ENDOMETRIOSIS	<1cm	1-3cm	>3cm
	Superficial	1	2	4
	Deep	2	4	6
OVARY	R Superficial	1	2	4
	Deep	4	16	20
	L Superficial	1	2	4
	Deep	4	16	20

	POSTERIOR CULDESAC OBLITERATION	Partial	Complete
		4	40

	ADHESIONS	<1/3 Enclosure	1/3-2/3 Enclosure	>2/3 Enclosure
OVARY	R Filmy	1	2	4
	Dense	4	8	16
	L Filmy	1	2	4
	Dense	4	8	16
TUBE	R Filmy	1	2	4
	Dense	4*	8*	16
	L Filmy	1	2	4
	Dense	4*	8*	16

*If the fimbriated end of the fallopian tube is completely enclosed, change the point assignment to 16.

Figure 25.5 American Fertility Society pathological classification of the severity of endometriosis (Revised American Fertility Society Classification of Endometriosis: 1985. *Fertility and Sterility* 1985; **43**:351–2. Reproduced with permission of the publisher, The American Fertility Society.)

anatomy of the pelvic organs is distorted, then an attempt at cure means an attempt at anatomical correction—an operation, either endoscopic (Chapters 21, 31, 39 and 40) or by laparotomy. Otherwise the traditional distinction between surgical and medical therapy does not give the best insights.

Removal or Destruction of Endometriotic Tissue

The efficacy of an operative, ablative approach depends on the assumption that enough abnormal tissue is destroyed or removed so that symptoms will disappear, and will not soon reappear. These symptoms may be clear cut, with immediate improvement either obvious or not (e.g. dyspareunia, dysmenorrhoea or dysfunctional uterine bleeding), or the symptom may need time and chance to be resolved (e.g. pregnancy among the infertile).

Serosal or ovarian lesions can be ablated by *electrocautery* (Chapter 37) or *laser vaporization* (Chapter 36) at the time of diagnosis at laparoscopy; ablation can be carried out after suppressive therapy (see below) has run its course without having produced lasting relief; or ablation can follow a course of suppressive therapy instituted in order to diminish extensive lesions to the point where it becomes practicable laparoscopically.

Conservative excision of endometriotic peritoneum or ovarian stroma, including ovarian chocolate cysts, can be carried out at laparotomy or at operative laparoscopy (Chapter 31). 'Conservative' here means that the uterus is conserved: the intention should be to remove all abnormal peritoneum or the operation may fail to relieve symptoms (Ranney, 1975). Incomplete operations are usually followed by a course of ovarian suppressive therapy. Because conservative operations are often intended to improve fertility it is especially important to safeguard against the development of adnexal adhesions (Jansen, 1988, 1991), insofar as this is possible (Chapter 41).

Withdrawal of Ovarian Support

The partly true deduction that endometriosis regresses during pregnancy led Kistner in the 1950s (Kistner, 1959) to propose that 'pseudopregnancy' with exogenous *progestogens* might be used to treat endometriosis. Progestogens or oestrogen–progestogen combinations act first by suppressing ovarian oestradiol secretion, particularly (and most effectively) the direct transudation of oestradiol across the wall of developing follicles into the peritoneal fluid bathing endometriotic lesions, and, second, by antagonizing the stimulatory effect of endogenous (or circulating exogenous) oestrogens on the lesions. Most modern contraceptive pills are too low in dosage thoroughly to inhibit follicle growth and thus reliably to withdraw the hormonal support upon which endometriotic lesions depend. Progestogen-only regimens are effective, and are especially useful for long-term treatment of teenagers yet to put their fertility to the test and for some older women while awaiting natural cessation of ovarian follicular function.

Other drugs are more effective at producing an amenorrhoeic state for initiating therapy and for reducing the size and extent of lesions in preparation for endoscopic ablation. *Danazol* inhibits ovarian oestradiol production more effectively than progestogens do and has the added advantage of blocking steroid receptors in endometriotic tissue (Dmowski, 1979). Long-acting agonistic analogues of gonadotrophic hormone releasing hormone (GnRH analogues) (Shaw *et al.*, 1983), such as buserelin, goserelin, leuprorelin and nafarelin, administered intranasally or by subcutaneous injection or monthly implantation, produce a state of hypogonadotrophic hypogonadism, achieving even lower levels of oestradiol in serum (and presumably in peritoneal fluid) than are seen with danazol; although there is probably no direct beneficial effect on endometriotic tissue, the endometriosis is as effectively suppressed. (These drugs should not be prescribed without a thorough understanding of their sometimes serious side-effects.)

Bilaterial ovariectomy and hysterectomy, accompanied by exogenous, systemic oestrogen replacement therapy, achieves the threefold benefit of dramatically lowering peritoneal fluid oestradiol levels, removing the target organ responsible for dysmenorrhoea and endometrial bleeding, and avoiding the systemic side-effects of ovarian progesterone or oral progestogens. Occasional patients with deep endometriosis not directly exposed to the peritoneal fluid (and thus presumably driven by circulating rather than peritoneal fluid oestrogens) may develop recurrences after bilateral ovariectomy, hysterectomy and oestrogen replacement therapy. But they are exceptions: most patients do not develop recurrences with exogenous oestrogen administration. If recurrences do occur, endoscopic approaches to residual endometriosis can then be considered.

These medical and surgical therapeutic approaches have in common the withdrawal of hormonal support from endometriotic lesions and foci, which either are left untouched or are known or thought to remain after attempts at ablation. The choice between drugs or ovariectomy is made according to the patient's needs and wishes. For the endoscopic surgeon, drug therapy with progestogens, danazol or GnRH analogues constitutes an important adjunct in preparing the pelvis for effective endoscopic ablation of extensive or substantial endometriotic lesions.

Symptomatic Approaches

Endometriosis is not a premalignant condition, so it does not need to be treated in its own right. It is the control of actual or expected symptoms that matters. Whereas, for example, the *oral contraceptive pill* in its modern, low-dose formulations does not reliably stop the progression of endometriosis, it can control dysmenorrhoea and menorrhagia—which may, in minimal cases or in older women, be enough. Although not to be especially encouraged, many operations for dyspareunia in the past involved *shortening the round ligaments* to correct retroversion of the uterus, which was a symptom-led approach, but which in practice often ignored the common endometriotic basis for the retroversion. *Uterine nerve ablation*, including presacral neurectomy, has better credentials for treating intractable dysmenorrhoea (Chapter 38). Dysfunctional uterine bleeding from endometriosis may respond to *hysteroscopic endometrial ablation* (Chapters 8–10).

Hysterectomy, unaccompanied by bilateral ovariectomy, is less obviously but just as legitimately classed as a symptomatic, non-curative operation. Dysmenorrhoea, abnormal uterine bleeding and, often, dyspareunia are controlled while ovarian function is preserved, but it is important to try and excise all endometriotic peritoneum or symptoms are likely to recur.

Lastly, one can take an active approach to the symptom of infertility by making use of *assisted conception* (Chapters 24 and 25). *In vitro* fertilization and gamete intrafallopian transfer (Jansen *et al.*, 1990) are generally at least as effective in mild to moderate endometriosis as in couples whose infertility is of other cause (ovarian endometriotic cysts, however, lead to lower rates of oocyte recovery and embryo transfer). The chance of success—although relatively good and with the expectation that pregnancy will later subdue the endometriosis—must be tempered by the knowledge that repeated cycles of ovarian stimulation unaccompanied by pregnancy will probably hasten the progression of the endometriosis.

References

American Fertility Society (1985) Revised American Fertility Society classification of endometriosis. *Fertility and Sterility* **43**:351–352.

Blumenkrantz MJ, Gallagher N, Bashore RA & Tenckhoff H (1981) Retrograde menstruation in women undergoing chronic peritoneal dialysis. *Obstetrics and Gynecology* **57**:667–670.

Buttram VC Jr (1979) Conservative surgery for endometriosis in the infertile female: a study of 206 patients with implications for both medical and surgical therapy. *Fertility and Sterility* **31**:117–123.

Chaterjee SK (1980) Scar endometriosis: a clinicopathologic study of 17 cases. *Obstetrics and Gynecology* **56**:81–84.

Czernobilsky B & Morris WJ (1979) A histologic study of ovarian endometriosis with emphasis on hyperplastic and atypical changes. *Obstetrics and Gynecology* **53**:318–323.

DiZerega GS, Barber DL & Hodgen GD (1980) Endometriosis: role of ovarian steroids in initiation, maintenance, and suppression. *Fertility and Sterility* **33**:649–653.

Dmowski WP (1979) Endocrine properties and clinical application of danazol. *Fertility and Sterility* **31**:237–251.

Dodge ST, Pumphrey RS & Miyazawa K (1986) Peritoneal endometriosis in women requesting reversal of sterilization. *Fertility and Sterility* **45**:774–776.

El-Mahgoub S & Yaseen S (1980) A positive proof for the theory of coelomic metaplasia. *American Journal of Obstetrics and Gynecology* **137**:137–140.

Halme J, Hammond MG, Hulka JF, Raj SG & Talbert LM (1984) Retrograde menstruation in healthy women and in patients with endometriosis. *Obstetrics and Gynecology* **64**:151–154.

Jänne O, Kauppila A, Kokko E *et al.* (1981) Estrogen and progestin receptors in endometriosis lesions: comparison with endometrial tissue. *American Journal of Obstetrics and Gynecology* **141**:562–566.

Jansen RPS (1986) Tubal resection and anastomosis. I. Sterilization-reversal. *Australian and New Zealand Journal of Obstetrics and Gynaecology* **26**:294–304.

Jansen RPS (1988) Early laparoscopy after pelvic operations to prevent adhesions: safety and efficacy. *Fertility and Sterility* **49**:26–31.

Jansen RPS (1991) Prevention of pelvic peritoneal adhesions. *Current Opinion in Obstetrics and Gynecology* **3**:369–374.

Jansen RPS & Russell P (1986) Nonpigmented endometriosis. Clinical, laparoscopic and pathologic definition. *American Journal of Obstetrics and Gynecology* **155**:1154–1159.

Jansen RPS, Anderson JC, Birrell WRS *et al.* (1990) Outpatient gamete intrafallopian transfer: 710 cases. *Medical Journal of Australia* **153**:182–188.

Jenkins S, Olive DL & Haney AF (1986) Endometriosis: pathogenetic implications of the anatomic distribution. *Obstetrics and Gynecology* **67**:335–338.

Kaplan CR, Eddy CA, Olive DL & Schenken RS (1989) Effect of ovarian endometriosis on ovulation in rabbits. *American Journal of Obstetrics and Gynecology* **160**:40–44.

Kerner H, Gaton E & Czernobilsky B (1981) Unusual ovarian, tubal and pelvic mesothelial inclusions in patients with endometriosis. *Histopathology* **5**: 277–283.

Kistner RW (1959) The treatment of endometriosis by inducing pseudopregnancy with ovarian hormones. A report of fifty-eight cases. *Fertility and Sterility* **10**:539–556.

Koninckx PR, Heyns W, Verhoeven G *et al.* (1980) Biochemical characterization of peritoneal fluid in women during the menstrual cycle. *Journal of Clinical Endocrinology and Metabolism* **51**:1239–1244.

Koninckx PR, Lesaffre E, Meuleman C, Cornillie FJ & Demeyere S (1991) Suggestive evidence that pelvic endometriosis is a progressive disease, whereas deeply infiltrating endometriosis is associated with pelvic pain. *Fertility and Sterility* **55**:759–765.

Kruitwagen RFPM, Poels LG, Willemsen WNP *et al.* (1991) Endometrial epithelial cells in peritoneal fluid during the early follicular phase. *Fertility and Sterility* **55**:297–303.

Lamb K, Hoffman RG & Nichols TR (1986) Family trait analysis: a case control study of 43 women with endometriosis and their best friends. *American Journal of Obstetrics and Gynecology* **154**:596–601.

Mahmood TA & Templeton A (1990) Pathophysiology of mild endometriosis: review of literature. *Human Reproduction* **5**:765–784.

Merrill JA (1966) Endometrial induction of endometriosis across Millipore filters. *American Journal of Obstetrics and Gynecology* **94**:780–790.

Murphy AA, Green WR, Bobbie D, dela Cruz ZC & Rock JA (1986) Unsuspected endometriosis documented by scanning electron microscopy in visually normal peritoneum. *Fertility and Sterility* 46:522–524.

Nisolle M, Paindaveine E, Bourdon A *et al.* (1990) Histologic study of peritoneal endometriosis in infertile women. *Fertility and Sterility* 53:984–988.

Novak ER & Hoge AF (1958) Endometriosis of the lower genital tract. *Obstetrics and Gynecology* 12:687–693.

Oliker AJ & Harris AE (1971) Endometriosis of the bladder in a male patient. *Journal of Urology* 106:858–859.

Ranney B (1975) The prevention, inhibition, palliation, and treatment of endometriosis. *American Journal of Obstetrics and Gynecology* 123:778–785.

Redwine DB (1987a) The distribution of endometriosis in the pelvis by age groups and fertility. *Fertility and Sterility* 47:173–175.

Redwine DB (1987b) Age-related evolution in color appearance of endometriosis. *Fertility and Sterility* 48:1062–1063.

Redwine DB (1988) Is 'microscopic' peritoneal endometriosis invisible? *Fertility and Sterility* 50:565–666.

Redwine DB (1989) Peritoneal blood painting: an aid in the diagnosis of endometriosis. *American Journal of Obstetrics and Gynecology* 161:865–866.

Redwine DB & Yocom LB (1990) A serial section study of visually normal pelvic peritoneum in patients with endometriosis. *Fertility and Sterility* 54:648–651.

Rosenfeld DL & Lecher BD (1981) Endometriosis in a patient with Rokitansky–Kuster–Hauser syndrome. *American Journal of Obstetrics and Gynecology* 139:105.

Russell P & Bannatyne P (1989) *Surgical Pathology of the Ovaries*, pp 171–187. Edinburgh: Churchill Livingstone.

Sampson JA (1940) The development of the implantation theory for the origin of peritoneal endometriosis. *American Journal of Obstetrics and Gynecology* 40:549–557.

Sanfilippo JS, Wakim NG, Schikler KN & Yussman MA (1986) Endometriosis in association with uterine anomaly. *American Journal of Obstetrics and Gynecology* 154:39–43.

Schifrin BS, Erez S & Moore JG (1973) Teen-age endometriosis. *American Journal of Obstetrics and Gynecology* 116:973–980.

Schweppe K-W, Wynn RM & Beller FK (1984) Ultrastructural comparison of endometriotic implants and eutopic endometrium. *American Journal of Obstetrics and Gynecology* 148:1024–1039.

Scott RB, TeLinde RW & Wharton LR (1953) Further studies on experimental endometriosis. *American Journal of Obstetrics and Gynecology* 66:1082–1103.

Shaw RW, Fraser HM & Boyle H (1983) Intranasal treatment with luteinising hormone releasing hormone agonist in women with endometriosis. *British Medical Journal* 287:1667–1669.

Simpson JL, Elias S, Malinak LR & Buttram VC Jr (1980) Heritable aspects of endometriosis. I. Genetic studies. *American Journal of Obstetrics and Gynecology* 137:327–331.

Simpson JL, Malinak LR, Elias S, Carson SA & Radvany RA (1984) HLA associations in endometriosis. *American Journal of Obstetrics and Gynecology* 148:395–397.

Stripling MC, Martin DC, Chatman DL, Vander Zwaag R & Poston WM (1988) Subtle appearance of pelvic endometriosis. *Fertility and Sterility* 49:427–431.

TeLinde RW & Scott RB (1950) Experimental endometriosis. *American Journal of Obstetrics and Gynecology* 60:1147–1173.

Vermesh M, Zbella EA, Menchaca A, Confino E & Lipshitz S (1985) Vesical endometriosis following bladder injury. *American Journal of Obstetrics and Gynecology* 153:894–895.

26

Diagnosis of Endometriosis: Laparoscopic Appearances

ANDREW S. COOK* AND JOHN A. ROCK‡

*Fertility Physicians of Northern California, Fertility and Reproductive Health Institute of Northern California, USA
‡Department of Gynecology and Obstetrics, The Union Memorial Hospital and Department of Gynecology and Obstetrics, The Johns Hopkins University School of Medicine, Baltimore, USA

Introduction

Endometriosis is a condition afflicting women in the reproductive age group. The correlation between endometriosis and both infertility and pain is well documented, but several aspects of this disease, including the pathophysiology and the most effective treatment, are not well understood. Current treatment modalities are based upon the premise that removal of endometriotic lesions will increase a patient's fecundity or decrease her pain (Adamson, 1991). The importance of a comprehensive understanding of the various appearances of endometriosis can not be understated, for effective surgical treatment cannot be achieved if the presence of the disease is not appreciated.

A non-invasive method to diagnose endometriosis is not currently available. The diagnosis of endometriosis is achieved through visual or histopathological documentation, the least invasive method of which is laparoscopic surgery. The magnification offered by the laparoscope may also aid in the diagnosis of endometriosis.

The skill of the surgeon is crucial to the accurate recognition of endometriosis. Use of the laparoscope has dramatically increased over the last couple of decades. Virtually all gynaecologists use the laparoscope to perform at least tubal sterilization.

Removal of ectopic endometriotic tissue is crucial for the successful treatment of endometriosis. Treatment of endometriosis involves two steps, visualization of endometriosis and subsequent removal of the lesion. The surgeon who does not routinely perform laparoscopic surgery will certainly diagnose typical endometriotic lesions, but is at an increased risk of missing a substantial amount of subtle endometriosis. Even an experienced laparoscopic surgeon who has treated hundreds of endometriosis patients can miss (7%) or underdiagnose (50%) a substantial number of patients (Martin et al., 1989). This level of diagnostic accuracy may reflect a small group of physicians with a special interest in the laparoscopic diagnosis and treatment of endometriosis. The diagnostic sensitivity, of all groups of physicians using laparoscopic surgery, correlates with the number of procedures performed. The physicians with the least number of cases, correctly identified endometriosis by visual identification in only 41% of the cases while physicians with the greatest case load displayed a sensitivity of 86% (Martin et al., 1990).

Analysis of normal appearing peritoneum with the scanning electron microscope has demonstrated endometriosis in up to 25% of cases (Murphy et al., 1986). Histologically, endometriosis has been shown in 13% of normal appearing peritoneum from patients with endometriosis and 6% from patients without endometriosis (Nisolle et al., 1990).

Systematic Approach to Evaluation of the Pelvis

The pelviscopic surgeon should adhere to a systematic and meticulous method of evaluating the pelvis to assure complete diagnosis of endometriosis. Prior to initiation of laparoscopy, a single tooth tenaculum is attached to the anterior lip of the cervix and an intrauterine cannula is placed into the uterus. Alternatively, a Humi cannula may be inserted. Following placement of the laparoscope and a suprapubic 5 mm probe, the surgeon should be careful not to rub the peritoneum with the probe while manipulating the pelvic organs. This can traumatize the peritoneum and cause micro-bleeding which is easily confused with atypical endometriosis. A thorough bimanual examination should be avoided for the same reason.

The laparoscope affords the surgeon the capability of minifying or magnifying the field of view, depending upon the proximity of the laparoscope to the tissue. Murphy et al. detail the correlation of the operating distance and the degree of magnification for several of the commonly used laparoscopes (Table 26.1). An increased operating distance results in minification and a panoramic view which provides an excellent overview of the pelvis but is not appropriate for diagnostic purposes. Near-contact laparoscopy, with the resulting magnification, has been suggested as the method of choice for meticulous analysis of the peritoneum for subtle abnormalities (Redwine, 1987a).

The development of high-resolution monitors and video cameras allows the surgeon to perform operative laparoscopy standing straight up while viewing the monitor rather than bending over the entire case peering directly through the laparoscope. There is some compromise in resolution, even with the best camera and monitor, in comparison to direct vision. Thus, evaluation of peritoneal abnormalities should be verified under direct vision to increase the sensitivity in detecting subtle lesions.

The upper abdomen including the right paracolic gutter, the liver, gallbladder, left paracolic gutter and the appendix should be assessed to rule out significant pathology prior to focusing on the pelvis. A panoramic view provides a general assessment of the pelvis. A detailed inspection of the pelvis is achieved under magnification with the laparoscope in close proximity to the peritoneum. The anterior compartment is evaluated with the assistant elevating the intrauterine cannula, displacing the uterus posteriorly. The anterior uterus, bladder flap, abdominal wall and both round ligaments are visually inspected. Adhesions are more likely to involve the left adnexa than the right as a result of the position of the sigmoid colon. The right fallopian tube, and ovary are inspected for the presence of endometriosis and adhesions, the latter of which may also represent endometriosis. An increase in the size of the ovary should alert the surgeon to the possibility of the presence of an endometrioma. Care must be taken during elevation of the ovary to avoid traumatizing the peritoneum overlying the board ligament with the blunt probe. Alternatively, atraumatic forceps may be used to grasp the ovarian ligament and elevate the ovary. The broad ligament underlying the left ovary, the uterosacral ligaments and the posterior cul-de-sac are inspected. A survey of the left adnexa and broad ligament completes the diagnostic portion of the laparoscopic surgery. If visually a diagnosis cannot be assigned with certainty, excision of the peritoneal abnormality or a representative biopsy should be taken for histological analysis.

Table 26.1 Hopkins' laparoscope: 10 mm with 3 mm operating channel

Working distance	Magnification		
	Wolf*	Olympus*	Storz*
3 mm	—	8.2	10
5 mm	—	5.7	6
10 mm	3.19	3.2	3
15 mm	—	2.2	2
20 mm	1.71	1.7	1.5
30 mm	—	1.2	1
50 mm	0.73	0.7	0.6

*Personal communication.
Reproduced with permission from Murphy (1992).

Anatomical Distribution of Endometriosis

Knowledge of the anatomical distribution of endometriosis will help the surgeon to focus on these areas of importance. The areas most commonly involved with endometriosis include the anterior and posterior cul-de-sac, ovaries, posterior broad ligaments and the uterosacral ligaments (Jenkins et al., 1986). Endometriosis involves the left side of bilateral pelvic structures more frequently than the right. The area of pelvic adhesions roughly correlates with the locations of endometriosis. The specific incidence of involvement by location, of 182 patients evaluated laparoscopically, is depicted in Table 26.2.

The anatomical distribution of endometriosis is evidently influenced by both uterine position and age. An anteverted uterus is more commonly associated with anterior compartment endometriosis than a retroverted uterus ($P<0.0005$) (Jenkins *et al.*, 1986). Posterior compartment disease is seen most commonly in patients with a posterior uterus but is observed, regardless of uterine position, in the majority of patients. Redwine (1987b) observed an age-related change in the anatomical distribution of endometriosis. The frequency of endometriosis involving the posterior cul-de-sac, uterosacral and broad ligaments decreased with age while involvement of the ovaries increased with age. The severity of endometriosis, as determined by the revised American Fertility Classification system, does not correlate with the amount of pain a patient experiences (Fedele *et al.*, 1990). Several recent studies have shown a correlation between the

Table 26.2 Implants and adhesions by anatomical location

Location	Implants		Adhesions	
	No. patients	%	No. patients	%
Anterior cul-de-sac	63	34.6	4	2.2
Posterior cul-de-sac	62	34.0	20	11.0
Right ovary	57	31.3	26	14.3
Left ovary	81	44.0	45	24.7
Right anterior broad ligament	2	1.1	2	1.1
Left anterior broad ligament	0	0	3	1.6
Right round ligament	1	0.5	2	1.1
Left round ligament	1	0.5	2	1.1
Right fallopian tube	3	1.6	20	11.0
Left fallopian tube	8	4.3	28	15.4
Right posterior broad ligament	39	21.4	30	16.5
Left posterior broad ligament	46	25.2	50	27.5
Right uterosacral ligament	28	15.3	5	2.7
Left uterosacral ligament	38	20.8	8	4.4
Uterus	21	11.5	6	3.3
Sigmoid	7	3.8	22	12.1
Right ureter	3	1.6	0	0
Left ureter	2	1.1	3	1.6
Anterior bladder flap	1	0.5	1	0.5
Small bowel	1	0.5	4	2.2
Anterior abdominal wall	0	0	3	1.6
Omentum	0	0	4	2.2

Reprinted with permission from the American College of Obstetricians and Gynecologists (*Obstetrics and Gynecology*, 1986, **67**, 335–338).

depth of infiltration and pelvic pain (Cornillie *et al.*, 1990; Koninckx *et al.*, 1991).

Laparoscopic Appearance of Endometriosis

Sampson (1921, 1924, 1927) used descriptive terms such as red raspberries, purple raspberries, blueberries, blebs, and peritoneal pockets in his original series of articles. Subsequent articles primarily emphasized the pigmented, blue or black 'powderburn' appearance of endometriosis. The concept of endometriosis as a uniform appearing pigmented lesion has permeated the psyche of the average gynaecologist to the point that this type of lesion is still referred to as typical endometriosis. In actuality, the subtle or non-pigmented form of endometriosis truly represents the majority of lesions (Redwine, 1987b).

Histologically, endometriosis is comprised of both endometrial glands and stroma. Visually, endometriosis presents a vast array of appearances. The gross appearance of endometriosis is a result of several factors, including the relative proportion of glands and stroma, amount of scarring, intralesional bleeding and quantity of haemosiderin. While the relative contribution of the above factors results in a continuum of visual appearances, the most commonly described types of endometriosis include scarred white lesions, strawberry-like reddish lesions, red flame-like lesions, reddish polyps, clear vesicular lesions, adhesions, peritoneal defects, yellow-brown patches and black puckered lesions.

Goldstein *et al.* (1980) described petechial and bleb-like endometriosis in adolescent patients. Jansen and Russell published a study in 1986 in which they performed 137 biopsies of abnormal appearing non-pigmented peritoneum in 77 patients. The idea that endometriosis could be found in lesions devoid of pigmentation, 'typical of this disease', was a departure from the contemporary thinking of the time. Endometriosis was histologically present on 53% of the biopsies which was significantly different from biopsies of normally appearing peritoneum which failed to detect endometriosis ($P=0.005$) (Jansen and Russell, 1986).

White opacified and red flame-like lesions most commonly (81%) represented endometriosis (Figure 26.1). Characteristically, white opacified peritoneum is peritoneal scarring which may be raised or thickened. Red flame-like lesions may be elevated. Glandular lesions contained endometriosis in 67% of the cases. Glandular lesions

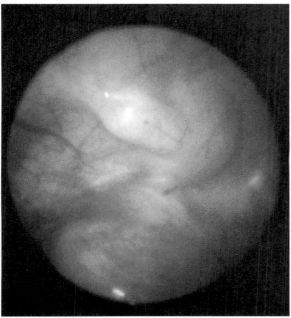

Figure 26.1 Fibrotic endometriosis in bladder peritoneum.

grossly appear the same as normal endometrium (e.g. at hysteroscopy). Subovarian adhesions, without peritubal adhesions typical of an infectious aetiology, represented endometriosis in two of the four cases. Other lesions which also contained endometriosis included yellow-brown peritoneal patches (47%), circular peritoneal defects (45%) and rarely, cribriform peritoneum (9%). Figure 26.2 depicts superficial yellow-brown

endometriosis. Vesicular excrescences which are loosely attached to the peritoneum represents a reaction to oil-based contrast medium.

Non-pigmented endometriosis progresses to pigmented endometriosis over time (Jansen and Russell, 1986). Second look laparoscopy in untreated patients 6–24 months following the initial surgery, documented pigmented lesions in areas which previously contained non-pigmented but abnormal peritoneum. Redwine's report suggested a progression of the visual appearance of endometriosis, from clear to red to white to black, with increasing age of the patient (Redwine, 1987a). Increasing age is associated with a decreasing incidence of subtle or atypical endometriosis and an increased incidence of 'typical' endometriosis, endometrioma and deeply infiltrating endometriosis (Koninckx et al., 1991).

Martin et al. pioneered the excisional techniques for the treatment of abnormal appearing peritoneum (Stripling et al., 1988; Martin et al., 1989). This provided the basis for extensive histological study of abnormal peritoneum and the delineation of a wide array of the appearances of endometriosis. The initial study described five different types of endometriotic lesions (puckered black, white, red, clear and pink lesions) in 109 patients (Stripling et al., 1988). Superficial clear papules of endometriosis are seen in Figure 26.3. Atypical endometriosis was noted in 55% of patients and was an isolated finding in 13% of the patients.

The puckered black lesion ('typical' endometriosis) is comprised of stroma, glands, fibromuscular scarring and intraluminal debris

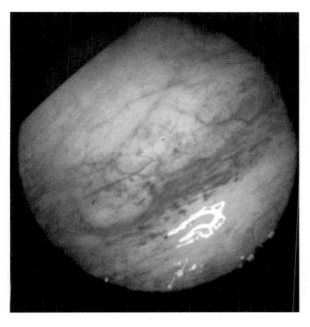

Figure 26.2 Superficial early confluent yellow-brown endometriosis.

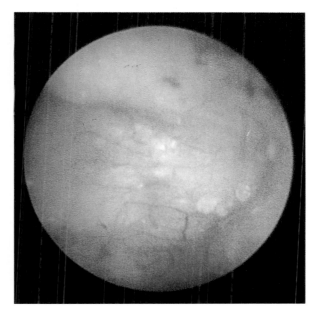

Figure 26.3 Superficial clear papules of endometriosis.

(Stripling *et al.*, 1988) (Figure 26.4). White endometriosis must be differentiated from postoperative scarring and from fibrotic adhesions resulting from inflammatory disease. Histologically, white endometriosis contains sparse glands and stroma, embedded in fibromuscular scar tissue. The red polypoid lesion is composed primarily of native appearing glands and stroma while flat red lesions are hypervascular. Deep endometriotic lesions may be associated with strawberry-like reddish areas. White scarred areas of endometriosis are frequently associated with strawberry-like reddish areas. The strawberry-like lesion may actually represent extension of deeper invasive lesions to the surface (Adamson, 1990). The amount of debris and intraluminal haemosiderin determines the intensity of coloration of brown and black lesions. In a subsequent study Martin *et al.* (1989) used up to 20 descriptive terms to characterize the appearance of endometriosis.

Allen and Masters (1955) described the presence of a peritoneal defect of the posterior aspect of the broad ligament in patients with pelvic pain. They postulated that the peritoneal defect was a result of trauma secondary to excessive motility of the uterus. It was not until later that the causal relationship between endometriosis and peritoneal defects was described (Chatman, 1981). Peritoneal defects frequently occur in areas of the pelvis which overlie loose connective tissue. The anatomical distribution of peritoneal defects is outlined in Table 26.3. Approximately 80% of peritoneal defects are associated with endometriosis, either on the border of the defect or in the defect itself (Chatman and Zbella, 1986).

Table 26.3 Anatomical distribution of defects

Location	Patients	%
Posterior cul-de-sac	19	31
Right broad ligament	18	29
Left broad ligament	18	29
Left uterosacral ligament	3	4
Right uterosacral ligament	2	3
Anterior cul-de-sac	2	3

Reproduced with permission of the publisher, The American Fertility Society, from Chatman and Zbella (1986).

Twenty-eight per cent of patients with endometriosis have peritoneal defects, which is significantly greater (*P*<0.005) than the 7% of patients with peritoneal defects in the general population (Chatman and Zbella, 1986). There is no correlation between the presence of peritoneal defects and the severity of endometriosis.

A 3-year prospective study of 643 consecutive laparoscopies demonstrated a highly significant correlation between pain and deeply infiltrating endometriosis (Koninckx *et al.*, 1991). When the depth of the endometriotic implant is taken into account, pelvic pain does not significantly correlate with the pelvic area or volume of endometriosis, nor with the presence or size of endometriomas. Deeply infiltrating endometriosis is found primarily in the rectovaginal septum and the uterosacral ligaments, and occasionally in the uterovesical fold. Visually these lesions appear as white plaques with puckered black spots or

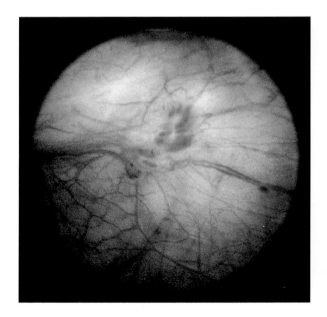

Figure 26.4 Classic 'powderburn' endometriosis.

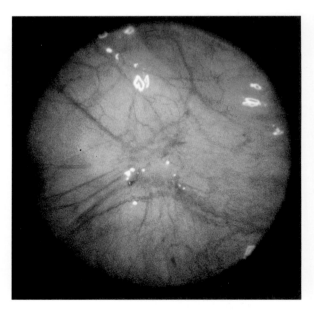

Figure 26.5 Invasive endometriosis with 'classical' lesions and fibrosis causing peritoneal contraction.

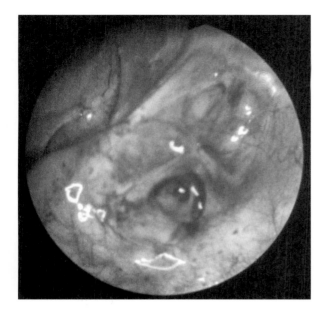

Figure 26.6 Deeply invasive fibrotic endometriosis causing marked peritoneal distortion.

isolated puckered black spots (Figures 26.5, 26.6). Some patients, particularly those with bowel involvement, deep endometriosis may present with retraction only. The diagnosis of deep endometriosis and evaluation of the extent of endometriosis is determined by palpation with the blunt probe and intraoperative rectovaginal examinations (Reich *et al.*, 1991). Endometriosis may be hard and sclerotic, which when retracted with a blunt probe causes movement of the surrounding tissue in block. The lesion should be resected and/or vaporized until soft, supple tissue is encountered. The tissue cannot be directly palpated, but with experience subtle differences in the consistency of the tissue can be appreciated visually. Surgical estimation of the depth of the lesion correlates well with histological findings (Cornillie *et al.*, 1990).

Not all abnormalities of the peritoneum represent endometriosis. Other lesions which may mimic endometriosis include old suture, residual carbon from laser surgery, splenosis, reaction to oil-based contrast medium, epithelial inclusion, Walthard rests, adrenal rests, secondary breast and ovarian cancer and inflammatory cystic inclusions (Jansen and Russell, 1986). Differentiation between atypical endometriosis and other lesions may be impossible visually but may be achieved histologically through excision or biopsy. An abnormality of the peritoneum, no matter what its size, shape, or appearance, should suggest the possibility of endometriosis. Biopsy of these atypical lesions often confirms the presence of disease.

Summary

The appearance of endometriosis is quite diverse, ranging from very subtle lesions which are difficult to visualize grossly, to the typical black, puckered 'powderburn' lesions. The subtle or atypical lesions probably represent a more active form of endometriosis. With increasing age, there is a progression to the less active 'typical' form of endometriosis. Retraction of the peritoneum may be the only sign of deeply infiltrating endometriosis. A combination of laparoscopy, palpation with the blunt probe and intraoperative rectovaginal examinations may be needed for the diagnosis of endometriosis. The ability to diagnose atypical and subtle appearances of endometriosis is directly related to the experience and skill of the surgeon.

References

Adamson GD (1990) Diagnosis and clinical presentation of endometriosis. *American Journal of Obstetrics and Gynecology* **162**:568–569.

Adamson GD (1991) Surgical and medical treatment of endometriosis. *Contemporary OB/GYN* **36**:48–63.

Allen WM & Masters WH (1955) Traumatic laceration of uterine support. *American Journal of Obstetrics and Gynecology* **70**:500–513.

Chatman DL (1981) Pelvic peritoneal defects and endometriosis: Allen–Masters syndrome revisited. *Fertility and Sterility* **36**:751.

Chatman DL & Zbella EA (1986) Pelvic peritoneal defects and endometriosis: future observations. *Fertility and Sterility* **46**:711–714.

Cornillie FJ, Oosterlynck D, Lauweryns JM & Koninckx PR (1990) Deeply infiltrating pelvic endometriosis: histology and clinical significance. *Fertility and Sterility* **53**:978–983.

Fedele L, Parazzini F, Bianchi S, Areaini L & Candiani GB (1990) Stage and localization of pelvic endometriosis and pain. *Fertility and Sterility* **53**:155–158.

Goldstein DP, DeCholnoky C & Eman J (1980) Adolescent endometriosis. *Journal of Adolescent Health Care* **1**:37.

Jansen RPS & Russell P (1986) Nonpigmented endometriosis: clinical, laparoscopic, and pathologic definition. *American Journal of Obstetrics and Gynecology* **155**:1154–1159.

Jenkins S, Olive DL & Haney AF (1986) Endometriosis: pathogenetic implications of the anatomic distribution. *Obstetrics and Gynecology* **67**:335–338.

Koninckx PR, Meuleman C, Demeyere S, Lesaffre E & Cornillie FJ (1991) Suggestive evidence that pelvic endometriosis is a progressive disease, whereas deeply infiltrating endometriosis is associated with pelvic pain. *Fertility and Sterility* **55**:759–765.

Martin DC, Hubert GD, Vander Zwaag R & El-Zeky FA (1989) Laparoscopic appearances of peritoneal endometriosis. *Fertility and Sterility* **51**:63–67.

Martin DC, Ahmic R, El-Zeky FA *et al.* (1990) Increased histologic confirmation of endometriosis. *Journal of Gynecologic Surgery* **6**:275–279.

Murphy AA (1992) Diagnostic and operative laparoscopy. In Thompson JD & Rock JA (eds) *TeLinde's Operative Gynecology*, pp 361–384. Baltimore: JB Lippincott Co.

Murphy AA, Green WR, Bobbie D, dela Cruz ZC & Rock JA (1986) Unsuspected endometriosis documented by scanning electron microscopy in visually normal peritoneum. *Fertility and Sterility* **46**:522–524.

Nisolle M, Paindaveine B, Boudon A *et al.* (1990) Histologic study of peritoneal endometriosis in infertile women. *Fertility and Sterility* **53**:984–988.

Redwine DB (1987a) Age-related evolution in color appearance of endometriosis. *Fertility and Sterility* **48**:1062–1063.

Redwine DB (1987b) The distribution of endometriosis in the pelvis by age groups and fertility. *Fertility and Sterility* **47**:173–175.

Reich H, McGlynn F & Salvat J (1991) Laparoscopic treatment of culdesac obliteration secondary to retrocervical deep fibrotic endometriosis. *Journal of Reproductive Medicine* **36**:516–522.

Sampson JA (1921) Perforating hemorrhagic (chocolate) cysts of the ovary. *Archives of Surgery* **3**:245.

Sampson JA (1924) Benign and malignant endometrial implants in the peritoneal cavity and their relationship to certain ovarian tumors. *Surgery, Obstetrics and Gynecology* **38**:287.

Sampson JA (1927) Peritoneal endometriosis due to dissemination of endometrial tissue into the peritoneal cavity. *American Journal of Obstetrics and Gynecology* **14**:422.

Stripling MC, Martin DC, Chatman DL, Vander Zwaag R & Poston WM (1988) Subtle appearance of pelvic endometriosis. *Fertility and Sterility* **49**:427–431.

27

Peritoneal Endometriosis: New Aspects in Two-dimensional and Three-dimensional Evaluation

M. NISOLLE, F. CASANAS-ROUX AND J. DONNEZ

Infertility Research Unit, Catholic University of Louvain, Brussels, Belgium

Endometriosis most commonly affects the pelvic peritoneum close to the ovaries, including the uterosacral ligaments, the ovarian fossa peritoneum, and the peritoneum of the cul-de-sac.

The increased diagnosis of endometriosis at laparoscopy may be explained by the increased ability to detect such subtle lesions due to the surgeon's experience. The greatest change was in the case of 'subtle' lesions, which increased from 15% in 1986 to 65% in 1988. The diagnosis of peritoneal endometriosis at the time of laparoscopy is often made by observation of typically puckered black or bluish lesions. There are in addition, numerous subtle appearances of peritoneal endometriosis. These lesions, frequently non-pigmented, were diagnosed as endometriosis following confirmation by biopsy by Jansen and Russell in 1986.

Typical Lesion

The typical peritoneal endometriotic lesion results from tissue bleeding and retention of blood pigment producing brown discoloration of tissue. Puckered black lesions are a combination of glands, stroma, scar and intraluminal debris (Figure 27.1).

Evolution

The macroscopic appearance of ectopic endometrium is probably dependent upon the lon-gevity of the process. Viable cells may implant and the initial appearance may be an irregularity or discoloration of the peritoneal surface (Figure 27.2)—the earliest sign being haemosiderin staining of the peritoneal surfaces. Initially, these lesions may appear haemorrhagic (Figure 27.3), but menstrual shedding from a viable endometrial implant initiates an inflammatory reaction which provokes a scarification process which in turn encloses the implants. The presence of entrapped menstrual debris is responsible for the typical black or bluish appearance. If the inflammatory process obliterates or devascularizes the endometrial cells, eventually this discoloration disappears. A white plaque of old collagen is all that remains of the ectopic implant. Scarring of the peritoneum around endometrial implants is a typical finding. In addition to encapsulating an isolated implant, the scar may deform the surrounding peritoneum or result in the development of adhesions.

Subtle Appearance

Sometimes the subtle endometriotic lesions can be the only lesions seen at laparoscopy. The subtle forms are more common and may be more active than the puckered black lesions (Table 27.1).

The non-pigmented endometriotic peritoneal lesions include the following:

1. White opacification of the peritoneum which

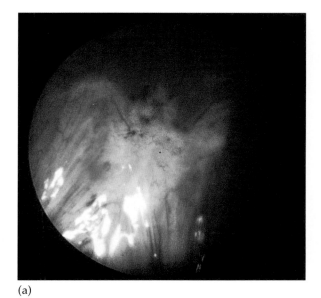

(a)

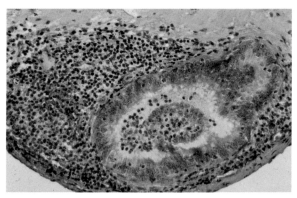

(b)

Figure 27.1 (a) Laparoscopical aspects: puckered black lesions. (b) Histology: combination of glands, stroma, scar and intraluminal debris (Gomori's trichrome × 110).

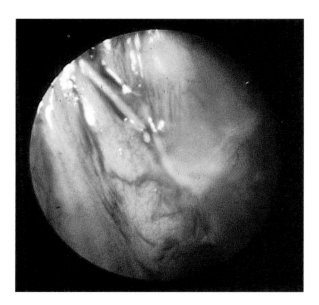

Figure 27.2 Yellow-brown patches of the peritoneum.

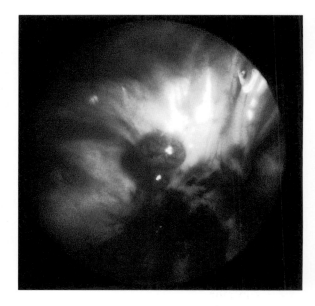

Figure 27.3 Red flame-like lesions of the peritoneum.

Table 27.1 Different appearances of peritoneal endometriosis

Typical aspect
Puckered black lesion
Subtle lesions
White opacification (Jansen and Russell, 1986)
Red flame-like lesion (Jansen and Russell, 1986)
Glandular excrescences (Jansen and Russell, 1986)
Subovarian adhesions (Jansen and Russell, 1986)
Yellow-brown peritoneal patches (Jansen and Russell, 1986)
Circular peritoneal defect (Chatman, 1981)
Petechial peritoneum (Nisolle *et al.*, 1990)
Hypervascularization areas (Nisolle *et al.*, 1990)

appears as peritoneal scarring or as circumscribed patches often thickened and sometimes raised. Histologically, white opacified peritoneum is due to the presence of an occasional retroperitoneal glandular structure and scanty stroma surrounded by fibrotic tissue or connective tissue.

2. Red flame-like lesions of the peritoneum or red vesicular excrescences affect more commonly, the broad ligament and the uterosacral ligaments. Histologically, red flame-like lesions and vesicular excrescences are due to the presence of active endometriosis surrounded by stroma.

3. Glandular excrescences on the peritoneal surface which in colour, translucency and consistency closely resemble the mucosal surface of the endometrium seen at hysteroscopy. Biopsy reveals the presence of numerous endometrial glands.

4. Subovarian adhesions or adhesions between ovary and peritoneum of the ovarian fossa which are distinctive from adhesions characteristic of previous salpingitis or peritonitis. Histologically, connective tissue with sparse endometrial glands is found.

5. Yellow-brown peritoneal patches resembling 'café au lait' patches. The histological characteristics are similar to those observed in white opacification, but in the yellow-brown patches the presence of the blood pigment—haemosiderin—among the stroma cells produces the 'café au lait' colour.

6. Circular peritoneal defects as described by Chatman (1981) when he reviewed the so-called Allen–Masters syndrome. Serial section demonstrates the presence of endometrial glands in more than 50% of cases.

7. Areas of petechial peritoneum or areas with hypervascularization were diagnosed as endometriosis in our recent study. These lesions resemble the petechial lesions due to manipulation of the peritoneum or to hypervascularization of the peritoneum. They most generally affect the bladder and the broad ligament, and histologically, red blood cells are numerous and endometrial glands are very rare.

Histological Study of Peritoneal Endometriosis

Typical

The morphological characteristics of peritoneal endometriosis were studied in 109 biopsies with histologically proven endometriosis (Nisolle et al., 1990). An endometriotic lesion was considered 'active' when typical glandular epithelium appeared as either proliferative or completely unresponsive to hormones, with typical stroma. Such a lesion was found in 76% of cases. Areas of oviduct-like epithelium with ciliated cells were demonstrated in 55% of peritoneal endometriotic foci. The epithelial height and the mitotic index were calculated in typical glandular epithelium. Epithelial height was measured with a micrometer and the mitotic index was calculated by counting mitotic figures per 2000 epithelial cells, as previously described. Their value was respectively 14.8 ± 3.2 μm and 0.6%.

Subtle Lesions

Confirmation of endometriosis in subtle lesions has been reported by Jansen and Russell (Chapters 25 and 26). Endometriosis was confirmed in 81% of white opacified lesions, 81% of red flame-like lesions, 67% of glandular lesions, 50% of subovarian adhesions, 47% of yellow-brown patches and 45% of circular peritoneal defects. Later, Stripling and colleagues (1988) confirmed endometriosis in 91% of white lesions, 75% of red lesions, 33% of haemosiderin lesions, and 85% of other lesions. In our study, we confirmed the presence of endometriotic lesions in non-pigmented lesions of peritoneum in more than 50% of cases.

Unsuspected Peritoneal Endometriosis

In a recent study (Nisolle et al., 1990), biopsies were taken from visually normal peritoneum of 32 women undergoing a laparoscopy for infertility and in whom neither typical nor subtle appearances of endometriosis were found. In another group of 52 women with apparent endometriosis, biopsies were also taken from visually normal peritoneum.

The peritoneum was considered as normal peritoneum if no lesion as described before was seen. Biopsy was taken from normal peritoneum of uterosacral ligaments.

Histological study revealed the presence of endometriotic tissue in two cases (6%) in the group of 32 infertile women without endometriosis. This rate was less than one-half the rate (13%) observed in normal peritoneum taken from women with visible endometriosis.

Identification of endometriosis in biopsy specimens from areas of normal peritoneum in patients with known endometriosis was reported by Murphy et al. (1986). By scanning electron microscopy, 25% of their specimens, which appeared normal by gross inspection, were found to contain evidence of endometriosis. In our study, by light microscopy, we reported a rate of 13%.

Moreover, histological study of biopsies from visually normal peritoneum in infertile women without any typical or 'subtle' endometriotic lesions revealed the presence of endometriosis in 6% of cases. Unsuspected peritoneal endometriosis can thus be found in visually normal peritoneum of infertile women with or without associated endometriosis. Although the rate (13%) in women with visible endometriosis was twice the rate observed in women without endometriosis, the difference was not significant. The size of endometriotic lesions in visually normal peritoneum (313 ± 185 μm) probably explains why the peritoneum had a normal aspect and why the lesion was not visible even though a meticulous inspection was made to identify small and non-haemorrhagic lesions.

The diagnosis of endometriosis in infertile women undergoing laparoscopy has increased. However, our data confirm that the operating surgeon missed the diagnosis in at least 6% of patients, despite the significant increase in the diagnosis and documentation of endometriosis.

Hormonal Independence

Using qualitative histochemistry, the microscopic changes (Vasquez *et al.*, 1984) present in endometrium have been observed in ectopic implants, but endometrial implants do not demonstrate the characteristic ultrastructural changes of normal endometrium. The fact that endometrial implants can undergo cyclical histological changes similar to those found in normal endometrium demonstrates that ectopic endometrium responds to gonadal hormones. But the majority of implants do not demonstrate histological changes synchronous with the comparable uterine endometrium (Roddick *et al.*, 1960). Some of the reasons are probably:

1. the deficiency in steroid receptors,
2. the influence of the surrounding scarification process,
3. the pressure atrophy,
4. the hormonal independence of ectopic endometrial glands.

The evaluation of steroid receptors in ectopic endometrial implants could be difficult because of the small number of glandular and stromal cells within the implant, and the heterogeneity of the tissue. While most implants can be demonstrated (Jänne *et al.*, 1981) to possess progesterone receptors, only 30% have oestrogen receptors. In the ovary, implants have far fewer oestrogen and progesterone receptors than does normal epithelium (Tamaya *et al.*, 1979; Bergqvist *et al.*, 1981). Castration, menopause, pregnancy or therapeutic suppression of gonadal function can dramatically alter the pattern of disease. We have recently shown (Nisolle *et al.*, 1988) that hormonal treatment is unable to eradicate endometriosis. Indeed both in peritoneal endometriosis and in ovarian endometriosis, microscopic examination of specimens (taken after 6 months of therapy) revealed a high incidence of active endometriosis without signs of degeneration. Mitotic activity was found, and this suggested the presence of hormonally independent glands in endometriotic foci.

New Histological Aspects of Endometriosis in Two-dimensional (2-D) Evaluation

Vascularization

Vascularization of endometriotic implants is probably one of the most important factors in the growth and invasion of endometrial glands into other tissue.

INFLUENCE OF GnRH AGONIST ON THE VASCULARIZATION OF TYPICAL PERITONEAL ENDOMETRIOSIS

The vascularization of peritoneal endometriosis and its modifications under hormonal therapy have been evaluated. A stereometric analysis was applied in order to study precisely the vascularization in typical peritoneal endometriotic foci.

Structure measurement was carried out according to Weibel's principles. A 2-D image analysis program set on a Vidas computer (Kontron Bildanalyse GmBH, Eching, Germany) was completed by the interactive counting of 262.144 points (Marchevsky *et al.*, 1987).

All endometriotic lesions ($n = 110$) (group I: without therapy, $n = 85$; group II: after a 12-week GnRH therapy, $n = 25$) were analysed field by field using the Axioskop light microscope. Histological structures of interest such as the stroma, the glandular epithelium and lumen and the capillaries were traced by a digitizer (Figure 27.4). Each different structure was discriminated and grey level images were transferred to binary images. The interactive measurements of the selected parameters—number of structures, area and perimeter of the structures per field—were appended and stored at the end of an existing data base.

The results concerning the capillaries are shown in Table 27.2. The number of capillaries per mm^2 of stroma, their mean surface and the surface ratio (capillaries/stroma) was calculated. There was no significant difference concerning the number of capillaries per mm^2 of stroma between the treated and untreated patients. However, in the treated group, their mean surface ($63 \pm 24\ \mu m^2$) was significantly different ($P < 0.001$) from the value observed in the untreated group ($113 \pm 8.1\ \mu m^2$). The capillaries/stroma ratio was significantly lower ($P < 0.002$) in the treated group (1.4%) than in the untreated group (2.5%).

Some morphological changes of endometriotic foci after hormonal therapy have previously been

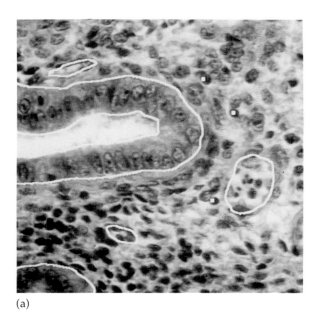
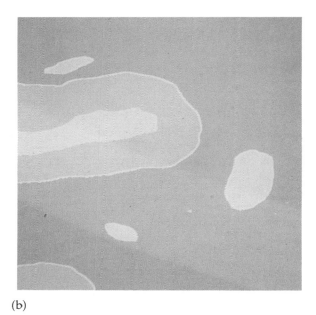

(a)

(b)

Figure 27.4 A 2-D image. (a) Histological structures are traced by a digitizer : glandular epithelium, lumen, stroma and capillaries. (b) Grey level image of the same field.

Table 27.2 Vascularization evaluation in typical endometriotic lesions

	Group I typical lesions (without therapy) $n = 85$	Group II typical lesions (after a 12-week therapy) $n = 25$
Number of capillaries/mm² stroma (M ± SD)	268	261
Capillaries mean surface (μm²) (M ± SD)	113 ± 81	65 ± 24*
Capillaries/stroma relative surface (%)	2.5	1.4**

*Significantly different $(P < 0.001)$ from non-treated lesions.
**Significantly different $(P < 0.02)$ from non-treated lesions.

described (Nisolle et al., 1988). The mitotic index has been found to be significantly reduced. One of our hypotheses concerning the mechanism of action was the reduction in the vascularization of stroma after GnRH agonist therapy. Macroscopically, preoperative hormonal therapy results in a reduction of pelvic vascularity and inflammation diagnosed at the time of the second look laparoscopy.

Our results demonstrated that there was a significant decrease in vascularization of the endometriotic foci after GnRH agonist therapy. This change was not due to a reduction in the number of capillaries in the lesion but to a decrease in the surface area of the vessels. Indeed, in the treated patients (group II) a predominance of smaller vessels was observed when compared with the untreated patients (group I). This vascularization decrease observed histologically was in accordance with the observations made by laparoscopy after hormonal therapy. Vascular effects of the GnRH agonist have also been demonstrated by Doppler on the uterine arteries (Matta et al., 1988). Probably the profound hypo-oestrogenic state induced by the GnRH agonist could also have an effect on the vascular compartment of the endometriotic stroma.

The reduction in the vascularization after hormonal therapy could explain the decrease in the inflammatory reaction observed around the endometriotic foci.

Vascularization Evaluation of Subtle Endometriotic Lesions

Vascularization has been evaluated in atypical lesions according to the previously described method.

The following subtle lesions have been evaluated: white opacification, yellow-brown lesions, red flame-like lesions, adhesions and glandular excrescences.

The results in this group, compared with typical black lesions ($n = 85$) are shown in Table 27.3. When compared to data on typical black lesions, significant differences were observed.

In white opacification and yellow-brown lesions, the number of capillaries/mm^2 was not significantly different from the number found in typical black lesions. However, their mean surface area (respectively 78 ± 42 μm^2 and 81 ± 28 μm^2) was significantly lower than the value observed in typical lesions.

In red flame-like lesions, the number of capillaries/mm^2 was not significantly different from typical lesions but the mean surface area was significantly higher.

In adhesions and in glandular excrescences, there was no significant difference in the number of capillaries/mm^2 compared with the number observed in other lesions, but the mean surface area was significantly lower than that observed in red flame-like lesions. The relative surface area of capillaries compared to stroma was respectively 2.5% (typical lesions), 2.0% (white opacification), 2.3% (yellow-brown patches), 3.1% (red flame-like), 2.7% (adhesions), 3.4% (glandular excrescences).

Hypothesis

Red flame-like lesions and glandular excrescences are probably the first stage of early implantation of endometrial glands and stroma. Their significantly higher vascularization is responsible for invasion. Indeed, mitotic activity has been proved to be related to the vascularization (Nisolle *et al.,* 1990). This could explain the growth and the aggressiveness of recently implanted endometrial cells. Thereafter, menstrual shedding from viable endometrial implants could initiate an inflammatory reaction which provokes a scarification process which encloses the implant. The presence of intraluminal debris is responsible for the typical black coloration of the same lesion. This scarification process is responsible for the reduction in vascularization as proved by the significant decrease in capillaries/stroma relative surface area (2.5% versus 3.1% and versus 3.4%).

Thereafter, the inflammatory process devascularizes the endometrial cells, and white plaques of old collagen are all that remain of the ectopic implant. The vascularization of this scarred endometriotic tissue was found significantly reduced in our study (relative surface area 1.5%). White opacification and yellow-brown lesions could be latent stages of endometriosis as suggested by the poor vascularization observed. They are probably non-active lesions which have been quiescent for a long time.

Three-dimensional (3-D) Architecture of Endometriosis

In order to elucidate further biological characteristics of peritoneal endometriotic lesions, for example how they develop stereologically *in vivo* and how glandular epithelium and stroma are related to the surrounding tissue, a newly developed stereographic computer technology was applied to the investigation of three-dimensional (3-D) architecture of peritoneal endometriosis. The histological features of the sections were displayed using an Axioskop microscope through a CCD 72 E camera on a TV monitor on which two-dimensional (2-D) figures drawn with a digitizer were superimposed using a computer (Vidas, Kontron Bildanalyse GmBH, Eching, Germany).

With this program, outlines of glandular struc-

Table 27.3 Comparison of vascularization in typical and subtle endometriotic lesions

	Puckered lesion $n = 85$	White opacification $n = 24$	Yellow-brown $n = 5$	Red flame-like $n = 12$	Adhesions $n = 17$	Glandular excrescences $n = 10$
Number of capillaries/mm^2 stroma (M $\pm$ SD)	268	213	324	173	185	181
Capillaries mean surface (μm^2)(M $\pm$ SD)	113 ± 81	$78 \pm 42^*$	$81 \pm 28^{**}$	$249 \pm 268^*$	149 ± 117	149 ± 98
Capillaries/stroma relative surface (%)	2.5	2.0	2.3	3.1	2.7	3.4

*Significantly different ($P < 0.001$) from typical lesions.
**Significantly different ($P < 0.02$) from typical lesions.

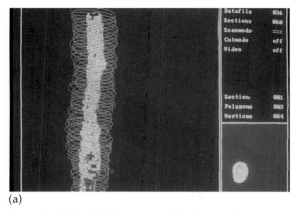
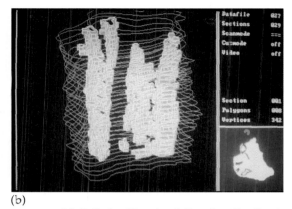

(a)   (b)

Figure 27.5 The 3-D image models displayed as a transparent structure. (a) Cylinder-like gland. Regular distribution of the glandular epithelium in the stroma. (b) Glands with ramifications. Luminal structures are interconnected.

ture and endometrial stroma in the serial histological sections were traced by the digitizer. All the serial outlines had been digitized and stored, and reconstructed (3-D) image models of these *in vivo* structures were displayed on the TV monitor. The 3-D reconstruction could generate a complete multicoloured model of the complex structure which could be rotated and viewed from any angle of orientation.

Recently, the first computer-stereographic study of endometriotic tissue has been reported describing the advantages of the computer-generated 3-D models of tissue structures (Donnez *et al.*, 1992). Our 3-D models showed realistic appearances of structures since the structures of the reconstructed models were coloured. Furthermore, the transparent display of our 3-D models was excellent for observation of their inside structures and the volumes of the reconstructed structures could be obtained by the computer-stereometry (Figures 27.5a and b).

The study demonstrates that two different types of peritoneal endometrial lesions may be differentiated:

1. a first type without ramification of the glands (Figure 27.5a);
2. a second type in which glands are ramified and seem more invasive through the stroma (Figure 27.5b).

From the stereographic findings (Donnez *et al.*, 1991) one may consider that the apparently multifocal occurrence (in 2-D) of glandular epithelium in one lesion is not confirmed by the 3-D study. Indeed, in each peritoneal lesion, epithelial glands are interconnected by luminal structures.

Further studies are needed in order to evaluate whether the two different types could be correlated either to the different degree of 'aggressiveness'

or to the different appearances of peritoneal endometriosis.

Conclusion

In this chapter, typical endometriosis and subtle appearances of endometriosis have been described not only macroscopically but also microscopically. Some new aspects in 2-D evaluation (vascularization) and in 3-D evaluation were studied in order to elucidate how peritoneal endometriosis stereogically develops *in vivo*. A hypothesis of evolution from early implantation to scarred peritoneum has been suggested according to the evolution of vascularization.

References

Bergqvist A, Rannevik G & Thorell J (1981) Estrogen and progesterone cytosol receptor concentration in endometriotic tissue and intrauterine endometrium. *Acta Obstetrica et Gynecologica Scandinavica* **101**:53–58.

Chatman DL (1981) Pelvic peritoneal defects and endometriosis; Allen–Masters syndrome revisited. *Fertility and Sterility* **36**:751–756.

Donnez J, Nisolle M & Casanas-Roux F (1992) Three dimensional architectures of peritoneal endometriosis. *Fertility and Sterility* **57**:980–983.

Jänne O, Kauppila A, Kokko E *et al.* (1981) Estrogen and progestin receptors in endometriosis lesions: comparison with endometrial tissue. *American Journal of Obstetrics and Gynecology* **141**:562–566.

Jansen RPS & Russell P (1986) Nonpigmented endometriosis: clinical laparoscopic and pathologic definition. *American Journal of Obstetrics and Gynecology* **155**:1154–1159.

Marchevsky AM, Gil J & Jeanty H (1987) Computerized interactive morphometry in pathology: current instrumentation and methods. *Human Pathology* **18**:320–331.

Matta WHM, Stabile I, Shaw RS & Campbell S (1988) Doppler assessment of uterine blood flow changes in patients with fibroids receiving the GnRH agonist buserelin. *Fertility and Sterility* **49**:1083–1085.

Murphy AA, Green WR, Bobbie D, de la Cruz ZC & Rock JA (1986) Unsuspected endometriosis documented by scanning electron microscopy in visually normal peritoneum. *Fertility and Sterility* **46**:522–524.

Nisolle M, Casanas-Roux F & Donnez J (1988) Histologic study of ovarian endometriosis after hormonal therapy. *Fertility and Sterility* **49**:423–426.

Nisolle M, Paindaveine B, Bourdon A *et al.* (1990) Histologic study of peritoneal endometriosis in infertile women. *Fertility and Sterility* **53**:984–988.

Roddick JW, Conkey G & Jacobs EJ (1960) The hormonal response of endometriotic implants and its relationship to symptomatology. *American Journal of Obstetrics and Gynecology* **79**:1173–1177.

Stripling MC, Martin DC, Chatman DL, Vander Zwaag R & Poston WM (1988) Subtle appearances of pelvic endometriosis. *Fertility and Sterility* **49**:427–431.

Tamaya T, Motoyaha T & Ohono Y (1979) Steroid receptor levels and histology of endometriosis and adenomyosis. *Fertility and Sterility* **31**:394–400.

Vasquez G, Cornille F & Brosens I (1984) Peritoneal endometriosis: scanning electron microscopy and histology of minimal pelvic endometriotic lesions. *Fertility and Sterility* **42**:696–703.

28

Laser Vaporization of Endometriosis

JOSEPH R. FESTE

Ob/Gyn Associates, Houston, Texas, USA

Introduction

One of the most common diseases amenable to treatment by laser laparoscopy is pelvic endometriosis. Because endometriosis is basically a disease of the peritoneal surface, it is easily treated with the laser. In the beginning, a surgeon's use of the laser laparoscope should be limited to treating only minimal and mild cases of endometriosis (stages I and II). With experience, the laser laparoscopist can safely and successfully treat moderate (stage III) and severe (stage IV) endometriosis with the laser laparoscope except when colon resection is required. Eventually, with careful use of either the operative laparoscope or the second-puncture probe, one can safely and adequately vaporize most visible endometriotic implants. Ideally, if endometriosis is diagnosed at laparoscopy performed for the evaluation of infertility or pelvic pain, it can be vaporized at the same time and the need for long-term medical therapy or subsequent major surgery is reduced.

General Considerations

Vaporization with laser energy offers several advantages over bipolar cautery or endocoagulation of endometriotic implants. With unipolar or bipolar cauterization, it is not possible to control the 'star burst' effect. Neither bipolar cautery nor endocoagulation provides a way to evaluate the depth of removal of the endometriotic implant, and thus a way to know at the time of the procedure whether the lesion has been completely destroyed. However, with the CO_2, argon and KTP lasers, the process of vaporization allows visualization of the three-dimensional boundaries of the lesion, thereby permitting its complete destruction and removal. In general, especially for the beginner, power densities between 2500 and 5000 W/cm² are used. Debulking endometriotic implants is best performed by using a continuous firing mode. But for lesions overlying a vital structure, the ureter, urinary bladder, colon, or larger blood vessels, single or repeat-pulse modes 0.05–0.1 seconds in duration provide safer vaporization. Pulses of this duration allow a 100–200 mm depth of vaporization, and thus substantially limit the depth of penetration. In addition, the intermittent blast of the laser decreases heat transfer, prevents damage to the underlying tissue, and prevents injury to vital structures. Single or repeat pulse modes are generally the safest modality for the novice CO_2 laser laparoscopist. Recently, use of high-power density superpulses has been advocated to vaporize peritoneal endometriosis. However, the potential depth of penetration dictates the need for extreme care when these settings are used. In most instances, the surgeon rapidly pulses the laser with the foot pedal in order to keep the depth of penetration under control. However, this technique should be used only by experienced surgeons.

The lesions of endometriosis are basically avascular. Therefore, haemostasis is a concern only in the underlying normal tissues. When an endometriotic implant is vaporized, the bubbling of old blood is seen first, followed by a curdy white material representing vaporization of the stromal layer. After the entire endometriotic lesion has been vaporized, retroperitoneal fat is encountered, and the appearance of the 'bubbling of water' confirms the complete vaporization of the lesion. The absorption of the CO_2 laser by water prevents deeper penetration of the laser beam for a few seconds after the endometriotic implant is vaporized.

Though they share some characteristics, such as avascularity, the endometriotic lesions vary considerably in appearance. The various forms of endometriosis are noted in Chapters 25 and 26. Whether it presents as a white scar-like lesion, a haemosiderin deposit, a bullous lesion or raised, red or port-wine coloured lesion, all of the peritoneal disease must be completely vaporized. As a matter of fact, the diffuse haemorrhagic deposits probably are the most active and produce significant pain and infertility. The tendency is to overlook these areas and look more intently for the textbook type of lesions. However, even the areas that appear to be only old scar tissue, especially after therapy with either danazol and a GnRH agonist for several months, should be completely vaporized. If left alone, these lesions are very likely in time to be activated by the influence of oestrogen and to become again symptomatic. Indeed some laser surgeons insist on at least two cycles without medical suppression for these areas to be reactivated and become macroscopically obvious (Evers, 1987). If the areas of vaporization are extensive and two lasered areas are in close proximity, the biodegradable graft, Interceed, should be used to minimize the development of adhesions postoperatively (Adhesion Barrier Study Group, 1989).

Techniques

Peritoneum and Soft Tissue

Usually, small implants can be excised, vaporized or coagulated. However, lesions > 3 mm deep have been reported in about 60% of patients in some series (Martin et al., 1989). For these deeper lesions, vaporization or excision should be taken down to the level of healthy tissue. The tissue distortion that occurs with vaporization techniques can be confusing, and deep lesions can

be missed. In some instances, it may be preferable to excise rather than vaporize the lesion (Martin and Vander Zwaag, 1987). This is particularly true when there are a multitude of lesions in the same area. Not only would excision be easier, but it would be safer if the point of dissection were over vital structures (Figure 28.1).

For excision, the lesion is outlined by cutting through the peritoneum and into the loose connective tissue with the laser. The underlying loose connective tissue and fat are noted and a blunt probe or irrigating solution is used to dissect through these layers. This technique is called 'hydrodissection' (Nezhat and Nezhat, 1989). Dissection with a blunt probe or irrigating solution is used in vascular areas to avoid inadvertently cutting across large vessels and is used in the broad ligament to push the ureter away from the peritoneum (Figure 28.2). Once tissue has been excised it is removed through the laparoscope. Tissue too large for removal through the trocar sheath is cut into smaller sections with scissors or removed by mini-laparotomy or colpotomy.

The advantages and disadvantages of excision are listed in Table 28.1. The method of removal of peritoneal implants should depend on the surgeon's own experience and skills. A superpulse or ultrapulse delivery mode can be used to decrease carbonization by facilitating rapid vaporization and reduction of the amount of lateral tissue desiccated or coagulated. Some authors recommend removal of the carbon by using pusher sponges (Taylor et al., 1986). However, one of the reasons for using the laser is that it coagulates while it cuts; removing the carbon

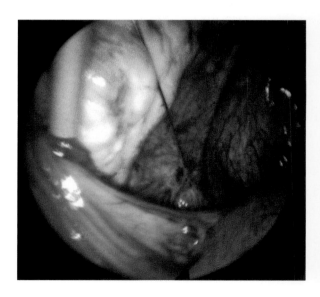

Figure 28.1 Excision of endometriosis implants over ureter.

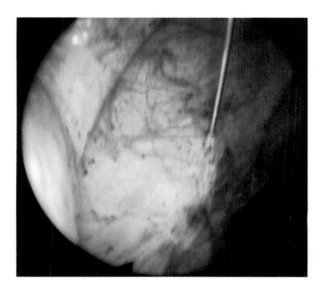

Figure 28.2 Hydrodissection with irrigating solution to lift the lesion off the ureter.

Table 28.1 Advantages and disadvantages of excisional method

Advantages
 Creates less smoke
 Leaves less carbon than vaporization
 Provides tissue for diagnosis

Disadvantages
 Removes unnecessary peritoneum
 Technically can be more difficult
 Slightly more time consuming

with a sponge defeats the purpose by wiping off the clots as well as creating microscopic bleeding. Instead, a strong stream of heparinized Ringer's lactate may be introduced through an irrigation probe to wash the carbon from the tissue. Even though carbon is inadvertently left behind, it will have no impact. The skilled surgeon learns to recognize residual carbon at a subsequent laparoscopy. Typically, it appears as a discrete, black speck that appears to have been imbedded in the peritoneum. There are no areas of scarring around the lesion and no signs of glandular tissue (Figure 28.3).

Bladder Lesions

Bladder lesions can be treated in much the same way as peritoneal disease if the lesions are on the surface of the peritoneum and no larger than 5 mm. If a patient has symptoms of haematuria without a definite bladder infection, cystoscopy should be performed. If the lesion involves the bladder mucosa or muscularis, excision should

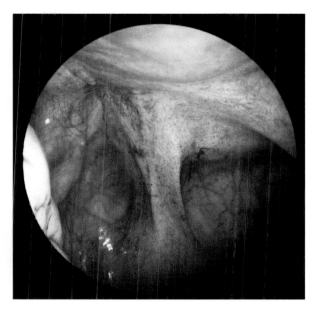

Figure 28.3 Carbon particles from residual vaporization of endometriosis.

be performed at laparotomy. All of the peritoneum overlying the bladder has been completely removed on several occasions. Over a period of 1–2 weeks, reperitonealization will take place and the peritoneum will be completely restored. However, the likelihood of development of extensive adhesions between the bladder and uterus is so great that it is necessary to take every precaution to prevent this from happening. I have used Interceed, the biodegradable cellulose made by Johnson & Johnson, to prevent formation of adhesions in this area (Adhesion Barrier Study Group, 1989). If adhesions are allowed to form, irritable bladder symptoms may follow.

Ureter and Uterine Vessels

It is imperative that the ureter and uterine vessels are identified prior to vaporization of endometrial implants in close proximity to their known location. In the case of a ureter, the peritoneum can be opened above the ureter in an area distal or proximal to the lesion. The path of the ureter can be traced simply by incising the peritoneum with a pair of micro-scissors or laser until the lesion is identified. With a blunt probe or hydrodissection, the ureter can easily be moved to the side before the lesion is vaporized. If the ureter or large vessel cannot be moved because of significant attachment to the peritoneum, laparoscopic removal should not be attempted. Laparotomy should be performed instead. Laparoscopic resection of a segment of ureter has been performed with a laparoscopic ureteral anastomosis. However, this approach cannot be recommended until there is more clinical evidence to show that the technique is safe and effective.

Cul-de-sac Disease

Most deep cul-de-sac dissections have been performed in the past by laparotomy. With the recent development of new instrumentation, it is now feasible to dissect the cul-de-sac by laparoscopy in most cases. It is extremely important for the patient who has any significant bowel symptoms, such as bleeding, pain with defecation, or rectal pressure, to undergo evaluation of the lower colon by barium enema and colonoscopy. Should there be involvement of the mucosa or muscularis, laparoscopic treatment should not be attempted. If the evaluation is negative, then the dissection can be performed.

For proper identification of the rectum and vagina, plastic probes should be inserted into each orifice and the cul-de-sac identified (Figure 28.4). Partial obliteration of the cul-de-sac may be even more difficult to deal with than complete obliteration caused occasionally by 'tenting up' of the serosa of the colon attached to the back of the vagina. Careful dissection with the laser will gradually separate the two structures. The probes will facilitate identification of the exact location of the vaginal and rectal mucosa (Figure 28.5). In cases of complete obliteration of the cul-de-sac, the probes are invaluable in preventing perforation of the colon. However, it is highly recommended that all patients with colon endome-

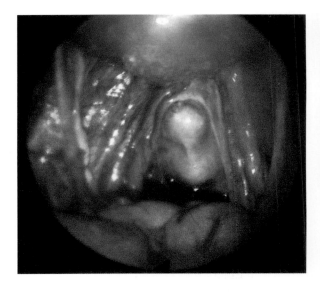

Figure 28.5 Rectal and vaginal probes in place during dissection of the cul-de-sac.

triosis have a thorough bowel preparation prior to the surgery.

As far as the proper selection of power density and wavelength, the choice most often is dependent upon the surgeon's experience. In the beginning, one should use low-power densities in the range of 2500–7000 W/cm². As a matter of fact, repeat pulses may be preferable when the laser is first used. After one is more familiar with the system and the effects on tissue, superpulses or ultrapulses with an average power of 10–30 W can be used. Care must be taken at these higher pulses to avoid entering the muscularis of the rectum. As noted, use of the rectal and vaginal probes will help to prevent such an accident.

Colon

A more extensive discussion of the treatment of colon disease can be found in Chapters 25 and 26. However, a few comments are in order regarding cases of superficial disease of the colon. A superficial lesion, involving the serosal surface only, can be easily removed with a superpulse laser beam of 5–10 W moved rapidly across the colon. As long as the muscularis is not entered, there is no need to close the defect. However, if the muscularis is entered, a 4-0 or 5-0 permanent suture should be used to close the defect. A physician who lacks the skill to place these small sutures by laparoscopy should not attempt laparoscopy but should perform laparotomy. Obstructing or concentric lesions generally should be approached by laparotomy. As noted in Chapter 37, instrumentation is available for

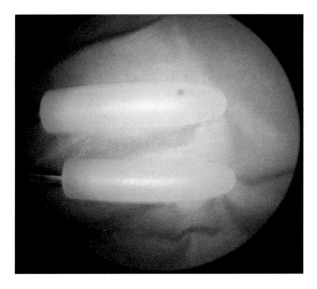

Figure 28.4 Rectal and vaginal probes used in identifying these cavities at laparoscopy.

laparoscopic segmental bowel resections. However, this procedure should only be attempted by an expert laparoscopic surgeon.

Other Areas

During the diagnostic portion of the laparoscopic procedure, care should be taken to look for endometriosis in unusual places such as in the canal of Nuck, pelvic brim, Allen–Master windows, serosal surface of the bowel, liver, diaphragm and fallopian tube. In most areas, except the diaphragm, the disease can easily be vaporized with a continuous mode at 8–10 W. When dealing with the round ligament as it enters the canal of Nuck, one must be certain to remove all of the disease. In some instances, endometriosis has been noted deep in the canal, and, indeed, occasionally is found under the inguinal ligament, preventing approach by laparoscopy but requiring direct access through the inguinal ligament itself.

The peritoneal defects, commonly known as Allen–Master defects or windows are frequently associated with endometriosis at their base (Figure 28.6). It is important in these cases to open the window and vaporize all the endometriosis within the defect. Actually, it is necessary to open the defect anyway because these defects apparently can cause pelvic pain or serve as an area for

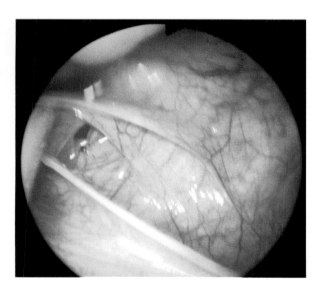

Figure 28.6 Allen–Master windows seen at laparoscopy to contain endometriosis.

collection of reflux menstrual blood. Should Sampson's theory be correct (Sampson, 1927), then this procedure theoretically would prevent recurrence of endometriosis in these areas.

Summary

The treatment of peritoneal endometriosis with lasers is the most suitable method available. The precision and accuracy of the laser beam and especially the 'what you see is what you get' concept of CO_2 laser vaporization, makes the wavelengths described in this chapter ideal for completely removing peritoneal endometriosis. Although this chapter is limited to peritoneal disease, the use of lasers is obviously very important in removing endometriosis of the ovary and deeply involved in the cul-de-sac. The value of the laser is limited only by the skill and efficiency of the surgeon.

References

Evers J (1987) The second look laparoscopy for the evaluation of the results of medical treatment of endometriosis should not be performed during ovarian suppression. *Fertility and Sterility* **47**:502–504.

Interceed (TC7) Adhesion Barrier Study Group (1989) Prevention of postsurgical adhesions by INTERCEED (TC7), an absorbable adhesion barrier: a prospective, randomized multicenter clinical study. *Fertility and Sterility* **51**:933–938.

Martin DC & Vander Zwaag R (1987) Excisional techniques with the CO_2 laser laparoscope. *Journal of Reproductive Medicine* **32**:753.

Martin DC, Hubert GD & Levy BS (1989) Depth of infiltration of endometriosis. *Journal of Gynecologic Surgery* **5**:55.

Nezhat C & Nezhat FR (1989) Safe laser endoscopic excision or vaporization of endometriosis. *Fertility and Sterility* **52(1)**:149–151.

Taylor MV, Martin DC, Poston W, Dean DL & Vander Zwaag R (1986) Effect of power density and carbonization on residual tissue coagulation using the continuous wave carbon dioxide laser. *Colposcopy and Gynecologic Laser Surgery* **2**:159.

Sampson J (1927) Peritoneal endometriosis due to menstrual dissemination of endometrial tissue into peritoneal cavity. *American Journal of Obstetrics and Gynecology* **14**:422.

29

Non-laser Resection of Endometriosis

DAVID REDWINE

2190 NE Professional Court Bend, Oregon, USA

Introduction

Endometriosis will frequently be encountered in
the endoscopic evaluation of pain or infertility,
although it is not always the sole cause of either
of these symptoms. Uncomplicated endometriosis
without pelvic distortion or ovarian endometriomas is being re-evaluated as a cause of infertility.
Although pain seems to be a more common and
more specific symptom of the disease, not all
pelvic pain is due to endometriosis. Usually
without realizing it, the clinician treating a patient
with endometriosis seeks one of two distinct
therapeutic end points: the successful treatment
of symptoms or the successful treatment of
disease. Although these end points seem separate
enough, the distinction blurs in clinical practice
and even research on the disease is hampered by
this lack of focus. The clinician must ask: am I
really treating the disease, or just its symptoms?
Successful treatment of symptoms may result from
any of several non-specific treatments which may
not have any effect on the disease, while successful
treatment of endometriosis requires that something physically destructive be done to the
disease.

Advantages of Non-laser Resection of Endometriosis over Medical Therapy

Medical therapy results in profound temporary
relief of hormonally responsive pain of any origin
while the patient is under therapy, but this does
not prove that all pain that is relieved is due to
endometriosis. Nor does relief of symptoms prove
that endometriosis is being effectively eradicated.
This non-specificity of medical therapy results in
a factitious magnification of apparent therapeutic
effect which has led a generation of gynaecologists
to believe that endometriosis might be eradicated
by medical therapy. Although by now there
should be abundant photomicrographic evidence
of endometriosis which is dead or dying as a
result of the presumed cytocidal effect of medical
therapy, the continued absence of such evidence
has remained glaringly apparent to the profession.
Indeed, the perception of improvement of endometriosis following medical therapy has been
based both on non-specific response of symptoms
and on the visual assessment at surgery done at
the conclusion of therapy. More recent studies of
medical therapy indicate a high persistence of
biopsy-proven disease at the end of therapy, even
in patients with minimal disease. Since all medical
therapy is based on the belief that pregnancy and
the menopause physically destroy endometriosis,
and since these beliefs were never scientifically
validated, the limitations of medical therapy come
as no surprise.

In contrast, surgeons have been removing
diseased tissue from the body for thousands of
years. Surgery is eminently understandable to
physicians as well as to patients in its mechanical
effects. Surgery eradicates the disease, and if
the clinician believes that the disease causes
symptoms, surgery will eradicate those as well.

Advantages of Non-laser Resection of Endometriosis over Laser Vaporization or Electrocoagulation

Although either laser vaporization or electrocoagulation is commonly used to treat endometriosis endoscopically, neither form of therapy returns a pathology report and the likelihood of failure of electrocoagulation is increased when more substantial disease of the uterosacral ligaments exists (Hasson, 1979). A surgeon employs the senses of sight and touch to ply his trade, and laser vaporization and electrocoagulation may compromise both of these senses. Neither laser vaporization nor electrocoagulation has been validated by long-term follow-up as being effective treatment resulting in eradication of endometriosis.

By contrast, laparoscopic excision of endometriosis provides a pathology report and allows excision of deeply invasive disease anywhere in the pelvis. Palpation and handling of the tissue with scissors and graspers results in tactile feedback which enhances surgery. Neither smoke nor heat is generated if electrodissection is not used, resulting in better vision and safer surgery. Every surgical technique normally used at laparotomy to treat endometriosis can be duplicated endoscopically with simple, inexpensive tools and using excisional techniques familiar to all gynaecological surgeons at laparotomy. Finally, laparoscopic excision of endometriosis by sharp dissection has a long-term record of efficacy which has been shown by life table analysis to result in effective treatment of endometriosis even in patients resistant to other forms of therapy (Redwine, 1991). Studies of laser vaporization and electrocoagulation have focused on symptom outcomes rather than long-term validation of disease destruction, reoperation, and rates of recurrence/persistence. This focus on symptom response rather than disease response makes it difficult to interpret the true efficacy of these modalities in the eradication of endometriosis.

Non-laser Resection of Endometriosis

Need for a Bowel Preparation

Certain symptoms and signs suggest the possibility of bowel involvement by endometriosis, and these patients should receive a bowel preparation before surgery. Rectal pain and rectal pain with defecation throughout the month suggest the presence of a rectal nodule of endometriosis. Previous surgery revealing bowel disease or obliteration of the cul-de-sac as well as tender nodularity of the cul-de-sac or uterosacral ligaments are signs suggesting the presence of intestinal involvement. Obliteration of the cul-de-sac is sometimes identified as 'severe cul-de-sac adhesions' or as 'adherence of the rectosigmoid colon to the uterus'. Thus, although a previous surgeon may have given a passing description of the morphological findings, the likely presence of a rectal nodule frequently escapes cognition. If a rectal nodule is present, this increases the likelihood of disease of the mid-sigmoid, terminal ileum, appendix or caecum.

Four litres of oral colonic lavage the afternoon before surgery followed by two enemas the evening before surgery results in a superb bowel preparation.

Patient Positioning for Surgery

The patient is placed in low lithotomy position with a retention catheter in the bladder. Because operative endoscopy can be a lengthy procedure, positioning of the legs is particularly important. If knee stirrups are used, extra thick padding is needed to avoid peroneal nerve paresis. To avoid patient hypothermia, a warming blanket can be placed under the patient, and blankets are placed around the upper torso, head and arms. The arms are ideally tucked along the side of the patient to allow full mobility by the surgeon and the assistant. Irrigation fluid can be passed through a blood warming coil. An intrauterine manipulator is placed for intraoperative manipulation, and the table is placed in steep Trendelenburg position.

Instrumentation

Non-laser resection of endometriosis requires the simplest of tools. After placing an intrauterine manipulator, a 10 mm operating laparoscope with a 3 mm operating channel accepting a 3 mm scissors is placed through an umbilical sheath. Laser laparoscopes are to be avoided, since they have a 5 mm air channel which reduces optical resolution and allows bothersome play in the shaft of the scissors during surgery. Two 5.5 mm trocars are placed lateral to the inferior epigastric vessels near the top of the pubic hair line with a suction–irrigator passing through the right lower quadrant sheath. A 3 mm atraumatic grasper passed through a stiffening sheath or a 5 mm grasper with fine teeth is passed through the left lower quadrant sheath. A bipolar coagulator, monopolar current which can be passed through the scissors, endoloop sutures and standard sutures with small needles used at laparotomy will allow almost any presentation of endometriosis to be treated laparoscopically. A high flow insufflator is helpful, but a video camera and monitor are unnecessary.

For the experienced laparoscopist, the scissors may be used with 70 W or more of cutting or 50 W of coagulating monopolar current. Monopolar scissors are the most versatile tool for resection of endometriosis, allowing various cutting or coagulating surfaces, sharp or blunt dissection, fulguration, increased ease of tissue handling, and tactile feedback. Instrument exchanges are decreased, and dissection is very fast and virtually bloodless. Cutting tissue is independent of the mechanical sharpness of the scissors. Finally and importantly, monopolar scissors are inexpensive.

Identification of Disease

Effective surgical treatment of endometriosis begins with accurate identification of disease. Inaccurate disease identification results in incomplete surgical treatment and confusion about the disease (Redwine, 1990). Some endometriotic lesions can change in appearance with advancing age (Redwine, 1987b; Koninckx et al., 1991). Laparoscopy (Vasquez et al., 1984; Redwine, 1988; Nisolle et al., 1990; Redwine and Yocom, 1990) combined with knowledge of the morphological characteristics of normal peritoneum (Redwine, 1988) appears to be more effective than laparotomy (Murphy et al., 1986) in identifying small lesions of endometriosis due to its magnifying effect in near-contact mode. Basic science studies of microscopic endometriosis predict that accurate identification of disease will result in complete removal of all disease in between 75 and 100% of patients.

The general gynaecologist will more frequently encounter endometriosis patients with pain than patients with infertility (Redwine, 1987a). Since invasive disease is strongly associated with the presence of pain (Koninckx et al., 1991), special attention must be paid to its appearance. Invasive disease is more likely to be undertreated than is superficial disease and frequently has a yellowish-white cast due to overlying fibrosis. Ironically, disease with such an appearance has been trivialized in the past as being 'burned out', when actually it represents highly active 'burned in' disease. Excision of endometriosis ensures that the

surgeon will encounter invasive retroperitoneal fibrotic disease and increases the likelihood of complete removal. Some innocuous-appearing lesions may at first appear to be superficial, but may invade well beyond the retroperitoneal fatty areolar tissue to involve major pelvic nerves or even the periosteum of the ilium (Redwine and Sharpe, 1990).

Techniques of Non-laser Excision of Endometriosis

Superficial Peritoneal Resection

Since most patients do not have severely invasive disease, this is the technique that is most commonly used. Because the peritoneum of the posterior pelvis is most commonly involved by endometriosis (Redwine 1987a), work should usually begin here. Otherwise, if the cul-de-sac is saved for last, bloody fluid from previous pelvic dissection may obscure this area. Wherever resection of endometriosis is performed, the tissue to be removed is elevated or dissected away from underlying vital structures and is pulled medially toward the centre of the pelvis during excision. During palpation with the graspers, small superficial lesions will be seen to slide easily over retroperitoneal vessels and can be grasped directly and elevated, then excised in only a few motions.

Deep Peritoneal Resection

When a lesion is larger, has fibrosis, or retroperitoneal invasion is suspected because vessels or the ureter cannot be seen, the peritoneum adjacent to the lesion should be nicked, and the hole grasped and elevated medially so the scissors can bluntly dissect the lesion away from underlying structures (Figure 29.1). Then, grasping either the lesion or the adjacent normal peritoneum as required, the line of incision can be extended around the lesion (Figure 29.2), with retroperitoneal dissection working toward the centre of the bottom of the lesion. It is only during retroperitoneal dissection that the invasiveness of endometriosis will be appreciated.

Resection of the Uterosacral Ligament

Either uterosacral ligament can be involved by invasive endometriosis with the volume of a

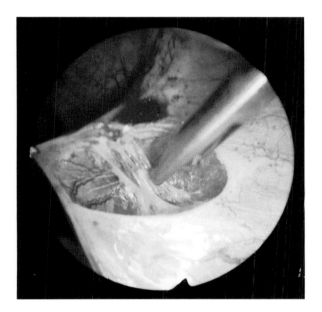

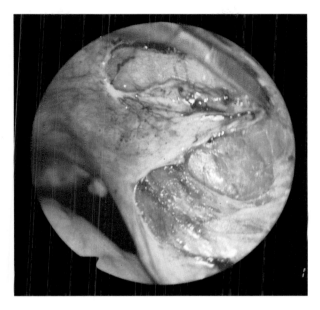

Figure 29.1 The peritoneum of the right broad ligament has been nicked with monopolar scissors using 70 W of cutting current, and the peritoneal incision has been enlarged. The graspers are pulling the peritoneum medially. Notice the reddish-white area of endometriosis above the tip of the scissors. Both electrosurgery and blunt dissection are used to undermine the peritoneum. There is little lateral thermal damage on the cut edge of the peritoneum. The monopolar scissors allow precise, bloodless dissection.

Figure 29.2 The peritoneal incision has been extended completely around the abnormal peritoneum. Although the graspers are drawing the tissue laterally, this is only to demonstrate that the lesion has been completely circumscribed by a line of incision. The peritoneum is pulled medially for the monopolar scissors to complete the dissection.

man's thumb, with fibrotic extension down to the sacrum. Resection of the entire uterosacral ligament is the only treatment that will ensure complete removal. To resect the uterosacral ligament, incise the peritoneum lateral and parallel to it (Figure 29.3). This incision over the adjacent broad ligament results in automatic retraction of the peritoneum with resultant visualization of the retroperitoneal structures. The ureter and uterine vessels can now be dissected bluntly laterally to ensure that they are not near the uterosacral ligament. The ligament can actually be partially undermined along much of its lateral length, and this will define much of the ensuing dissection. With bulky invasive disease, fibrosis will extend laterally to involve the ureter or branches of the uterine vessels descending along the lateral vaginal wall. In this case the dissection must begin in uninvolved peritoneum more posteriorly along the broad ligament with the dissection working around the ureter toward the uterosacral ligament. Just medial to the point where the uterine vessels cross the ureter are the inferior branches of the uterine vessels.

Blunt dissection alternating with meticulous use of bipolar or monopolar current is necessary to separate the uterosacral ligament from these vessels (Figure 29.4). If bleeding is encountered, it can be safely controlled with unipolar or bipolar coagulation because the dissection at this point is well medial to the previously identified ureter. Once the lateral margin of the uterosacral ligament has been dissected away from these branches of the uterine vessels, a peritoneal incision is made medial and parallel to the ligament. Next, the insertion of the uterosacral ligament into the posterior cervix is divided with unipolar coagulating current or with bipolar coagulation followed by scissors transection. The uterosacral ligament is grasped and dissected off of the pelvic floor using a combination of sharp, blunt and electro-dissection (Figure 29.5). As the dissection retreats from the area of the cervix and the endometriotic invasion is completely undermined, it will be seen that the uterosacral ligament becomes less dense and spreads out into the surrounding perirectal connective tissue. At this distal point the ligament is transected and removed.

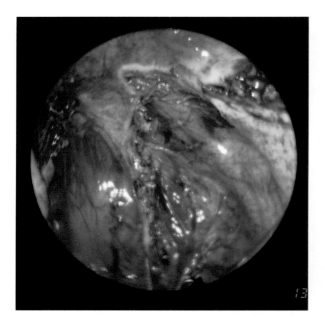

Figure 29.3 An incision has been made with the monopolar scissors lateral and parallel to the right uterosacral ligament. No peritoneal resection has been performed yet. Notice the large area of invasive endometriosis of the right uterosacral ligament. This had resulted in such traction and distortion of the peritoneum that the lateral incision resulted in a quite wide automatic separation of the peritoneum in this area.

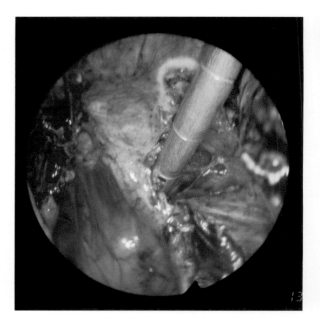

Figure 29.4 A blunt probe is used behind the insertion of the uterosacral ligament in the posterior cervix to separate the ligament from the vessels just lateral to it. In this area, damage to vessels is more likely than damage to the ureter, which lies further laterally. After the ligament is isolated, it is transected with the monopolar scissors and then dissected off of the pelvic floor using blunt dissection, sharp dissection and electrosurgery.

Ureterolysis and Angiolysis

Retroperitoneal fibrosis associated with invasive endometriosis will commonly invest the ureters and occasionally the internal iliac vessels and their branches. In these situations, gentle mechanical dissection is required in order to ensure complete removal of disease. An uninvolved area of normal peritoneum is chosen adjacent to the lesion, then grasped and elevated. The 3 mm graspers allow just the outer layers of peritoneum to be grasped so the ureter will not tent up into the area of surgery. The elevated peritoneum is then nicked with the scissors. The scissors are inserted retroperitoneally and undermine the peritoneum, bluntly separating it from the underlying vital structures. The peritoneal incision can then be extended along the lesion. This further exposes the retroperitoneal space, and the ureter must be identified. In thin patients, the peristalsis may be quite obvious, while further gentle blunt dissection may be required to identify the ureter in other patients. Although it is taught at laparotomy that the ureter is commonly found attached to the peritoneum that is dissected medially off the pelvic sidewall, the laparoscopic perspective is different. With laparoscopic sur-

gery, the peritoneum directly over the ureter is more commonly incised first, and the ureter will often be seen to lie directly beneath the area of dissection in the visual axis of observation. The graspers can now alternately grasp either the peritoneum or the ureter as the scissors bluntly dissect the ureter out of the fibrosis. Occasional short bursts of monopolar coagulating current will bloodlessly transect peritoneal vessels. It is occasionally necessary to lay the ureter completely bare from the pelvic brim to the uterine vessels. In rare instances the uterine vessels must be sacrificed with bipolar coagulation or endoloops in order to dissect the ureter completely out of investing fibrosis which may extend toward the base of the bladder.

Retroperitoneal fibrosis resulting from invasive endometriosis can pass the ureter to involve the large pelvic blood vessels, most commonly the branches of the internal iliac artery. The thinner-walled veins fortunately lie deeper along the pelvic sidewall and it is rarely necessary to operate around them. The rigidity of the arteries and the fact that they are less commonly involved with severe fibrosis than is the ureter makes the dissection easier, since an artery is a more stable

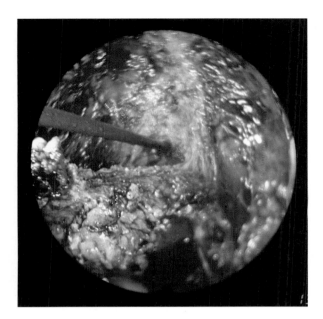

Figure 29.5 The right uterosacral ligament occupies the left quadrant of the frame and is being drawn to the left across the pelvis by graspers attached to the top of the ligament which has been separated from the posterior cervix. Notice the thick nodularity along the length of the ligament. The long probe is developing the rectovaginal septum to ensure separation of the rectum from the ligament. Once this is done, the ligament can be transected on the pelvic floor and removed.

structure than the ureter. Still, it is necessary to proceed with caution in this area. The use of monopolar coagulation current along the sidewall will occasionally result in stimulation of the muscles controlled by the unseen obturator or femoral nerves. While this does not seem to result in any deficit whatsoever, it is prudent to switch to bipolar coagulation if this recurs often.

Ovarian Endometriosis

Small areas of superficial ovarian endometriosis can be excised by cutting the cortex around the lesion and then undermining the cortex with the scissors. This results in removal of more normal ovarian tissue than laser vaporization or electro-coagulation, although an occasional intraovarian accumulation of bloody fluid may be encountered which initially was not visually apparent. To preserve ovarian tissue, it would be more prudent to fulgurate or vaporize larger superficial lesions and probe the interior of the ovary with a needle to search for underlying chocolate cysts (Candiani *et al.*, 1990). Many red superficial lesions are

nothing but haemorrhagic adhesions, while not all chocolate cysts are endometriotic (Sampson, 1921).

Endometriotic cysts are frequently adherent to the pelvic sidewall, uterus or sigmoid colon at points of previous rupture and contiguous endometriosis. When dealing with such cysts, the likelihood of endometriosis in the opposing structure should be considered and dealt with by deep peritoneal resection techniques. Endometriotic cysts frequently rupture during surgical treatment. After irrigation and suction of the cyst fluid, the edge of the cyst wall is grasped and the scissors are used bluntly to dissect away the normal ovarian cortex. If the edge of the cyst wall is indistinct and cannot be grasped easily, the scissors can be used to cut along the normal ovarian cortex adjacent and parallel to the open edge of the cyst cavity. This incision is carried just to the fibrotic capsule of the cyst. The graspers now may grasp a small 'handle' of ovarian cortex attached to the edge of the cyst, allowing a more positive purchase and facilitating the dissection. The endometriotic cyst is then dissected out of the ovarian stroma (Figure 29.6). It is occasionally necessary to coagulate bleeders at the base of the cyst. Suture of the cyst wall is not recommended, since this may result in an increase of adhesions.

Endometriosis of the Large Bowel

In descending order, the most common sites of intestinal involvement by endometriosis are the

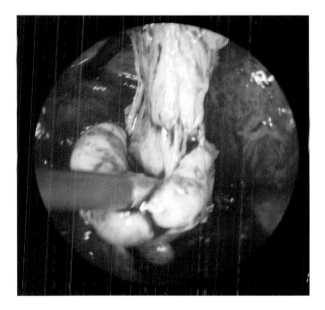

Figure 29.6 The fibrotic capsule of an ovarian endometrioma is being stripped bluntly out of the body of the ovary.

rectum, sigmoid, ileum, caecum and appendix. The large bowel is composed of four layers: the serosa, outer longitudinal muscularis, inner circular muscularis, and mucosa. The serosa does not extend below the peritoneal reflection. Endometriosis almost never penetrates into the bowel lumen, and intestinal diagnostic studies will fail to detect most cases of intestinal disease (Redwine and Sharpe, unpublished data). Many invasive bowel lesions have a yellowish, fibrotic appearance which blends well with the bowel wall. For ease of identification, it is helpful to palpate the bowel wall with the graspers, or to slide a ring forceps up and down the bowel to identify a mass effect. If laparoscopic bowel surgery is anticipated, antibiotic prophylaxis and preoperative osmotic bowel evacuation are prudent in case the lumen is entered. Small, superficial lesions may be excised by serosal resection and suturing the bowel wall is not necessary.

The layers of the bowel wall allow partial thickness resection of larger lesions. The scissors cut through the serosa and muscularis to a depth sufficient to allow the lesion to be undermined. This will occasionally require exposure of the mucosa. In many cases, the lesion can then be dissected off the bowel wall without penetration of the lumen. The dissection planes offered by the layers of muscularis result in a clean, almost bloodless dissection, but the surgeon can easily dissect too far past the lesion, so a three-dimensional awareness of the extent of the lesion is necessary at all times. The defect in the bowel wall is then closed with interrupted 3-0 silk sutures. If extension of disease and its accompanying fibrosis extend to the submucosa, the dissection will frequently enter the bowel lumen. This allows the extent of the lesion to be palpated through the mucosa. The ring forceps in the bowel creates a dependent space within the bowel where the remaining bowel preparation fluid can collect. As a result, spillage of bowel contents into the pelvis is uncommon. If spillage occurs, copious irrigation is used after closure of the bowel. Full thickness defects can be repaired with a mucosal stitch of running 3-0 chromic followed by interrupted 3-0 silk to close the muscularis and serosal layers. If multiple full thickness resections are anticipated, each defect should be closed before the next is created so as to limit bowel spillage.

Although not previously emphasized in the literature, obliteration of the cul-de-sac is highly predictive of the presence of disease invading the wall of the rectum, as well as invasive disease of the uterosacral ligaments and the hidden cul-de-sac. Many clinicians may observe 'dense cul-de-sac adhesions' or 'the rectum adherent to the posterior cervix' without realizing that their next thought should be that the wall of the rectum is probably involved with endometriosis. Surgical treatment of the obliterated cul-de-sac involves more than an attempt at mechanical separation of the rectum from the cervix. It includes the psychic recognition of the need to remove all invasive endometriosis. This will frequently require an *en bloc* resection of the uterosacral ligaments, posterior cervix, cul-de-sac, as well as the rectal nodule. If the ovaries are involved by large endometriomas adherent to the pelvic sidewalls, consideration should be given to proceeding with a laparotomy rather than continuing with laparoscopy. This is because ovarian and pelvic sidewall involvement by endometriosis, combined with treatment of the obliterated cul-de-sac, will result in a lengthy surgery which may be beyond the physical and mental capacities of the average gynaecologist.

Laparoscopic surgical treatment of the obliterated cul-de-sac involves specific steps which are consistently reproducible and which will allow an experienced laparoscopist to complete this surgery successfully. These surgical steps include: lateral isolation of the uterosacral ligaments, transverse incision across the cervix above the adherent bowel, intrafascial dissection down the cervix toward the rectovaginal septum, medial isolation of the uterosacral ligaments by development of the rectovaginal septum, transection of the uterosacral ligaments at their insertion into the posterior cervix, mobilization of the rectum by transection of the lateral rectal attachments and *en bloc* resection of the mobilized mass. This may result in partial thickness, full thickness, or segmental resection and end-to-end anastomosis of the bowel. Deep partial and full thickness resections are repaired as discussed above.

Segmental bowel resection with end-to-end anastomosis is occasionally required for large nodules or multiple nodules along a length of bowel (Redwine and Sharpe, 1991). Two transabdominal stay sutures are used to stabilize and suspend the bowel wall just above and below the point of initial transection. The bowel is transected proximal to the lesion and the proximal segment is retracted against the abdominal wall with a stay suture to avoid spillage. The distal cut edge is elevated with the other stay suture, and the open bowel is closed with an endoloop in order to avoid unnecessary spillage. The bowel is separated from the mesentery by electrosurgical methods. The surgeon works by looking 'down the barrel' of the bowel (which is held closed by the endoloop) immediately adjacent to the bowel wall. A ring forceps in the bowel allows intraoperative manipulation and also results in evacuation of residual liquid bowel preparation material. Bipolar coagulation and mechanical division with scissors or division with monopolar scissors can be used to isolate the segment to be removed. Once the segment has been sufficiently isolated, the bowel wall distal to the second proposed transection line is grasped with a grasper or stay suture. The bowel is transected distally and the segment is extracted transanally. A distal purse-string suture of 3-0 prolene or an endcloop is applied and an end-to-end anastomosis (EEA) stapler is inserted transanally and into the proximal segment. The proximal purse-string suture or endoloop is applied, then the stapler is closed and fired to complete the anastomosis. The pelvis is filled with fluid and air is injected through a sigmoidoscope to check for leaks. If bubbles are seen, interrupted 3-0 silk suture is used to reinforce the bowel wall until the leak is stopped.

Complications

The potential complications of laparoscopic surgery include those specific to laparoscopy (injuries caused by trocar insertion, insufflation of carbon dioxide or patient positioning) and those common to laparotomy treatment (bleeding, infection, damage to internal organs and resulting reoperation). Among 359 patients undergoing laparoscopic excision of endometriosis by sharp dissection, only two significant complications were noted, both in association with management of severe adhesions (Redwine, 1991). Among 16 more recent patients undergoing full thickness bowel resection (including three undergoing segmental resection and end-to-end anastomosis), there have been no clinical leaks, infectious complications related to bowel surgery, or reoperations. As with laparotomy, intraoperative recognition of unanticipated injury to adjacent vital structures allows them to be repaired primarily at that time, with little serious consequence (Gomel and James, 1991). Unrecognized surgical injury, however, can lead to postoperative morbidity or mortality soon after the completion of surgery.

If a small hole is created in the unprepared bowel, colostomy should not be performed. Instead, a small defect should be closed laparoscopically with interrupted 3-0 silk, and the resulting integrity of the bowel should be checked by underwater air pressure examination. Copious intraoperative irrigation should be performed and postoperative prophylactic antibiotics should be given for approximately 24 hours. If laparotomy and colostomy were to be summarily performed, this would usurp the highly likely probability that the patient would do well with a simple laparoscopic repair as well as lead to a later laparotomy for closure of the colostomy.

Perioperative Patient Management

Modern laparoscopic surgery is major surgery which bears little resemblance to a 10 minute diagnostic laparoscopy with might have been performed in 1970. The notion that most laparoscopic surgery can be performed on an out-patient basis is unreasonable. Unanticipated admission to the hospital following out-patient surgery has been found to be most strongly associated with the use of general anaesthesia and the performance of laparoscopy (Gold et al., 1989). Hospital surgical committees should require minimal recovery criteria to have been met before discharging patients from out-patient surgical centres. These should include cessation of vomiting, demonstrated ability to retain both liquids and pain medication by mouth, and the ability to ambulate to the bathroom with minimal assistance. Patients are frequently discharged too early with unrelenting nausea and vomiting and are unable to retain oral fluids and pain medications. Advanced laparoscopic surgery most commonly results in a hospitalization of 24 hours or less, although laparoscopic segmental bowel resection may require hospitalization of up to 5 days.

Full activities may be resumed by 3 weeks in most patients, while intercourse should be delayed for 5 weeks, especially in patients with cul-de-sac or uterosacral ligament resections. The first two menstrual flows may be unusually painful, and some patients may require 4 months to appreciate the full extent of pain relief.

Patient Outcome

Life table analysis of long-term rates of reoperation and recurrent diagnosis of endometriosis after non-laser resection indicate a maximum occurrence of new disease of 19%, achieved in the fifth postoperative year (Redwine, 1991). Most reoperated patients had no endometriosis, and when disease was present, it was always superficial and minimal in amount. This low rate of recurrence is identical to that found following laparotomy (Wheeler and Malinak, 1986), and is apparently a conseqeunce of the non-spreading nature of endometriosis which has been demonstrated by two studies (Redwine, 1987a; Koninckx et al., 1991). Adhesion formation was more likely to occur following surgery on or around the ovaries, while reformation of adhesions was quite common.

Complete surgical eradication of endometriosis is possible, and this will result in pain relief in patients whose pain is due to endometriosis. If pain persists, this does not necessarily indicate a failure of surgical therapy to eradicate endometriosis. Instead, persistent pain indicates the need for more specificity in determining preoperatively which types of pain are more likely to be due to endometriosis.

References

Candiani, GB, Vercellini P & Fedele L (1990) Laparoscopic ovarian puncture for correct staging of endometriosis. *Fertility and Sterility* **53**: 994–997.

Gold BS, Kitz DS, Lecky JH *et al.* (1989) Unanticipated admission to the hospital following ambulatory surgery. *Journal of the American Medical Association* **262**: 3008–3010.

Gomel V & James C (1991) Intraoperative management of ureteral injury during operative laparoscopy. *Fertility and Sterility* **55**: 416–419.

Hasson HM (1979) Electrocoagulation of pelvic endometriotic lesions with laparoscopic control. *American Journal of Obstetrics and Gynecology* **135**: 115–119.

Koninckx PR, Meuleman C, Demeyere S, Lesaffre E & Cornillie FJ (1991) Suggestive evidence that pelvic endometriosis is a progressive disease, whereas deeply infiltrating endometriosis is associated with pelvic pain. *Fertility and Sterility* **55**: 759–765.

Murphy AA, Green WR, Bobbie D *et al.* (1986) Unsuspected endometriosis documented by scanning electron microscopy in visually normal peritoneum. *Fertility and Sterility* **46**: 522–524.

Nisolle M, Paindaveine B, Bourdon A *et al.* (1990) Histologic study of peritoneal endometriosis in infertile women. *Fertility and Sterility* **53**: 984–988.

Redwine DB (1987a) The distribution of endometriosis in the pelvis by age groups and fertility. *Fertility and Sterility* **47**: 173–175.

Redwine DB (1987b) Age related evolution in color appearance of endometriosis. *Fertility and Sterility* **48**: 1062–1063.

Redwine DB (1988) Is 'microscopic' peritoneal endometriosis invisible? *Fertility and Sterility* **50**: 665–666.

Redwine DB (1990) The visual appearance of endometriosis and its impact on our concepts of the disease. *Progress in Clinical and Biological Research* **323**: 393–412.

Redwine DB (1991) Conservative laparoscopic excision of endometriosis by sharp dissection: lifetable analysis of reoperation and persistent or recurrent disease. *Fertility and Sterility* **56**: 628–634.

Redwine DB & Sharpe DR (1990) Endometriosis of the obturator nerve. *Journal of Reproductive Medicine* **35**: 434–435.

Redwine DB & Sharpe DR (1991) Laparoscopic segmental resection of the sigmoid colon for endometriosis. *Journal of Laparoendoscopic Surgery* **1**: 217–220.

Redwine DB & Yocom LB (1990) A serial section study of visually normal pelvic peritoneum in patients with endometriosis. *Fertility and Sterility* **54**: 648–651.

Sampson JA (1921) Perforating hemorrhagic (chocolate) cysts of the ovary. *Archives of Surgery* **3**: 245–323.

Vasquez G, Cornillie F & Brosens I (1984) Peritoneal endometriosis: scanning electron microscopy and histology of minimal pelvic endometriotic lesions. *Fertility and Sterility* **42**: 696–703.

30

Laparoscopic Treatment of Advanced Endometriosis

DAN C. MARTIN

Reproductive Surgery, 910 Madison Avenue, Memphis, Tennessee, USA

Introduction

Superficial endometriosis can be destroyed by coagulation while infiltrating lesions require dissection, vaporization or excision. Although the depth is related to the size for infiltrating lesions, endometriosis is flattened against the cyst wall in large ovarian endometriomas and does not infiltrate more than 1.5 mm. Thus, exploration, examination and coagulation of the inner lining of even large endometriomas is capable of destroying the endometriosis that lines these.

Equipment

Bipolar electrosurgical, thermal coagulation, laser coagulation, laser vaporization have all been used to destroy endometriotic lesions without sending these for pathological confirmation. However, excisional techniques have resulted in increased awareness and increased documentation of the various forms of endometriosis and increase the potential for complete removal of the disease (Martin and Vander Zwaag, 1987; Redwine, 1987, 1991; Martin et al., 1989b). Excisional technique can be performed using scissors, lasers, or electrosurgical knives as a cutting instrument and using bipolar coagulation or mechanical occlusive devices for haemostasis. Although each of these techniques has their own proponents, all of these appear to result in appropriate patient care.

Continued investigation is needed to determine if there is equipment that is the best for a given problem (Martin, 1991b). At present, it seems reasonable to conclude that the equipment that appears the most useful to the surgeon is the one that he or she is most familiar with.

Ovarian Endometriomas

Smaller ovarian endometriomas can be biopsied and then the base coagulated or vaporized. Endometriomas that are larger than 2 cm require more extensive preoperative preparation and discussion. The larger these are, the greater the chance of finding unexpected cancer (Maiman et al., 1991; Schwartz, 1991a). In addition, those greater than 5 cm are more technically difficult to control as the walls collapse and overlap in the operative field (Martin, 1990). Large endometriomas can require 2–5 hours to remove through the laparoscope. Treatment of these can be drainage, biopsy and coagulation or stripping (Semm and Friedrich 1987). An intermediate approach is to stage this with a limitation of the degree of treatment at first operation, use of postoperative medical suppression, monitoring by sonogram and being prepared to perform a subsequent operative laparoscopy in order to remove any residual endometriosis.

The easiest approach is to drain the ovarian cyst, take representative biopsies and then coagulate the remnant wall with bipolar coagulation or with laser (Martin and Diamond, 1986; Brosens and Puttemans, 1989). Once the cyst has been drained and lavaged, endometriomas generally have a red or red and brownish mottled appearance on a white fibrotic background. A more uniform brownish appearance is present when these are the residual of haemorrhagic corpus luteum. Both endometriomas and haemorrhagic corpora lutea have a significant amount of haemosiderin and this cannot be used as a part of the histological differentiation (Martin and Berry, 1990). Biopsies are most commonly positive when these are taken from the red ridges. The brownish areas are commonly haemosiderin-laden and the cellular architecture is not recognizable.

The stripping technique (Semm and Friedrich, 1987) is begun by aspirating or by opening and draining the cystic ovary. Once it is opened and drained, the inner wall is inspected. If there are areas that appear suspicious for cancer, these can be biopsied and a frozen section performed. The opening is generally on the dependent or the broad ligament side in order to lessen the chance of midpelvic or bowel adhesions. The wall of the endometrioma is then grasped and slowly peeled away from the healthy ovary. A relaxing incision into the healthy ovary sometimes facilitates this stripping. In addition, dissection with water solutions may help develop the plane of dissection. If the cyst is large and the capsule is adherent near the hilar vessels, the cyst wall can be amputated away from the hilar vessels and then the endometriosis coagulated over this area. Coagulation is effective as the depth of infiltration of endometriosis in the capsule has not been more than 1.5 mm even when the endometriomas are large (Martin, 1990).

Staging the operation may be advantageous and may avoid unnecessary damage to the ovaries. When the ovarian endometriomas are stripped, the specimen commonly includes a thin wall of healthy ovary. Stripping a large endometrioma may remove so much healthy ovarian tissue that the ovary is destroyed. Drainage, biopsy and coagulation allow these endometriomas to shrink in size and potentially avoids further surgery. The disadvantage is that anything short of complete stripping of the internal wall may increase the chance of missing a small focal cancer. After the initial surgery, medical suppression is used and the patients followed by sonography. If there is no evidence of persistence, the medication is stopped and the patients are observed. If persistence occurs, a second laparoscopy is performed and the cyst stripped or coagulated at that time.

Sutures are not used and adhesions have not been a problem (Martin, 1990, 1991a; Diamond et al., 1991). This is compatible with other studies (Brumsted et al., 1990: De Leon et al., 1990; Meyer et al., 1991; Nezhat et al., 1991b).

When there is great concern regarding the possibility of ovarian cancer on the basis of sonographic appearance or of tumour markers (Schwartz, 1991b), then oophorectomy is indicated. If this is to be performed at laparoscopy, spill should be avoided. This can be accomplished by first dissecting the ovary off of its vessels (Figures 30.1–30.7) and off the lateral sidewall and then placing it in a bag. The neck of the bag is closed and pulled through a small incision. With the neck of the bag in an extra-abdominal position, the cyst is then drained. This will generally collapse the cyst so that it can be pulled through the previous trocar incision. Alternately, a morcellator can be placed in the bag and the cyst morcellated while in the bag. This is based on techniques used for nephrectomy by urologists.

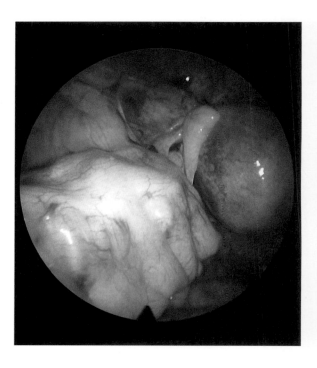

Figure 30.1 The first patient had persistent left adnexal pain and tenderness following a previous attempt at laparoscopic resection of left broad ligament endometriosis. At the first operation, the ureter was not recognized and the procedure was discontinued. The left tube and ovary are hidden behind the sigmoid colon which is adherent to the left tube and ovary with what appears to be congenital bands and/or adhesions from her endometriosis.

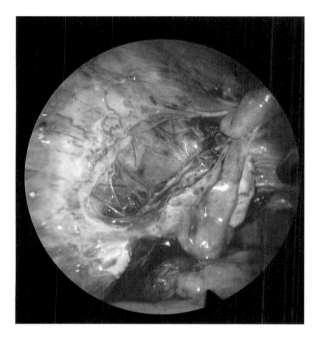

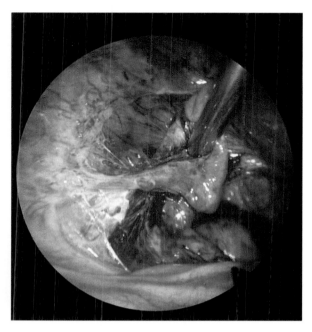

Figure 30.2 The sigmoid colon has been freed off the left tube and ovary and an initial incision made into the left broad lateral to the tube. This portion of the dissection of the infundibulopelvic ligament and ovarian vessels has been done with the CO_2 laser in a superpulse mode.

Figure 30.4 Both the lateral and medial leaves of the broad ligaments have been dissected in order to visualize the infundibulopelvic ligament with the ovarian vein and artery. The ureter has been identified in the lower portion of the field. To this point, all dissection has been performed with the CO_2 laser. Bipolar coagulation and endoloops will be used for haemostasis from the ovarian vessels while bipolar coagulation alone will be used to remove the pedicles from the uterus.

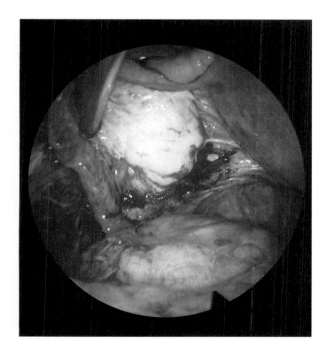

Figure 30.3 Dense adherence of the tube, ovary, broad ligament and uterosacral ligament are seen in the area overlying the ureter.

Deep Infiltration

Although coagulation is effective on lesions less than 2 mm, deep lesions with infiltration ≤3 mm were seen in 60% of patients (Martin et al., 1989a) and greater than 6 mm in 9–38% of patients (Koninckx et al., 1991). These deeper lesions require techniques designed for this depth. Although vaporization can be used to remove these lesions, vaporization of larger lesions create a significant amount of smoke. With deep lesions and when carbon accumulates, residual endometriosis is found in association with the carbon and residual of the previous vaporization (Martin and Diamond, 1986; Martin, 1990).

Excision has been more reliable for removing these lesions (Figures 30.8–30.11). This has been performed with electrosurgery and scissors (Redwine, 1990) and with lasers (Martin and Vander Zwaag, 1987; Nezhat et al., 1989; Cornillie et al., 1990; Koninckx et al., 1991). In addition to scissors or laser as an incising instrument, fluid

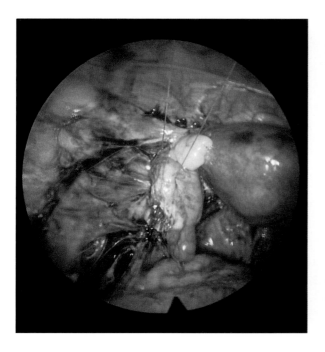

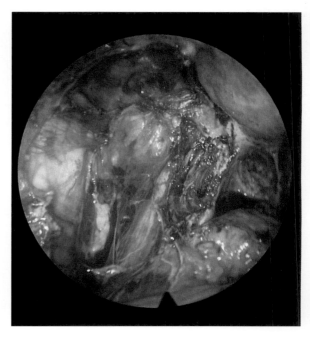

Figure 30.5 The infundibulopelvic ligament has been coagulated at three points and then cut. An endoloop tie has been placed over the ovarian vascular pedicle.

Figure 30.7 Once the ureter was dissected out of the area of the surgical resection, bipolar coagulation and scissors were used for haemostasis prior to resecting the tube and ovary from the uterus. Compare the tissue distortion of the uterosacral in this figure with the lack of tissue distortion following CO_2 laser lysis and initial dissection in Figure 30.2.

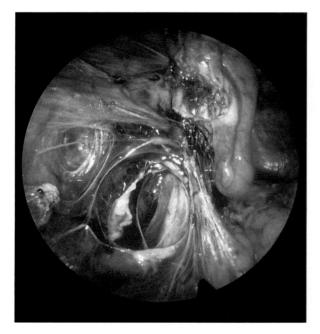

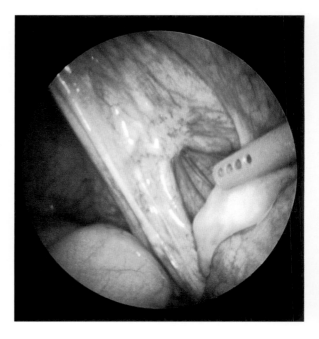

Figure 30.6 The ureter, uterosacral, broad ligament and ovary are densely adherent in the middle of the picture. This area was dissected using a blunt probe and hydrodissection.

Figure 30.8 In the second patient, peritoneal involvement of the broad ligament overlying the ureter is seen on the right.

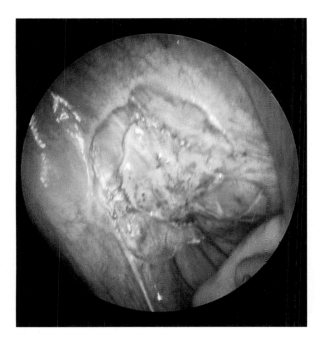

Figure 30.9 The initial part of the dissection is to outline the lesion using the CO_2 laser in superpulse.

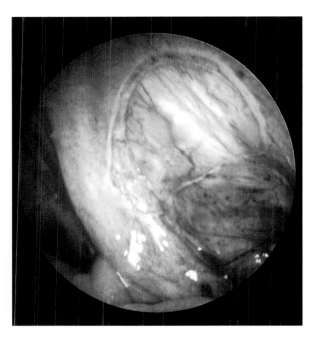

Figure 30.11 The appearance after this resection shows a very thin white rim of coagulation at the perimeter but the remainder of the tissue is healthy with no evidence of damage to the underlying structures.

Bladder and Ureteral Involvement

The majority of lesions overlying the ureter and bladder are in the peritoneum and loose connective tissue and are not adherent to the urinary structures. Sharp dissection with laser, electrosurgery or scissors combined with blunt dissection using probes or hydrodissection (Nezhat and Nezhat, 1989) is used to separate the endometriosis from the underlying structures. If the bladder or ureter does not push away easily, dissection can result in immediate opening or delayed perforation. Avoid difficult dissection unless prepared to manage the possibility of this type of damage.

Unintended ureteral injury has been corrected laparoscopically (Gomel and James, 1991) and uretero-neocystostomy has been performed (Nezhat et al., 1991a). Furthermore, urologists have performed lymph node dissections and radical prostatic resections under laparoscopic control.

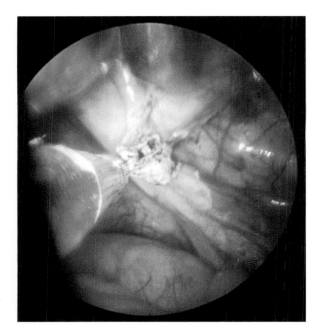

Figure 30.10 The lesion is grasped and pulled medially and then the CO_2 laser used to dissect through loose connective tissue. If the lesion is pulled further to the midline, fluid solutions will be placed to use as a backstop.

solutions and blunt probes are used for mechanical dissection. A combination of various mechanical, electrosurgical and laser techniques provides a more comprehensive approach than relying on only one of these techniques.

Rectosigmoid Infiltration

Infiltration of the rectosigmoid is suggested by a palpable mass on rectal examination, rectal bleeding at the time of menses, persistent pain following laparoscopic removal of recognized lesions, and pain on defecation. Palpation of this area requires close attention to the presence of tenderness, particularly when extending lateral to the bowel and toward the sacral margins. With the deep uterosacral margins involved, lesions can extend around and behind the rectosigmoid. As this type of surgery has a distinct chance of rectosigmoid resection and anastomosis, a gynaecologist or general surgeon familiar with deep bowel surgery is needed. Although this chapter will discuss laparoscopic management of these lesions, they are more commonly managed by laparotomy. This is particularly true with those where the infiltration is lateral to the bowel and is more palpable than visual.

As long as the lesions can be delineated by visualization and by mechanical palpation, these can be resected laparoscopically. However, large lesions can be missed at laparoscopy but palpated at laparotomy. In addition, the three mesenteric nodules and approximately 50% of the appendiceal involvements in my series were missed at laparoscopy but picked up by palpation at laparotomy. The technical aspects of laparoscopic resection and suturing are easier to overcome than the lack of palpation and manual control.

In preparation for deep resection, a combination of mechanical and antibiotic bowel preparation is used. For those gynaecologists who do their own bowel surgery, this will be their routine bowel preparation. If the gynaecologist is using a general surgeon as a consultant, the bowel preparation should be that of the general surgeon. Self blood-banking is encouraged as these procedures can last 3–5 hours and, if deep vessels are encountered, blood loss can be slow but substantial.

In controlling these deep resections, the use of intrauterine, intravaginal and rectal manipulators are helpful (Reich *et al.*, 1991). Reich uses a combination of a Sims curette in the uterus, a sponge on ring forceps in the vagina and a rectal probe in the rectosigmoid area. The rectal probe is a modified 81 French probe. The use of a 25 mm rectal dilator as a probe for distension is discussed later in this chapter.

The initial dissection is to resect the posterior uterine, cervical and uterosacral margins down to the level of the rectovaginal septum. If the rectovaginal septum is free of disease, healthy fat and loose connective tissue will be entered and then the mass is developed laterally and toward the rectal margin. If there is vaginal involvement, laparoscopic colpotomy (Davis and Brooks, 1988; Martin, 1988) is used to remove the vaginal

component and to reach the healthy rectovaginal septum.

The posterior cervix is hard to distinguish from the infiltrating endometriosis and careful palpation of this area is needed to limit the amount of healthy cervix which is removed. Frequent palpation, both vaginal and rectal, can help maintain the orientation which is frequently lost during these deep dissections. If the vagina is entered, two wet 4 × 4 sponges are placed in the vagina in order to stop the gas from escaping and to maintain the pneumoperitoneum for the laparoscopy.

An initial series of five patients had anterior rectus wall resection with removal of as much of the component as could be recognized laparoscopically but without full thickness resection. All five of these have subsequently had exploratory laparotomy for residual disease. The largest area which had been missed was a linear area along the anterior wall of approximately 2 cm in length and 1 cm in diameter. These techniques are currently used on small lesions with preparation for full thickness resection and/or laparotomy if needed (Figures 30.12–30.19). Rectal probes are used to help identify residual endometriosis as demonstrated in Figures 30.13–30.17.

For those surgeons who plan to do full thickness resections, Reich reports that using the surgeon's or assistant's finger in the rectum helps identify the extent. Three of Reich's first 236 patients have had full thickness resection with laparoscopic suturing (Reich *et al.*, 1991). I have used an alternate approach for suturing these areas. When

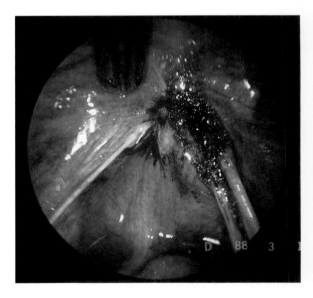

Figure 30.12 In the third patient, a large lesion of the right uterosacral and mid cul-de-sac has pulled the rectum into the cervix. Dissection will proceed as covered in the text.

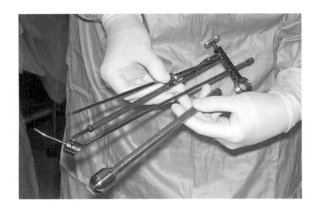

Figure 30.13 The equipment used for this type dissection includes Valtchev uterine mobilizer in order to flex the uterus and the 25 mm EEA (end-to-end anastomotic) dilator in order to distend and define the rectal wall.

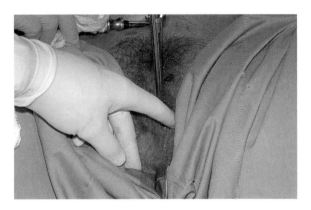

Figure 30.14 The rectal dilator is placed into the rectum and then the gloves are changed.

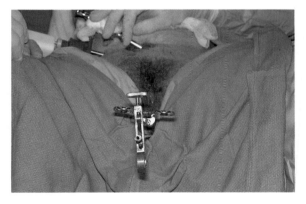

Figure 30.15 The rectal probe is then draped separately in order to avoid contaminating the remainder of the operating field.

there has been full thickness involvement in the rectosigmoid or low sigmoid, I have pulled these through a colpotomy incision and sutured these vaginally. When the entrance has been at the mid or high sigmoid, a mini-laparotomy has been used with the bowel moved into this area under

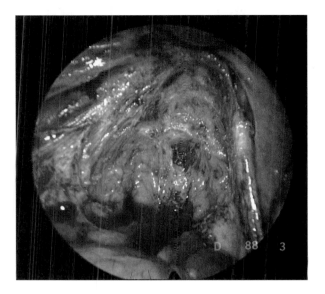

Figure 30.16 Once the resection is complete, the pelvis appears to be free of disease and the rectosigmoid has been freed into a posterior position. This picture is taken with the rectal probe out of position so that there is no distension of the rectum. The location of the rectum becomes easier when the rectal probe is placed as seen in Figure 30.17.

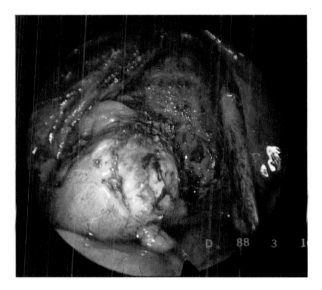

Figure 30.17 With pressure from the rectal probe, residual disease is seen on the right outer margin of the rectosigmoid. Further dissection was needed to remove this part of the lesion. At the end of this dissection, the rectal probe showed no evidence of full thickness perforation. Air can also be injected into the rectum with the rectum under water to check for air leak. However, in spite of testing for perforation, these can still occur as a delayed affect if there is significant compromise to the rectal wall or rectal vasculature.

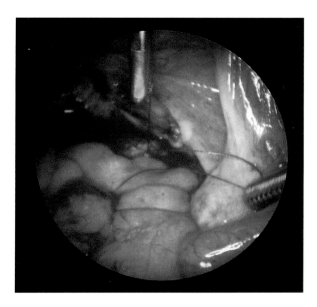

Figure 30.18 The fourth patient had partial resection of the muscularis. Intracorporeal suturing technique was used to oversew this area.

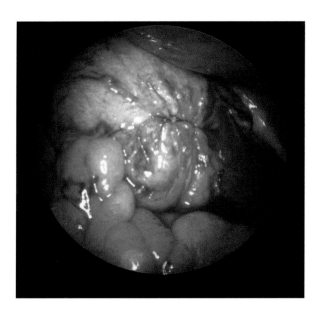

Figure 30.19 At the end of the suturing, the muscularis layers are closed and healthy non-damaged tissue is noted at the margin.

laparoscopic control for suturing. These have been performed in one patient with a 1 cm rectosigmoid nodule and two additional patients where the bowel was densely adherent to the ovary and was entered in the process of freeing these from the ovary. In these three patients, an attempt at dissection and resection had been abandoned at a first operation followed by subsequent informed consent and preparation for bowel surgery.

Using cul-de-sac resection techniques, Reich has reported a 76% pregnancy rate in patients with partial cul-de-sac obliteration and a 72%

pregnancy rate in patients with complete cul-de-sac obliteration. When broken down by staging, he reported a 100% pregnancy rate in stage II, 75% in stage III, and 70% in stage IV (Reich *et al.*, 1991).

Using similar techniques, Redwine has performed resections that have included a segmental resection and anastomosis of the mid-sigmoid. He concluded that if the patient had meticulous removal of all endometriosis and continued to be symptomatic, other causes should be considered. In addition, repeat operations were unproductive and patients with persistent pain appeared to benefit from radical surgery (Redwine, 1991; Redwine and Sharpe, 1991). Nezhat has adapted these techniques to perform deep rectal resection and anastomosis (Nazhat *et al.*, 1991b).

Laparotomy

Laparotomy is still the standard for surgical therapy of deep and bowel endometriosis. At laparotomy, palpation, delicate handling of deep tissue and multilayered closures are enhanced. Open surgery is used when these characteristics are needed. This appears most useful when patients have deep rectal involvement which is palpated in the office, deep extension lateral to the rectum extending toward the sacrum and/or persistent pain following initial laparoscopic resection.

Complications

The major difficulty with deep infiltration involves determining the depth and involvement of other structures such as the ureter, bowel and bladder. Complications have included ureteral lacerations corrected at laparoscopy, bowel lacerations corrected at laparoscopy, bowel lacerations with laparotomy and colostomy, bladder peritoneal fistulas, ureteroperitoneal fistulas and delayed rectal perforation (Martin and Diamond, 1986; Gomel and James, 1991).

Conclusions

The laparoscopic treatment of endometriosis is not limited by the stage or volume of the disease.

However, extensive laparoscopic treatment can require significantly more time than the same procedure at laparotomy and laparoscopy compromises palpation and delicate handling. These factors and a patient's desires regarding surgery must be balanced in order to come to a reasonable plan of approach for a given clinical situation.

References

Brosens IA & Puttemans P (1989) Double-optic laparoscopy. Salpingoscopy, ovarian cystoscopy and endo-ovarian surgery with the argon laser. *Baillière's Clinical Obstetrics and Gynaecology* 3: 595–608.

Brumsted JR, Deaton J, Lavigne E & Riddick DH (1990) Postoperative adhesion formation after ovarian wedge resection with and without ovarian reconstruction in the rabbit. *Fertility and Sterility* 53: 723–726.

Cornillie FJ, Oosterlynck D, Lauweryns JM & Koninckx PR (1990) Deeply infiltrating pelvic endometriosis: histology and clinical significance. *Fertility and Sterility* 53: 978–983.

Davis GD & Brooks RA (1988) Excision of pelvic endometriosis with the carbon dioxide laser laparoscope. *Obstetrics and Gynecology* 72: 816–819.

De Leon FD, Edwards M & Heine MW (1990) A comparison of microsurgery and laser surgery for ovarian wedge resections. *International Journal of Fertility* 35: 177–179.

Diamond MP, Daniell JF, Johns DA *et al.* (1991) Postoperative adhesion development after operative laparoscopy: evaluation at early second-look procedures. *Fertility and Sterility* 55: 700–704.

Gomel V & James C (1991) Intraoperative management of ureteral injury during operative laparoscopy. *Fertility and Sterility* 55: 416–419.

Koninckx PR, Meuleman C, Demeyere S, Lesaffre E & Cornillie FJ (1991) Suggestive evidence that pelvic endometriosis is a progressive disease, whereas deeply infiltrating endometriosis is associated with pelvic pain. *Fertility and Sterility* 55: 759–765.

Maiman M, Seltzer V & Boyce J (1991) Laparoscopic excision of ovarian neoplasms subsequently found to be malignant. *Obstetrics and Gynecology* 77: 563–565.

Martin DC (1988) Laparoscopic and vaginal colpotomy for the excision of infiltrating cul-de-sac endometriosis. *Journal of Reproductive Medicine* 33: 806–808.

Martin DC (1990) Therapeutic laparoscopy. In Martin DC (ed) *Laparoscopic Appearance of Endometriosis*, 2nd edn, vol. I, pp 21–29. Memphis Resurge Press.

Martin DC (1991a) Laparoscopic appearance of ovarian endometriomas. In Pitkin RM & Scott JR (eds) *Clinical Obstetrics and Gynecology*, pp 452–459. Philadelphia: JB Lippincott.

Martin DC (1991b) Tissue effects of lasers. *Seminars in Reproductive Endocrinology* 9(2): 127–137.

Martin DC & Berry JD (1990) Histology of chocolate cysts. *Journal of Gynecologic Surgery* 6: 43–46.

Martin DC & Diamond MP (1986) Operative laparoscopy: comparison of lasers with other techniques. *Current Problems in Obstetrics, Gynecology, and Fertility* 9: 563–601.

Martin, DC & Vander Zwaag R (1987) Excisional techniques for endometriosis with the CO2 laser laparoscope. *Journal of Reproductive Medicine* 32: 753–758.

Martin DC, Hubert GD & Levy BS (1989a) Depth of infiltration of endometriosis. *Journal of Gynecologic Surgery* 5: 55–60.

Martin DC, Hubert GD, Vander Zwaag R & El-Zeky FA (1989b) Laparoscopic appearance of endometriosis. *Fertility and Sterility* 51: 63–67.

Meyer WR, Gainger DA, DeCherney AH Lachs MS & Diamond MP (1991) Ovarian surgery on the rabbit: effect of cortex closure on adhesion formation and ovarian function. *Journal of Reproductive Medicine* 36: 639–643.

Nezhat C & Nezhat FR (1989) Safe laser endoscopic excision or vaporization of peritoneal endometriosis. *Fertility and Sterility* 52: 149–151.

Nezhat C, Crowgey SR & Nezhat F (1989) Videolaseroscopy for the treatment of endometriosis associated with infertility. *Fertility and Sterility* 51: 237–240.

Nezhat C, Pennington E, Nezhat F & Silfen SL (1991a) Laparoscopically assisted anterior rectal wall resection and reanastomosis for deeply infiltrating endometriosis. *Surgical Laparoscopic Endoscopy* 1: 106–108.

Nezhat C, Silfen S, Nezhat F & Martin D (1991b) Surgery for endometriosis. *Current Opinion in Obstetrics and Gynecology* 3: 385–393.

Redwine DB (1987) Age-related evolution in color appearance of endometriosis. *Fertility and Sterility* 48: 1062–1063.

Redwine DB (1990) Laparoscopic excision of endometriosis (LAPEX) by sharp dissection. In Martin DC (ed) *Laparoscopic Appearance of Endometriosis*, 2nd edn, Vol. I, pp 9–19. Memphis: Resurge Press.

Redwine DB (1991) Conservative laparoscopic excision of endometriosis by sharp dissection: life table analysis of reoperation and persistent or recurrent disease. *Fertility and Sterility* 56: 628–634.

Redwine DB & Sharpe DR (1991) Laparoscopic segmental resection of the sigmoid colon for endometriosis. *Journal of Laparoendoscopic Surgery* 1: 217–220.

Reich H, McGlynn F & Salvat J (1991) Laparoscopic treatment of cul-de-sac obliteration secondary to retrocervical deep fibrotic endometriosis. *Journal of Reproductive Medicine* 36: 516–522.

Schwartz PE (1991a) An oncologic view of when to do endoscopic surgery. *Clinical Obstetrics and Gynecology* 34: 467–472.

Schwartz PE (1991b) Ovarian masses: serologic markers. *Clinical Obstetrics and Gynecology* 34: 423–432.

Semm K & Friedrich ER (1987) *Operative Manual for Endoscopic Abdominal Surgery.* Chicago: Year Book Medical Publishers.

31

Laparoscopic Treatment of Bowel Adhesions (Enterolysis)

JAMES F. DANIELL

2222 State Street Suite A, Nashville, TN, USA

Introduction

Bowel adhesions which form following intraperitoneal trauma of many causes, can be associated with obstruction, intermittent ileus, or chronic abdominal pain (Weibel and Majno, 1973; Alexander-Williams, 1987). In the past, bowel adhesions were usually only lysed when producing severe symptoms, or bowel obstruction. In addition, it was considered ill advised to attempt laparoscopy in patients with a history of previous bowel obstruction or suspected omental or bowel adhesions (Cook, 1977). Now, with the greater interest in operative laparoscopy, better equipment, and excellent training, both general surgeons and gynaecologists are aggressively exploring methods to lyse bowel adhesions via laparoscopy. This chapter will review our experiences, techniques, and results for treating bowel adhesions via the laparoscopic approach.

History

A few general surgeons have been active in laparoscopy for over a decade, performing appendectomy (De Kok, 1977; Semm, 1983; Schreiber, 1987) and enterolysis (Kjer, 1987), with good reported results. However, only with the advent of laparoscopic cholecystectomy have North American general surgeons widely accepted laparoscopy (Reddick et al., 1989). As general surgeons embrace laparoscopy, they are also beginning to consider that bowel adhesions may cause chronic pain in addition to obstructive symptoms. Finally, some of these general surgeons are starting to recommend and perform laparoscopic enterolysis for patients with adhesions and abdominal pain.

Gynaecologists have long noted that postsurgical adhesions are a common finding at laparoscopy (Daniell and Pittaway, 1983; DeCherney and Mezer, 1984; Diamond et al., 1984). Often these patients are asymptomatic, but certain patients have pain localized in areas overlying known intra-abdominal adhesions. Laparoscopic enterolysis has been reported, specifically following appendectomy (Kleinhaus, 1984) or open pelvic surgery in females with postsurgical adhesions and lower abdominal pain (Goldstein et al., 1979; Kresch and Seifer, 1984; Rapkin, 1986; Kjer, 1987). Initially, techniques for managing bowel adhesions laparoscopically were simple blunt lysis, electrosurgery, or sharp dissection. More recently, lasers, including the CO_2 laser (Sutton and MacDonald, 1990) and fibreoptic lasers (Daniell, 1989), have been reported to successfully accomplish enterolysis at laparoscopy.

Armamentarium Available for Laparoscopic Enterolysis

All of the standard methods for adhesiolysis used at laparotomy can now be applied laparoscopically. Initially, these included sharp and blunt dissection in combination with traction. More recently, the use of irrigation fluids under pressure has proved to effectively separate tissue planes and to allow lasers or electrosurgical energy to be safely applied laparoscopically for adhesiolysis (Daniell, 1989). Both unipolar and bipolar cautery can be used laparoscopically to deal with adhesions. However, electrosurgical energy is dangerous when used contiguous to the bowel. It is now possible using fine needle electrodes to dissect laparoscopically closer to the bowel than was possible in the past. The CO_2 laser, which has been investigated for laparoscopic use for over a decade, allows vaporization close to the bowel with minimal lateral thermal effect (Sutton and MacDonald, 1990). However, the CO_2 laser can be associated with significant bleeding, generates intraperitoneal smoke, and cannot be used under fluids. More recently, fibreoptic lasers such as the potassium–titanyl–phosphate (KTP) have all been used laparoscopically for many procedures, including enterolysis (Daniell, 1989). Because of its deep thermal effects, the neodymium:yttrium–aluminium–garnet (Nd:YAG) laser is probably not appropriate for enterolysis except if used with expensive synthetic sapphire tips. Fibreoptic laser energy can be delivered under fluids, which effectively eliminates lateral heat transfer from the areas of planned impact to the adjacent bowel. This reduces risk of thermal damage to the bowel as well as allows working in a wet field without smoke generation during aquadissection.

Even more recently, titanium clips, which can be placed directly on the bowel serosa without damage (except for direct pressure), have become available for laparoscopy. Special microtipped scissors for laparoscopy now allow fine sharp dissection close to bowel serosa. Finally, the argon beam coagulator (ABC), which allows a non-touch mode of electrosurgical energy, is undergoing clinical investigations for laparoscopic use (Daniell et al., 1991). The ABC allows almost instantaneous haemostasis and can be used in a wet field with no smoke production. It can penetrate tissues 2–3 mm (Bard Electro Medical Systems, 1988), so it must be used judiciously on the bowel serosa. It can be very effective for accomplishing haemostasis during laparoscopic dissection for enterolysis.

It should be emphasized that laparoscopic enterolysis is an advanced operative laparoscopic procedure and should only be attempted by persons comfortable with multiple punctures and skilled in using multiple systems of laparoscopic surgery.

Patient Evaluation and Selection for Laparoscopic Enterolysis

The relationship of chronic abdominal pain to adhesions is very difficult to evaluate scientifically. There are many patients who have extensive abdominal adhesions, and no symptoms whatever. There are also patients with marked localized pain that appears to be related to intra-abdominal adhesion formation. Exactly why some patients have pain secondary to adhesions while others do not, remains an enigma. Thus, it is important to practise extensive preoperative evaluation and counselling before undertaking attempts at laparoscopic enterolysis.

Most patients referred for an attempt at laparoscopic enterolysis give a history of multiple previous laparotomies with previous adhesiolysis having already been performed by laparotomy, with persistence of symptoms. The patients often have been evaluated by multiple physicians, including internists, gastroenterologists, general surgeons, and psychologists or psychiatrists. Unfortunately, no specific diagnostic tests available to physicians can confirm or rule out abdominal adhesions. Thus, accurate diagnosis can only be made by direct intraperitoneal visualization. It is common for patients referred to us to have had extensive work-ups, including MRI, CT scan, upper GI, barium enema, and colonoscopy, with the final conclusion of their physicians being that there is no pathology. The patient is then referred to a pain centre or psychologist or psychiatrist for chronic pain management. Many of these patients have functional overlay and/or psychological problems, but the majority of symptomatic patients with a history of adhesions at previous laparotomy will be found to have abdominal adhesions at laparoscopy.

These patients with chronic pain are usually very frustrated with their previous medical care, and require careful preoperative counselling and consultation. It is important to warn patients that undertaking a laparoscopy with a history of probable bowel adhesions is risky, and may lead to immediate laparotomy because of bowel damage, intraperitoneal bleeding, or inability to correct the pathology encountered. It is important to stress to patients and their families that clinical results of laparoscopic enterolysis are not good in all cases. The patient must make the final decision whether to accept the risks associated with attempted operative laparoscopy in these situations, as opposed to the alternative of coping with chronic pain, intermittent obstruction, or other symptoms.

As general surgeons more widely accept the value of laparoscopy, many patients who in the past have suffered with undiagnosed chronic abdominal pain will be correctly diagnosed as having postsurgical adhesions. These patients can then be given the opportunity to consider laparoscopy as an alternative to no treatment, chronic narcotic use, or repeated laparotomies. Conventional wisdom among surgeons in the past was only to offer enterolysis if the patient was obstructed. In our opinion, this leaves many symptomatic patients in a very difficult medical situation. Certainly there is much data to confirm that any abdominal surgical procedure can result in postoperative adhesions following open and laparoscopic surgery (Diamond et al., 1991). Thus, physicians should always consider abdominal adhesions when evaluating abdominal pain in patients with previous abdominal surgery of any type.

Preoperative Preparation of the Patient for Surgery

We feel that laparoscopic enterolysis is always risky, and should only be performed either with a general surgeon as co-surgeon, or available for immediate assistance if needed. Preferably, the patient should consult with this general surgeon preoperatively, so rapport can be established and the patient can be clearly aware of the potential for open bowel surgery, including possible resection and/or temporary diversion. Our method of preoperative bowel preparation consists mainly of 24 hours of clear liquids, with an enema at home the night before surgery. Occasionally, preoperative antibiotics will be given orally by the consulting general surgeon, but usually we only give them intravenously immediately prior to surgery. All patients must give preoperative consent for possible immediate laparotomy, including all potential procedures that might occur. Ideally, blood should be available, with self-donation preferable.

Operating Room Preparation for Laparoscopic Enterolysis

Since every laparoscopy performed for enterolysis may end up a laparotomy, it is mandatory that

operating room personnel be prepared for possible laparotomy. Equipment for video monitoring, for open laparoscopy, and a full complement of operative instruments, including aquadissection systems and lasers (if used by the surgeon), should be available. These procedures often involve more than three punctures. Thus, the surgeon should always request skilled assistants experienced at operative laparoscopy for these difficult operations. To attempt this type of operative procedure without video control is very difficult, because the assistant must have adequate visibility to provide the delicate traction, countertraction, and exposure that is necessary during dissection. Anaesthesia should be aware that this may potentially be a long procedure, and plan accordingly. The supine position is usually best, since the patient's thighs may hinder laparoscopic manipulations in the dorsal lithotomy position. In females, a uterine elevator or sponge stick in the vagina will aid manipulation during surgery. If necessary, the urinary bladder can be distended with methylene blue dye, and/or fibreoptic ureteral stents can be placed if dissection involves the ureters or bladder.

Technique of Establishing Entry into the Abdomen for Laparoscopic Enterolysis

Establishing pneumoperitoneum for initial visualization of the peritoneal cavity is particularly dangerous in patients who have multiple scars from previous laparotomies and thus may have intestine adherent to the abdominal wall. The three methods for accomplishing this are open laparoscopy, preliminary insertion of a Veress needle to accomplish pneumoperitoneum, or direct trocar insertion with insufflation of gas after initial visualization with the laparoscope. We feel that the latter choice has no place in cases of laparoscopic enterolysis because of the high risk of impaling adherent loops of bowel with the larger trocar. Open laparoscopy can certainly be performed and has been described extensively in the past (Hasson, 1971). Our preference is to attempt Veress needle placement at least 2 inches (5 mm) away from any skin incision. The Veress needle is inserted using standard methods, and CO_2 is infused, at pressures under 20 mmHg. If satisfactory pneumoperitoneum can be established, a 5 mm trocar is inserted and a 5 mm diagnostic laparoscope passed through this initial trocar for initial inspection of the peritoneal cavity. If successful pneumoperitoneum cannot be established, so-called 'finger laparoscopy' can be attempted. With this technique, a mini-lap incision is made, and the index finger is inserted and used to bluntly dissect away any structures that are adherent to the parietal peritoneum in the area of the small incision. Once this area is dissected, a trocar can be placed and the laparoscope introduced.

Each case of laparoscopic enterolysis is different, and thus placement of extra trocars varies, depending on the fixation of adhesions and/or bowel to the abdominal wall and patterns in which this fixation occurs. Enterolysis and adhesiolysis basically are the same, the difference being to be careful to distinguish fatty omentum from actual bowel serosa. Omentum or bowel fat is most often adherent to the parietal peritoneum, but occasionally loops of intestinal serosa may be directly attached.

The basic dissection principle is the same as for laparotomy, the difference being that one must work through fixed locations and from a distance. Once the initial visualization of the bowel and its distortion is assessed, a decision is made for placement of extra trocars. There is no standard location for the extra trocars. This depends upon the location of adhesions and the surgeon's plan for lysis. For instance, if the transverse colon is adherent to the umbilicus, but a free space is seen in the right lower quadrant, a second 5 mm trocar could be placed there and instruments passed for initial manipulation and dissection. It is rarely possible to accomplish enterolysis effectively with only two probes. Thus, safe enterolysis usually requires at least four trocar sites. This allows one for visualization, one for retraction, one for countertraction, and one for dissection. Most of the dissection can be done using 5 mm ports, particularly if a low light video camera with good resolution is used (Circon ACMI, Santa Barbara, California). If necessary, a 5 mm trocar site can be enlarged to 10 mm to introduce an operating scope which allows instruments to pass down the line of sight, thus allowing dissection without introducing another trocar.

It will be necessary to change the view of the operator to successfully visualize all areas of adhesions. This can be easily accomplished by placing the 5 mm laparoscope through the different ports, and thus interchangeably operating from a different angle. This initially can be somewhat difficult with the video monitor, since most physicians are accustomed to working from one location. The surgeon may find it necessary to change his position around the operating table to maintain orientation and good

hand–eye coordination. For instance, for dealing with adhesions beneath the umbilicus, placing the laparoscope suprapubically and looking upwards would give a good view of those adhesions. Then accessory probes through each lateral mid-abdomen could allow effective access for safe dissection.

Method for Enterolysis

Our basic technique for enterolysis is to identify the bowel and omentum and carefully dissect these from the peritoneum, trying to occlude large vessels as they are encountered. This may require the use of laparoscopic clips, electrosurgical, or laser energy. Pretied suture loops can be used for haemostasis in larger pieces of omentum, but it is better to occlude each vessel haemostatically before it is separated, as the layers of fat are initially dissected from the abdominal walls.

In females, particularly after hysterectomy, adhesions may adhere to the vaginal cuff and bladder peritoneum and along the lateral pelvic sidewalls. A most difficult problem in females is the ovarian remnant syndrome (Utian *et al.*, 1978), in which a residual portion of ovary is often buried retroperitoneally, with the colon adherent to it encompassing the entire area in a mass. Recurrent ovarian function in this fixed area often causes lower abdominal pain in many of these cases. Dissection in this area is particularly tedious and requires an understanding of the anatomy, a willingness to dissect the ureter and vessels retroperitoneally, as well as patience, adequate experience, and the proper equipment.

Our primary method for enterolysis is to use 5 mm atraumatic alligator grasping forceps to grab either bowel or omentum, and then attempt blunt dissection and aquadissection with a disposable 5 mm suction–irrigation probe through which we pass a 600 μm KTP/YAG fibre (Figure 31.1). KTP laser energy is used to vaporize thicker

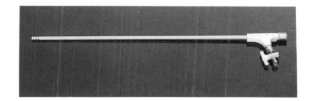

Figure 31.1 The 5 mm disposable suction–irrigation probe used for aquadissection, smoke and fluid suction and blunt dissection is shown here. A 600 μm fibreoptic laser fibre can be passed through the inner channel for tissue vaporization during irrigation.

bands, and the blunt probe through which it passes is used for aquadissection via a disposable suction–irrigation system (PumpVac Plus, Marlow Medical, Willoughby, Ohio) (Figure 31.2). This is accomplished while maintaining traction and countertraction with atraumatic graspers. If bleeding cannot be controlled with the KTP laser, endoloop sutures can be placed or laparoscopic clips can be placed using a disposable 10 mm clip applier (US Surgical, Norwalk, Connecticut). Since March, 1991, we have used the argon beam coagulator with a setting of 40–80 W to coagulate bleeding omental vessels in a smokeless non-touch technique using a prototype 10 mm disposable laparoscopic probe (Birtcher Medical Systems, Irvine, California). Copious volumes of warmed heparinized Ringer's (5000 units heparin per litre) are used during the procedure, for both aquadissection and irrigation.

Complications of Laparoscopic Enterolysis

There are obvious risks associated with attempting laparoscopic enterolysis. These include immediate bowel perforation, bleeding that cannot be controlled laparoscopically, injury to the bowel wall that results in delayed perforation, ileus, peritonitis, or failure of resolution of the patient's symptoms. This last problem is not a complication,

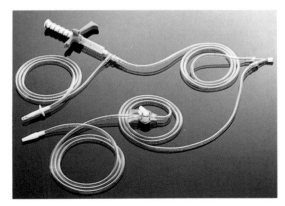

Figure 31.2 This disposable suction–irrigation system for laparoscopic enterolysis has many advantages. The vacuum syringe allows the scrub nurse instantaneously to vary the volume and pressure of fluid used for aquadissection. The valve allows venting of smoke or fluids simultaneously via wall suction. The inflow tubing attaches to a bag of heparinized Ringer's (5000 units/litre) which can be attached to the operating table since pressure or gravity is not needed to accomplish irrigation via the vacuum syringe.

but reflects the inability to adequately lyse adhesions that are symptomatic or early post-surgical readhesion formation.

Methods to Reduce Postsurgical Adhesions Formation at Laparoscopic Enterolysis

There is much data in the gynaecological literature addressing postsurgical adhesion formation after laparotomy. Recent data suggest that laparoscopic surgery also has a high risk of producing postsurgical adhesions, including both recurrence of old adhesions and *de novo* adhesions, no matter what type of surgical techniques are used (Diamond *et al.*, 1991). Thus, we should expect that after laparoscopic enterolysis, adhesions may re-form postoperatively. Methods hopefully to reduce this readhesion formation include use of heparinized Ringer's, careful placement of Interceed (Ethicon, Somerville, New Jersey) intraperitoneally over raw areas, and consideration for early second look laparoscopy after laparoscopic enterolysis.

There is a large body of literature addressing prevention or reduction of postsurgical adhesions in gynaecology, but at present, nothing has proven to be clinically effective. The natural history and evolution of adhesion formation after abdominal surgery is still poorly understood in humans. Careful surgical techniques that limit tissue trauma and bleeding, and which minimize the raw tissue left intraperitoneally are probably the most important factors in reducing postsurgical adhesion formation. At present, it seems overly aggressive to routinely recommend early second look laparoscopy for all patients who have undergone laparoscopic enterolysis. However, in those patients who do not report improvement in their abdominal pain 6 weeks after extensive enterolysis via laparoscopy, discussion with the patient about possible second look laparoscopy should be considered.

Presently, sodium hyaluronate, which is the natural lubricant found in our body joints, is being evaluated for its potential to reduce postsurgical adhesions. Whether this substance will be found to be of benefit is unknown at this time, as randomized prospective clinical trials using early second look laparoscopy are just beginning to evaluate its effectiveness for reducing postsurgical adhesions.

Results of Laparoscopic Enterolysis

The actual results of laparoscopic enterolysis are difficult to evaluate scientifically, because it requires direct subsequent intraperitoneal observation, or alternatively accepting patients' subjective opinions of their clinical improvement. Our initial report retrospectively questioned 42 patients who had undergone at least three previous laparotomies and underwent subsequent laparoscopic enterolysis with fibreoptic laser energy (Daniel, 1989). In that series, 67% of the patients stated that their symptoms were improved when they responded to a questionnaire sent at least 6 months after their laparoscopic enterolysis. Fourteen patients were not improved, and ten of those subsequently underwent laparotomy because of persistence of pain, known intraperitoneal adhesions, and inability to cope with their pain in non-surgical fashions.

Sutton and MacDonald (1990) in a subsequent report of laparoscopic adhesiolysis using the CO_2 laser as the primary method of dissection, reported 84% improvement in 65 patients with abdominal pain and adhesions without endometriosis. They concluded that laparoscopic adhesiolysis was effective therapy and not mere placebo effect. They also noted that controversy still exists concerning the relationships between abdominal pain and intra-abdominal adhesions.

North American general surgeons have not yet published data on their experience with laparoscopic enterolysis, because of the short time over which they have been attempting these procedures. However, personal communication with general surgeons practising laparoscopic enterolysis in our area reveals that two-thirds of their patients obtain satisfactory results with this therapy for abdominal pain related to postsurgical bowel adhesions.

The Future of Laparoscopic Enterolysis

As more general surgeons become skilled at laparoscopy, more patients who have bowel adhesions will probably be offered laparoscopic treatment if they are symptomatic. Concomitantly, gynaecologists who are also becoming more aggressive at laparoscopy, will find it easier to recruit general surgeons to assist them with laparoscopic enterolysis. One of our problems several years ago was to recruit a general surgeon to assist us at attempts at laparoscopic enterolysis.

The difficulties in finding a general surgeon willing to assist at laparoscopy are thankfully now gone for gynaecologists. In the future, both gynaecologists and general surgeons will more aggressively treat bowel and other intra-abdominal adhesions laparoscopically as they are encountered. Thus, more data will hopefully come forth from both gynaecologists and general surgeons based on their experiences dealing with bowel adhesions at laparoscopy.

Animal work in various models will also hopefully be reported, from both the general surgical and gynaecological investigators. This should lead to better instrumentation and techniques for successfully dealing with bowel adhesions laparoscopically, as well as better training for trainee laparoscopists. Patients should benefit from this 'minimally invasive surgery' as treatment for symptomatic bowel adhesions compared to the previously required major open abdominal laparotomy. Whether the long-term benefits to patients will be greater than the increased numbers of patients undergoing laparotomy for complications at attempted laparoscopic enterolysis remains to be seen.

All laparoscopists should carefully explore the potential for incorporating laparoscopic enterolysis into their practices. Only those laparoscopists who feel very comfortable with aggressive laparoscopic surgery, take the time to acquire the proper training and skills, and practise good patient selection and counselling, should attempt these potentially risky procedures. Much work is needed in carefully controlled animal studies, and both prospective and retrospective analysis of clinical data before firm conclusions can be drawn concerning the efficacy of laparoscopic enterolysis. We encourage all interested endoscopists to join us in evaluating this complicated and difficult medical problem exploring the role that laparoscopy plays in the management of intra-abdominal adhesions.

References

Alexander-Williams J (1987) Do adhesions cause pain? *British Medical Journal* **294**: 659.

Bard Electro Medical Systems, Inc. (1988) System 6000 argon beam coagulator tissue effects. Technical document. Bard Electro Medical Systems, Inc. Englewood, Colorado.

Cook WA (1977) Needle laparoscopy in patients with suspected bowel adhesions. *Obstetrics and Gynecology* **49**: 105–106.

Daniell JF (1989) Laparoscopic enterolysis for chronic abdominal pain. *Journal of Gynecologic Surgery* **5**: 61.

Daniell JF & Pittaway DE (1983) The role of laparoscopic adhesiolysis in an *in vitro* fertilization program. *Fertility and Sterility* **40**: 49.

Daniell JF, Fisher B & Alexander W (1992) Laparoscopic evaluation of the argon beam coagulator — initial report. *Journal of Reproductive Medicine* (in press).

DeCherney AH & Mezer HC (1984) The nature of posttuboplasty pelvic adhesions as determined by early and late laparoscopy. *Fertility and Sterility* **41**: 643.

De Kok H (1977) A new technique for resecting the non-inflamed not-adhesive appendix through a mini-laparotomy with the aid of the laparoscope. *Archivum Chirurgicum Neerlandicum* **29**: 195–197.

Diamond MP, Daniell JF, Feste J, McLaughlin D & Martin DC (1984) Pelvic adhesions at early second-look laparoscopy following carbon dioxide laser surgery procedures. *Infertility* **7**: 39–44.

Diamond MP, Daniell JF, Feste J & Martin DC (1991) Postoperative adhesion development after operative laparoscopy: evaluation at early second-look procedures. *Fertility and Sterility* **55**: 700–704.

Goldstein DP, DeCholnoky C, Leventhal JM & Emans SJ (1979) New insights into the old problem of chronic pelvic pain. *Journal of Pediatric Surgery* **14**: 675.

Hasson HM (1971) Modified instrument and method for laparoscopy. *American Journal of Obstetrics and Gynecology* **110**: 886–887.

Kjer JJ (1987) Laparoscopy after previous abdominal surgery. *Acta Obstetrica et Gynecologica Scandinavica* **66**: 159.

Kleinhaus S (1984) Laparoscopic lysis of adhesions for postappendectomy pain. *Gastrointestinal Endoscopy* **5**: 304.

Kresch AJ & Seifer DB (1984) Laparoscopy in 100 women with chronic pelvic pain. *Obstetrics and Gynecology* **64**: 672.

Rapkin AJ (1986) Adhesions and pelvic pain: a retrospective study (1986). *Obstetrics and Gynecology* **68**: 13.

Reddick EJ, Olsen D, Daniell J et al. (1989) Laparoscopic laser cholecystectomy. *Laser Medicine and Surgery News and Advances* 38–40.

Schreiber J (1987) Early experience with laparoscopic appendectomy in women. *Surgical Endoscopy* **1**: 211–216.

Semm K (1983) Endoscopic appendectomy. *Endoscopy* **15**: 59–64.

Sutton C & MacDonald R (1990) Laser laparoscopic adhesiolysis. *Journal of Gynecologic Surgery* **6**: 155.

Utian WH, Katz M, Davey DA & Carr PJ (1978) Effect of premenopausal castration and incremental doses of conjugated equine estrogens on plasma follicle-stimulating hormone, luteinizing hormone, and estradiol. *American Journal of Obstetrics and Gynecology* **132**: 297–302.

Weibel MA & Majno G (1973) Peritoneal adhesions and their relation to abdominal surgery. *American Journal of Surgery* **126**: 345.

32

Prevention of Adhesion Reformation

LISA BARRIE SCHWARTZ* AND MICHAEL P. DIAMOND‡

*Yale University School of Medicine, New Haven, CT, USA
‡Vanderbilt University Medical Center, Nashville, TN, USA

Introduction

Despite the recent surge of information on pelvic adhesive disease available in the literature, postoperative development of pelvic adhesions remain a constant source of frustration to the reproductive pelvic surgeon. Their presence has been implicated as a cause of infertility, pelvic pain, and small bowel obstruction, and, in addition, has mechanically interfered with the potential improvement in fertility following reproductive pelvic surgery. The aetiology of adhesive disease includes previous surgical trauma, pelvic infections, haemorrhage, and other types of peritoneal irritation such as foreign body reactions (i.e. talcum powder from surgical gloves, fluff from gauze pads, fibres from torn paper drapes, and reactive suture materials) and endometriosis. The combination of blood with a tissue injury is more likely to lead to adhesion formation.

The mechanism of adhesion formation has been described as a variation of the normal peritoneal healing process, and is likely to stem from suppressed endogenous fibrinolytic activity due to inhibition of plasminogen activator activity (PAA). Thus, fibrin deposits formed as a part of the inflammatory response to peritoneal injury persist (instead of being resorbed due to the function of PAA) and subsequently become infiltrated by fibroblasts forming fibrous adhesions. Factors known to inhibit PAA include tissue ischaemia (i.e. crushing, ligating, or stripping peritoneum), surgical trauma (i.e. devascularization, necrosis), and grafting or suturing tissue or other materials to peritoneal defects. Thus, it is not surprising that these factors are thought to stimulate postoperative adhesion development.

Adhesion Reformation versus *de novo* Adhesion Formation

Adhesion reformation refers to new postoperative adhesions located at the same site as the adhesions that were lysed at the initial operative procedure, whereas *de novo* adhesion formation refers to newly formed adhesions present at a location which did not have adhesions at the time of the initial surgical procedure. Although current data suggest that adhesion formation and reformation differ, the pathophysiology of reformation and *de novo* formation has not yet been well elucidated. However, adhesion reformation is considered to be more difficult to prevent.

In a multicentre study (Diamond *et al.*, 1991), the frequency and severity of adhesion reformation and *de novo* adhesion formation following laparoscopic surgery was assessed in 51 women. Although the mean adhesion score had decreased by 50% ± 4% at second look laparoscopy (SLL) within 12 weeks of the initial operative laparoscopy procedure, 96% of women still had pelvic adhesions. Adhesion reformation was noted in all these women (41% were filmy and avascular; 61% were dense and vascular). *De novo* adhesion formation occurred in only 16% of women.

Likewise, another group (Nezhat et al., 1990) evaluated 157 women at SLL after laparoscopic surgery and noted the occurrence of adhesion reformation but no de novo adhesion formation. Thus, there remains a high incidence of adhesion development following operative laparoscopy, with de novo adhesion formation probably less of a problem. Therefore, the focus of this review will be the methods currently available to prevent adhesion reformation following gynaecological endoscopy.

Laparoscopy versus Laparotomy

In a series of reports in which SLL was employed after reproductive pelvic surgery performed at laparotomy, pelvic adhesions were noted in 56–100% of women (Diamond et al., 1987; Diamond, 1988; Raj and Hulka, 1982; Surrey and Friedman, 1982; Daniell and Pittaway, 1983; DeCherney and Mezer, 1984; Diamond et al., 1984a; McLaughlin, 1984; Pittaway et al., 1985; Trimbos-Kemper et al., 1985).

To assess whether the method of entry into the abdominal cavity would alter postoperative adhesion development, Filmar and coworkers, in 1987, compared postoperative adhesion formation following standard uterine injury at laparoscopy versus laparotomy in the rat model, and reported no significant difference between the two groups. In contrast, Luciano and colleagues, in 1989, reported fewer adhesions following laparoscopy compared with laparotomy in the rabbit uterine horn model. Thus, the animal literature contains conflicting reports on whether endoscopic surgery will reduce postoperative adhesions.

Unfortunately, the question of whether laparoscopic procedures would be less likely than laparotomy to lead to postoperative pelvic adhesions has not been adequately studied clinically, probably because of difficulties with proper randomization and control. Postulations such as less tissue drying, tissue manipulations, foreign bodies, and lack of trauma from packing the bowel at laparoscopy need to be further investigated.

Microsurgery

The backbone of the tenets of gynaecological microsurgery rests on the use of proper precise

surgical techniques aimed at minimizing adverse factors that suppress endogenous PAA and lead to adhesion formation. In addition to using the microscope or loupes for magnification (which allows the use of fine microsurgical instruments and fine suture of low tissue reactivity), this also involves minimizing tissue handling and trauma, meticulous haemostasis with pinpoint electrocautery, frequent irrigation to prevent tissue drying, precise reapproximation of tissue without tension, elimination of foreign bodies, avoidance of tissue devitalization, and excising rather than incising adhesions. General surgical principles should also include avoiding crushing instruments, irrigating rather than sponging, and eliminating the application of devascularized tissue grafts. When possible, the use of a small, fine-calibre tapered atraumatic needle is recommended. Smooth-tipped forceps should be used whenever possible to avoid crushing the tissue. A suction apparatus that does not allow delicate tissue to be sucked into the lumen should be used. Woven material should be avoided since it has been shown to cause adhesions due to serosal abrasion. Moist packs are preferable to dry ones.

Careful attention to the choice of suture material is necessary. Catgut sutures are classically the most reactive types and should be avoided when performing reproductive gynaecological surgery. Polyglycolic acid (Dexon) and polyglactin (Vicryl) reportedly produce much milder foreign body reactions. Multifilament suture reportedly causes more inflammation than monofilament suture. Polydioxanone (PDS), a synthetic absorbable monofilament suture, has been shown by some investigators to cause fewer adhesions than multifilament suture (DeCherney and Laufer, 1983), although others were unable to confirm this difference (Neff et al., 1985).

However, meticulous microsurgical technique does not appear to be the sole panacea, since use of these principles in six different studies still resulted in 56–100% of patients found to have postoperative adhesions at SLL (Raj and Hulka, 1982; Surrey and Friedman, 1982; Daniell and Pittaway, 1983; McLaughlin, 1984, Pittaway et al., 1985; Trimbos-Kemper et al., 1985); although one study reported improved postoperative pregnancy rates after lysis of adhesions using microsurgical (57%) versus macrosurgical (25%) techniques (Diamond, 1979).

Laser Surgery

Use of the laser during reproductive pelvic surgery hypothetically enables more precise incisions, reduced tissue handling and bleeding, and shorter operating time, which has been suggested to cause less tissue trauma and, therefore, reduced adhesion formation. The carbon dioxide laser is currently most frequently used, but the argon, potassium–titanyl–phosphate (KTP 532), and neodymium: yttrium–aluminium–garnet (Nd:YAG) lasers are becoming more popular.

However, like microsurgery, results from laser surgery have also been disappointing with regard to eliminating postoperative adhesion formation. Between 57% and 86% of patients were found to have postoperative adhesions at the time of SLL despite the initial use of the laser in the pelvic surgical procedure (Diamond et al., 1984a,b; McLaughlin, 1984; Diamond and DeCherney, 1987). In another study, there was no difference found in adhesion reformation following laser surgery versus electrosurgery (Tulandi, 1987).

SLL

The use of SLL following pelvic surgery to assess the pelvis and treat postoperative adhesions has not been thoroughly investigated. Hypothetical potential benefits of SLL include providing post-surgical pelvic assessment, evaluating operative techniques and perioperative therapies, and enhancing initial surgery with the implementation of operative laparoscopic techniques. Several investigators have reported adhesions at early SLL to be predominantly fine, filmy, avascular, and easy to lyse with less blood loss than the adhesions found at late SLL which are thick, dense, and more vascular (Surrey and Friedman, 1982; Daniell and Pittaway, 1983; DeCherney and Mezer, 1984; Diamond et al., 1984a; McLaughlin, 1984; Trimbos-Kemper et al., 1985; Diamond and DeCherney, 1987).

Pregnancy rates following SLL were found to be 52% at early SLL versus 17% at late SLL by one group (Surrey and Friedman, 1982), but, in contrast, equal rates were found in both groups in other studies (Raj and Hulka, 1982; DeCherney and Mezer, 1984).

Morbidity, inconvenience, discomfort, and expense have been arguments against the use of SLL to evaluate and treat postoperative adhesive disease. However, the most important question with regard to early SLL has yet to be resolved, namely whether performance of this procedure improves efficacy (i.e. pregnancy rate, pain reduction, etc).

Adjuvants

Adjuvants have been widely used for attempts at postoperative adhesion reduction. There are numerous uncontrolled, non-uniform studies reported in the literature with conflicting results, and the efficacy of adjuvant usage remains inconclusive. Adhesions can be reduced by adjuvants that intervene at various steps in the adhesion-formation cascade to decrease the initial inflammation, prevent coagulation, stimulate PAA, mechanically separate injured peritoneal surfaces, or inhibit fibroblastic proliferation.

Reduction in the inflammatory response is achieved with corticosteroids, non-steroidal anti-inflammatory drugs (NSAIDs), and antihistamines such as promethazine. Steroid use can be complicated by immunosuppression causing infections and wound dehiscence. Progestins also have immunosuppressive effects causing decreased antibody production and vascular permeability and increased degradation of granulation tissue. Anticoagulants and fibrinolytic agents have been used to prevent persistence of the fibrinous mass, but require high doses with haemorrhagic complications. Perioperative prophylactic antibiotics are commonly used despite a lack of studies. Intravenous doxycycline to empirically treat Chlamydia and other infectious organisms is currently a popular regimen. More recently there have been promising reports on pentoxifylline, a methylxanthine derivative, to reduce postoperative adhesion reformation in animal models by interfering in multiple steps of the adhesion development process (Steinleitner et al., 1990).

Use of intra-abdominal instillates and barriers to mechanically separate adjoining raw peritoneal surfaces during the healing process has been extensively studied in both animals and humans. Instillates are thought to prevent early fibrinous adhesion formation by separating raw surfaces by the mechanisms of hydroflotation (increasing intraperitoneal volume by third spacing of fluid into the abdominal cavity) and siliconization (coating tissue surfaces which reduces direct apposition of traumatized structure). Hyskon, consisting of 32% dextran 70 (200 ml) has been the most widely used intra-abdominal instillate during pelvic laparotomy or laparoscopy, although studies present inconsistent results. Although shown to be beneficial in most animal models, results of human trials have been variable. Of the four clinical trials, Hyskon was beneficial in two (Adhesion Study Group, 1983; Rosenberg and Board, 1984) and non-beneficial in two (Jansen, 1985; Larsson et al., 1985). Risks, although rare, include fluid imbalance with its sequelae, pseudo-pulmonary embolus (symptoms due to diaphragmatic irritation), anaphylaxis, serum sickness, and wound separation. Other types of intra-abdominal instillates include saline, mineral oil, silicone, povidone, vaseline, crystalloid solutions, and carboxymethylcellulose (CMC) (Diamond *et al.*, 1988a). Use of the rabbit uterine horn model has shown CMC, a viscous hydroscopic fluid, to reduce mean adhesion reformation scores (from 3.96 in the control group to 2.15 in the CMC-treated group) (Diamond *et al.*, 1988b). More recently, preliminary studies have shown poloxamer 407 (a biocompatible polymer existing as a liquid at room temperature a solid at body temperature) to reduce adhesion reformation in the animal model (Steinleitner *et al.*, 1991).

Both endogenous tissues and exogenous materials have been used as barriers to adhesion formation. Devascularized tissue grafts are no longer used since they actually increase postoperative adhesion formation. Use of material barriers (i.e. metal, plastic, rubber) has also been abandoned since a second procedure is usually necessary to remove them. In addition, foreign

body reactions can be precipitated by synthetic materials. The haemostatic agents Surgicel, Gelfoam, and Gelfilm have been used as barriers. Interceed (TC7), an absorbable barrier, is a distant cousin of Surgicel. Specifically designed for adhesion reduction, Interceed is an oxidized regenerated cellulose in a knitted weave differing from Surgicel in the degree of oxidation, porosity, density, and weave. Interceed gelates on raw peritoneum to form a continuous surface within 8 hours, preventing fibrin band formation and subsequent fibroblast invasion. Other possible biochemical effects have not yet been explored. Haemostasis must be meticulous before applying Interceed since the presence of blood significantly reduces its ability to minimize subsequent adhesion formation. Although the majority of studies have been performed using the rabbit uterine horn model, to date there is one prospective randomized multicentre clinical trial confirming the safety and efficacy of Interceed (Interceed [TC7] Adhesion Barrier Study Group, 1989). The rabbit pelvic sidewall/uterine horn model has also been used to evaluate the ability of the Gore-tex surgical membrane, an inert,

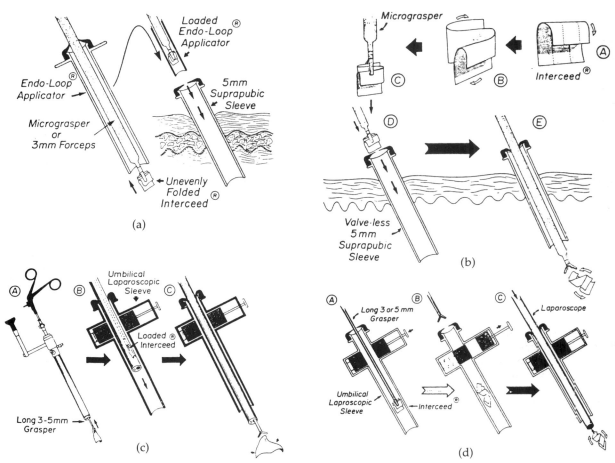

Figure 32.1 Laparoscopic application of Interceed. Top row: with (a) or without (b) an endoloop applicator through the suprapubic sleeve. Bottom row: through the umbilical sleeve (c,d). From Azziz *et al.* (1991), with permission.

non-reactive polytetrafluoroethylene used as a synthetic pericardial membrane for over 10 years, to reduce adhesions (Boyers et al., 1988).

A recent prospective, multicentre trial showed the ability of Interceed to be safely and easily applied at laparoscopy (Azziz et al., 1991). An average of two pieces were placed per patient with an average time required per piece of 2 minutes, 40 seconds. The material was successfully placed through either the umbilical sleeve (using a grasper) or the suprapubic sleeve (using either a grasper or an endoloop applicator) (Figure 32.1).

Summary

The reproductive pelvic surgeon continues to face the persistent problem of adhesion reformation interfering with the postoperative results of reproductive pelvic surgery. Prevention is of paramount importance, and should be strived for by carefully applying the combined armamentarium of microsurgical principles, laser surgical equipment, and adjuvant usage.

Although adhesion reformation is reduced when these agents are used, elimination has not yet been achieved. Thus, there remains room for further improvement in therapy. A better understanding of the pathophysiology, especially at the molecular level, may lead to new future developments.

References

Adhesion Study Group (1983) Reduction of postoperative pelvic adhesions with intraperitoneal 32% dextran 70: a prospective randomized clinical trial. Fertility and Sterility **40**: 612–619.

Azziz R, Murphy AA, Rosenbery SM et al. (1991) Use of an oxidized regenerated cellulose absorbable adhesion barrier at laparoscopy. Journal of Reproductive Medicine **36**: 479–482.

Boyers SP, Diamond MP & DeCherney AH (1988) Reduction of postoperative pelvic adhesions in the rabbit with Gore-tex surgical membrane. Fertility and Sterility **49**: 1066–1070.

Daniell JF & Pittaway DE (1983) Short-interval second-look laparoscopy after infertility surgery. A preliminary report. Journal of Reproductive Medicine **28**: 281–283.

DeCherney A & Laufer N (1983) The use of a new synthetic monofilament suture, polydioxanone (PDS), for surgery. Fertility and Sterility (abstract) **39**: 401.

DeCherney AH & Mezer HC (1984) The nature of posttuboplasty pelvic adhesions as determined by early and late laparoscopy. Fertility and Sterility **41**: 643–646.

Diamond EE (1979) Lysis of postoperative pelvic adhesions in infertility. Fertility and Sterility **31**: 287–295.

Diamond MP (1988) Surgical aspects of infertility. In Sciarra JW (ed) Gynecology and Obstetrics, pp 1–23. Philadelphia: Harper and Row.

Diamond MP & DeCherney AH (1987) Pathogenesis of adhesion formation/reformation: application to reproductive pelvic surgery. Microsurgery **8**: 103–108.

Diamond MP, Daniell JF, Feste J et al. (1984a) Pelvic adhesions at early second look laparoscopy following carbon dioxide laser surgical procedures. Infertility **7**: 39–44.

Diamond MP, Daniell JF, Martin DC et al. (1984b) Tubal patency and pelvic adhesions at early second-look laparoscopy following intraabdominal use of the carbon dioxide laser: initial report of the intraabdominal laser study group. Fertility and Sterility **42**: 717–723.

Diamond MP, Daniell JF, Feste J et al. (1987a) Adhesion reformation and de novo adhesion formation after reproductive pelvic surgery. Fertility and Sterility **47**: 864–866.

Diamond MP, DeCherney AH, Linsky CB et al. (1988a) Assessment of carboxymethylcellulose and 32% dextran 70 for prevention of adhesion in a rabbit uterine horn model. International Journal of Fertility **33**: 278–282.

Diamond MP, DeCherney AH, Linsky CB et al. (1988b) Adhesion reformation in the rabbit uterine horn model: 1. Reduction with carboxymethylcellulose. International Journal of Fertility **33**: 372–375.

Diamond MP, Daniell JF, Johns DA et al. (1991) Adhesion formation and reformation after operative laparoscopy: assessment at early second-look procedures. Fertility and Sterility **55**: 700–704.

Filmar S, Gomel V & McComb PF (1987) Operative laparoscopy versus open abdominal surgery: a comparative study on postoperative adhesion formation in the rat model. Fertility and Sterility **48**: 486–489.

Interceed (TC7) Adhesion Barrier Study Group (1989) Prevention of postsurgical adhesions by interceed (TC7), an absorbable adhesion barrier: a prospective randomized multicenter clinical study. Fertility and Sterility **51**: 933–938.

Jansen RPS (1985) Failure of intraperitoneal adjuncts to improve the outcome of pelvic operations in young women. American Journal of Obstetrics and Gynecology **153**: 363–371.

Larsson B, Lalos O, Marsk L et al. (1985) Effect of intraperitoneal instillation of 32% dextran 70 on postoperative adhesion formation after tubal surgery. Acta Obstetrica et Gynecologica Scandinavica **64**: 437–441.

Luciano AA, Maier DB, Koch EI et al. (1989) A comparative study of postoperative adhesions following laser surgery by laparoscopy versus laparotomy in the rabbit model. Obstetrics and Gynecology **74**: 220–224.

McLaughlin DS (1984) Evaluation of adhesion reformation by early second-look laparoscopy following microlaser ovarian wedge resection. *Fertility and Sterility* **42**: 531–537.

Neff MR, Holtz GL & Betsill WL (1985) Adhesion formation and histologic reaction with polydioxanone and polyglactin suture. *American Journal of Obstetrics and Gynecology* **51**: 20–23.

Nezhat CR, Nezhat FR, Metzger DA *et al.* (1990) Adhesion reformation after reproductive surgery by videolaseroscopy. *Fertility and Sterility* **53**: 1008–1011.

Pittaway DE, Daniell JF & Maxson WS (1985) Ovarian surgery in an infertility patient as an indication for a short-interval second-look laparoscopy: a preliminary study. *Fertility and Sterility* **44**: 611–614.

Raj SG & Hulka JF (1982) Second-look laparoscopy in infertility surgery: therapeutic and prognostic value. *Fertility and Sterility* **38**: 325–329.

Rosenberg SM & Board JA (1984) High-molecular weight dextran in human infertility surgery. *American Journal of Obstetrics and Gynecology* **48**: 380–385.

Steinleitner A, Lambert H, Kazensky C *et al.* (1990) Pentoxifylline, a methylxanthine derivative, prevents postsurgical adhesion reformation in rabbits. *Obstetrics and Gynecology* **75**: 926–928.

Steinleitner A, Lambert H, Kazensky C *et al.* (1991) Poloxamer 407 as an intraperitoneal barrier material for the prevention of postsurgical adhesion formation and reformation in rodent models for reproductive surgery. *Obstetrics and Gynecology* **77**: 48–52.

Surrey MW & Friedman S (1982) Second-look laparoscopy after reconstructive pelvic surgery for infertility. *Journal of Reproductive Medicine* **27**: 658–660.

Trimbos-Kemper TCM, Trimbos JB & van Hall EV (1985) Adhesion formation after tubal surgery: results of the eight-day laparoscopy in 188 patients. *Fertility and Sterility* **43**: 395–400.

Tulandi T (1987) Adhesion reformation after reproductive pelvic surgery with and without the carbon dioxide laser. *Fertility and Sterility* **47**: 704–706.

Hysteroscopic Surgery

33

Initiating a Hysteroscopic Programme and Hysteroscopic Instrumentation

MICHAEL S. BAGGISH

Ravenswood Hospital Medical Center, Chicago, Illinois, USA

Introduction

Increasingly, direct visual examination of the uterine cavity has been taken up by gynaecologists in place of blind or indirect evaluation methods. The advantages of seeing the pathology with one's own eyes are many:

1. The most appropriate diagnosis is likely to be made.
2. An accurate assessment of the pathology may be done prior to treatment.
3. A record of the examination may be accomplished by still or video photography.
4. The initial investigation may be completed quickly within the office or out-patient clinic setting.
5. Capital expenditure of equipment is relatively small.

During the past decade and continuing into the 1990s the number of diagnostic and operative hysteroscopy seminars have quadrupled and have enjoyed excellent attendance. For example, at the annual meeting of the American College of Obstetricians and Gynecologists a large number of postgraduate courses are offered. Over the last 5 years dedicated hysteroscopy courses have enjoyed either the best or second best attendance of all such courses and have been amongst the earliest to fill up.

A pattern for learning these techniques has emerged. The prospective student should plan to learn during a didactic conference the details of anatomy, pathology, optics, instrumentation, principles of diagnostic and operative techniques. Practical 'hands on' experience is essential to learn how to manipulate the instruments and apply the lessons learned during the didactic sessions. I prefer to use heifer uteri in these laboratories, since they provide an accessible, reasonable model of the human uterus and are easily distended with water delivered by pump or syringe. Generally a 2-day experience of combined didactics and laboratory sessions is sufficient to provide the practitioner with a suitable introduction to hysteroscopy. Clearly, as with any endoscopic technique, practice by doing simple, uncomplicated normal intrauterine assessment is the key to subsequent skilful operative hysteroscopic procedures. I recommend that the novice perform at least 50 diagnostic hysteroscopies prior to attempting the simplest operative procedure. Orientation within the uterus, particularly when doing hysteroscopy under direct video monitoring, is vitally important, since complications experienced during difficult operative procedures most frequently relate to loss of orientation within the uterus with resultant perforation or/and deep myometrial penetration.

The critical passage from a high level of confidence, performing diagnostic hysteroscopy then progressing to skilful operative hysteroscopy, must be attained gradually by planned steps, starting with the easiest intrauterine manipulations and advancing to difficult procedures. The greatest levels of skill are required for extraction of submucous myomas and treating extensive uterine adhesions. Simultaneous laparoscopy should be performed when operative hysteroscopy carries a risk of uterine perforation, e.g. septum resection. Again the beginner should never attempt to begin intrauterine surgery before gaining suitable diagnostic experience on a large number of patients.

Initiation of a hysteroscopic programme should therefore progress in a logical fashion. Both office and operating room plans will be offered below. As with other endoscopic techniques, familiarity with instruments and distending media as well as techniques are crucial to success.

Instrumentation

Any skilled craftsman, whether that person be a carpenter, musician or surgeon, must acquire the best tools to do the job properly. Although saving money where appropriate is meritorious, cutting corners with precision instruments will in the long run prove wasteful. The old adage 'you get what you pay for' fortunately or unfortunately holds true when selecting surgical instruments. The best rule is to buy the very best equipment that one can afford. It is infinitely better to purchase less equipment rather than to sacrifice quality.

Telescopes

The most important piece of equipment for the performance of hysteroscopy is the lens or telescope. The optics as well as the fibreoptic illumination bundles are packaged together in this single instrument. Most rigid telescopes range in diameter from 2 mm to 4 mm (o.d.). The best light shower and optical resolution are likely to be found in 4 mm (o.d.) instruments. Although flexible telescopes are now finding their way into the market place, they suffer from inferior resolution compared to rigid equipment. The most convenient length for the hysteroscopic telescope is 35 cm. Shorter instruments offer no advantage and some distinct disadvantages when coupled to operative sheaths. The telescope consists of three major parts:

1. the magnifying eyepiece;
2. the transmitting lens system;
3. the objective lens (Baggish *et al.*, 1989).

The most commonly used terminal objective

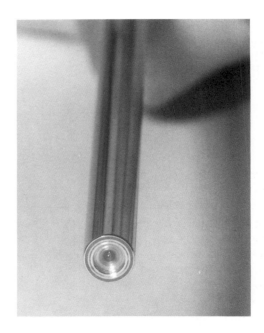

Figure 33.1 4 mm 0° telescope. The optics and fibreoptic light bundles are contained within the stainless steel skin.

lenses provide a straight on view (0°) or offset view (30°). Selection of the lens is a matter of personal preference, but for the best panoramic operative view the 0° lens is recommended, particularly when using laser fibres, flexible or semi-rigid operating accessories. Rigid lenses are fragile and must be handled with due care to avoid injury. Rough handling, steam autoclaving, improper liquid disinfection, inadequate cleaning will shorten the life of the telescope and require expensive repairs as well as system down-time. A properly cared for lens will last a lifetime and provide excellent service over and over again. I prefer to clean the telescope myself and to place it in its proper storage container after finishing each case. I am then assured that the instrument will function properly for the next procedure. Located just below the eyepiece is the fibreoptic coupling connection. At this location the fibreoptic cable joins the telescope. Each lens manufacturer has a unique coupling. Several companies supply attachments which permit a variety of cables to join their particular instrument. The latter is an advantage since any light generator and light cable can be used with a given telescope.

Fibreoptic Light Cable

Fibreoptic cables transmit intense cold light to the telescope and form a conduit which connects the high-intensity (heat-producing) generator to the telescope. The cable is filled with many

Figure 33.2 The lens consists of an objective lens, transmitting lens system and eyepiece.

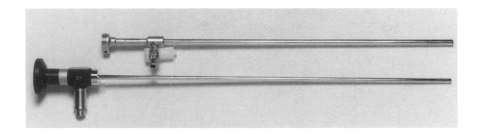

incoherent drawn-out glass fibres, capable of conducting light from the generator to the terminus of the cable. Obviously these cables are fragile and can be easily damaged if not handled gingerly. Inspection of the end of the cable will readily determine whether fibres or groups of fibres have been broken. These are indicated by dark spots in an otherwise intense light shower. Inspection of the periphery of the cable in a darkened room can also reveal fibre disruption. This appears as light transmission through the sides of the cable. Poor light at the end of the telescope is almost always due to a damaged cable. The only alternative to substandard light is to replace the cable. Cables should be disinfected by soaking in Cidex (glutaraldehyde) for 15–20 minutes, followed by thorough washing in sterile water. At the end of the case, the fibre should be washed again, resoaked and cleansed again with water. The cable should then be stored dry in a protective container.

Light Generator

Several varieties of light generators are offered in the equipment market place. These range from simple and inexpensive tungsten light generators (US $500–700) to costly xenon generators (US $2000–5000). For office use a simple apparatus will suffice; however, hysteroscopy performed in the operating room under video control demands intense light. Xenon (300 W) generators produce white light which is most favourable when coupled with endoscopic television cameras (Baggish, 1992). Characteristically the simpler tungsten light generators produce an orange tinted light which creates a rather poor colour on the video monitor. Between the two aforesaid types of generators are the 250 W metal halide generators. These produce intense light which is adequate for video images but characteristically give off a bluish tinge. Since the light bulbs in all these generators produce a lot of heat, a fan is built in to the cabinet to dissipate the heat and prolong bulb life. Should the fan become defective and not work properly, bulbs, which in fact cost $100 or more, will burn out prematurely. Light generators and fibreoptic cables may be used interchangeably for hysteroscopy or laparoscopy. Obviously the more powerful generators are required for laparoscopy. All generators should be appropriately grounded and should be periodically inspected (and indexed) by biomedical engineering for low frequency electrical leakage.

Hysteroscopic Sheaths

Two general categories of sheaths are utilized for hysteroscopic procedures: diagnostic and operating. A sheath is required for panoramic hysteroscopy in order to serve as a conduit through which to instil the distending medium into the uterine cavity. The diagnostic sheath fulfils this singular requirement and measures approximately 5 mm in outer diameter (when coupled to a 4 mm telescope). The sheath is essentially a hollow stainless steel tube equipped with a proximal port through which the distending medium is injected. The telescope must couple tightly to the sheath with a sufficient seal to prevent medium leakage at the telescope/sheath interface. The objective lens of the telescope should fit precisely flush with the end of the sheath to produce an unobstructed view. Therefore each given manufacturer's lens must

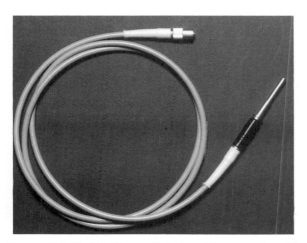

Figure 33.3 Flexible fibreoptic light cable transmits cold light from the generator to the lens.

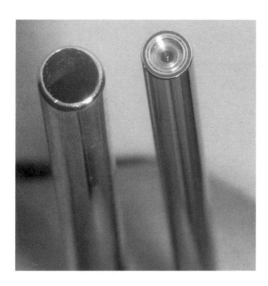

Figure 33.4 The 5 mm diagnostic sheath easily passes through the cervix and serves as a conduit for the distending medium.

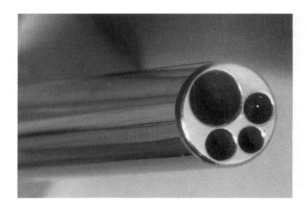

Figure 33.5 Isolated channel sheath. The large channel houses the telescope; the two operating channels support 2.5 French instruments. The lowest channel transmits the distending medium.

correspondingly be matched to the same manufacturer's sheath. Unfortunately each coupling mechanism differs amongst the variety of individual hysteroscopes, which prevents interchanging lenses and sheaths. A 5 mm sheath ordinarily will allow passage through nulliparous cervices without resorting to dilatation. They are therefore ideally suited to office hysteroscopy. Hysteroscopic sheaths are sturdy and stand up to routine handling. They may be steam autoclaved. Obviously they should be thoroughly flushed and cleansed after usage and stored away clean. The stopcock mechanism should be disassembled, cleaned, lubricated and reassembled after each usage. The stopcock should be turned to the opened position when stored. I prefer to clean the sheath with a long handled wire brush, flush with sterile water and blow air through the sheath to dryness. From time to time the sheath as well as the shaft of the telescope should be polished with a high quality metal cleansing compound.

Two types of operative sheaths are currently manufactured—single cavity and multi-channel operating sheaths. Both types of operating sheaths measure 7.5–8.5 mm in outer diameter and require some mechanical dilatation of the cervix to gain entry into the uterine cavity. Single channel sheaths share the cavity space between the telescope, operative accessory instruments, usually flexible or semi-rigid, and the distending medium. Two intake ports (opposite each other) are connected to the sheath and permit instillation of the medium from either side. These do not allow flushing of the uterine cavity. Recently some of these sheaths have been fitted with a

second sheath which allows return of the medium, i.e. continuous flushing of the cavity, but which increases the diameter of the sheath. Some of the single cavity sheaths are constructed with a terminal deflecting bridge which allows some angulation of operating instruments. The bridge is controlled by two small wheel-like levers attached to the proximal portion of the sheath. Operating tools, e.g. scissors, graspers, biopsy forceps, fibres and electrodes, gain entrance to the sheath's interior by an operating port, again located at the proximal portion of the sheath, either at the 12 or 6 o'clock position. Rubber caps or nipples must be fitted onto this entry port to prevent leakage of the medium when an operating tool is in place. The greatest disadvantages of the single cavity sheath are:

1. Inability to place instruments accurately into a given location within the uterine cavity, even when equipped with the rather cumbersome bridge device.
2. Inability to routinely flush the cavity unless equipped with an oversheath.
3. Limitation to the insertion of one operating tool.

The multi-channel operating sheath was invented specifically to overcome the deficiencies cited above. First the multi-channel sheath has four isolated channels (Baggish, 1988). The large 4.5 mm channel accommodates the optics and light bundles, i.e. the telescope. A separate channel serves for the instillation of the distending media. Two 2.5 mm operating channels may be used for a variety of purposes (Baggish, 1983). Two operating tools may be inserted simultaneously, e.g. grasping forceps may be placed

Figure 33.6 Panoramic view of multi-channel operating sheath, 8 mm o.d.

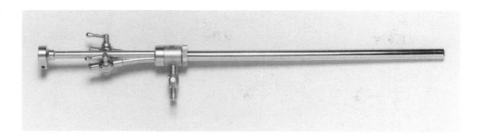

into position to grasp on to the end of a polyp, thereby putting traction on the tissue while through the other channel scissors or laser fibre may be inserted to cut the polyp off at the base. Alternatively an aspiration cannula may be inserted through one channel to keep the operating field clear of blood and debris, while the cutting instrument is simultaneously placed into the second channel. Obviously many different permutations of instrumentation may be selected. Of great advantage is the ability to flush the uterus continuously during the operation by attaching a suction to one operating channel and using the opposite channel to place the surgical device. Finally, the design of the multi-channel sheath allows instruments to be placed anywhere within the uterine cavity. In its normal position the instruments are easily able to reach the posterior wall of the uterus, while rotation of the sheath 180° brings the instruments to the anterior wall. Alternating right and left operating channels locates the instrument to either the left or right walls of the patient's uterus respectively. The author prefers the multi-channel sheath for all intrauterine operations because of its cited advantages. Additionally, separate sheaths are specifically designed to accept 0° or 30° telescopes. Finally, the medium intake port swivels to allow medium to be instilled equally easily from the operator's right or left side.

Brief mention should be made of infrequently used specialized sheaths. These sheaths have relatively large rigid operating devices incorporated into their construction, e.g. scissors located at the 12 o'clock position at the terminus of the sheath. They must be used in conjunction with a 30° telescope. The handle of the sheath is scissor-like and allows for the opening and closing of the terminal device. The disadvantages of these sheaths are:

1. All surgery must be done close-up and is therefore highly magnified.
2. The sheath is difficult to insert through the cervix.
3. The entire sheath must be removed when changing instruments.
4. Flushing the cavity is precluded.

Operating Accessories

Operating tools are a vital part of hysteroscopy. Without them therapeutic measures would be impossible by the transcervical approach. Most of the mechanical instruments measure 2 mm in diameter and 35 cm in length. They are either flexible or semi-rigid and by their very nature are somewhat delicate. The most common operative tool are the *scissors*, which are used to cut lesions such as adhesions, septae, polyps or myomata. The flexible scissors are less likely to be broken by torque whereas the semi-rigid instruments provide greater stability for direction as well as the actual sectioning of tissue. The semi-rigid instrument is susceptible to breakage at the point where the shaft joins the handle. Another useful conventional tool is the alligator *grasping forceps*. These are commonly used to hold onto and extract severed tissues. The *biopsy forceps* are really too small to obtain suitable samples of tissue. Recently Cook OB/GYN Instrument Company marketed a series of very useful and disposable hysteroscopic accessories. The Cook 2.3 mm *aspirating cannula* is probably the single most valuable tool the surgeon has in his catalogue of instruments. This simple aspirating device allows debris to be sucked out of the cavity, rendering a clear view of the field. This manoeuvre is essential for the performance of safe operative hysteroscopy. When combined with dual operating channel sheaths, aspiration may be continuously carried out in a fashion analogous to sponging or suctioning during a laparotomy. *Hysteroscopic needles* with varying sized tips may be used to manipulate intrauterine structures as well as to serve as a conduit for the injection of vasoconstrictive drugs. Recently Cook developed a hysteroscopic *myoma screw* which can be locked into a submucous myoma and permits easy manipulation of the mass, while it is being cut off. Various types of *electrical loops* and *needles* will soon appear on the market.

Nipples and Plugs for the Operating Channel

In the past the only gasket available to cover the operating channel, preventing leakage of medium

Figure 33.7 Two semi-rigid operating tools which gain entrance into the uterine cavity via the operating channel.

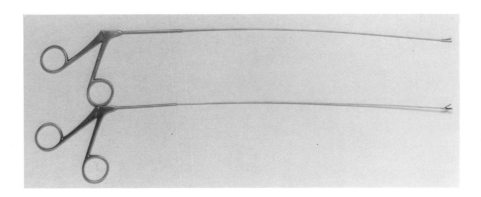

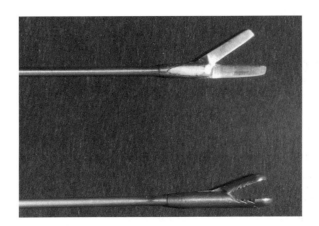

Figure 33.8 Close-up view of semi-rigid scissors and alligator grasping forceps.

does not leak as do the urological nipples. Operating instruments may be conveniently moved in and out, similar to the action of a trombone slide. This permits operations to be performed relatively close to or distant from the objective end of the telescope, i.e. either highly magnified or in the panoramic view.

Instruments for Medium Instillation

Several pieces of equipment are now available to facilitate the injection of distending media. These are discussed in detail in Chapter 36 by Ray Garry.

Hyskon Pump

Hyskon (32% dextran 70) is a highly viscid, crystal clear medium which does not mix with blood, is non-electrolytic and is well suited for both diagnostic and operative hysteroscopy. Although there is little difficulty injecting this material through operative sheaths, pressures of over 700 mmHg are required to drive it through the narrow clearance of a 5 mm diagnostic sheath. For this reason a pump assist is very useful. The

when operating tools were inserted was the simple urological rubber nipple. Not uncommonly these nipples become dislodged during the operation, causing the medium to leak out and the uterine cavity to collapse around the operating device. Cook OB/GYN offers a Luer-lock type plastic cap which locks onto the metal fitting of the operating channel (Baggish and Baltoyannis, 1988). This plug cannot become dislodged and

Figure 33.9 Cook OB/GYN hysteroscopic accessories (from above): hysteroscopic injection needles, aspirating cannula, medium injection tube, and leaf valve hysteroscopic plugs.

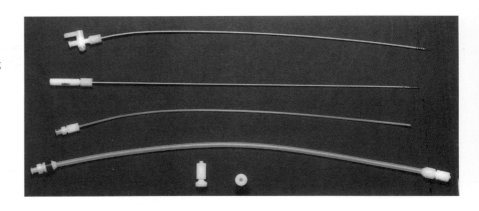

Figure 33.10 Close-up view of hysteroscopic injection needles 18 and 22 gauge.

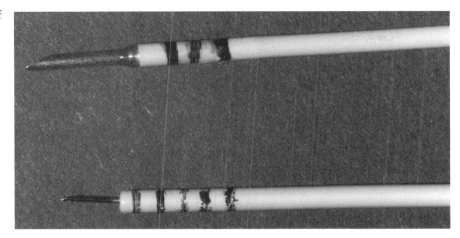

Figure 33.11 Dual channel hysteroscopic sheath. Each operating channel is 2.3 mm in diameter. The overall diameter of the sheath is 8 mm.

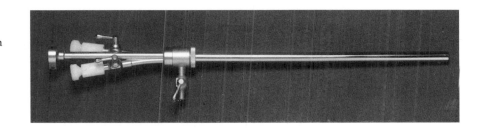

axiom of equating excellence with simplicity holds in this instance. Cook OB/GYN produces a simple hand-held screw device which permits a substantial mechanical advantage for injecting Hyskon via a 60 ml syringe and through a diagnostic sheath. This device is simple to use and very safe. In contrast Hyskon pumps driven by carbon dioxide gas have proved to be complicated, expensive and unsafe in actual practice.

Low Viscosity Liquid Pumps

With the use of continuous flow resectoscopes and multi-channel sheaths, pumps which deliver saline, lactated Ringer's solution and glycine at high flow rates facilitate surgery by constantly

exchanging these blood miscible solutions. Although a 3 litre plastic bag compressed with a blood pressure cuff can deliver the medium satisfactorily, the advent of variable pressure and flow pumps has offered greater sophistication and flexibility to such a system. Several machines are now available on the market. The outflow from the pump is attached to the inflow port of the hysteroscopic sheath, i.e. in infusion. A suction pump withdraws the flushed uterine fluid via the outflow port thereby completing a circuit and maintaining a clear operative field of view.

Video Equipment

Modern operative hysteroscopy is performed most advantageously utilizing a direct video camera

Figure 33.12 Hand-operated Hyskon pump.

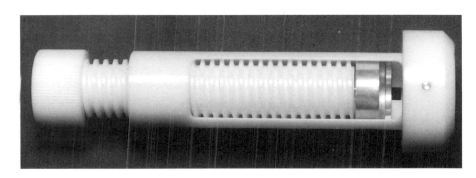

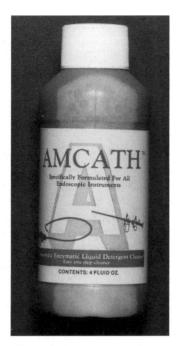

Figure 33.13 Proteolytic enzyme wash removes residual Hyskon from instruments.

hook-up to the eyepiece of the telescope. The advantages of this approach are multiple:

1. greater magnification for the surgeon;
2. elimination of optical risk for the surgeon when using a laser as the operative tool;
3. provision of visibility (operative field) for assistants and support personnel;
4. production of a permanent record of the operation.

The newer endoscopic video cameras offer high resolution as well as miniature composition. The better cameras provide the ability to change lens focal distance either by unscrewing and replacement or by zooming. This is an advantage because a lens with a 25 mm focal point will permit a wider viewing angle compared to a highly magnified 35 mm lens. Regardless of which video camera is selected, the prospective purchaser should be assured that the apparatus can be safely soaked in a cold sterilization liquid, e.g. Cidex. The video camera should be coupled to an appropriate high definition video monitor. These monitors range in size from 12 to 27 inches. Generally the smaller monitors produce an overall clearer picture (12–14 inch).

Office Hysteroscopy

Diagnostic hysteroscopy is ideally suited to the office environment. Entry into the uterus can be

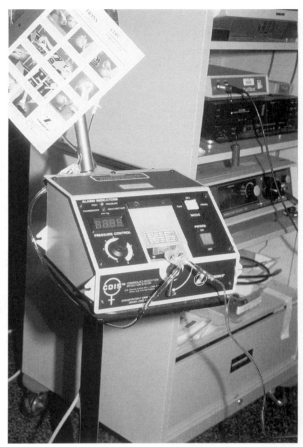

Figure 33.14 Electric low-viscosity-medium hysteroscopic pump. This type of pump maintains flow rate and enough pressure to keep the uterine cavity distended for operative hysteroscopy.

accomplished with minimal discomfort by means of the 5 mm (o.d.) instrument. Here the organization of instrumentation is of prime importance if one desires to launch a programme successfully. I recommend securing a three-tier stainless steel cart mounted on wheels. The top shelf of the cart is reserved for the telescope, sheath, connecting tubing, tenaculum, syringes and solutions. The middle shelf is dedicated for the hysteroscopic CO_2 insufflator. The bottom shelf houses the fibreoptic light generator as well as fibreoptic cables. The advantage of the above set-up is that everything is located in one place and is always ready and accessible for use.

Without doubt, the most appropriate medium for office hysteroscopy is carbon dioxide (CO_2). In order to carry out CO_2 hysteroscopy safely, a specially designed insufflator, i.e. one flowing at the rate of ml/min, must be used. Contemporary units read out data digitally. Obviously the most important information is flow rate and intrauterine pressure. The former should never exceed 100 ml/min and the latter should never exceed 150 mmHg. The advantages of CO_2 as a distending medium relate to its convenience, neatness and clarity. Although CO_2 is ideal for diagnostic hysteroscopy, it is inferior when compared to liquid media for operative hysteroscopy.

One word of warning will be given here; CO_2 instilled into the uterus by means other than the type of insufflator mentioned above can result in disastrous embolism and death for the patient. If the proper equipment is not at hand then hysteroscopy should not be carried out.

Special Instruments

Fibreoptic Laser

Lasers enjoy certain unique properties which make them useful for hysteroscopic surgery (Baggish, 1983, 1989; Baggish and Baltoyannis, 1988). The laser which is currently most suitable for intrauterine procedures is the neodymium: YAG (Nd:YAG) laser. Nd:YAG lasers range in power outputs from 20 to 100 W. Most equipment suitable for hysteroscopic operations will put out approximately 60–100 W of power. The Nd:YAG laser operates in the near infrared (invisible) part of the spectrum at approximately 1064 nm and is conveniently transmitted by fine fibres to the operative site. These bare fibres range in diameter between 600 and 1200 µm. In no circumstances whatsoever should a coaxial or gas cooled fibre be used for operative hysteroscopy. Recently silicone extruded or sculpted fibres have appeared in the market place. These fibres' terminal portions are available in several shapes, e.g. ball, conical, wedge, and tend to concentrate the Nd:YAG laser energy. Laser fibres may be used in the contact or non-contact position. Interestingly, penetration in the non-contact mode is deeper and less predictable than when the fibre touches the surface. Since the Nd:YAG laser acts by front scatter, the amount of coagulation injury to the tissue tends to be 4–5 times greater beneath the surface as compared to the visible surface wound since laser energy is not conducted through tissue as is electricity. The lesions produced are more predictable. Similarly the 1064 nm wavelength is practically ideal since it penetrates all liquid media safely and instantaneously.

Resectoscope

The resectoscope is the same instrument used by urologists for many years to do transurethral prostatectomy and bladder tumour resection. The instrument consists of a double sheath equipped with inflow port (inner sheath) and outflow port (outer sheath) (Baggish, 1989). The sheath is specifically designed to slide an insulated electrode out from the terminus of the inner sheath and then back into the same sheath. The telescope is situated in the same inner sheath cavity and looks out to the end of the electrode. Various designs of the electrode, e.g. cutting loop, roller ball, are available. The advantage to the resectoscope lies in the large surface area of the cutting and/or coagulating electrode. Additionally the utilization of the apparatus within the uterus requires less hand–eye coordination than does the manipulation of a laser fibre. The disadvantages of the instrument are: a diminished visual field because of the space occupied by the electrode in front of the lens; difficulty entering small or angulated spaces, e.g. the cornu; and necessity to use monopolar electrical current for the energy source. Most of the accidents and complications associated with the resectoscope relate to the latter, i.e. high-frequency electrical leakage injuries.

Documentation of Data

A major component of learning a new technique is to record what one sees and does. This process is particularly important with an eye to obtaining proficiency with hysteroscopy. The video recorder is an excellent device to reach this end. A simple ½ inch recorder is satisfactory if editing is not to be done, whereas ¾ inch recording is best suited if editing and future generations of tape are desired. Following a diagnostic or operative procedure, the tape should be reviewed to evaluate the appearance of normal and abnormal structures; to see how manipulations of the hysteroscope exposed pathology, and to determine the effectiveness of operative techniques. If a video recording system is not at hand, then documentation should be made in a diary for the operator's benefit. The colour and contour of the endometrium should be noted and later correlated with the pathology; the various portions of the uterine body should be clearly identified on entrance and exiting. The configuration of the cornu and tubal ostia should be recorded. The central pillar-like structure formed by the fused Müllerian ducts should be identified and variations noted; this frequently is confused with a septum (Baggish, 1990).

The recording should take place immediately after the operation in order to derive any benefit. Interestingly the compulsion to write down the hysteroscopic findings reinforces the visual experience and solidifies the learning process.

Finally, if equipment is to retain functionality with longevity, the gynaecologist must learn to take apart and service his/her own hysteroscopic instruments.

In summary, a successful hysteroscopic programme depends in order of importance on: a well trained endoscopist, extensive diagnostic experience, graded operative hysteroscopic experience, high quality instrumentation, organization and appropriate documentation. Success demands persistence and repetition. As with all other things, short cuts frequently lead to retracing of steps already taken.

References

Baggish MS (1983) New instruments and techniques for hysteroscopy. *Contemporary Obstetrics and Gynecology* **22**: 67.

Baggish MS (1988) A new laser hysteroscope for Nd-YAG endometrial ablation. *Lasers in Surgery and Medicine* **8**: 99.

Baggish MS (1989) Update on hysteroscopes. *Contemporary Obstetrics and Gynecology* **34**: 125.

Baggish MS (1990) Endoscopic laser surgery. In Baggish MS (ed) *Clinical Practice at Gynecology*, Vol 2, pp 187–205. New York: Elsevier.

Baggish MS (1992) Hysteroscopy. In Thompson D & Rock J (eds) *Telinde's Operative Gynecology*, 6th edn. Philadelphia: Lippincott (in press).

Baggish MS & Baltoyannis P (1988) New techniques for laser ablation of the endometrium in high risk patients. *American Journal of Obstetrics and Gynecology* **159**: 287.

Baggish MS, Barbot J & Valle RF (1989) *Diagnostic and Operative Hysteroscopy*, pp 58–65. Chicago: Year Book.

34

Diagnostic Hysteroscopy: Technique and Documentation

KEES WAMSTEKER* AND SJOERD DE BLOK‡

Hysteroscopy Training Centre, Haarlem, The Netherlands

*Department of Obstetrics and Gynaecology, Spaarne Hospital, Haarlem, The Netherlands
‡Onze Lieve Vrouwe Gasthuis, Amsterdam, The Netherlands

Introduction

For many decades the diagnosis of intrauterine disorders has been performed by dilatation and curettage (D & C) and hysterography. The relatively thick myometrial wall allows the 'blind', sharp scraping of the endometrium from its substratum, usually without permanent damage to the mucosa or the entire organ itself.

For the diagnosis or exclusion of endometrial cancer and hyperplasia D & C has appeared to be very effective. However, after the development of appropriate techniques for hysteroscopic visualization of the uterine cavity (Edström and Fernström, 1970; Lindemann, 1971), D & C appeared to be especially unreliable for the diagnosis of benign intrauterine tumours. Direct visual inspection of the uterine cavity revealed endometrial polyps, submucous fibroids and also synechiae, which D & C had completely failed to disclose.

In addition, hysteroscopic endosurgery has been developed to a level that enabled the endosurgical treatment of almost all these disorders with minimally invasive therapy, requiring no or very short hospitalization.

Hystero(salpingo)graphy (HSG) is mainly used in infertility patients for detection of intracavitary and tubal pathology. The technique used is of great importance for the reliability of the results. Comparison with hysteroscopic examination has demonstrated both false-positive and false-negative results of the HSG findings of the uterine cavity.

Hysterographic filling defects can only be suggestive of intrauterine disorders and warrant further diagnosis. Hysteroscopy has appeared to be the most reliable method to determine the nature of intracavitary HSG abnormalities and to define the necessity for treatment. HSG is useful as a screening method, but it should be kept in mind that it does not exclude intrauterine or (peri)tubal pathology.

Indications

Abnormal Uterine Bleeding

Abnormal uterine bleeding is the most common complaint of patients consulting the gynaecologist and provides the most frequent indication for hysterectomy. Especially in these cases dilatation and curettage (D & C) has been the diagnostic method of choice for many decades. However, for the diagnosis of non-malignant intrauterine pathology, such as endometrial polyps (Figure 34.1) and intrauterine fibroids (Figure 34.2), which may cause uterine bleeding disorders, D & C has appeared to be unreliable (Wamsteker, 1977, 1984a; Gimpelson and Rappold, 1988; Loffer, 1989; Motashaw and Dave, 1990).

Direct hysteroscopic inspection with adequate distension and visualization discloses almost

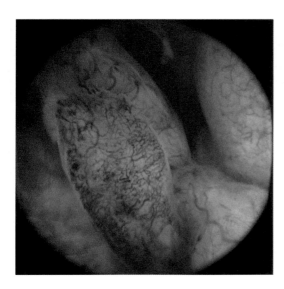

Figure 34.1 Endometrial polyp with atypical vessel structure.

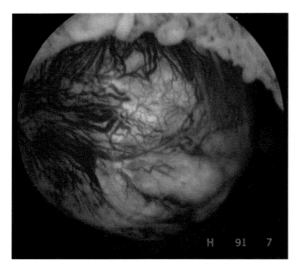

Figure 34.2 Submucous fibroid with typical stretched and dilatated capsular vessels.

every intrauterine abnormality with high accuracy. Additionally, it enables the exact localization of the pathology and the determination of its intracavitary extent. However, the diagnosis of endometritis and adenomyosis are not yet able to be made by hysteroscopic criteria.

For histological examination selective samples of any abnormal tissue can be obtained by visually controlled biopsies. A significant percentage of benign intrauterine pathology, disclosed with hysteroscopic diagnosis in patients with abnormal uterine bleeding, can be treated with minimally invasive transcervical hysteroscopic endosurgery.

As the majority of intrauterine disorders, resulting in abnormal uterine bleeding in the

reproductive phase of life, the climacteric and the post-menopausal period, are benign types of pathology, the D & C can no longer solely hold its position as the primary diagnostic method in patients with abnormal uterine bleeding. Today in almost all these cases, ambulatory or out-patient hysteroscopy with visually directed biopsies or directed curettage is to be recommended as the diagnostic method of choice.

With the recently developed continuous flow (CF) technique the surface structure of the endometrium can be observed with very low intrauterine pressure, which prevents compression of the soft tissue of the mucosa and also reduces the transtubal flow of the distension medium. Extensive studies have not indicated any negative effect of abdominal spill of the gas or liquid, used for distension of the uterine cavity in panoramic hysteroscopy, in cases of endometrial cancer (Wamsteker, 1977).

Johnson (1973) studied 764 patients with endometrial cancer stage I and II with a follow-up of between 5 and 14 years. In all patients the diagnosis was made by curettage and in 606 patients a hysterography had been performed before and sometimes also during the treatment. In 158 patients no hysterography had been performed. The percentage of tumour recurrences and/or distant metastases was 30% in the non-hysterography group and 24% in the hysterography group. There was no significant difference in the localization of the recurrences in both groups. In the hysterography group abdominal spill of the contrast medium occurred in 72% and intravasation in 29% of the cases. The relation of tubal spill and recurrences or metastases could be studied in 592 patients. Tubal spill of the contrast medium occurred in 77% and intravasation in 28% of the patients who did not develop recurrences or metastases. In the patients with recurrences or metastases tubal spill occurred in 60% and intravasation in 31%. From this study the abdominal spill of fluid, applied under pressure in the uterine cavity in endometrial carcinoma, does not seem to have a negative effect on the prognosis.

In addition, the intra-abdominal spread of intrauterine particles has also been demonstrated during D & C (Barents and van der Kolk, 1975), which apparently does not seem to increase the occurrence of recurrences or metastases in endometrial cancer. During curettage and even during bimanual palpation in patients with endometrial cancer tumour cells also have been demonstrated in the inferior vena cava and the vena cubiti (Roberts et al., 1960).

In any case, review of the literature does not

indicate that hysteroscopy with abdominal spill of the distension medium should be considered to be more hazardous in cases of endometrial cancer than D & C alone.

Although D & C will seldom fail to disclose endometrial cancer (Figure 34.3) and hyperplasia, hysteroscopic investigation additionally enables the early detection of small endometrial cancers and the determination of the localization, size and extent of the neoplasia and/or its precursors. Notwithstanding the above-mentioned considerations it seems to be sensible to recommend the reduction of transabdominal spill of the distension medium as much as possible in these cases. This could be realized by reduction of the intrauterine working pressure during the hysteroscopic examination in suspected cases.

Specific indications for hysteroscopic diagnosis in patients with abnormal uterine bleeding are:

- hypermenorrhoea,
- menorrhagia,
- metrorrhagia,
- intermenstrual bleeding,
- postmenopausal bleeding.

In cases of cervical dysplasia or malignancy accurate *in vivo* diagnosis on a cellular level can be performed with contact microcolpohysteroscopy (Hamou, 1981). However, experience with the determination of cytological pathology is a prerequisite for this technique.

Infertility

Hysteroscopic diagnosis and treatment has appeared to be very important in patients with

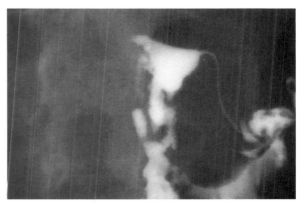

Figure 34.4 Hysterosalpingogram with intrauterine filling defects caused by intrauterine adhesions grade III (ESH classification).

infertility or recurrent pregnancy loss. The method should be considered complementary to hysterosalpingography (HSG) rather than competing with it in these patients.

Intrauterine filling defects identified by HSG (Figure 34.4) always require diagnostic hysteroscopy to confirm or exclude pathology and to determine the nature of an abnormality and the possibilities for transcervical endosurgical treatment. In case the filling defects are caused by intrauterine adhesions (Figure 34.5), for which treatment by hysteroscopy is the method of choice, any other 'blind' intrauterine procedure can even deteriorate the possibilities for hysteroscopic treatment by creating a false route or perforation and reducing the amount of residual normal endometrium which is required for adequate regeneration after synechiolysis.

The diagnosis of intrauterine adhesions (IUA)

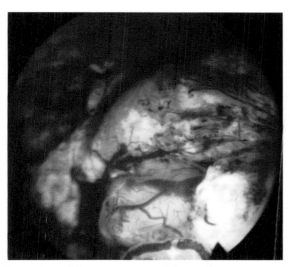

Figure 34.3 Adenocarcinoma of the endometrium with irregular surface with necrosis and dilatated, tortuous vessels.

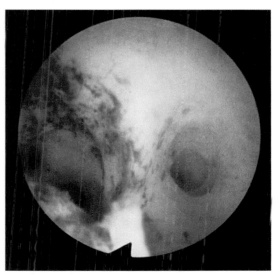

Figure 34.5 Intrauterine adhesions grade III (ESH classification).

can only be made with certainty by hysteroscopy (March, 1989), and the extent of the adhesions should be evaluated with hysteroscopy and HSG. To be able to compare the results of treatment and to determine the therapeutic regimen, the adhesions should be classified from the hysteroscopic and HSG findings according to the IUA classification of the European Society of Hysteroscopy (ESH) (Table 34.1) (Wamsteker, 1984b). In some cases the initial classification has to be changed during treatment.

Submucous fibroids can be a reason for infertility or pregnancy loss (Kistner, 1971; Wallach, 1979). They generally cause abnormal uterine bleeding, but may also be asymptomatic and may only present themselves as intracavitary filling defects during HSG in infertility patients. In these cases hysteroscopic diagnosis will disclose the nature and extent of the pathology and the possibilities for endosurgical treatment (Figure 34.6). To be able to determine the (endo)surgical technique to be chosen, the classification for submucous fibroids of the European Society of Hysteroscopy, according to their intramural extent (Table 34.2) can be used. This classification should

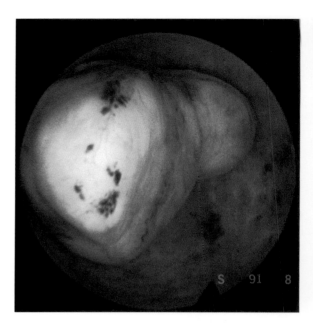

Figure 34.6 Submucous fibroid without intramural extension (type 0, ESH classification).

Table 34.2 ESH classification of submucous fibroids

Type	Degree of intramural extension
0	No intramural extension
I	Intramural extension $< 50\%$
II	Intramural extension $\geq 50\%$

Wamsteker K (1990), Hysteroscopy Training Centre, Spaarne Hospital, Haarlem, The Netherlands.

be part of the presurgical appraisal of these intrauterine tumours in infertility patients. Submucous fibroids without or with only limited intramural extension should be treated with endoresection as soon as the diagnosis has been made, as with increasing size of the fibroid(s) endoresection will become more difficult.

Other intrauterine disorders that may interfere with fertility and may cause bleeding abnormality are endometrial polyps, endometrial hyperplasia and endometritis. An abnormal uterine bleeding pattern in patients with infertility and ovulatory cycles always warrants diagnostic hysteroscopy. Hysteroscopy also offers the possibility to obtain visually directed biopsies for study of the endometrial structure and cyclic development.

It is questionable whether diagnostic hysteroscopy should be performed early in the work-up of every infertility patient. The results do not seem to justify this policy as intrauterine disorders are rather seldom the primary cause of the infertility (Wamsteker, 1977; Surrey and Aronberg, 1984). In case of concomitant bleeding abnormality

Table 34.1 ESH classification of intrauterine adhesions (IUA)

Grade	Extent of intrauterine adhesions
I	Thin or filmy adhesions Easily ruptured by hysteroscope sheath alone Cornual areas normal
II	Singular firm adhesions Connecting separate parts of the uterine cavity Visualization of both tubal ostia possible Cannot be ruptured by hysteroscope sheath alone
IIa	Occluding adhesions only in the region of the internal cervical os Upper uterine cavity normal
III	Multiple firm adhesions Connecting separate parts of the uterine cavity Unilateral obliteration of ostial areas of the tubes
IIIa	Extensive scarring of the uterine cavity wall With amenorrhoea or pronounced hypomenorrhoea
IIIb	Combination of III and IIIa
IV	Extensive firm adhesions with agglutination of uterine walls At least both tubal ostial areas occluded

Wamsteker K (1982/1989), Hysteroscopy Training Centre, Spaarne Hospital, Haarlem, The Netherlands.

or a history of a complicated intrauterine procedure, however, hysteroscopy is indicated.

Laparoscopy for infertility reasons should always be combined with hysteroscopy. This combination could also be performed instead of hysterosalpingography, providing for a complete investigation of the anatomy of the internal genital organs in specific cases.

In cases of recurrent pregnancy loss hysteroscopy is indicated to exclude or diagnose intrauterine causes, such as congenital uterine malformation, intrauterine adhesions or submucous fibroids, and to determine the possibilities for treatment with transcervical endosurgery.

Specific indications for diagnostic hysteroscopy in infertility patients are:

- abnormal uterine bleeding,
- history of complicated intrauterine procedures or uterine surgery,
- abnormalities of the uterine cavity or intrauterine filling defects with hysterosalpingography,
- together with laparoscopy, if no hysteroscopy has been performed before,
- infertility with unknown cause,
- unsuccessful IVF-ET, if no hysteroscopy has been performed before.

Other indications

SECONDARY DYSMENORRHOEA

As secondary dysmenorrhoea quite often appears to be caused by intrauterine disorders like submucous fibroids, endometrial polyps or intrauterine adhesions, hysteroscopic diagnosis should be performed in these cases primarily.

'MISSING' INTRAUTERINE CONTRACEPTIVE DEVICE (IUCD)

If the retrieval threads of an IUCD are not visible, its proper location can be determined by ultrasonography. In case ultrasonography indicates abnormal position or if the IUCD has to be removed, hysteroscopy is the method of choice to visualize its complete or partial intrauterine position and to remove the IUCD safely under direct visual control.

COMPLICATED INTRAUTERINE MANIPULATIONS RELATED TO PREGNANCY

As most cases of intrauterine synechiae have their origin in instrumental intrauterine manipulations related to pregnancy, it may be worthwhile to

perform diagnostic hysteroscopy 6 weeks or 2 months after such procedures. Grade I (Figure 34.7) or grade II intrauterine adhesions (ESH classification, Table 34.1) have appeared to be present rather frequently and should be treated as soon as possible to prevent fibrotic extension of the adhesions. Intrauterine adhesions appear to tend to extend and to become more firm in the course of time. Early diagnosis and treatment appears to enhance the fertility prognosis.

Puerperal curettages for persisting bleeding or partially retained placenta and repeat evacuation after incomplete abortion curettage are especially notorious for the development of intrauterine adhesions.

CONTROL OF INTRAUTERINE ENDOSURGERY

The results of intrauterine endosurgery should always be evaluated with a control hysteroscopy 2 or 3 months after the procedure to determine the healing of the endometrium, to exclude residual pathology and to remove adhesions, if present.

Instrumentation

The instruments needed for diagnostic hysteroscopy depend on the hysteroscopic technique to be used. These techniques can be divided into contact and panoramic hysteroscopy, which again

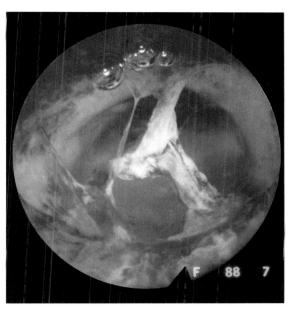

Figure 34.7 Fragile intrauterine adhesions grade I (ESH classification).

is to be subdivided into flexible and rigid hysteroscopy.

Contact Hysteroscopy

Contact hysteroscopy originally referred to hysteroscopy without uterine distension with a special contact hysteroscope (Barbot *et al.*, 1980; Baggish and Barbot, 1983). The intrauterine structures are examined in direct contact with the tissue. This technique has almost completely been abandoned in modern hysteroscopy.

Today contact hysteroscopy is mainly used with magnification for experimental studies of endometrial and endocervical vascular patterns and cellular structures, mostly in combination with panoramic hysteroscopy. The Storz contact microhysteroscope I with magnification up to 150 ×, can be used to that purpose both for panoramic and contact hysteroscopy and is especially useful for examination of the ecto- and endocervix in cases with cervical dysplasia (Hamou, 1981) and for endometrial dating studies.

Some hysteroscopes, primarily designed for panoramic hysteroscopy, are equipped with a telescope that can also be used with magnification in contact mode. As these techniques only have limited applicability in routine gynaecological practice, they will not be further discussed in detail in this chapter.

Panoramic Hysteroscopy

The most generally applied method for diagnostic hysteroscopy is panoramic hysteroscopy with distension of the uterine cavity. Panoramic diagnostic hysteroscopy can be performed with rigid or flexible hysteroscopes.

FLEXIBLE HYSTEROSCOPES

For diagnostic purposes a 3.6 mm flexible hysteroscope can be used, which is equipped with a 1.2 mm channel for CO_2 gas or irrigation fluid. The honeycomb structure of the image, caused by the fibreoptic image transmission, however, reduces the resolution and the sharpness of the image. For this reason visualization with the 3.6 mm flexible hysteroscopes can not compete with the performance of rigid hysteroscopes, but the instrument can be very useful in routine office procedures without any anaesthesia.

For much better imaging qualities and biopsies, a 5 mm flexible hysteroscope (Figure 34.8) can be used for diagnostic and minor intrauterine or Nd:YAG laser procedures.

The tip of flexible hysteroscopes can be bent and manipulated manually at the eyepiece portion. The direction of view is 0° with a viewing field of 120°. The tip can be bent up to 100° or 120° in either direction. These properties enable excellent visualization of the cornual areas and the tubal orifice. Flexible biopsy forceps can be used with the 2.2 mm working channel.

RIGID HYSTEROSCOPES

For diagnostic purposes different rigid hysteroscope systems are available. They are all equipped with a 30° foreoblique telescope for adequate visualization of the cornual areas and the uterine cavity in ante- or retroverted uterine position.

The diagnostic hysteroscopes can be divided into single flow (SF) and continuous flow (CF) hysteroscopes.

Single Flow (SF) Hysteroscopes

The outer sheath of single flow hysteroscopes leaves a channel for CO_2 gas or fluid irrigation. There is no separate channel for outflow of the distension medium.

The outer diameter of the hysteroscope depends on the telescope diameter:

- 3 mm 30° foreoblique telescope and 4 mm outer sheath,
- 4 mm 30° foreoblique telescope and 5 mm outer sheath.

The standard hysteroscope for panoramic diagnostic hysteroscopy with excellent visualization properties both in direct viewing and videoendoscopy is the 5 mm hysteroscope (Figure 34.9).

In some cases these hysteroscopes are supplied with a separate single flow 6 or 7 mm operating sheath for biopsies or minor intrauterine procedures. However, the performance of continuous

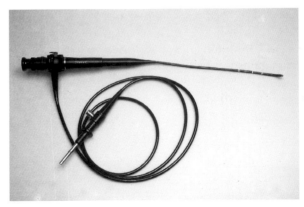

Figure 34.8 Five mm flexible fibreoptic hysteroscope.

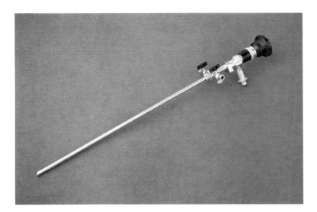

Figure 34.9 Single flow diagnostic hysteroscope with a 4 mm 30° foreoblique telescope and a 5 mm outer sheath.

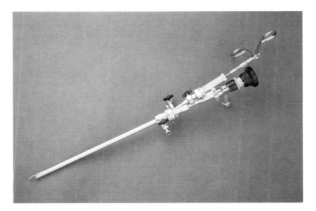

Figure 34.10 Continuous-flow Olympus hysteroscope with a 4 mm 30° foreoblique telescope, a 7 mm outer sheath and a 5 Fr biopsy forceps; the in- and outflow channels are completely separated.

flow operating hysteroscopes is so much better than that of single flow operating hysteroscopes, that the latter should be considered obsolete.

Continuous Flow (CF) Hysteroscopes
The new generation of continuous flow hysteroscopes from Olympus are equipped with completely separated in- and outflow channels for the distending medium and a round outer sheath for optimal fitting in the internal cervical os. They can be used with gaseous or liquid distension media, but are especially suitable for the use of low viscosity fluids, which can not be applied with single flow hysteroscopes. Clear irrigating fluid can continuously flush the viewing tip of the telescope and the field of vision, as cloudy fluid is evacuated through the separate outflow channel. The 4 mm 30° foreoblique telescope is equal to the one used with the single flow 5 mm hysteroscopes.

For diagnostic purposes the telescope is equipped with an inner sheath and a 7 mm outer sheath, which also provides for a working channel for a biopsy forceps, high-frequency electroprobes and 400 or 600 μm Quartz laser fibres (Figure 34.10).

The continuous flow hysteroscope can be used in diagnostic procedures:

- in cases with blood and/or mucus in the uterine cavity,
- in cases with impaired visualization due to cervical leakage with the single flow diagnostic hysteroscopes,
- for visually controlled biopsies,
- in general anaesthesia.

Techniques

The techniques for diagnostic hysteroscopy differ for the different distension media: CO_2 gas, high-viscosity fluids (HVF) and low-viscosity fluids (LVF).

Some general rules, however, hold for all techniques:

1. The hysteroscope should always be introduced into the uterine cavity under direct visual control.
2. The hysteroscope should never be advanced towards the fundal area without adequate visualization or uterine distension, as this can cause bleeding, endometrial damage, false passage formation and eventually perforation.
3. To benefit from the advantages of the 30° telescope the hysteroscope should be rotated in combination with horizontal and vertical movements.

Distension media and the hazards associated with either use are discussed in Chapter 36 by Ray Garry and Chapter 45 by Bruno van Herendael.

Distension Media

CO_2 gas and Hyskon™ are the most frequently applied distension media in diagnostic hysteroscopy with single flow hysteroscopes. CO_2 gas has to be administered by means of a special insufflator, designed according to the safety precautions for use in hysteroscopy (Figure 34.11). The complete system must be gas-tight as gas leakage will result in frustrating procedures. The highly viscous Hyskon™, a 32% dextran 70 in dextrose 5% solution, is very effective for

Figure 34.11 CO_2 insufflator for hysteroscopy; the flow rate can be set with a maximum of 100 ml/min; the intrauterine pressure is limited to 200 mmHg.

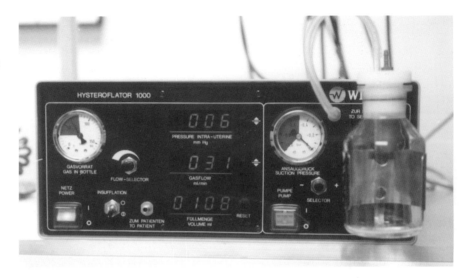

diagnostic procedures because of its rinsing effect, but should be 10% diluted with saline or dextrose 5% for use in 4 or 5 mm diagnostic hysteroscopes to enhance its flow through the hysteroscope.

Low viscosity fluids like sorbitol 4%, glycine 1.5% and dextrose 5% should only be used with a continuous flow hysteroscope and a pressurized delivery system in specific circumstances and for biopsies and minor intrauterine procedures.

Method

Diagnostic hysteroscopy can easily be performed on an ambulant basis with local anaesthesia. In uncomplicated pure diagnostic procedures with the 4 or 5 mm hysteroscope quite often no anaesthesia is required at all. We prefer the application of an intra- and paracervical block with a 1% local anaesthetic in all cases. The anaesthetic is injected at 10 and 2 hours intracervical and at 5 and 7 hours paracervical. Our choice for the anaesthetic is prilocaine. Great care should be taken to prevent intravascular injection of the local anaesthetic in all cases.

Useful premedication in ambulant or outpatient procedures without or with local anaesthesia has appeared to be a prostaglandin-synthetase inhibitor orally 2 hours before the procedure to prevent uterine contractions during dilatation of the uterine cavity and 0.5 mg atropine i.m. 15 min before the procedure to prevent vagal reactions. If necessary the internal cervical os should be dilatated with half-size Hegar dilators.

Patients should preferably be scheduled in the proliferative phase of the menstrual cycle. In case of actual uterine bleeding a continuous flow hysteroscope with liquid distension medium should be used.

Minor Intrauterine Procedures

In a significant number of cases minor intrauterine diagnostic or therapeutic interventions can be performed during a diagnostic procedure. These can be: biopsies, polypectomy, synechiolysis or focal coagulation. To this purpose a diagnostic set of instruments should include an operating hysteroscope with working channel and operating instruments. Preferably this should be a continuous flow hysteroscope (Figure 34.12). Because of

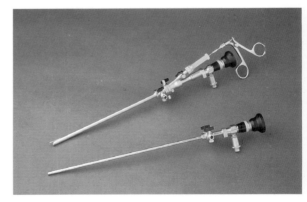

Figure 34.12 Hysteroscope set for diagnostic hysteroscopy: a 5 mm single flow hysteroscope and a 7 mm continuous-flow hysteroscope with 5 Fr biopsy forceps.

the excellent performance of these instruments with low-viscosity fluid distension in difficult diagnostic procedures and minor endosurgical interventions, low-viscosity fluids with delivery system should be available in an out-patient diagnostic hysteroscopy unit.

Documentation

The most frequently used method for documentation of endoscopic findings are written reports with or without drawings. Advantages of these methods are that the report can be made immediately after the procedure and stored in the patient's record.

However, the description of all endoscopic findings can be very difficult and may not always be clear or understandable for others. On the other hand, the preparation of good quality drawings is very time-consuming and highly dependent on the artistry of the surgeon.

Hysteroscopic findings should be described schematically, mentioning both negative and positive findings at the different levels of the uterine cavity: endocervical canal, internal cervical os, isthmus, fundal and both cornual areas and tubal ostia. Tubal flow of the distension medium should be evaluated and reported. The aspect of the endocervical mucosa and the endometrium should be described. A preprinted diagram of the uterus with transections at different levels can be very useful for immediate documentation in patient records.

It is beyond doubt that pictures of good quality say much more than written reports or poor drawings, and modern technology and instrumentation has tremendously simplified the means of obtaining image records in endoscopy at constant high quality. Good visual image documentation with photography or video recording is of utmost importance for teaching and education, and for evaluation of the results of treatment and comparison of different techniques.

Storage and retrieval of hard copy material always has been one of the main drawbacks in these methods of documentation. Optical disc recorders coupled with computer systems solve these problems with very high storage capacity and instantaneous computerized retrieval possibilities. However, this equipment is still rather expensive.

In hysteroscopic photography and video documentation the complete imaging and documentation system can be considered to be an 'imaging chain', from light source up to film or videotape (Figure 34.13) (Wamsteker, 1989). The end result relies upon the quality of each individual component of the chain. Each connection in the chain reduces the quality, non-fitting connections being extremely detrimental to the process.

In photography five technical parts with five different connections (optical, magnetic and/or electronic) have to be in good order to complete the chain through the uterus to documentation. Video recording requires six or seven technical parts with seven or eight connections. Because of the relative complexity of these systems the separate parts need to be compatible to reach the optimal end result. As industrial equipment often does not fit well with components from other brands, the matching of different brands should be investigated thoroughly before buying equipment.

The light source is of great importance for the quality of the image. As hysteroscopy today preferably is being performed as video endoscopy, with the video camera coupled directly to the eyepiece of the hysteroscope, a high-capacity light source is a must in the hysteroscopic equipment. The capacity should be ≥ 300 W. Most of these light sources are also suitable for photography

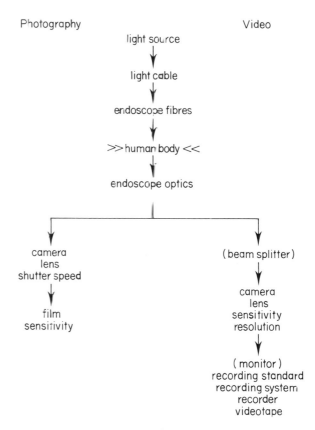

Figure 34.13 The 'imaging chain' in photography and video documentation in endoscopy.

and video recording. The light intensity and/or film speed and exposure time in photography is generally automatically regulated by the light source. If not, an automatic camera is required, in which case the light intensity from the light source must be high enough to prevent long exposure times, causing blurred pictures.

The quality of the light conducting cables is very important and should be the first thing checked in bad documentation results. Fibreoptic and fluid light cables are available. Fluid cables are less flexible than the fibre ones, but have a somewhat increased light transmission. In case of fluid leakage they are worthless. Fibreglass cables should be checked regularly for ruptured fibres, as this significantly reduces the light transmission. Olympus light guide cables have condenser lenses built into the fibre cable in order to improve the focus of the light at the light source–light cable and the light cable–hysteroscope connections, which produces a higher light intensity.

With the new Olympus CLV-S light source (Figure 34.14), which has a special 'high-intensity' mode, special light guide cables have to be used with a filter. Normal light cables would burn immediately in the high-intensity mode. The performance of this light source in hysteroscopic imaging and documentation is excellent and fully automatic.

The condition of the telescope is another important factor in the 'imaging chain'. Damage in the light conducting fibres or the optical lens system of the telescope will result in bad imaging and documentation quality. This can be brought about by lens fractures after dropping, fluid in

the telescope due to leakage or steam sterilization of non-autoclavable telescopes.

A factor that is not directly equipment-related is the intrauterine environment. In whitish atrophic endometrium both the imaging and documentation will always be excellent, due to the bright picture. In a uterine cavity with blood, the dark blood will absorb much of the light and this will significantly reduce the quality of photographic pictures and video recordings. In these cases flushing of the uterine cavity or the use of continuous flow hysteroscopes is to be preferred for documentation.

The final sections of the 'imaging chain' will be discussed separately for photography and videorecording.

Photography

For hysteroscopic photography a 35 mm single-lens mirror reflex camera with TTL, 'through-the-lens' exposure metering is preferred (Figure 34.15). This camera can only be used for endoscopic photography and is unsuitable for general use because the usual ground-glass focusing screen has been replaced by a clear glass screen. Standardized adapters between camera and hysteroscope are available. For external flash generators only a non-automatic camera body can be used. Some automatic flash generators require an automatic camera body (light measurement in the camera body), while others will cope with a non-automatic body (light measurement in the lens) (Figure 34.16). Accessory equipment for cameras includes: motor drive winder for film advance

Figure 34.14 High-power light source for video imaging and photography in hysteroscopy; special light guide cables must be used in the high-intensity mode.

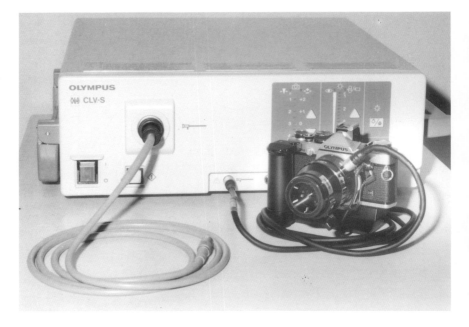

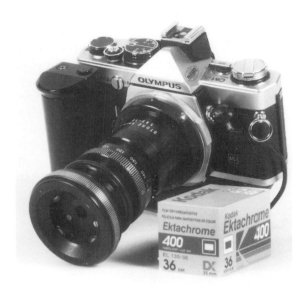

Figure 34.15 Automatic mirror reflex camera body with motor drive winder for film advance, record data-back and zoom lens.

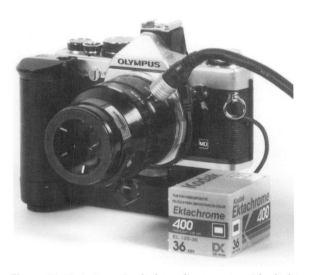

Figure 34.16 Automatic light adjustment with light measurement in the camera lens; a non-automatic camera body can be used.

and record data-back for superimposition of different items of information.

The quality of the lens of the camera is a very important feature in hysteroscopic photography. The aperture of the lens is calibrated in F-stops. The lower the F-number, the larger the lens opening (more light), but the less the depth of field. The focal length of the lens (f in mm) determines how much of the frame of the 35 mm film is exposed (Marlow, 1989). Some manufacturers provide zoom lenses with a focal length of 70–140 mm.

The film to be used should be a colour-slide

film balanced for electronic flash, the so-called 'daylight' film, emphasizing the blue-light spectrum with temperatures between 5000 and 6100 K. The best results are obtained with professional films. However, these films must be stored at ≤ 13°C and be removed from the refrigerator 1 hour before use. For good results processing should be performed as soon as possible after use (Marlow, 1983).

Film sensitivity is designated by the ASA (American Standards Association), DIN (German equivalent) or ISO (comparable to ASA) number. For hysteroscopic photography ASA 400 provides the best results. Films with increased sensitivity may be used in situations with low light intensity, but will reduce the definition of the image.

It is very important to take many pictures, but to only choose the best few for filing.

Video Documentation

With the introduction of miniature electronic chip cameras the possibilities for video imaging and recording in endoscopy have increased enormously. Both in hysteroscopy and laparoscopy direct viewing through the endoscope has largely been replaced by video endoscopy, in which the surgeon works from the video screen. Facilitated by this development video recording in specific cases will increasingly become a routine procedure.

VIDEO STANDARDS

Many different norm-standards exist all over the world (Wamsteker, 1989). The most important of these are:

1. The PAL standard (phase alternating line) used in Western Europe (except for France), most countries in the Far East, most African countries, Australia and New Zealand).
2. The NTSC standard (National Television Standard Committee), also referred to as 'never the same colour' because of its colour instability, used in Northern America, Japan, some South American and Asian countries.
3. The SECAM standard (Séquentiel Couleur a Mémoire), used mainly in France and Eastern Europe and also in some African and some Asian countries.

Most professional equipment in Europe can be used for either PAL or SECAM and recently videoplayers and monitors are available that are also suitable for NTSC. For translation of videotapes from PAL to NTSC, or vice versa, special norm-translation equipment is always necessary. The most important differences between PAL and NTSC are different colour coding and different number of image lines (PAL/SECAM 625 lines; NTSC 525 lines). PAL is more expensive, but has a higher stability and a true colour reproduction, while NTSC has colour instability due to atmospheric interferences and other disturbances. Using videotape recordings in different countries requires knowledge of the used video standard and, if applicable, norm-translation into the appropriate standard.

VIDEO SYSTEMS

Not only different, incompatible video standards complicate international video communication and exchange. The various recording systems and tape formats are also incompatible (Gisolf, 1987). Professional quality required 2 or 1 inch tape width for a long time, but more recently also 0.75 inch U-matic 'SP high-band' recording (also called BVU) with U-matic SP tapes is accepted as professional (or broadcast) system. U-matic SP recordings are not compatible with U-matic low-band recorders (no colour reproduction). The most recent Sony recorders, however, can accept both U-matic SP and low-band tapes (Sony VO-9600P recorder (Figure 34.17) and Sony VP-9000P player). Recording with 0.75 U-matic low-band is considered semi-professional.

Another professional system is the Betacam or Betacam SP system, which takes a 0.5 inch Betamax casette tape in special recording mode. A comparable professional 0.5 inch VHS counterpart is the M2 format. In 0.5 inch VHS also a (semi)professional system is available, the Super-VHS (S-VHS) recorders and tapes with a higher horizontal resolution of 400 lines (standard VHS approximately 250 lines).

For video recording in hysteroscopy of professional quality and at reasonable costs 0.75 inch U-matic SP high-band is to be preferred. At least 0.75 inch U-matic low-band should be used for recordings to be edited. For routine use standard 0.5 inch VHS or S-VHS is acceptable. If editing is required anyway, the VHS tape should be upgraded to 0.75 inch U-matic SP high-band, Betacam SP or even 1 inch and edited at this format. After editing the mastertape can be translated to VHS again. Editing in the normal VHS format will give too much loss of quality. At this moment not enough experience is available with the 8 mm format (V8) to comment on its use in hysteroscopic documentation and editing capabilities.

VIDEO CAMERA

An important breakthrough in the use of video in endoscopy has been the development of the so-called CCD (Charge-Coupled Device) or 'chip' camera (Figure 34.18). It is referred to as a 'chip' because of its basic form as a small silicon wafer. The CCD is an integrated circuit image sensor and depends on the sensitivity of silicon to light. Light striking a silicon device decreases the electrical resistance of the silicon and generates current carriers. The photosensitive silicon elements store and transfer information as packets of electrical charge, which can be amplified. Individual picture elements are called 'pixels' and the number of pixels determines the sensitivity and resolution (Sivak, 1986). The way the electrical charges are moved on the device is called 'charge-coupling'.

Figure 34.17 Sony VO-9600P U-matic recorder; can be used for SP high-band and low-band recordings.

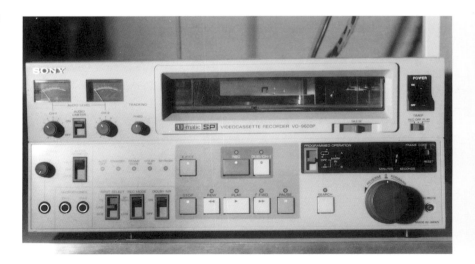

Figure 34.18 CCD video camera for endoscopy.

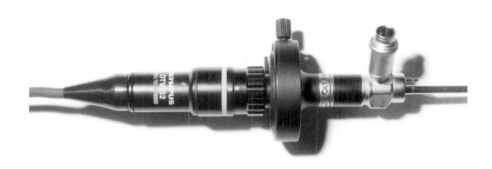

CCD video cameras are very small and light in weight, have a high sensitivity and relatively high resolution and can be immersed in disinfecting solutions. The cameras are connected with a cable to a camera control unit (CCU), which regulates light adjustment (via light source) (auto or manual), colour adjustment and (auto) white balance.

Most modern cameras have auto gain control, which can compensate for the reflections of very bright sites of the image. Most modern video light sources do have an automatic brightness control function in combination with the camera. The camera can be mounted directly on the ocular end of the hysteroscope (video endoscopy) or with a beam splitter, that also enables direct viewing through the hysteroscope.

Video endoscopy refers to a *method*, while the name video endoscope refers to an *instrument*. Electronic video endoscopes, with a CCD chip at the distal end of a flexible hysteroscope and mainly used in gastroenterology, are not available for hysteroscopy and will most probably never be competitive with the optical rigid telescopes, due to the required limitation of the diameter.

MONITOR

High quality professional RGB monitors should be used. They must be equipped with the same norm-standard as used in the video imaging system. Most modern professional monitors are multi-norm and can be used with PAL, NTSC and SECAM standards.

Some companies recommend their own special monitors, which does not seem to provide specific advantages.

RECORDER

As stated before, a good quality recording system for hysteroscopy is the 0.75 inch U-matic low-band system. For very high quality, professional recordings 0.75 inch U-matic SP high-band (BVU) should be used. The most widely used U-matic video recorders are the Sony VO-5600 (0.75 inch U-matic low-band) and the Sony VO-5600P (0.75 inch U-matic SP high- and low-band, see Figure 34.17). For routine use any good quality VHS recorder can be applied. Of course the norm-standard again has to match the one used in the video imaging system.

VIDEO PRINTING

High quality video printers, like the Sony UP-5000P with about 10–12 dots/mm, provide an excellent alternative to hard-copy photography. Printouts can be used for patient records and are of much better quality than the hard copies of presently available instant photography cameras.

HIGH-FREQUENCY INTERFERENCE

Several hysteroscopic surgical techniques are performed with high-frequency current. The frequency of the current has to exceed a lower frequency limit to avoid muscle and nerve stimulation and is usually in the range of 300 kHz to 2 MHz. As these frequencies are situated within the bandwidth of every video imaging system, this can cause electromagnetic interference to a video imaging system in use during electrosurgery (Flachenecker, 1987). The video system has, therefore, to be electromagnetically shielded, or the high-frequency power of the electrosurgical unit must be reduced. Both techniques are applied in the more recently developed equipment.

Summary

Technological developments and new techniques have made hysteroscopy with visually directed biopsies the method of choice for diagnosis of intrauterine disorders in patients with abnormal uterine bleeding and infertility. The method can easily be performed on ambulant or out-patient basis and can almost completely replace diagnostic D &C in these cases.

The performance of continuous flow hysteroscopes with low-viscosity fluid distension has appeared to be a major breakthrough in diagnostic hysteroscopy as it enables excellent intrauterine visualization in cases where the former single flow instruments failed. With this technique minor intrauterine endosurgical interventions have also become easy, routine procedures.

Diagnostic hysteroscopy further opens the way to minimally invasive and preserving transcervical endosurgery. Modern hysteroscopy is to be performed as video endoscopy with a CCD video camera directly coupled to the ocular of the hysteroscope. High quality documentation with photography or video recording has come into the sphere of routine hysteroscopic practice.

References

Baggish MS & Barbot J (1983) Contact hysteroscopy. *Clinical Obstetrics and Gynecology* **26**: 219–241.

Barbot J, Parent B & Dubuisson JB (1980) Contact hysteroscopy: another method of endoscopic examination of the uterine cavity. *American Journal of Obstetrics and Gynecology* **136**: 721–726.

Barents JW & van der Kolk G (1975) Iatrogene migratie van cellen en weefselelementen bij curettage. *Nederlands Tijdschrift voor Geneeskunde* **119**: 229–232.

Edström K & Fernström I (1970) The diagnostic possibilities of a modified hysteroscopic technique. *Acta Obstetrica Gynecologica Scandinavica* **49**: 327–330.

Flachenecker G (1987) High frequency interference: basic electrotechnical principles. In Wamsteker K, Jonas U, van der Veen G & van Waes PFGM (eds) *Imaging and Visual Documentation in Medicine*, pp 85–94. Amsterdam: Excerpta Medica.

Gimpelson RJ & Rappold HO (1988) A comparative study between panoramic hysteroscopy with directed biopsies and dilatation and curettage. *American Journal of Obstetrics and Gynecology* **158**: 489–492.

Gisolf AC (1987) Video systems: fighting the chaos. In Wamsteker K, Jonas U, van der Veen G & van Waes PFGM (eds) *Imaging and Visual Documentation in Medicine*, pp 85–94. Amsterdam: Excerpta Medica.

Hamou J (1981) Microhysteroscopy: a new procedure and its original applications in gynecology. *Journal of Reproductive Medicine* **26**: 375.

Johnson JE (1973) Hysterography and diagnostic curettage in carcinoma of the uterine body. *Acta Radiologica Supplement* **326**: 1–79.

Kistner RW (1971) *Gynecology: Principles and Practice.* 764 pp. Chicago: Year Book Medical Publishers.

Lindemann HJ (1971) Eine neue Untersuchungsmethode für die Hysteroskopie. *Endoscopy* **4**: 194–199.

Loffer FD (1989) Hysteroscopy with endometrial sampling compared with D & C for abnormal uterine bleeding. *Obstetrics and Gynecology* **73**: 16–20.

March CM (1989) Hysteroscopy for infertility. In Baggish MS, Barbot J & Valle RF (eds) *Diagnostic and Operative Hysteroscopy*, pp 136–146. Chicago: Year Book Medical Publishers.

Marlow JL (1983) Endoscopic photography. *Clinical Obstetrics and Gynecology* **26**: 359–365.

Marlow JL (1989) Hysteroscopic photography. In Baggish MS, Barbot J & Valle RF (eds) *Diagnostic and Operative Hysteroscopy*, pp 215–222. Chicago: Year Book Medical Publishers.

Motashaw ND & Dave S (1990) Diagnostic and therapeutic hysteroscopy in the management of abnormal uterine bleeding. *Journal of Reproductive Medicine* **35**: 616–620.

Roberts S, Long L, Jonasson O *et al.* (1960) The isolation of cancer cells from the bloodstream during uterine curettage. *Surgery, Gynecology and Obstetrics* **111**: 3–11.

Sivak MV (1986) Video endoscopy. *Clinics in Gastroenterology* **15**: 205–234.

Surrey MW & Aronberg S (1984) Hysteroscopic diagnosis of abnormal uterine bleeding: a clinical study. In Siegler AM & Lindemann HJ (eds) *Hysteroscopy, Principles and Practice*, pp 121–122. Philadelphia: JB Lippincott.

Wallach EE (1979) Evaluation and management of uterine causes of infertility. *Clinical Obstetrics and Gynecology* **22**: 43–60.

Wamsteker K (1977) Hysteroscopie. PhD thesis. University of Leiden.

Wamsteker K (1984a) Hysteroscopy in the management of abnormal uterine bleeding in 199 patients. In Siegler AM & Lindemann HJ (eds) *Hysteroscopy, Principles and Practice*, pp 128–131. Philadelphia: JB Lippincott.

Wamsteker K (1984b) Hysteroscopy in Asherman's syndrome. In Siegler AM & Lindemann HJ (eds) *Hysteroscopy, Principles and Practice*, pp 198–203. Philadelphia: JB Lippincott.

Wamsteker K (1989) Documentation in laparoscopic surgery. In Sutton CJG (ed) *Baillière's Clinical Obstetrics and Gynaecology* **3**: 625–647. London: Baillière Tindall.

35

Rigid and Flexible Optical Systems for Hysteroscopy

E. CORNIER

Clinique du Trocadero 75116, Paris

Since 1805 an increasing number of conditions have been treated due to the ability to observe the uterine cavity. At the beginning of the nineteenth century, it was a rigid tube (Bozzini), a mirror, and candle light. In 1879 Nitze closed the tube with lenses and placed the light at the proximal end of the endoscope (Nitze, 1879).

The greatest advance was the invention of electricity in 1907 and later Charles David placed a lamp at the distal end (David, 1908).

The next problem to be solved was distension of the uterus. During the early part of the twentieth century Schröder found that an intrauterine pressure of 25–35 mmHg was enough to distend the uterine cavity. This was achieved by a water column of 65–95 cm above the uterus (Schröder, 1934).

The use of the quartz fibre improved the optical systems, and the fibreglass systems have allowed the so-called cold light supply since 1965. The Hopkins system, replacing the glass lenses by air between two quartz rods, gives a better transmission of light and reduces the size of the endoscope to allow a wider angle of view to the front of the lens.

Nevertheless, at the end of the 1970s some problems remained. The diameter of the instrument was too large and needed cervical distension and a portio adapter. The observation of the cervical canal was then not feasible.

The first aim of hysteroscopy was a better diagnostic approach to be performed under local or general anaesthesia in operating theatres. Because of its rigidity and the presence of the portio adapter, the instrument did not always allow the observation of the edges and corners of the uterus.

In the 1970s, although Neuwirth was beginning the removal of leiomyomas with a 9 mm rigid resectoscope (Neuwirth, 1983), and Mohri had begun with transuterine tuboscopy, the average gynaecologist did not have easy access to operating instruments. When pathological disease had been observed a so-called 'directed curettage' was recommended.

The first steerable hysteroscope was then designed by Brueschke and Wilbanks (1974), with a rigid light guide and a flexible distal steerable end. It was supposed to facilitate tubal catheterization and controlled biopsy. Unfortunately this delicate instrument had a 9 mm diameter and remained experimental.

At the beginning of the 1980s, Hamou developed an excellent small 4 mm optical system, fitted into a 5 mm sheath mainly for observation and diagnostic purposes (Hamou and Taylor, 1979). At the same time we tried the gastroenterologist's flexible endoscope (duodenocholedochoscope—5 mm) for the purpose of developing an operating instrument. As it had a 2.2 mm inner channel, this instrument could carry flexible forceps for biopsy, flexible loops in order to remove polyps as well as catheters for fallopian tubes.

As there has been much progress in optical fibres, the flexible systems may become more popular now and they will continue to develop and give new possibilities to hysteroscopy.

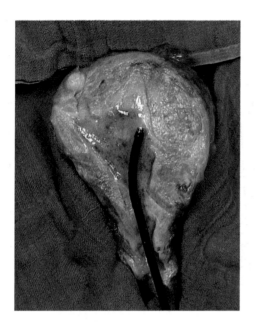

Figure 35.1 A 4.9 mm hysteroscope in the uterus.

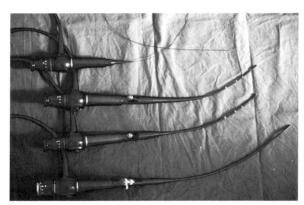

Figure 35.2 From top, down: choledochoduodenoscope used as a 5 mm hysteroscope, 1980; the flexible hysteroscope, 4.9 mm, field of view 120°, observation depth 2–50 mm, bending section 120° up and down, instrument channel 2.2 mm, two-point discrimination 10 μm; the flexible diagnostic hysteroscope, 3.6 mm diameter, field of view 90°, observation depth 1–50 mm, bending section 100° up and down, inner channel 1.2 mm; the tuboscope, outer diamter 0.5 mm, field of view 55°, observation depth 2–30 mm, no bending section, no inner channel (placed in a 1 mm irrigation catheter).

The Principles of the Flexible Endoscopes

The flexible endoscope has three main parts. A compact one hand control unit fits the inside of the left hand, leaving the right one free for advancement of the tube or other operations. The distal part has a multidirectional bending system.

Its rigidity and flexibility varies with the different medical applications.

The insertion tube is the flexible part of the instrument. The characteristics of the optical fibres (10 μm resolution power) have to be compared with the human eye resolution power of 75 μm, an operative microscope with a resolution power of 15 μm and a rigid hysteroscope, 17 μm to 5 μm.

As there is no additional outer sheath, cleaning and disinfection is easy. Immediately after each examination the instrument is washed with a cotton swab and soap solution. A special brush is passed through the irrigation operative channel and then washed with a syringe containing the soap solution. The endoscope is then placed into the disinfection solution for 20 minutes.

The physician who is accustomed to rigid endoscopes will initially be disorientated when using the flexible hysteroscope. The speculum is positioned and the uterine cervix is disinfected. The left hand holds the eyepiece and lever which is manipulated with the thumb. The right hand holds the distal end of the endoscope. It guides it gently into the external os of the cervix, while the left hand bends the distal part with the thumb. The distal lens of the endoscope has a 0° frontal view. The progression into the cervix and uterus is made with observation of the channel and the centre of the endoscopic image. The distal lens of the instrument is held against the internal cervical os, carefully aligned with the isthmus uteri. The operator waits for spontaneous

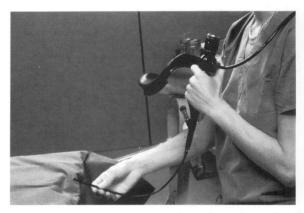

Figure 35.3 A good position for hysteroscopy. The head, the neck and the back of the operator will remain in a good anatomical position during the examination of all parts in the uterus. The operator moves his left arm from left to right. The endoscope will turn clockwise in his right hand and inside the uterus. If the operator moves his left thumb on the angle lever at the control section, the movement inside the uterus will be a circle.

relaxation of the muscle. The wide angle and bending permits observation and operation into the cervico-isthmic canal and uterus—visualization of the internal os gives no special problem.

For office procedure and observation a 3 mm flexible endoscope is used. Penetration into the uterine cavity is easy and painless in almost all young women. In atrophic postmenopausal women dilation to a 3 mm Hegar after local anaesthesia is necessary. For operating procedures, a 5 mm flexible hysteroscope is used. Penetration into the uterine cavity occurs easily in 70% of cases, but in 20% of cases one has to wait 60–120 seconds before uterine relaxation occurs, and in 10% of cases the operator will dilate the cervical canal. In these cases a dilation up to 7 mm is necessary to allow the blood to escape out of the cervix along with the distension medium.

As with some rigid optics, a lateral indentation in the image indicates the site of entry of ancillary instruments. With the 3 mm diagnostic hysteroscope the introduction of tiny biopsy forceps is possible but of limited interest.

With the 2.2 mm channel of the 5 mm operative hysteroscope we can introduce biopsy forceps, or other strong forceps for removal of foreign bodies, one can put in place a Nd:YAG laser fibre, a small 0.8 mm baby scope for tubal catheterization and observation, an electric needle for electrocautery and some other instruments.

Results

The results of hysteroscopic investigations and operative procedures with rigid scopes will be explained in other parts of this book. With flexible instruments the results will be separated between diagnostic and operative procedures.

About 600 hysteroscopies have been performed for *diagnostic purposes* with the diagnostic 3 mm flexible hysteroscope. No anaesthesia or premedication was given, and hysteroscopy is performed at the end of a normal gynaecological examination. No special reference to the menstrual cycle was required. CO_2 was used as the distension medium. The duration of the examination was about 2 minutes (120 seconds). Except for pathological isthmic or uterine stenoses, it was successful in 96% of cases.

After the report of the examination has been made, and the patient still lying on the examination table, an endometrial biopsy is performed. For the purposes of obtaining a histological specimen we use the 3 mm endometrial Cornier pipelle. The use of the pipelle after a flexible 3 mm hysteroscopy is always feasible, but sometimes one has to evacuate the remaining bubble before applying a negative pressure. The value of this instrument is now very well documented. The results of combination of these two methods during a single gynaecological examination allows a combined diagnostic examination with no requirement for analgesia or X-rays. The combination with echography makes hysterosalpingography unnecessary except in cases of infertility when the fallopian tubes have to be evaluated.

The catheterization of the fallopian tubes with a 0.5 mm flexible endoscope into a 1 mm catheter is feasible, but it requires general anaesthesia. In our experience, the visualization is still too imprecise for routine diagnostic purposes.

The disadvantages of the flexible endoscope are their expense which is double that of the rigid ones, and less brightness and a smaller image. But as the optical resolution is now very near to that of rigid hysteroscopes the diagnostic capability is excellent. The technique for introduction of this hysteroscope is completely different from that of a rigid one. But it seems that as soon as experience has been acquired it will be much simpler, because of its flexibility and smaller diameter. It will also be a less painful and a quicker out-patient procedure requiring no anaesthetics.

The Operative Hysteroscope

After 10 years of experimental work it is now possible to separate the indications for rigid operative hysteroscopes and for flexible operative hysteroscopes. The flexible operative hysteroscope has an outer diameter of 4.9 mm versus 8–10 mm for the operative rigid sheaths. The cervix then has to be dilated forcibly. Two complications may occur:

1. perforation of the isthmus,
2. cervico-isthmic incompetence.

These two complications have had bad consequences during pregnancy. For this reason the flexible hysteroscope, introduced without any dilation, should be used as much as possible in young and infertile patients. It is now evident that big polyps and fibroids are more easily treated with resectoscopes although small polyps or fibroids (less than 1 cm) can be resected with the flexible hysteroscope and Nd:YAG laser energy. In the case of infertility it seems better to use the flexible instrument to cut uterine septae and synechiae and to catheterize the tube.

The long-term results of Nd:YAG laser intrauterine procedures were published in 1990 (Cornier, 1990). In a cohort of 144 women, endometrial ablation with Nd:YAG and flexible endoscopy was performed in 44 women; 42 had a one-stage procedure and 2 a two-stage procedure. The minimum duration of the operative follow-up is 18 months. Twenty-four patients became amenorrhoeic and 15 others had scanty menses which lasted only for a short duration. Three patients had a poor operative result and hysterectomy was performed, two others were lost to follow-up. A total of more than 200 procedures have now been performed for these indications. No uterine perforation or other complications have occurred.

The long-term results (more than 18 months) seem to be better than after a partial endometrial ablation. Because of the absence of deep destruction by electrosurgery, the uterine mucosa grows again normally in more than 50% of cases and menses return. Hysterographic documentation shows that uterine ischaemia is the means by which the treatment is effective with the laser. After months and years the treated corpus uteri shrinks progressively—the untreated cervix remains as normal.

Endometrial Ablation

The results seem better after complete resections. But how does complete electroresection or roller coagulation work? Is it a cervico-isthmic synechia or is it complete destruction of the hyperplastic endometrium? What are the long-term results and how many accidents occur? Published results suggest that the Nd:YAG laser used for haemostatic endometrial ablation is a safer instrument than electricity. The flexible hysteroscope makes the work easier than with the rigid hysteroscope.

But the absence of a continuous irrigation system makes the procedure difficult and the new rigid hysteroscopes with a specially adapted sheath for continuous flow and laser operations will have to be compared with the flexible.

Fibroids

The destruction of fibroids by photocoagulation has been performed since 1984. In 28 cases with

more than 18 months of follow-up, heavy bleeding ceased in 18 women and the menses were reported as normal. This 64% long-term success is not very different from the published success rates (long-term follow-up) after endometrial resection. Results are more difficult to analyse in cases of multiple intrauterine pathology. In more than 33% of these 144 cases, fibroids are associated with mucosal hyperplasia, polyps, or mural adenomyosis and hypervascularization.

Association of resection and photocoagulation could be the best method to stop heavy bleeding. It becomes increasingly obvious that rigid scopes can perform better than the flexible ones in these cases because of blood obscuring the operator's vision.

Infertility—Synechiae and Septae

The advantages of flexible endoscopy lie in cases of infertility, especially for tubal catheterization and section of septae or synechiae. As has been demonstrated at open surgery, uterine septae should not be resected, but cut. This can be achieved with scissors, or an electric needle guided down a rigid hysteroscope. But the same results, without any isthmic and cervical uterine dilation can also be achieved with an electric needle placed in the operative channel of the flexible hysteroscope. The operation must be guided by transabdominal echography. The Nd:YAG laser fibre can be used for the same purpose. In the case of synaechiae the technique we use is exactly the same. The abdominal ultrasound guidance is a significant improvement of the technique and avoids a laparoscopy and enables the surgeon to leave a 1.5 cm margin of safety of uterine wall at the uterine fundus.

Seventy-three patients have been treated for uterine adhesions by these methods (electricity or Nd:YAG). Twenty-four had filmy adhesions, 39 thick adhesions and 10 very dense and severe adhesions. Twenty-three of the filmy adhesions became pregnant (10 had miscarriages) and 34 of the thick adhesions, but only 3 of the severe. Cutting these severe adhesions was always possible but as they were very extensive we were worried about perforation and stopped the procedure in 5 cases (4 laparotomies, 2 pregnancies). No intrauterine device was left in place and conception was attempted as soon as possible.

Only in cases of thick or severe adhesions and in the absence of pregnancy 4–6 months later was second look hysteroscopy recommended. In these cases recurrence was observed in 50% and treated again if possible.

The flexible hysteroscope seems to be a much more delicate instrument than the rigid one in these cases. Because of its length and flexibility it makes echographic control at the same time much simpler.

The same results have been obtained with uterine septae. Twelve septae with more than 3 cm of length and in-patients with a history of premature labour have been treated (five with electrosurgery, seven with Nd:YAG laser). Ten have had after this procedure at least one healthy live birth, although the pregnancies were between 32 (two cases) and 39 weeks. None of these patients had had a baby before.

In two cases (one without echographic control during procedure, one with echography but the patient had undergone a uteroplasty previously) a dehiscence of the fundus uteri had been observed and an emergency caesarean section was necessary.

The Future

As technology progresses endoscopes are now connected to video systems. It allows better operator comfort, together with printing facilities for documentation. In the near future, the video endoscopes put the video camera (micro-CCD) at the tip of the flexible endoscope. Will the future video hysteroscope be flexible or rigid? Or semi-flexible? This will certainly depend on the aim of these endoscopes. Small diameter diagnostic hysteroscopes (with or without endosonographic system) will develop with flexible instruments.

References

Brueschke EE & Wilbanks (1974) A steerable fibreoptic hysteroscope. *Obstetrics and Gynecology* **44 (2)**: 273–278.

Cornier E (1990) Traitement des metrorrages par hysteroscopie operation et laser Nd:YAG. *Contraception Fertilité et Stérilité* **18–12**: 1111–1117.

David C (1908) L'endoscopie uterine. G. Jacques Edit. No. 112. Thèse Paris.

Hamou J & Taylor P (1979) Panoramic contact and microhysteroscopy. *Current Problems in Obstetrics and Gynecology* **2**: 3.

Neuwirth RS (1983) Hysteroscopic management of symptomatic submucous fibroids. *Obstetrics and Gynecology* **62**: 509.

Nitze M (1879) *Über eine neue Beleuchtung Methode der Höhlen des menschlichen Körpers*, pp 851–858. Wien: Medizinische Presse.

Schröder C (1934) Über den Ausbau und die Leistungen der Hysteroscopie. *Archiv für Gynaekologie* **156**: 407.

36

Distension Media and Fluid Systems

RAY GARRY

Women's Endoscopic Laser Foundation, South Cleveland Hospital, Middlesbrough, UK

Introduction

Continuous crystal clear vision is an essential prerequisite for safe and satisfactory hysteroscopy. The uterine walls are normally in apposition and to visualize the cavity, the walls must be separated by infusing a suitable medium under pressure.

Distension Media

Carbon Dioxide

The cavity may be distended with gas or fluid. For diagnostic hysteroscopy, particularly in the out-patient or office environment, gaseous distension media are usually preferred. The use of carbon dioxide was first described by Rubin (1925) and it is now much the most frequently used gas. It is preferred because of its ready availability and convenience. It is the least messy of the available agents. CO_2 infused under pressure tends to flatten the endometrium and gives excellent visibility. It has virtually the same index of refraction as air and excellent photographs can be obtained with this medium.

A continuous flow is necessary to replace gas lost through the tubes, around the hysteroscope and absorbed into the uterus. The rate of flow must be carefully controlled for deaths have occurred from gas embolism. Intravasation can occur and bubbles of gas have been detected

moving in the pelvic vessels during simultaneous hysteroscopy and laparoscopy (Donnez, 1989). The risk of gas embolism is proportional to the flow rate of the infused gas. Lindemann *et al.* (1976) demonstrated in a series of experiments in dogs that flow rates below 200 ml/min were associated with minimal changes in pulse rate and breathing. Flow rates above 400 ml/min were associated with tachypnoea and arrhythmias and rates of 1000 ml/min were associated with death within 60 seconds. Physiological mechanism can cope with the transport of 150 ml of CO_2 per minute without risk of embolism or metabolic disturbances. Hulf *et al.* (1979) have shown no changes in electrocardiograms, P_{CO_2} or pH during CO_2 hysteroscopy with controlled rates of CO_2 flow. It is essential to use an infusion apparatus specifically designed for hysteroscopy. The maximum flow rate must be fixed at not more than 100 ml/min and a flow rate of 40 ml/min is usually adequate. Equipment designed for laparoscopy permit flow rates of 3000–4000 ml per minute and must <u>never</u> be used for hysteroscopy.

The principal disadvantage of CO_2 as a distension medium is the tendency for troublesome gas bubbles to form. These are particularly likely to occur when the gas mixes with blood and can obscure vision. These bubbles can usually be avoided with good technique. Blood and mucus should be carefully cleansed from the cervical os with a dry swab and detergent skin cleansing agents should be avoided. The hysteroscope should be advanced slowly under direct vision after creating a series of microcavities just ahead of the tip of the hysteroscope. The instrument can, in this manner, be kept in the centre of the canal and introduced into the uterine cavity without damaging the cervical mucosa which is the usual source of bleeding.

Most workers use CO_2 hysteroscopy only for diagnostic purposes, because bleeding and smoke can seriously impair vision during surgical manipulations. Gallinat et al. (1989), however, also uses CO_2 during Nd:YAG laser ablation of the endometrium. He believes this is safer than fluid distension of the uterus because CO_2 avoids the potentially serious risk of fluid overload and he has designed a closed-circuit system to filter out smoke and plume produced during the ablation which are discussed in Chapter 9.

High-viscosity Fluids

Dextran 70 (Hyskon) has a molecular weight of 70 000 and is a mixture of 32% dextran in 10% dextrose. It is a thick viscous fluid which is electrolyte free, non-conductive, and biodegradable. It was first used as a distension agent for diagnostic hysteroscopy by Edström and Fernström (1970) because it is optically clear and immiscible with blood. Baggish (1989) also considers it to be the best medium for operative hysteroscopic surgery because of its optical clarity, immiscibility with blood and because its consistency reduces the risk of extravasation into the uterine circulation. A pool of static dextran will remain optically clear for longer than a similar pool of a low molecular weight fluid and in such circumstances may be the preferred agent.

Dextran 70 is, however, a difficult medium to work with. Its high viscosity makes continuous infusion difficult, and a laborious and labour-intensive system of intermittent instillation and extraction with large syringes is required. Some force is required for this instillation and unless specially modified tubing is used, accidental disconnection of the tubing with consequent spraying of the sticky material is quite common. When dextran 70 dries it sets solid. If the equipment is not immediately and thoroughly washed in hot water, switches and taps will jam and expensive equipment can readily be ruined. When used with instruments producing high local temperatures, dextran 70 can caramelize and the dark brown colour may impair vision.

Dextran 70 is hydrophilic and when infused into the circulation its high molecular weight pulls with it at least six times its own volume of fluid. Fluid overload and pulmonary oedema may occur. Cases of non-cardiogenic pulmonary oedema have also been described following the use of dextran 70 during hysteroscopy (Zbella et al., 1985; Leake et al., 1987). It is suggested that in such cases the dextran 70 may have a direct toxic effect on the pulmonary capillaries resulting in extravasation and interstitial pulmonary oedema. Jedeikin et al. (1990) have described a case of disseminated intravascular coagulopathy and adult respiratory distress syndrome complicating dextran 70 hysteroscopy. Rare but potentially fatal anaphylactic reactions to dextran 70 have also been described (Borten et al., 1983), the incidence of such life-threatening complications is between 0.069% and 0.008%.

Low-viscosity Fluids

A uterine cavity distended with a stagnant pool of low-viscosity fluid will initially be clear but will soon become cloudy because of the accumulation of small particles of endometrial debris which are dislodged during hysteroscopic manipulation. As such fluids are also readily miscible with blood any oozing will further cloud the fluid and impair vision. If the fluid is repeatedly replaced and a continuous flow of the fluid under pressure is established, bleeding will be prevented by a 'tamponade' effect and the endometrial debris will be flushed out, thereby maintaining continuous clear vision. Under these circumstances clear fluids are the simplest, most convenient and cheapest media for hysteroscopy.

5% Dextrose in Water

Goldrath et al. (1981) in his early cases of Nd:YAG laser ablation of the endometrium used 5% dextrose as the uterine distension medium but in several cases he observed dilutional hyponatraemia as an additional feature complicating fluid overload. As this substance has no clinical advantages over 0.9% sodium chloride solution but has this significant additional risk of dilutional electrolyte disturbance its use can no longer be recommended.

1.5% Glycine

When electrical energy is used inside the uterine cavity it is essential to use a distension fluid which is electrolyte free. Glycine has been widely used for this purpose by urologists during transurethral resection of the prostate. It is optically clear and non-haemolytic and does not conduct electricity Excessive absorption of such an electrolyte-free solution can be associated with hyponatraemia and haemolysis. Magos *et al.* (1991) reported the systemic effects of the absorption of up to 4350 ml of glycine. A fall in serum sodium to 107 mmol/l (normal 140 mmol/l) was noted in one case and this was associated with a significant rise in lactate dehydrogenase which is a marker of red cell breakdown. Glycine is metabolized in the liver and its breakdown can also be associated with an increase in ammonia radicals producing confusion, coma and death. Several deaths have occurred in Europe following intravasation of 1.5% glycine.

Sorbitol

Sorbitol is a non-conducting 3% sugar solution. It is optically clear and is being used as an alternative to glycine. It is hyperosmolar (165–180 mosmol) and excessive absorption can produce disturbances in blood glucose levels and diabetic features as well as overload and electrolyte disturbances.

0.9% Sodium Chloride

Normal saline is optically clear, cheap and readily available. The concentration of electrolytes in this fluid approximate to that in blood and it is metabolically inert. Excess intravasation is not associated with any major electrolyte or metabolic disturbances and any fluid overload can rapidly be reversed with diuretic therapy alone. Ringer's solution is even more physiological with additional potassium radicals added but is less freely available and in practice offers only theoretical advantages over normal saline.

Summary of Distension Media

CO_2 is the most convenient and least messy of the distension media to use. It is useful for diagnostic procedures and is particularly suitable for out-patient and office investigations. Operative manipulations provoking bleeding and the production of smoke and bubbles during ablation impair vision and make CO_2 less suitable for operative hysteroscopy. Dextran 70 is difficult to work with and is associated with rare but serious complications. Sorbitol and glycine can both produce severe electrolyte and metabolic disturbances when absorbed in excess and are not recommended for routine use except when more physiological fluids are contraindicated. In prac-

tice this means that such fluids should only be used when electrical energy is being used inside the cavity during electroresection or roller-ball ablation. In all other circumstances 0.9% sodium chloride infused in a continuous manner is the distension fluid of choice.

Infusion Systems

Hysteroscopes

When Goldrath first attempted Nd:YAG laser ablation he used a hysteroscope with an operating channel and a single channel which he used for infusion of the distending fluid. There was no outflow channel available and fluid could only escape around the barrel of the hysteroscope. To ensure this occurred it was necessary to widely dilate the cervix. Many difficulties encountered during hysteroscopic surgery are caused by using inadequate or inappropriately designed equipment. It is now clear that good operating conditions require the medium inside the cavity to be replaced at very frequent intervals and this can best be produced with a closed-circuit, continuous-flow system.

The uterine resectoscope is very closely modelled on the resectoscope used to perform transurethral resection of the prostate. Urologists have had many years in which to recognize the need for, and to develop such a continuous-flow system. Many resectoscopes have a continuous-flow facility usually in the form of an outer sheath which surrounds the hysteroscope. With this arrangement fluid is infused into the cavity down the central barrel of the hysteroscope and leaves via the outer sheath. It is essential that the inflow and outflow channels are completely separate, communicating only at the distal end of the hysteroscope barrel.

Endometrial ablation using the Nd:YAG laser was first described in 1981. The early hysteroscopes used for this operation were slightly modified cystoscopes and were not specifically designed for the purpose. Many of the models still on the market are not suitable for laser hysteroscopy. Most operating hysteroscopes have at least two taps at the proximal end but in many instances these taps communicate in the common barrel. In these circumstances irrigation of the cavity is impaired. Hysteroscopes with completely separate fluid inflow and outflow channels are to be preferred. Such a hysteroscope has been designed by Baggish and offers improved fluid circulation with consequent improved visibility (Figure 36.1). When a satisfactory continuous circuit is established inside the hysteroscope it is no longer necessary to dilate the cervix excessively and indeed it is better to restrict dilatation to that which will ensure a water-tight fit between the canal and the hysteroscope. Such a fit is facilitated if the outer barrel of the hysteroscope is round in cross-section. There seems little reason to continue to make hysteroscopes with an oval cross-section designed more to match the shape of the male urethra than the circular shape of both the cervical canal and the uterine dilators.

Fluid Instillation

The potential cavity inside the uterus requires the application of pressure to separate the walls. The minimum pressure required to produce a satisfactory degree of distension is usually about 40–50 mmHg but can vary considerably. This can be achieved with:

1. *Syringes.* One or two large capacity syringes can be used to maintain uterine distension. Such a system is labour intensive and relatively uncontrolled as neither the flow rate nor the pressure inside the cavity is known.
2. *Hydrostatic pressure.* A bag of infusion fluid suspended 60 cm above the uterus will enter the cavity with a pressure of about 45 mmHg. Varying the height of the bag above the patient will clearly alter this infusion pressure. This is a simple and inexpensive system for controlling the inflow pressure.
3. *Pressure cuff.* A suitably designed pressure cuff can be placed around the soft-walled infusion bag and the cuff inflated to a suitable level. Infusion rates can be varied by altering the pressure in the cuff.
4. *Simple pump.* The tubing from the infusion bag

can be led through a simple roller pump. The rate of infusion can be altered by varying the speed of rotation of the pump. A constant flow of fluid for a given pump rate will be produced regardless of the outflow resistance.
5. *Pressure-controlled pump.* Various methods of limiting the pressure that a pump can produce have been devised. Quinones has described a compact regulating-compression apparatus which is favoured by Magos and others and Hamou (Hamou Hysteromat, K. Storz, Tuttlingen, Germany) has developed a pressure-limited rotary pump which in a modified form is much favoured by the author (Figure 36.2).

It was soon appreciated that an inherent problem of infusing fluid into the uterine cavity under pressure was that a proportion of that fluid could be absorbed from the cavity into the systemic circulation. Goldrath in this first paper on Nd:YAG laser ablation reported several cases of pulmonary oedema and almost every subsequent worker has described similar complications. In a recent series of 859 cases of endometrial laser ablation Garry et al. (1991) reported a mean fluid deficit of 1350 ml. In an earlier series Davis (1989) describes a case in whom more than 12 litres of fluid entered the circulation.

Various approaches to minimizing such fluid absorption have been proposed (Table 36.1). Goldrath, because he only had available a hysteroscope with a single channel available for fluid, found it necessary to recommend hyperdilatation of the cervix to allow fluid to escape from the cavity. This did provide the simplest form of safety valve to minimize the risk of excess intrauterine pressure. Lomano (1988) and Loffer (1987) both suggested that 'blanching' the surface of the endometrium rather than 'dragging' the laser fibre across and into the endometrium might minimize damage to the uterine vessels and hence

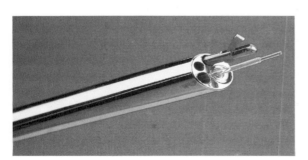

Figure 36.1 Weck–Baggish hysteroscope with an optic and three separate operating channels.

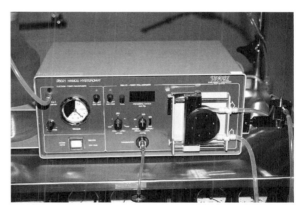

Figure 36.2 Hamou Hysteromat with a rotary pump connected to an integral pressure transducer.

Table 36.1 Suggested methods for reducing fluid absorption during endometrial laser ablation

Year	Author	Cervical dilatation	Infusion	Outflow	Medium	Laser method
1981	Goldrath *et al.*	Wide	Syringe	Free	Saline	Dragging
1987	Loffer	Minimal	BP cuff	Free	Saline	Blanching
1988	Baggish & Baltoyannis	Minimal	Syringe	Syringe	Hyskon	Dragging
1988	Lomano	Wide	?	Free	Saline	Blanching
1989	Grochmal*	Minimal	BP cuff	Suction	Saline	Dragging
1989	Davis (a)	Wide	Pump	Free	Saline	Dragging
	(b)	Minimal	Gravity	Pump	Saline	Dragging
1991	Garry *et al.*	Minimal	Hamou pump	Free	Saline	Dragging

* Personal communication.

reduce fluid absorption. Baggish and Baltoyannis (1988) advocated the use of the highly viscous dextran 70 which appeared to enter the circulation less easily. The author (Garry *et al.*, 1991) has suggested that the use of a Hamou hysteromat pressure-controlled pump can be associated with a marked reduction in fluid absorption.

Of the various systems for infusing fluid into the uterus, some deliver fluid at a constant rate of flow irrespective of the resistance inside the uterus. Syringes and simple roller pumps are examples of such a constant flow, variable pressure system. Other systems provide a fixed head of pressure which results in a variable flow rate into the uterus depending on the resistance in the infusion circuit. Gravity feed and pressure-limited pumps are examples of this constant pressure-variable flow rate system.

In general, the main advantage of a continuous flow system is that excellent vision will be continuously maintained. Providing the outflow channel remains patent such a system ensures that there will always be adequate flow to wash out debris and adequate pressure to maintain a tamponade effect and prevent bleeding into the cavity. The disadvantage of such a system is that the flow continues irrespective of outflow resistance and in some circumstances the intra-uterine pressure levels can rise in an uncontrolled way and may become unacceptably high. This may result in excessive absorption of the distending medium into the systemic circulation.

The advantage of a continuously limited fixed pressure system is that fluid absorption will be minimized. The disadvantage of this system is that as the preset pressure level is approached the rate of flow gradually slows and the flow stops completely when the limit is reached. This slow or stagnant fluid pool rapidly clouds and vision is soon impaired.

The ideal fluid distension system should be an amalgamation of both these systems. The pressure should be limited to prevent excess fluid absorption but set at a level just below the threshold at which absorption occurs. By maintaining the pressure at this highest possible level the resultant flow of fluid should be maintained at a rate sufficient to flush out debris and maintain optimum visual conditions.

Factors Influencing Fluid Absorption

The first 105 patients on whom we performed endometrial laser ablation in South Cleveland Hospital had uterine distension produced with a simple continuous flow pump. The mean fluid absorption measured in this group was 1386 ml. In the next 92 cases the pump was replaced by a Hamou Hysteromat with a preset maximum pressure level. Using such a continuous pressure system the mean absorption fell to 209 ml, a reduction of 85% in mean volume absorbed. We had demonstrated that control of the intrauterine pressure profoundly influenced the amount of fluid absorbed.

To investigate in more detail the factors influencing fluid absorption we developed a system to measure intrauterine pressure directly. The pressure was measured by inserting a semi-rigid catheter down one channel of a Weck–Baggish hysteroscope (Linvatec, North Carolina, USA). This hysteroscope has two operating channels angled only slightly from the midline and with a three-way tap one of these channels can accommodate both the path for fluid infusion and the fluid filled catheter (Figure 36.3). The fluid in the recording catheter is maintained at a pressure of 300 mmHg so there is no flow into this catheter. The end of the catheter was

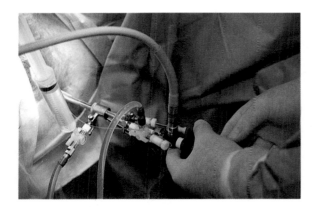

Figure 36.3 Weck–Baggish hysteroscope with a laser fibre in the left operating channel, a three-way tap for fluid inflow and a pressure-recording catheter in the right channel and a three-way tap for reverse flushing on the outflow channel.

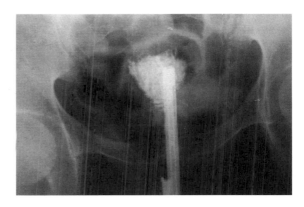

Figure 36.4 An X-ray of the uterine cavity at the end of endometrial laser ablation with the uterine pressure set at 80 mmHg. Note the multiple irregularities caused by the laser furrows and that at this pressure all the dye is retained inside the uterine cavity.

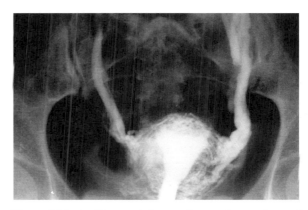

Figure 36.5 An X-ray of the uterine cavity at the end of endometrial ablation with the uterine pressure set at 160 mmHg. Note that much of the radio-opaque material has left the cavity and is outlining the pelvic venous system, a typical finding in a 'high-pressure' absorption situation.

connected to a pressure transducer and a pressure monitoring system. Using this system we can observe the effects of varying intrauterine pressure on volume of fluid absorbed. We can also take X-ray hysterograms at specific intrauterine pressures and demonstrate visually the effect of such pressure changes.

In a prospective randomized trial we demonstrated in a group in whom the fluid was infused with a simple continuous-flow pump that the mean volume of fluid absorbed was 1255 ml and in the group in whom the intrauterine pressure was directly measured and carefully controlled the mean fluid volume absorbed was zero. The intrauterine pressure rose to a mean maximum value of 136 mmHg in the simple pump group and to 70 mmHg in the pressure controlled group (Hasham, 1992). We noted that fluid absorption appeared to occur in an 'all or nothing' manner, i.e. if the intrauterine pressure remained below a critical level no fluid absorption occurred and if the pressure rose above that critical value absorption occurred which seemed then unrelated to any further increases in pressure. This critical level appeared to be related to the mean arterial blood pressure (MAP). This conclusion based on our pressure studies was confirmed by our hysterosalpingogram observations. X-rays taken at any pressure level below the MAP at the completion of an ablation showed the radio-opaque dye confined to the uterine cavity (Figure 36.4). X-rays taken at any level above the mean arterial blood pressure showed dye freely entering the uterine capillaries and venous system, producing remarkably symmetrical venograms of the pelvic system (Figure 36.5).

We demonstrated that even small changes in uterine pressure would affect the passage of the radio-opaque dye. Pressures 5 mmHg below the mean arterial pressure resulted in the dye staying in the cavity and values 5 mmHg above MAP resulted in the dye entering the venous system. The mean arterial pressure under anaesthesia is usually around 75–85 mmHg and fluid absorption does not usually occur with intrauterine pressures of that level. We, however, demonstrated that in a patient with abnormally low MAP of 52 mmHg an intrauterine pressure of 70 mmHg provoked a fluid deficit of 830 ml and conversely in two hypertensive patients with MAP respectively of 130 and 135 mmHg, intrauterine pressure levels of 120 mmHg were associated with no fluid absorption. We conclude that the mean arterial pressure reflects the intrinsic resistance of the superficial layers of a given uterus to fluid intravasation. Maintaining intrauterine pressure below that level is usually associated with zero fluid absorption.

Once appropriate inflow and outflow rates are established the intrauterine pressure usually remains at a steady level. The levels of the intrauterine pressure and the MAP can be recorded at 5 minute intervals, and in the normal situation the IUP should remain below the MAP. Continuous pressure monitoring did, however, on some occasions demonstrate a sudden, unexpected, and at times marked elevation in the intrauterine pressure levels. The almost invariable explanation for such rises in pressure was complete or partial obstruction of the outflow channel by particles of endometrial debris (Figure 36.6). Such obstructions produce a reduction in outflow with a subsequent build-up of intrauterine pressure. If recognized the obstruction can easily be freed by flushing with a syringe attached to the outflow channel. Such reverse flushing rapidly restores the uterine pressure to normal levels. We believe that, in an otherwise steady state, obstruction to the outflow channel is the principal cause of unexpected 'high-pressure' fluid absorption.

We feel that careful control of intrauterine pressure prevents most but not all cases of excess fluid absorption. Using this system of direct pressure measurement and control in 23 consecutive cases of endometrial laser ablation we obtained a zero fluid absorption in 21 cases. In one case with an unusually large cavity containing a pedunculated fibroid it was necessary to deliberately keep the intrauterine pressure above the MAP to ensure adequate visualization and in this case 1000 ml fluid deficit was noted. In the final case in this small series the procedure appeared to be technically uncomplicated and the IUP remained below the MAP and indeed fell as

the procedure progressed. In spite of this a fluid deficit of 1200 ml was observed. An X-ray hysterogram taken at the completion of this procedure gave a clue to the cause of this 'low-pressure' absorption. The X-ray was taken at a pressure below the MAP but dye entered the uterine veins. The hysterogram was not, however, the typical symmetrical pattern and demonstrated only one side of the vascular tree (Figure 36.7). We have found that such asymmetrical venograms are consistently associated with cases of 'low-pressure' absorption and they seem to demonstrate a direct communication between the uterine cavity and a major uterine vessel.

This uncommon 'low-pressure' absorption occurred unpredictably and was difficult to study until we started to take endometrial laser biopsies. During the development of this technique to take full thickness endometrial biopsies with the YAG laser prior to endometrial laser ablation we noticed that every time we took such a biopsy we observed the same type of 'low-pressure' absorption. This occurred even when pressure control and fluid management were otherwise satisfactory. X-ray hysterograms demonstrated that these biopsies penetrate deeply into the myometrium and can often be shown to enter major intrauterine vessels directly. As the pressure in the uterine veins is no more than 20 mmHg and the pressure in the cavity inevitably in excess of 45 mmHg fluid will inevitably be forced into the circulation from the cavity. We therefore suggest that this 'low-pressure' absorption is produced during endometrial ablation when the laser fibre or the resectoscope is taken too deeply into the myometrium, thereby producing a fistula between the large myometrial veins and the uterine cavity. It does not occur when tissue destruction is confined to the superficial layers of

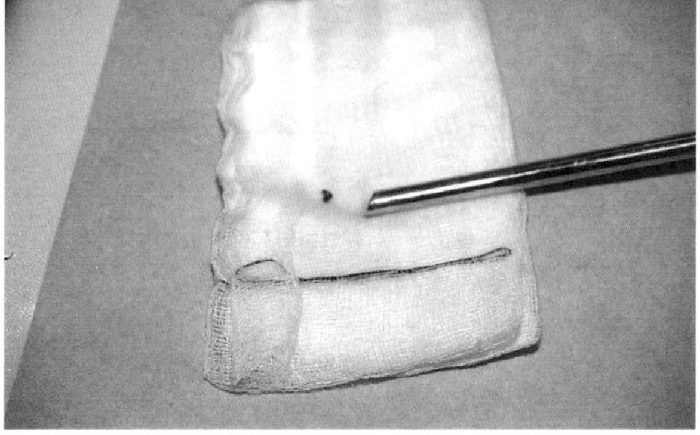

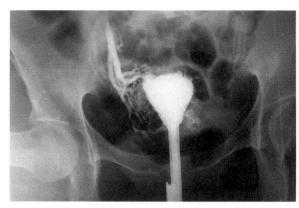

Figure 36.6 A particle of debris obstructing the outflow channel during an endometrial laser ablation.

Figure 36.7 An X-ray hysterogram of a patient with 'low-pressure' absorption showing an asymmetrical venogram demonstrated at an IUP of 75 mmHg.

the uterine wall. Good technique, removing sufficient but not too much tissue, will minimize the risk of this type of fluid absorption.

In summary we believe that four main factors determine the amount of fluid absorbed from the uterine cavity during hysteroscopic surgery and they are:

1. the level of the intrauterine pressure,
2. the level of the mean arterial blood pressure,
3. the patency of the outflow channel of the hysteroscope,
4. the depth of penetration of the uterine instruments.

The superficial layers of the uterine cavity seem to prevent ingress of fluid into the systemic circulation until the pressure in the uterine cavity exceeds a value equal to the mean arterial pressure. When damage to the uterus is confined to the superficial layers absorption is dependent on a simple pressure equation. If the MAP exceeds the IUP no absorption will occur. To ensure that this happens in practice it is necessary to ensure that the level of the intrauterine pressure is always less than the mean arterial pressure by limiting the infusion pressure. To avoid any resultant slowing and ultimate stagnation and consequent clouding of the fluid pool, it is necessary to ensure that the outflow channel remains patent at all times. To prevent direct entry into the major intramyometrial veins it is necessary to use correct techniques to restrict the depth of penetration of the laser fibre or the resectoscope. With good control of the factors mentioned above other factors such as the size of the cavity, duration of the procedure, state of the endometrium do not seem to be important.

Summary

For optimal hysteroscopic surgery it is important to use an operating hysteroscope with separate channels for fluid inflow and outflow and to establish a closed continuous-flow circuit with a water-tight seal between the cervix and the hysteroscope. The intrauterine pressure should be measured and carefully controlled, complete patency of the outflow channel should be maintained, and a high fluid flow rate established. The laser fibre or the resectoscope wire should remove all the endometrium but should not penetrate too deeply into the myometrium. If these principles are followed it is demonstrably possible to perform operative hysteroscopic surgery with continuous crystal clear vision and minimal fluid absorption.

References

Baggish MS (1989) Distending media for panoramic hysteroscopy. In Baggish MS, Bardot J & Valle RF (eds) *Diagnostic and Operative Hysteroscopy*, pp 89–101. Chicago: Year Book Medical Publishers Inc.

Baggish MS & Baltoyannis P (1988) New techniques for laser ablation of the endometrium in high risk patients. *American Journal of Obstetrics and Gynecology* 159: 287–292.

Borten M, Seibert CP & Taymor ML (1983) Recurrent anaphylactic reaction to intraperitoneal dextran-75 for the prevention of postsurgical adhesions. *Obstetrics and Gynecology* 61: 755–757.

Davis JA (1989) Hysteroscopic endometrial ablation with the neodymium-YAG laser. *British Journal of Obstetrics and Gynaecology* 96: 928–932.

Donnez J (1989) Instrumentation. In Donnez J (ed) *Laser Operative Laparoscopy and Hysteroscopy*, pp 207–221. Leuven: Nauwelaerts Printing.

Edström K & Fernström I (1970) The diagnostic possibilities of a modified hysteroscopic technique. *Acta Obstetrica et Gynecologica Scandanavica* 49: 327–329.

Gallinat A, Lueken RR & Moller CP (1989) *The Use of the Nd:YAG Laser in Gynecological Endoscopy*. Laser Brief 14 Munich: MBB-Medizintechnik GmbH.

Garry R, Erian J & Grochmal S (1991) A multicentre collaborative study into the treatment of menorrhagia by Nd–YAG laser ablation of the endometrium. *British Journal of Obstetrics and Gynaecology* 98: 357–362.

Goldrath MH, Fuller T & Segal S (1981) Laser photovaporization of the endometrium for the treatment of menorrhagia. *American Journal of Obstetrics and Gynecology* 140: 14–19.

Hasham F, Garry R, Kokri MS et al. (1992) Fluid absorption during laser ablation of the endometrium in the treatment of menorrhagia. *British Journal of Anaesthesia* (in press).

Hulf JA, Corall IM, Knights KM et al. (1979) Blood carbon dioxide changes during hysteroscopy. *Fertility and Sterility* 32: 193–196.

Jedeikin R, Olsfanger D & Kessler I (1990) Disseminated intravascular coagulopathy and adult respiratory distress syndrome: life threatening complications. *American Journal of Obstetrics and Gynecology* 162: 44–45.

Leake JF, Murphey AA & Zacur HA (1987) Noncardiogenic pulmonary edema: a complication of operative hysteroscopy. *Fertility and Sterility* 48: 497–499.

Lindemann HJ, Mohr J, Gallinat A et al. (1976) Der Einluss von CO_2-gas während der Hysteroscopie. *Geburtshilfe und Frauenheilkunde* 36: 153–156.

Loffer FD (1987) Hysteroscopic endometrial ablation with Nd–YAG laser using a non-contact technique. *Obstetrics and Gynecology* 69: 6679–6689.

Lomano JM (1988) Photocoagulation of the endometrium with the Nd–YAG laser for the treatment of menorrhagia. *Journal of Reproductive Medicine* **31**: 148–150.

Magos AL, Baumann R, Lockwood GM *et al.* (1991) Experience with the first 250 endometrial resections for menorrhagia. *Lancet* **337**: 1074–1078.

Rubin IC (1925) Uterine endoscopy, endometroscopy with the aid of uterine insuflation. *American Journal of Obstetrics and Gynecology* **10**: 313–315.

Zbella EA, Moise J & Carson SA (1985) Noncardiogenic pulmonary edema secondary to intrauterine instillation of 32% dextran 70. *Fertility and Sterility* **43**: 479–480.

37

Hysteroscopic Metroplasty

NAOMI WHITELAW

Department of Obstetrics and Gynaecology, Royal Surrey County Hospital, Guildford, UK

The septate uterus is associated with a 20% reproductive failure rate (Rock and Jones, 1977). Traditionally, where a septate uterus has been identified as the cause of reproductive failure, surgical correction has been by the abdominal route by either the classic Strassman operation or a variation of that procedure (Jones, 1977). However, such procedures involve lengthy anaesthesia with the potential for surgical complications such as infection requiring antibiotic therapy, or even haemorrhage necessitating blood transfusion. Postoperative adhesions or tubal occlusion secondary to the surgery carried out could render the woman infertile, thus worsening the prognosis of the initial reproductive problem. Chervenak and Neuwirth (1981) were the first to show that certain Müllerian fusion defects are amenable to hysteroscopic surgery when they described hysteroscopic resection of a uterine septum using fine microscissors placed adjacent to the hysteroscope. Microscissors can be employed through the operating channel of the hysteroscope (Daly et al., 1983) as can the urological resectoscope to cut the intrauterine septum (DeCherney and Polan, 1983). Resection of intrauterine septae has also been described using the neodymium:yttrium–aluminium–garnet laser (Nd:YAG) (Donnez and Nisolle, 1989) potassium–titanyl–phosphate laser (KTP) (Daniell et al., 1987) and the argon laser (Candiani et al., 1991).

Operative Technique and Management

Before commencing operative resection it is essential that the precise Müllerian abnormality is well defined. Only septate uteri (complete or incomplete) are amenable to this type of hysteroscopic surgery. Hysteroscopic resection of a bicornuate or didelphys uterus is contraindicated because of the potential for breaching the myometrium and entering the abdominal cavity with associated risks of damage to pelvic viscera and major vessels. Before the advent of operative hysteroscopy, the accuracy of preoperative diagnosis of uterine anomalies was not critical because they were repaired in the same way, therefore simple hysterosalpingography sufficed (Reuter et al., 1989). However, in order to make the differential diagnosis, hysterosalpingography or hysteroscopy combined with laparoscopy is required, although Reuter et al. (1989) suggest that hysterosalpingography in conjunction with pelvic ultrasound increases non-invasive accuracy of diagnosis.

Such procedures can be performed under general anaesthesia or under local anaesthesia, the latter providing an additional safety factor in laser hysteroscopic surgery where the conscious patient will experience pain sensation should the laser energy encroach on the sensitive uterine serous peritoneum (Dequesne, 1992).

Concurrent laparoscopy at the time of hysteroscopic resection is strongly recommended. Laparoscopic observation enables the hysteroscopic surgeon to be reassured that the uterus is free of all contact with the pelvic viscera and vessels at all times. Should the myometrium be breached, the procedure can be stopped immediately before irreparable harm is done.

If scissors are employed for resection, then a standard irrigating fluid can be used as the uterine distending medium (dextran 70, 5% or 10% dextrose in water, 0.9% sodium chloride, 5% dextrose in 0.9% sodium chloride, 1.5% glycine and Ringer's lactate solution). Each of these has their advantages and disadvantages (Kershaw and Van Boven, 1992) but if the electrosurgical resectoscope is used, glycine or sorbitol is the preferred medium. Uterine septae are usually considered to be relatively avascular structures so the theoretical risk of fluid overload should be considerably less than that associated with total endometrial resection; nevertheless, fluid overload associated with hyponatraemia, haemolysis and mild disseminated intravascular coagulation has been reported with this particular procedure (D'Agosto et al., 1990).

In view of the avascularity of the septum, pretreatment with danazol or LHRH analogues is not required. Both tubal ostia should be visualized by the operator before commencing the procedure, and the septum should be kept in view at all times. Irrespective of the method employed, the section of the septum is commenced from the inferior margin of the septum and carried cephalad until flush with the surrounding endometrium. Using the cutting loop or right-angled needle electrode of the resectoscope or a 'touch' technique for the fibreoptic lasers, the septum is shaved away by simple advancement of the resecting instrument, keeping both tubal ostia and the septum in view at all times. If microscissors are employed, progressive horizontal cuts are made in the midline. The procedure is considered complete when a normal uterine cavity is obtained and the hysteroscope can be moved freely from one tubal ostium to the other.

Initially only partial septal defects were treated hysteroscopically, but recently, successful hystero- scopic treatments of complete septal uterine defects have been carried out. Rock et al. (1987) have described a one-stage method where the other cervical os is occluded with the balloon of a Foley catheter in order to prevent the loss of the distending medium and resection of the septum is performed distal to the cervix. Donnez and Nisolle (1989) have described a two-stage method where the cervical septum is incised with the carbon dioxide laser until the lower portion of the uterine septum is visible. Two months later, Nd:YAG laser resection of the uterine septum is then carried out.

The insertion of an intrauterine device and postoperative hormone treatment does not appear to confer any extra benefit (Vercellini et al., 1989; Candiani et al., 1990b) although performed in many instances (Donnez and Nisolle, 1989; Dequesne, 1992).

Comment

DeCherney et al. (1986) reported on 72 patients out of 103 who successfully underwent hysteroscopic resection of intrauterine septae with a subsequent 86% pregnancy rate, which approximates to that achieved after abdominal surgery (Thompson, 1985). Where there has been resection of a complete cervical and uterine septum, prophylac- tic cervical cerclage may need to be considered (Donnez and Nisolle, 1989).

Hysteroscopic incision would appear to be the treatment of choice for the septate uterus associated with reproductive failure (DeCherney et al., 1986; Valle and Sciarra, 1986; March and Israel, 1987; Daly et al., 1989). Postoperative morbidity and discomfort are considerably reduced and there is less adhesion formation because the peritoneum is not opened. Hystero- scopic division of the uterine septum has no effect on subsequent vaginal delivery as the myometrium is not transected, so there is no need for caesarean section which would be considered necessary by most (Sant-Cassia et al., 1985; Donnez and Nisolle, 1989; Dequesne, 1992) although by no means all authors (Candiani et al., 1990a), had conventional uterine reconstructive surgery been performed. The choice of instrument depends in part on operator preference and availability. The resectoscope has the advantages of being relatively inexpensive, readily available and simple to operate with good results. Micro- scissors are also an economic and effective instrument for the treatment of the septate uterus. There is a high initial cost with lasers, hence laser treatment of the septate uterus will probably be limited to those centres already using a laser on a large number of other endoscopic procedures. The only randomized study to date to compare the surgical and anatomical results of septal incision by microscissors versus laser did not confirm any advantage of the latter instrument (Candiani et al., 1991). The argon laser was chosen for the study because of its endometrial sparing, whereas the power of the beam of the Nd:YAG laser can effectively ablate endometrium, although the latter is the choice of many operators including ourselves (Donnez and Nisolle, 1989; Dequesne, 1992) for performing laser incision of the uterine septum. Although bleeding from the incised septum is minimal, arteriolar bleeding is often present when the cephalad part of the septum is performed, being a physiological sign that the myometrium has been reached. In such instances the coagulation power of the laser would seem to be an advantage but was not confirmed by Candiani *et al.* (1991) in their study. More recently, transcervical metroplasty has been successfully carried out under ultrasound control (Querleu *et al.*, 1990), the advantage being that concomitant laparoscopy is not required. However, concern about blindly traumatizing the endometrium with this procedure has been raised (Dabirashrafi and Moghadami-Tabrizi, 1991).

Conclusions

The hysteroscopic treatment of septate uteri associated with reproductive failure, whether by microscissors, resectoscope or laser, is a simple and effective method of managing this condition, without resorting to major surgery and is associated with lower morbidity and postoperative sequelae.

References

Candiani GB, Fedele L, Parazzini M & Zamberletti D (1990a) Reproductive prognosis after abdominal metroplasty in bicornuate or septate uterus: a life table analysis. *British Journal of Obstetrics and Gynaecology* **97**: 613–617.

Candiani GB, Vercellini P, Fedele L *et al.* (1990b) Repair of the uterine cavity after hysteroscopic septal incision. *Fertility and Sterility* **54**: 991–994.

Candiani GB, Vercellini P, Fedele L *et al.* (1991) Argon laser versus microscissors for hysteroscopic incision of uterine septa. *American Journal of Obstetrics and Gynecology* **164**: 87–90.

Chervenak FA & Neuwirth RS (1981) Hysteroscopic resection of the uterine septum. *American Journal of Obstetrics and Gynecology* **141**: 351–353.

Dabirashrafi H & Moghadami-Tabrizi N (1991) Establishing the accuracy of ultrasound-guided transcervical metroplasty. *Fertility and Sterility* **56**: 152–153.

D'Agosto J, Ali NMK & Maier D (1990) Absorption of irrigating solution during hysteroscopic metroplasty. *Anesthesiology* **72**: 379–380.

Daly DC, Tohan N, Walters C & Riddick DH (1983) Hysteroscopic resection of the uterine septum in the presence of a septate cervix. *Fertility and Sterility* **39**: 560–562.

Daly DC, Maier D & Soto-Albers C (1989) Hysteroscopic metroplasty: six years' experience. *Obstetrics and Gynecology* **73**: 201–205.

Daniell JF, Osher S & Miller W (1987) Hysteroscopic resection of uterine septi with visible light laser energy. *Colposcopy and Gynecological Laser Surgery* **3**: 217–220.

DeCherney AH & Polan ML (1983) Hysteroscopic management of intrauterine lesions and intractable uterine bleeding. *Obstetrics and Gynecology* **61**: 392–397.

DeCherney AH, Russell JB, Graebe RA & Polan ML (1986) Resectoscopic management of mullerian fusion defects. *Fertility and Sterility* **45**: 726–728.

Dequesne J (1992) Laser hysteroscopic surgery and focal ablation of the endometrium. In Sutton CJG (ed) *Lasers in Gynaecology*, pp 184–186. London: Chapman & Hall.

Donnez J & Nisolle M (1989) Operative laser hysteroscopy in mullerian fusion defects and uterine adhesions. In Donnez J (ed) *Laser Operative Laparoscopy and Hysteroscopy*, pp 249–261. Leuven: Nauwelaerts Printing.

Jones HW (1977) Surgery of the double uterus. In Mattingly RF (ed) *Te Linde's Operative Gynecology*, p 309. Philadelphia: JB Lippincott Company.

Kershaw EJ & Van Boven MJ (1992) Laser safety: hazards and precautions. In Sutton CJG (ed) *Lasers in Gynaecology*, pp 238–246. London: Chapman & Hall.

March CM & Israel R (1987) Hysteroscopic management of recurrent abortion caused by the septate uterus. *American Journal of Obstetrics and Gynecology* **156**: 834–842.

Querleu D, Brasme TL & Parmentier D (1990) Ultrasound-guided transcervical metroplasty. *Fertility and Sterility* **54**: 995–998.

Reuter LK, Daly DC & Cohen SM (1989) Septate versus bicornuate uteri: errors in imaging diagnosis. *Radiology* **172**: 749–752.

Rock JA & Jones HW (1977) The clinical management of the double uterus. *Fertility and Sterility* **28**: 798–806.

Rock JA, Murphy AA & Cooper WH (1987) Resectoscopic technique for the lysis of a class V complete uterine septum. *Fertility and Sterility* **48**: 495–497.

Sant-Cassia LJ (1985) Recurrent abortion. In Studd JWW (ed) *Progress in Obstetrics and Gynaecology*, Vol 5, pp 248–258. Edinburgh: Churchill Livingstone.

Thompson JD (1985) Surgery for anomalies of mullerian ducts. In Mattingly RF (ed) *Te Linde's Operative Gynecology*, p 345. Philadelphia: JB Lippincott Company.

Valle RF & Sciarra JJ (1986) Hysteroscopic treatment of the septate uterus. *Obstetrics and Gynecology* **67**: 253–257.

Vercellini P, Fedele L, Arcaini L, Rognoni MT & Candiani GB (1989) Value of intrauterine device insertion and estrogen administration after hysteroscopic metroplasty. *Journal of Reproductive Medicine* **34**: 447–450.

38

Trans-cervical Resection of the Endometrium (TCRE)

J.A. MARK BROADBENT AND ADAM L. MAGOS

Minimally Invasive Therapy Unit, University Department of Obstetrics and Gynaecology, The Royal Free Hospital, London

Introduction

Until recently, hysterectomy has been the only surgical treatment of menorrhagia available to the many women that present with this problem. Approximately one-third of gynaecological consultations are accountable to menorrhagia and 60% of these culminate in hysterectomy as a definitive treatment within 5 years of presentation (Coulter et al., 1991). Medical treatment of this condition is either ineffective or poorly tolerated due to side-effects which has resulted in hysterectomy becoming the most frequently performed major surgery in women of reproductive age.

Transcervical resection of the endometrium (TCRE) is one of the alternatives to hysterectomy, and, like other techniques such as laser ablation of the endometrium, relies on the production of a type of therapeutic Asherman's syndrome (1950) within the uterine cavity resulting in amelioration of menstrual symptoms.

Origins of Resectoscopic Surgery within the Uterus

The beginning of surgical procedures within the uterine cavity using a urological resectoscope took place in 1978, when Neuwirth described the resection of submucous fibroids in women with abnormal bleeding. If focal operative procedures were possible, why not more extensive intrauter-ine surgery involving the whole of the uterine cavity? This notion was touched upon in a review article by Neuwirth in 1983, namely the destruction of the entire uterine cavity by the systematic shaving of the endometrium as far as the isthmus with the cutting loop of the resecting hysteroscope (Amin and Neuwirth, 1983). In the same year, the Americans DeCherney and Polan (1983) reported their experience with resectoscopic electrocoagulation of the endometrium as *emergency* treatment of intractable and life-threatening uterine haemorrhage, unyielding to other therapies, in 11 women who were deemed unfit for hysterectomy. This series was updated 4 years later and included 21 patients, all but three suffering from either blood dyscrasias or other serious illnesses, who were treated with either endometrial diathermy or resection and followed up for a maximum of 6 years (DeCherney et al., 1987). The results were most impressive: 18 of the 19 who survived their underlying medical condition were amenorrhoeic and only one required further treatment.

The French master of hysteroscopy, Jacques Hamou, introduced endometrial resection to Paris in 1985, modifying the technique somewhat. The Americans had been using dextran 70 for uterine distension whereas Hamou suggested using non-viscous fluids, such as 1.5% glycine solution, as a more manageable alternative for both distension and irrigation. He also initiated the use of the continuous-flow resectoscope, as developed by Hallez et al. (1987), for easier and safer fluid control. Of more importance than these technical modifications was his suggestion that what has come to be known as *partial endometrial resection* be used in otherwise healthy women with menorrhagia as an alternative to hysterectomy, aiming at making menstruation light enough to be acceptable but not to suppress periods completely. Hamou justified incomplete excision by a fear that resection down to the endocervix would lead to cervical stenosis, and the fact that Parisian women wanted to continue with their periods provided that they were light. Hamou demonstrated his new technique in Oxford, UK in 1988, following which the more extensive procedure of *total endometrial resection* was developed (Magos *et al.*, 1989b). In effect, this is the gynaecologist's version of transurethral resection of the prostate (TURP) and so the term 'transcervical resection of the endometrium' (TCRE) was coined.

Technique

A 26 French gauge unmodified continuous-flow resectoscope fitted with a 4 mm forward-oblique telescope and 24 French gauge cutting loop is generally used to perform TCRE. Distension of the uterine cavity, via the inner inflow sheath, is required to allow access to the fundal and cornual regions. An intrauterine pressure of 80–120 mmHg is usually needed; collapse of the uterine cavity occurs if the pressure is too low and renders resection unsafe whilst the consequence of too high a pressure is excessive absorption of the irrigation fluid with the potential for fluid overload. Uterine distension can be achieved by simple gravity and the additional help of a sphygmomanometer cuff inflated around the bag of irrigant. It is more convenient to use one of the commercially available irrigation pumps, such as the Quinones pump or the Hamou Hysteromat. Flux of irrigant through the uterine cavity is achieved by continuous suction via the outer sheath of the resectoscope, usually with a negative pressure of −50 mmHg. If the flux of irrigant is insufficient to maintain a clear view of the uterine cavity then the rate of suction can be increased. Resection should never be attempted in the absence of a clear view of the uterine cavity, the ability to control uterine distension and irrigation accurately being paramount to patient safety.

The resectoscope handle mechanism can be either active or passive and we prefer to use the passive mechanism. When using this, the cutting loop sits inside the sheath at rest so there is no obstruction to the endoscopic view when inspecting the uterine cavity. Also, accidental trauma is less likely than when using a permanently exposed loop. The depth of cut of the loop is 3–4 mm, which means that, ideally, resection should be performed immediately after menstruation when the endometrial thickness is of the order of 3 mm. From an administrative point of view, this is very difficult and so an endometrial suppressant, such as danazol or a gonadotrophin releasing hormone agonist, can be used to this effect. We prefer to treat our patients with danazol at a dose of 200 mg t.d.s. for 6 weeks prior to surgery, a regimen which has been shown to produce a thin, atrophic endometrium (Jeppsson *et al.*, 1984) that is ideally suited to endometrial resection. This has the added advantage of making the endometrium less 'fluffy' and less likely to block the outflow holes of the outer sheath and restrict clear vision. It must also be remembered that glandular elements are almost invariably present deep in the myometrium and resection should therefore include 2.5–3 mm of myometrium as well (Reid and Sharp, 1988). Video monitoring is used with advantages in terms of operator comfort, operative field magnification, theatre staff interest, and not least to facilitate teaching.

Using a blended cutting and coagulating current of 75–125 W, submucous myomata can be easily resected if indicated, followed by the systematic excision of the endometrium, including the superficial layer of the myometrium. The obvious circular myometrial fibres are used to judge the depth of resection, care being taken not to cut too deeply into the myometrium as this may result in haemorrhage or perforation. A slightly forward-angled loop is used to resect the fundal region, the conventional loop being used for the remainder of the uterine cavity. When performing partial TCRE the endometrium is resected to within 0.5–1 cm of the isthmus, and for total TCRE the entire endometrial cavity is resected. The resected tissue can be removed using a flushing curette or polyp forceps and sent for histological examination. The uterine cavity is then reinspected for residual endometrium which may have been missed during the initial resection, and bleeding points can be coagulated. This ability to visually confirm the completeness of surgery is a major advantage of hysteroscopic techniques, particularly endometrial resection.

Anaesthesia

The autonomic nerve supply of the uterus renders it relatively insensitive to touching, cutting or burning. Minor hysteroscopic procedures, using relatively narrow endoscopic instruments, have already been described under local anaesthesia combined with sedation (Cornier, 1986; Hallez *et al.*, 1987), but we have found that TCRE, using a wider instrument, can also be carried out without recourse to general anaesthesia (Magos *et al.*, 1989a). Patient preference is usually the deciding factor as to which mode of anaesthesia is used and about one-third of our patients choose to avoid general anaesthesia. Medically unfit patients also benefit from the decreased hazards associated with local anaesthesia.

Our current regimen involves admitting the patient in time for premedication with oral temazepam 20 mg and rectal diclofenac 100 mg 1 hour prior to surgery. Once in the operating suite, anxiolysis and light sedation are produced using small doses of intravenous midazolam, systemic analgesia with incremental doses of intravenous fentanyl, and finally local anaesthesia with a combination of para- and intracervical and intrauterine lignocaine/adrenaline mixture, the latter injected under direct vision using the resectoscope. Heart rate, electrocardiogram and arterial oxygen saturation are monitored continuously, and facial oxygen is given routinely. Patients remain fully cooperative during surgery and some choose to watch their operation on the video monitor.

Postoperative recovery is rapid and within 3–4 hours most patients are fit for discharge from hospital. This technique is tolerated very well, to the extent that of those patients who require retreatment almost all choose to have the second procedure performed under sedation. The combination of TCRE with local anaesthesia avoids the two most important hazards of hysterectomy, major abdominal surgery and general anaesthesia, especially important for those patients with menorrhagia for whom hysterectomy is considered undesirable, dangerous or impossible (Lockwood *et al.*, 1990).

Results

The following discussion on the results of endometrial resections is based on the experience reported in the detailed published series, of which there are only five (Magos *et al.*, 1989a, 1991; Hill and Maher, 1990; Maher and Hill, 1990; Derman *et al.*, 1991; Pyper and Haeri, 1991). In the series by Derman *et al.*, the effect of endometrial ablation on menstruation is not reported in detail and

concentrates on hysteroscopic myomectomy. It is important to realize that follow-up data for this procedure, as treatment for menorrhagia, is at present limited to just over 3 years.

Treatment Criteria

Our treatment criteria for TCRE are outlined in Table 38.1. Appropriate patient selection is important with regard to the success of any surgical intervention. Treatment criteria will change as more experience is gained. We believe that these criteria will help to identify those women who are most likely to benefit from this procedure, whilst remembering that treatment failure and surgical complications are likely to increase if less stringent criteria are used.

Rutherford *et al.* (1991) have estimated that up to 58% of women currently being treated by hysterectomy for menstrual abnormalities may be suitable for this treatment, including those women with moderately sized uterine myomata. This is an advantage over other methods of endometrial ablation which are generally restricted to the treatment of dysfunctional uterine bleeding.

Careful counselling is mandatory prior to surgery, especially with regard to the risks of the procedure, the likelihood of menstrual improvement, the risk of pregnancy, and perhaps the most important, the lack of knowledge regarding possible long-term effects. It is important that the patient's expectations of surgery correlate with the expected results.

Surgery

Most patients (95.2%) choose to undergo total resection of the endometrium. Failure to complete intended hysteroscopic surgery is unusual, and in our experience less than 5% of those requesting

Table 38.1 Treatment criteria for transcervical resection of the endometrium

Menstrual problems justifying hysterectomy
Symptoms resistant to medical therapy
Uterine size smaller than the equivalent of a 12 week pregnancy (or uterine cavity < 10 cm in length)
Submucous fibroids < 5 cm diameter
Benign endometrial histology
Completed family
No other gynaecological problems indicating alternative surgery (e.g. prolapse, endometriosis, cervical intra-epithelial neoplasia)
Thoughtful counselling

total TCRE had surgery abandoned before completion (Magos et al., 1991). Difficulty in dilating the cervix enough to introduce the resectoscope rarely occurs. Other reasons include inability to visualize the entire uterine cavity often because of fibroids, an 'unprepared' endometrium that is thick and difficult to resect, and operative complications such as perforation of the uterus or fluid overload necessitating cessation of surgery.

Operating Time

Hysteroscopic experience is by far the greatest determinant of duration of surgery, shorter operating times being associated with the greater hysteroscopic experience, the so-called learning curve. Maher and Hill (1990) report actual resection times of 15–45 minutes which compares well with our average operating of 33.6 minutes, uncorrected for teaching (Magos et al., 1991). The presence of fibroids and other intrauterine pathology and the lack of preoperative endometrial preparation have been found to increase operating time (39.0 versus 32.0 minutes and 36.9 versus 31.9 minutes respectively) (Magos et al., 1991).

Fluid Balance

Fluid dynamics during surgery depend on influencing factors such as endometrial preparation, tubal patency, concurrent hysteroscopic myomectomy, and duration of surgery, as well as intrauterine pressure. In our experience, the large range of values means that these factors did not produce statistically significant differences, but, to give an example, the volume of fluid absorbed by those patients who did not have endometrial preparation, had patent tubes, had concurrent hysteroscopic myomectomy performed, and in whom surgery took more than 40 minutes was 697 ml (range 100–2300), compared with 125 ml (range 0–250) for those having had endometrial preparation, had been sterilized, had a normal uterine cavity, and in whom surgery took less than 20 minutes. Overall, the average amount of glycine solution absorbed was just under 500 ml and it is our practice to stop surgery when the total volume of fluid absorbed during surgery exceeds 2 litres to prevent any serious sequelae (Table 38.2).

Histological Examination of Resected Endometrium

It is difficult to remove all the resected endometrial tissue from the uterine cavity, so our average of

Table 38.2 Guidelines for the management of fluid absorption during hysteroscopic surgery using electrolyte-free aqueous solutions (e.g. 1.5% glycine)

Volume absorbed	Effect	Action
< 1000 ml	Well tolerated by healthy patients	Continue surgery
1000–2000 ml	Mild hyponatraemia likely	Complete surgery as quickly as possible
> 2000 ml	Severe hyponatraemia and other disturbances likely	Stop surgery

6.67 g (range 0.98–43) of tissue is an underestimate of the total amount of endometrium resected. Endometrium that was preoperatively treated with danazol was usually reported as being 'basal', 'inactive' or 'atrophic'. Recently, it has been suggested that LHRH agonists are the most, danazol the next, and progestogens the least effective at thinning the endometrium (Brooks et al., 1991).

The angle at which the endometrial chipping is resected varies and this makes the assessment of the amount of myometrium present in the surgical specimen difficult, as is determining the presence of adenomyosis. However, typically over 75% (range 10–100) of the surgical specimen is reported as consisting of myometrium, adenomyosis being reported as present in 12% of cases (Magos et al., 1991).

Concurrent Operative Procedures

Of all the women at risk of pregnancy who underwent endometrial resection in our series only 14% requested laparoscopic sterilization. Whilst menstrual abnormality and concurrent gynaecological pathology may indicate the need for hysterectomy, this is not always necessary. The combination of endometrial resection and other minimally invasive techniques is preferable to hysterectomy for some women and we have used operative laparoscopy to treat endometriosis and ovarian cysts.

Postoperative Recovery

Recovery following endometrial resection is generally rapid and uneventful, making it ideally

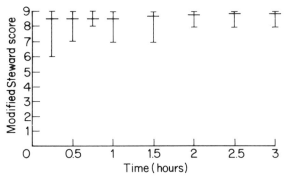

Figure 38.1 Recovery after transcervical resection of the endometrium performed under local anaesthesia and intravenous sedation as assessed by a modified Steward score. The bars refer to the mean and range. The modified Steward score is from 0–9 where 9 represents being wide awake. If required the scoring system is as follows:

Consciousness

Fully awake, eyes open, conversing	4
Lightly asleep, eyes open intermittently	3
Eyes open on command or in response to name	2
Responds to ear pinching	1
Does not respond	0

Airway

Opens mouth or coughs or both on command	3
No voluntary cough but airway clear without support	2
Airway obstructed on neck flexion, clear on extension	1
Airway obstructed without support	0

Activity

Raises one arm on command	2
Non-purposeful movement	1
Not moving	0

suited to day-case surgery. If performed under local anaesthesia and sedation, postoperative recovery is exceptionally rapid (Figure 38.1), patients being fit for discharge within a few hours. Whatever the mode of anaesthesia, hospitalization is short and recovery fast (Table 38.3) (Maher and Hill, 1990; Magos *et al.*, 1991).

Table 38.3 Postoperative recovery following transcervical resection of the endometrium

Postoperative hospital stay (days)	0.79	(0–13)
Duration of bleeding (days)	12.1	(1–42)
Duration of discharge (days)	12.0	(0–120)
Return to normal domestic activities (weeks)	1.30	(0–4)
Return to work (weeks)	2.12	(0–6)

Reproduced with permission from *The Lancet* 1991; **337**: 1074–1078.

Postoperative vaginal loss is rarely heavy, although bleeding can last for weeks. Typically, bleeding is reported for just under 2 weeks tailing off into an abnormal discharge which again lasts for about 2 weeks. So far we have not had any women with secondary haemorrhage.

Effects on Menstruation

The effects that endometrial resection has on menstruation have not been widely published in the literature to date. Some series (Derman *et al.*, 1991) not only do not give detailed accounts of the effects on menstruation but do not distinguish between endometrial resection and hysteroscopic myomectomy. Under these circumstances the results are very difficult to interpret. Further difficulties arise when comparing the results of different series because of differences in resecting techniques used (total versus partial), the inconsistent use of pre- and postoperative hormonal suppression, different levels of experience with operative hysteroscopy, and differing durations of follow-up. The results of some of the larger series (published and unpublished) are summarized in Table 38.4.

The rates of amenorrhoea reported range from 6 to 59%, which seems somewhat inconsistent. This highlights the difficulties already mentioned in comparing results from different series. Some authors give postoperative hormonal suppression which is likely to improve the incidence of amenorrhoea, although whether this is a long-term effect is not yet known. Maher and Hill (1990) report a relatively low incidence of amenorrhoea (21%) as do Pyper and Haeri (1991), but this is largely explained by their reluctance to resect into the endocervical canal for fear of uncontrollable haemorrhage and possible cervical stenosis (not substantiated by others). Roller-ball electrocoagulation in this area should overcome this potential risk, and is now being employed by Maher and Hill who expect to see an improvement in their results.

What is evident from the results of these series is that up to 97% of patients experience an improvement in their symptoms, whatever the technique of endometrial resection. Where resection has failed to alleviate symptoms, it is unnecessary to resort to hysterectomy. Repeat resection is an effective and safe option in these cases, providing a successful menstrual outcome in about 80% (Magos *et al.*, 1991). Indeed, Pyper and Haeri (1991) report one case where a total of three endometrial resections were performed before a satisfactory result was achieved.

Table 38.4 Menstruation and further surgery after transcervical resection of the endometrium

Series	Maher & Hill (1990)	Magos et al. (1991)	Pyper & Haeri (1991)	Shaxted (unpublished)	Holt (unpublished)
Number of patients	100*	250	80	274	350
Menstrual result					
Amenorrhoea	21%	27–42%†	6–8%†	59%‡	42%‡
Improved	95%	92%	81%	91%	97%
Not improved	3%	8%	19%	9%	3%
Further surgery					
TCRE	3 (3%)	16 (7%)	15 (19%)	N/A	8 (2%)
Hysterectomy	0 (0%)	10 (4%)	4 (5%)	N/A	11 (3%)

* Two patients lost to follow-up.
† Amenorrhoea rate after total TCRE dependent on time after surgery.
‡ Some given medroxyprogesterone acetate post-operatively (Depo-Provera).
N/A, Data not available.

Our results of 250 patients followed for up to 2.5 years have been analysed in more detail and are shown in Figures 38.2–38.5. Over 90% reported lighter, shorter, and less painful periods and satisfaction rates were consistently over 80%. Whilst subjective impressions by the patient are important, confirmation by objective measurement of menstrual blood loss (MBL) showed that 24 of the 25 (96%) patients monitored after total TCRE had measurements well within the normal MBL range (< 80 ml/cycle) (Figure 38.6). The results after partial TCRE were not as impressive despite favourable subjective impressions from the patients. It seems that the amount of residual endometrium at the end of surgery is critical. Less satisfactory results were found in women under the age of 35 years, though the results of surgery were not influenced by the presence of fibroids.

Effects on the Uterine Cavity

The effects of TCRE on the uterine cavity when assessed by hysteroscopy at 3 and 12 months post-resection are marked funcal fibrosis and occasionally total obliteration of the uterine cavity. Histological examination of tissue biopsies from the uterine wall showed, perhaps surprisingly, the presence of microscopic deposits of endometrium in 25% of amenorrhoeic women. This is in keeping with Asherman's first description of his syndrome (Asherman, 1948) and has obvious implications for the management of the menopause in these patients with respect to the use of hormone replacement therapy.

Ultrasonographic examination of the uterus shows no change in the total volume, but a definite shrinkage of the uterine cavity, from an

Figure 38.2 Menstrual flow after transcervical resection of the endometrium.

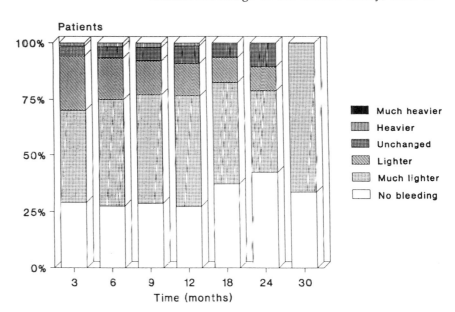

Figure 38.3 Menstrual duration after transcervical resection of the endometrium.

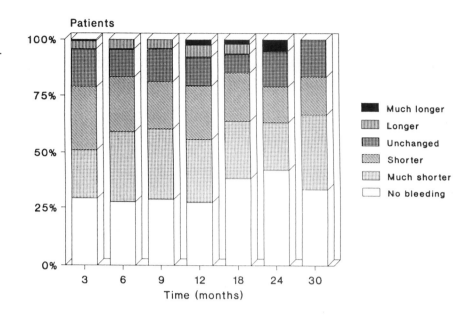

Figure 38.4 Menstrual pain after transcervical resection of the endometrium.

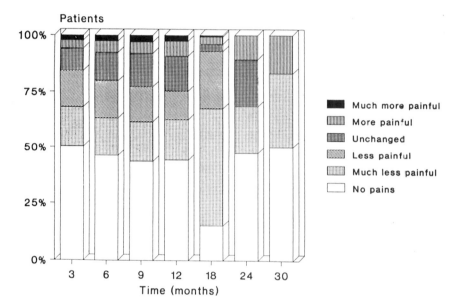

average of 3 ml to 1 ml, presumably a consequence of the fibrosis (unpublished observations).

Long-term Outcome

The effects of total TCRE in the long term have not yet been assessed. With the introduction of any new surgical procedure, the interest generated by impressive short-term results can overshadow the importance of careful assessment of long-term outcome, not only with respect to effect on menstruation, but also, for example, the chance of unwanted pregnancy or potential malignant change within the uterine cavity. For instance, a recent large retrospective comparison of transurethral resection of the prostate with open prostatectomy showed a small but significantly increased

risk of death from cardiovascular causes for up to 8 years following the endoscopic procedure (Roos *et al.*, 1989). Obviously, this cannot be directly applied to hysteroscopic endometrial surgery, but it serves to illustrate the potential for long-term problems which may not be predictable from the short-term experience. This possibility must be conveyed to the patient.

Complications of Transcervical Resection of the Endometrium

Potential benefits of surgery must be balanced with the potential hazards, and nowhere is this more important than when a new technique or

Figure 38.5 Patient satisfaction of menstrual effects following transcervical resection of the endometrium.

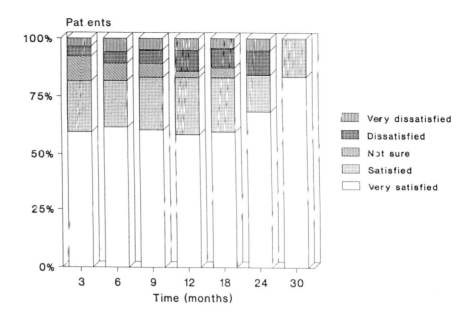

Figure 38.6 Actual menstrual blood loss (MBL) after transcervical resection of the endometrium.

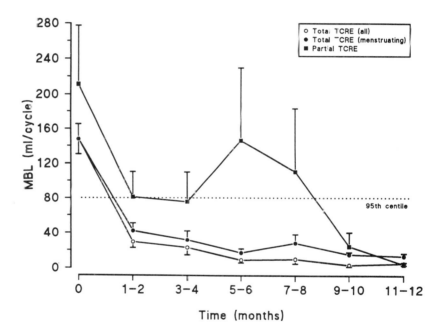

procedure is introduced. Assessment of the complications of new procedures in isolation is important but more pertinent is a comparison with the procedure it is replacing.

Hysterectomy has a low but definite mortality rate of 6/10 000 when performed for benign disease, but the associated morbidity is far more prevalent. Dicker *et al.*'s large American audit (1982) reports startlingly high morbidity rates of 24.5/100 and 42.8/100 for vaginal and abdominal hysterectomies respectively. Recognized long-term morbidity such as cardiovascular disease (Centerwall, 1981) urinary and bowel dysfunction (Taylor *et al.*, 1989), and premature ovarian failure (Siddle *et al.*, 1987) are equally worrying. This needs to be kept in mind when assessing new hysteroscopic procedures.

Uterine Perforation

Uterine perforation and fluid overload are probably the most potentially dangerous complications following TCRE (Table 38.5). Uterine perforation was documented in our initial series using the resectoscope (Magos *et al.*, 1989b), as well as with other methods of endometrial ablation such as laser vaporization (Goldrath *et al.*, 1981). In our later series there were four uterine perforations (1.6%), and this correlates with other reports of between 1 and 3.7% when using the resectoscope (Maher and Hill, 1990; Magos *et al.*, 1991; Pyper and Haeri, 1991; Sturdee and Hoggart, 1991) and with the 1.5% rate reported by Macdonald and Phipps (1992) following their anonymous postal questionnaire surveying nearly 3000 resection

Table 38.5 Potential complications of endometrial resection

Intra-operative	Postoperative	
	Short term	Long term
Uterine perforation	Infection	Recurrence of symptoms
Fluid overload	Haematometra	Pregnancy
Primary haemorrhage	Secondary haemorrhage	(Uterine malignancy)
Gas embolism	Cyclical pain	
	Treatment failure	

procedures. It was noted in our series (Magos et al., 1991) that the uterine perforations occurred during the first 57 procedures and it was concluded that this complication is very much related to the experience of the operator. This observation was confirmed by Macdonald and Phipps (1992) who reported that 33% of uterine perforations occurred during the operator's first procedure and 52% during the first five procedures.

The mode of perforation is an important factor with regard to the consequences of this complication. Uterine perforation occurring during instrumentation of the uterus, whether during cervical dilatation, insertion of the resectoscope or when using polyp forceps or the flushing curette to evacuate the endometrial chippings, is unlikely to result in damage to the intra-abdominal viscera or blood vessels, hence laparoscopic inspection of the abdomen and pelvis will suffice. However, perforation occurring whilst the resectoscope is in use can easily damage adjacent structures such as bowel, bladder, large vessels and even ureters, and under these circumstances laparotomy is essential.

It can be difficult to diagnose uterine perforation, or put another way, it can be easy to miss. Visualization of the bowel or peritoneum through the hysteroscope is pathognomonic, but uterine perforation should also be suspected if there is a sudden absorption of uterine irrigant or if the abdomen becomes unduly distended. Under these conditions the procedure should be stopped and perforation excluded before recommencing. This complication occurs most commonly at the thinnest part of the uterine wall, namely the cornual regions of the uterine cavity, unfortunately the most difficult area to resect. Using the roller-ball to electrocoagulate this area may help to reduce but not eliminate the incidence of perforation, especially for the less experienced.

Fluid Overload

Of all complications, most attention has been focused on the risks of fluid overload as a result of absorption of the uterine distension/irrigation fluid. The use of non-electrolytic solutions such as 1.5% glycine for electrosurgery and the relatively non-compliant nature of the myometrium requiring high pressures to achieve uterine distension predispose to the absorption of large quantities of irrigant fluid producing what is known to the urologists as the transurethral resection (TUR) syndrome. This potentially lethal condition, with a spectrum of signs and symptoms including hyponatraemia, hypertension, congestive cardiac failure, neurological symptoms, haemolysis and coma, demands careful monitoring of fluid balance.

The dilutional effect of fluid absorption during endometrial resection using 1.5% glycine solution as the uterine irrigant has been reported in detail (Baumann et al., 1990; Boto et al., 1990). Detectable falls in haemoglobin and serum albumin concentrations do occur, but of greater clinical importance is the fall in serum sodium concentration which is directly proportional to the volume of irrigant absorbed (Figure 38.7). This dilutional effect can result in large fluctuations in electrolytes during surgery, which is particularly noticeable following perforation of the uterus (Figure 38.8).

In view of the potential seriousness of fluid overload with its sequelae we now have guidelines concerning fluid balance (Table 38.2) which are strictly adhered to, thereby eliminating the problem as surgery is abandoned well before there is any danger to the patient. Fluid balance measurements are made at frequent intervals and again at the end of surgery and the balance calculated. More refined methods of continuous monitoring using intravascular electrodes or 'tagged' glycine are currently being evaluated, although whether they will prove to be more effective or safer remains to be seen.

What has become evident from our initial studies (Magos et al., 1991) is that it is possible to identify women at increased risk of absorbing excessive volumes of irrigant solution: these are women who have patent fallopian tubes, have had no endometrial preparation preoperatively, and have uterine fibroids. It may be advisable to avoid this group of patients when first attempting endometrial resection.

Uterine Haemorrhage

Uterine haemorrhage is a surprisingly uncommon complication of endometrial resection considering

Figure 38.7 The relationship between plasma sodium concentration and the volume of 1.5% glycine solution absorbed. From *Lancet* (1990) i: 44, with permission.

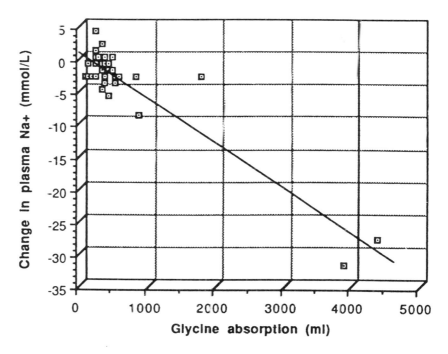

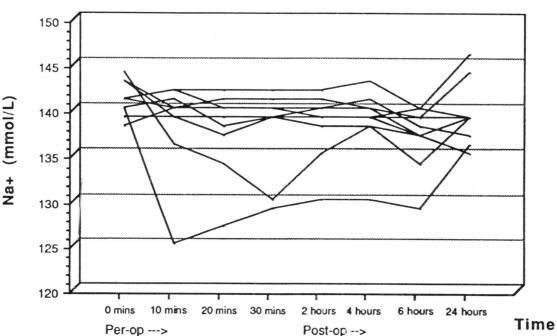

Figure 38.8 Changes in plasma sodium concentrations during and after transcervical resection of the endometrium when using 1.5% glycine solution for uterine distension. From *Progress in Obstetrics and Gynaecology* (1991), Vol. 9, J. Studd (ed.), with permission from Churchill Livingstone.

the vascularity of the uterus. Avoiding deep resection into the myometrial vascular bed is fundamental to avoiding this problem. Bleeding points may be cauterized using electrocoagulation under direct vision, but if bleeding persists tamponade of the uterine cavity is usually effective, using a 30 ml Foley catheter balloon for 6–8 hours. Endometrial preparation with gonadotrophin releasing hormone agonists or danazol may reduce the vascularity of the uterus

and hence the risk of haemorrhage, and rollerball electrocoagulation of the cervical canal may help prevent bleeding from this area.

Gas Embolism

Gas embolism has been reported as a complication of both laser endometrial ablation (Baggish and Daniell, 1989), being fatal on two occasions, and endometrial resection (Wood and Roberts, 1990). Air embolism can occur when an open vein is exposed to air at a greater pressure than that in the vein, such as when the operating site is raised above the level of the heart. Wood and Roberts (1990) suggest the use of positive pressure ventilation rather than spontaneous breathing during anaesthesia and not using the head-down position for nursing peri- and postoperative patients. Similarly, the use of irrigation pumps that employ air at pressure for delivery of the uterine irrigant should always have an air trapping system in use. Although a rare complication of endometrial resection, it should not be forgotten.

Infection

Assessing the true incidence of primary and secondary infection following endometrial resection has proved difficult, mainly because of the vague associated symptomatology occurring following discharge from hospital. However, in view of the potential risk of infection from instrumentation of the uterine cavity and intraperitoneal leakage of uterine irrigant trans-tubally, we would encourage the use of antibiotic prophylaxis until more information is available.

Haematometra and Cyclical Pain

The risk of cervical stenosis causing haematometra following total endometrial resection is more theoretical than real, and in fact, to our knowledge has never yet been described. Haematometra can occur following endometrial resection but is usually localized to the fundal area. The presence of haematometra may be suspected with symptoms of cyclical or constant pain and is readily diagnosed by ultrasonography. The haematometra is released by re-resecting and hence opening the uterine cavity. Whether this particular complication can be prevented by postoperative probing of the uterine cavity, as practised by some, remains to be seen.

Cyclical lower abdominal pain can occur following endometrial resection, even in the absence of haematometra, and this pain can be worse than menstrual pains reported prior to surgery. Asherman described this phenomenon in his report on intrauterine synechiae (Asherman, 1950), and it is likely to be a consequence of small islands of endometrium becoming buried within the myometrium, resulting in adenomyosis. This complication is difficult to treat; simple analgesia is often inadequate in severe cases, laparoscopic uterine nerve ablation may be an option but has not yet been adequately assessed, and ultimately hysterectomy may be required in the most severe cases.

Pregnancy

Both intrauterine and tubal pregnancies have been reported following endometrial resection. Most intrauterine pregnancies are terminated or spontaneously abort; however, uneventful term pregnancies have also been reported with no apparent fetal or placental complications (Maher and Hill, 1990) but there have been isolated cases of fetal growth retardation and fetal abnormality (Whitelaw and Sutton, 1993).

The risk of pregnancy following endometrial resection has not yet been quantified. It is important that preoperative counselling makes this clear and that appropriate contraceptive advice is given, offering those at risk the option of being sterilized.

Treatment Failure and Recurrence of Symptoms

Satisfactory menstrual results can be expected in 80–90% of patients following endometrial resection. Treatment failure therefore occurs only in a small minority. Recurrence of symptoms following successful surgery is relatively uncommon, most women benefiting from surgery in the early postoperative period continuing to do so. In our series, one patient who became amenorrhoeic following total endometrial resection relapsed 2 years later when her symptoms of menorrhagia recurred, but this is highly unusual. Those patients experiencing treatment failure or recurrence of symptoms can be safely retreated with a second resection procedure, or hysterectomy if requested.

Uterine Malignancy

There is no reason to believe that endometrial resection, or endometrial ablative techniques *per se*, should result in an increased risk of uterine malignancy. What is of greater concern is the possibility of malignancy arising in buried islands of residual endometrium and presenting at a later stage than would be expected. As yet, this is still a theoretical risk.

If the question of hormone replacement therapy arises then we would advocate the use of combined hormone replacement as endometrial glands and stroma may be present even in those women who have become amenorrhoeic following endometrial resection. Under these circumstances, the possibility of endometrial atypia and even malignancy may occur with the use of unopposed oestrogen therapy.

Comparison of Endometrial Ablation Techniques

Other endometrial ablative techniques include laser ablation, radiofrequency-induced thermal ablation (RITEA) and 'roller-ball' electrocoagulation (RBE). Taking into account that TCRE is a more recent procedure with a shorter follow-up than laser ablation, the efficacy in treating abnormal menstruation in terms of amenorrhoea and hypomenorrhoea is comparable. This is probably true for RITEA, although it must be emphasized that the use of this technique is limited to treating dysfunctional uterine bleeding, that is, those cases that have an essentially normal uterine cavity in terms of size and shape. All the techniques of endometrial ablation have their advantages and disadvantages, and the choice of technique is somewhat dependent on availability of equipment and preference of the individual surgeon performing the operation. We believe TCRE to be the preferred surgical option in terms of faster operating time, the ability to deal effectively with abnormally enlarged cavities and submucous fibroids, and the lesser capital outlay and maintenance of the equipment. TCRE is the only technique which provides an operative specimen for histological assessment. Pertinent to this advantage, a recent case report describes a woman who was found to have a small focus of endometrial carcinoma in the resected chippings which had been missed both by hysteroscopy and endometrial sampling preoperatively (Dwyer and Stirrat, 1991). Ultimately, the best technique is the one that the surgeon feels most confident with.

Conclusion

The emergence of a safe and effective surgical alternative to hysterectomy is undoubtedly attractive enough to dramatically change everyday gynaecological practice. The advantages to the patient and the health service in terms of shorter hospitalization, faster recovery, reduced discomfort and disfigurement, and impressive financial savings (Rutherford and Glass, 1990) speak for themselves. It is important, however, before the widespread introduction of endometrial ablative techniques, that a scientific comparison with the 'gold standard', hysterectomy, is performed. Controlled trials are now underway in several centres, including a multicentred study coordinated from our unit in London. The medium- and long-term effects and morbidity are are as yet unknown, and until they are the full facts regarding endometrial ablation cannot be given to the patients.

Acknowledgements

The authors gratefully acknowledge the information supplied by Mr Edward Shaxted, Consultant Obstetrician and Gynaecologist at Northampton, England, and Mr Eddie Holt, Consultant Obstetrician and Gynaecologist at Reading, England.

References

Amin HK & Neuwirth RS (1983) Operative hysteroscopy utilizing dextran as distending medium. *Clinical Obstetrics and Gynecology* 26: 277–284.

Asherman JG (1948) Amenorrhoea traumatica atretica. *Journal of Obstetrics and Gynaecology of the British Empire* 55: 23–30.

Asherman JG (1950) Traumatic intra-uterine adhesions. *Journal of Obstetrics and Gynaecology of the British Empire* 57; 892–896.

Baggish MS & Daniell JF (1989) Catastrophic injury secondary to the use of coaxial gas-cooled fibres and artificial sapphire tips for intrauterine surgery. *Lasers in Surgery and Medicine* 9: 581–584.

Baumann R, Magos AL, Kay JDS & Turnbull AC (1990) Absorption of glycine irrigating solution during transcervical resection of the endometrium. *British Medical Journal* 300: 304–305.

Boto TCA, Fowler CG, Cockroft S & Djahanbakch O (1990) Absorption of irrigating fluid during transcervical resection of endometrium. *British Medical Journal* 300: 748–749.

Brooks PG, Serden SP & Davos I (1991) Hormonal inhibition of the endometrium for resectoscopic endometrial ablation. *American Journal of Obstetrics and Gynecology* 161: 1601–1608.

Centerwall BS (1981) Premenopausal hysterectomy and cardiovascular disease. *American Journal of Obstetrics and Gynecology* 139: 58–61.

Cornier E (1986) Traitement hysterofibroscopique ambulatoire des metrorragies rebelles par laser Nd:YAG.

Journal de Gynécologie, Obstétrique et Biologie de la Reproduction **15**: 661–664.

Coulter A, Bradlow J, Agass M, Martin-Bates C & Tulloch A (1991) Outcomes of referrals to gynaecology outpatient clinics for menstrual problems: an audit of general practice records. *British Journal of Obstetrics and Gynaecology* **98**: 789–796.

DeCherney AH & Polan ML (1983) Hysteroscopic management of intrauterine lesions and intractable uterine bleeding. *Obstetrics and Gynecology* **61**: 392–397.

DeCherney AH, Diamond MP, Lavy G & Polan ML (1987) Endometrial ablation for intractable uterine bleeding: hysteroscopic resection. *Obstetrics and Gynecology* **70**: 668–670.

Derman SG, Rehnstrom J & Neuwirth RS (1991) The long-term effectiveness of hysteroscopic treatment of menorrhagia and leiomyomas. *Obstetrics and Gynecology* **77**: 591–594.

Dicker RC, Greenspan JR, Strauss LT *et al.* (1982) Complications of abdominal and vaginal hysterectomy among women of reproductive age in the United States. *American Journal of Obstetrics and Gynecology* **144**: 841–848.

Dwyer NA & Stirrat GM (1991) Early endometrial carcinoma: an incidental finding after endometrial resection. Case report. *British Journal of Obstetrics and Gynaecology* **98**: 733–734.

Goldrath MH, Fuller TA & Segal S (1981) Laser photovaporization of endometrium for the treatment of menorrhagia. *American Journal of Obstetrics and Gynecology* **140**: 14–19.

Hallez J-P, Netter A & Cartier R (1987) Methodical intrauterine resection. *American Journal of Obstetrics and Gynecology* **156**: 1080–1084.

Hill DJ & Maher PJ (1990) Intrauterine surgery using electrocautery. *Australian and New Zealand Journal of Obstetrics and Gynaecology* **30**: 145–146.

Jeppsson S, Mellquist P & Rannevik G (1984) Short-term effects of danazol on endometrial histology. *Acta Obstetrica et Gynecologica Scandinavica* **123**: 41–44.

Lockwood M, Magos AL, Baumann R & Turnbull AC (1990) Endometrial resection when hysterectomy is undesirable, dangerous or impossible. *British Journal of Obstetrics and Gynaecology* **97**: 656–658.

Macdonald R & Phipps J (1992) Endometrial ablation: a safe procedure. *Gynaecological Endoscopy* **1**: 7–9.

Magos AL, Baumann R, Cheung K & Turnbull AC (1989a) Intra-uterine surgery under intravenous sedation: an out-patient alternative to hysterectomy. *Lancet* **ii**: 925–926.

Magos AL, Baumann R & Turnbull AC (1989b) Transcervical resection of the endometrium in women with menorrhagia. *British Medical Journal* **298**: 1209–1212.

Magos AL, Baumann R, Lockwood GM & Turnbull AC (1991) Experience with the first 250 endometrial resections for menorrhagia. *Lancet* **337**: 1074–1078.

Maher PJ & Hill DJ (1990) Transcervical endometrial resection for abnormal uterine bleeding—report of 100 cases and review of the literature. *Australian and New Zealand Journal of Obstetrics and Gynaecology* **30 (4)**: 357–360.

Pyper RJD & Haeri AD (1991) A review of 80 endometrial resections for menorrhagia. *British Journal of Obstetrics and Gynaecology* **98**: 1049–1054.

Reid PC & Sharp F (1988) Hysteroscopic Nd:YAG endometrial ablation: an *in vitro* and *in vivo* laser–tissue interaction study. Abstract. *IIIrd European Congress on Hysteroscopy and Endoscopic Surgery*, Amsterdam, p 70.

Roos NP, Wennberg JE, Malenka DJ *et al.* (1989) Mortality and reoperation after open and transurethral resection of the prostate for benign prostatic hyperplasia. *New England Journal of Medicine* **320**: 1120–1124.

Rutherford AJ & Glass MR (1990) Management of menorrhagia. *British Medical Journal* **301**: 290–291.

Rutherford AJ, Glass MR & Wells M (1991) Patient selection for endometrial resection. *British Journal of Obstetrics and Gynaecology* **98**: 228–230.

Siddle N, Sarrel P & Whitehead MI (1987) The effect of hysterectomy on the age of ovarian failure: identification of a subgroup of women with premature loss of ovarian function and literature review. *Fertility and Sterility* **47**: 94–100.

Sturdee D & Hoggart B (1989) Problems with endometrial resection. *Lancet* **337**: 1474.

Taylor T, Smith AN & Fulton PM (1989) Effect of hysterectomy on bowel function. *British Medical Journal* **299**: 300–301.

Whitelaw N & Sutton C (1993) Nine years experience of endoscopic surgery in a District General Hospital. In Sutton CJG (ed.) *New Surgical Techniques in Gynaecology*. Carnforth, Lancs: Parthenon Publishing.

Wingo PA, Huezo CM, Rubin GL *et al.* (1985) The mortality risk associated with hysterectomy. *American Journal of Obstetrics and Gynecology* **152**: 803–808.

Wood SM & Roberts FL (1990) Air embolism during transcervical resection of endometrium. *British Medical Journal* **300**: 945.

39

Endometrial Electroablation

THIERRY G. VANCAILLIE

Center for Gynecologic Endosurgery, Texas, USA

Introduction

Although most gynaecologists view electrocoagulation of the endometrium as 'new' and 'innovative', the actual history of this technique stretches back over half a century. In 1948, Baumann reported a high degree of success with the technique and, indeed, this mode of therapy was extremely popular in Germany, Austria and the Netherlands (Bardenheuer, 1937; Baumann, 1948)—this, despite the fact that the necessary technology was, at that time, virtually in its infancy. Surgeons in those days used a 5–8 mm steel ball electrode on a 20 cm long insulated shaft, employing the electrode in a blind fashion, using no anaesthesia of any kind. Such a procedure would hardly be acceptable today! Despite these handicaps, Baumann, reporting on 387 cases treated in this manner over a period of 10 years, experienced an astoundingly low failure/complication rate of only 3.4% (Table 39.1).

Economic and political change often result in dramatic shifts in therapeutic modalities, but nowhere is this influence more apparent than in the history of endometrial electrocoagulation. Born in a time of economic hardship and high-risk anaesthesia and fostered during the wartime shortage of hospital beds, the technique foundered in the relative affluence of the 1950s, because of the unjustified association with the use of X-rays or radium for 'menolysis' which were subsequently found to cause secondary malignancies. Furthermore, the fashionable trend at that time was to extend the limits of invasive

surgery. Proponents of electrocoagulation, such as Baumann, continued to defend the technique— but their 'voice in the wilderness' went unheeded. As the rise–fall–rise course of this modality appears to have been largely determined by extrinsic factors, the student of history may justifiably ask what shift in economic, political or social factors has produced the recent resurgence of interest in this form of therapy. Certainly the current economic climate plays a role, but I think the increasingly greater involvement of the patient in the decision-making process probably is the decisive factor, along with greater awareness on the part of both the physician and the patient concerning any possible undesirable secondary effects of clinical interventions. Although the old reports made no mention concerning possible secondary malignancy following electroablation, and although conclusions of this sort dare not be hastily drawn, there has indeed been no reported carcinogenesis—leading the clinician to a kind of cautious optimism.

Patient Selection

Electroablation is ideally suited for the treatment of bleeding which is excessive, rather than irregular. Surgery will reduce the amount of bleeding, but will not necessarily correct the erratic pattern of metrorrhagia. Endometrial carcinoma and other, less common conditions, remain

Table 39.1 Complications and failures after electrocoagulation of the endometrium as reported by Baumann (1948)

Indication	Number	Early comp.	Late comp.	Early hyst.	Late hyst.	Repeat el.
Metrorrhagia	324	2	1	2	1	2
Myoma	58	3	0	0	2	0
Postmenopause	5	0	0	0	0	0
Total	387	5	1	2	3	2
%	100.0	1.3	0.26	0.52	0.78	0.52

Comp., complication; hyst., hysterectomy; el., electrocoagulation.

the purview of other therapeutic modalities. The ideal candidate for electroablation is a multiparous woman with a uterus of normal size and heavy, but regular, bleeding, in whom sterilization has already been accomplished by previous tubal ligation. Early reports on this technique pointed out that greatest success was achieved in perimenopausal dysfunctional bleeding.

Reduction or complete elimination of menstrual bleeding is accompanied by certain beneficial side-effects. Dysmenorrhoea is usually diminished concomitant with reduction of flow. A reduction in premenstrual symptoms has been reported (Lefler, 1989; Lefler and Lefler, 1991) and the incidence of pelvic inflammatory disease or its recurrence may be reduced as well. An additional benefit of electroablation is that this technique offers both the patients and the surgeon a physiological indicator of its success—namely amenorrhoea.

If the objective of electroablation is actually one of its beneficial side-effects, the clinician's goal should be that of complete amenorrhoea. However, the subject should be reviewed thoroughly with the patient, to decide whether or not complete amenorrhoea is the goal. It is the experience of the writer that long-term persistence of amenorrhoea cannot be forecast with 100% certainty, and this fact should be made absolutely clear to the patient when she is counselled preoperatively, lest there be subsequent disappointment and misunderstanding.

Can endometrial ablation ever be a reliable alternative technique for sterilization? The answer depends on many factors, most of them related to the armamentarium of the surgeon's experience, skills and education. With advancing experience, the clinician will become more adept at predicting which patient will become reliably amenorrhoeic. Implementation of additional techniques and skills, e.g. hysteroscopy, will enable the operator to ensure amenorrhoea in a particular patient. The surgeon who has mastered only roller-ball

ablation is unnecessarily restricted. Obviously a thorough knowledge and understanding of the endocrinology and pharmacology of the lower genital tract is imperative. It hardly need be mentioned that patients should be absolutely certain they wish no future fertility; however, this decision is one that is often heavily influenced by years of menstrual problems.

Patient Counselling

Expectations

Because of the sometimes variable outcome, it is essential that patients considering or intending to undergo electrocoagulation of the endometrium be counselled thoroughly to prevent subsequent misunderstanding and/or disappointment. Those patients suffering from excessive menstrual flow will obtain relief from the procedure, whether or not total amenorrhoea is obtained. However, patients with other complaints, often multiple and minor, may be less enthusiastic about the outcome, if their prospects are not explained thoroughly and in detail prior to the surgery. Available information may be summarized for the patient as follows:

- Menstrual flow will be reduced in almost all (> 90%) cases.
- Post-surgical bleeding pattern is unpredictable.
- True dysmenorrhoea will almost certainly be reduced parallel to the reduction in menstrual flow; however, minor cramping similar to that of dysmenorrhoea may persist, even if amenorrhoea is obtained and there is no haematometra.
- Pelvic pain other than that of true dysmenorrhoea (e.g. endometriosis), but which the patient has mistakenly thought to be

dysmenorrhoea, will remain unchanged. Further examination and possible intervention (e.g. laparoscopy) may be needed to obtain a definitive diagnosis and/or relief.

• PMS (Lefler, 1989; Lefler and Lefler, 1991) symptoms are relieved, in the author's experience, only when total amenorrhoea is obtained. Obviously, progesterone-influenced symptoms, such as bloating and breast tenderness, will remain relatively unrelieved. Psychosomatically, the patient may obtain relief from the 'vicious circle' of PMS symptoms when the physical signs of the menstrual cycle are eliminated. Additionally, some women with PMS feel better in anticipation of the surgery, perhaps as a result of their decision to take further control of their lives by finally 'doing something about it'.

Complications

Preoperative hormonal treatment may result in side-effects such as hot flushes, but these are generally well-tolerated in the patient who has received adequate counselling. The more serious complications are:

• Intravasation
• Uterine perforation
• Electrosurgical accidents
• Excessive uterine bleeding
• Pregnancy

INTRAVASATION

Intravasation always occurs! No control system exists that can totally eliminate this danger. Intravasation occurs because tissue and capillary pressures (≤ 15 mmHg) are less than the pressure needed to distend the uterine cavity adequately (35 mmHg). The goal of the surgeon and his supporting operating room staff is, therefore, not elimination of intravasation, but its control within acceptable limits. Patients with normal metabolic functions should experience no difficulty with a fluid load of 1000 ml, and can tolerate even larger volumes. On the other hand, compromised patients such as those undergoing renal dialysis, will be unable to handle even a slight increase in vascular volume because of the resultant hyponatraemia and hypokalaemia. A brush-up course in electrolyte homeostasis would be helpful to the clinician, to assist him coping with the problems inherent in fluid overload. (Distension media are discussed in another chapter.) Only the salient points will be mentioned here.

Hyskon and similar hyperosmolar media cause haemodilution, not by direct fluid overload, but by osmosis. Diuretics are of no effect, because these macromolecules do not pass the renal filter. Indeed, diuretics may cause paradoxical hypervolaemia, because of the increased loss of free water in the presence of continued osmotic pressure.

Early on, we used Hyskon, because this was the medium with which we had had the most experience, but it quickly became apparent that accidents resulting from intravasation were a major problem with this medium. The three most serious accidents occurred when Hyskon was being used as the distension medium. Aspiration pneumonia occurring in one patient undoubtedly came about as a result of her altered cognitive state due to hyponatraemia. Careful monitoring of electrolytes can avoid this major complication. Two other patients, with sickle cell trait, suffered a haemolytic crisis. Clearly, the complication rate with Hyskon is too high and macromolecular media are unsuitable for use with the resectoscope.

Hypoosmotic, non-conductive media such as sorbitol (with or without mannitol) and glycine are current favourites. Preoperative serum electrolyte values should always be obtained, to screen for borderline low values that can be corrected prior to surgery. Ingestion of a potassium-rich diet prior to operative hysteroscopy is also helpful, and should be routinely prescribed.

When fluid overload does occur, diuresis can be initiated by use of diuretics (furosemide, USA; frusemide, UK). Sorbitol admixed with mannitol will initiate diuresis by itself. All diuretics result in sodium and potassium loss and replacement should be initiated at the time of diagnosis, rather than waiting for values to drop below normal. For example, an i.v. infusion of Ringer's lactate with added potassium (e.g. 4 mEq/100 ml) at a rate of 50 ml/h can be administered. When fluid overload of ≥ 1000 ml occurs, it is advisable to monitor serum electrolyte values until excess fluid has been filtered out. Note that, at the time of diagnosis (usually toward the end of the procedure), peripheral serum values may still be normal, due to a latency period in redistribution of fluids. Although an increase in diuresis in the patient is certainly welcome at this time, concomitant loss in sodium and potassium is also increased.

A thorough understanding of the dynamics of electrolyte balance is essential in the immediate postoperative period. A patient may appear to be doing fine following a procedure, and be allowed to go home 2 hours later. Upon arriving home, she may experience malaise and nausea or even become disoriented. Such an experience will leave the patient and her family with unpleasant recollections of the surgery, to say the least. Moreover, more serious complications, such as aspiration pneumonia, could ensue, especially if the patient's state of consciousness is affected.

Fluid overload is less likely to occur if only a large contact electrode, such as the roller, is employed during the procedure, because tissue is coagulated rather than cut, sealing rather than severing the vessels. However, if such a large contact electrode is used improperly it may slowly burn a path into the uterine wall, opening venous sinuses in the process.

To summarize, fluid balance must be monitored at all times and under all circumstances. An easy way to accomplish this is to recover the distension fluid, using direct aspiration under low negative pressure, collecting the recovered fluid in containers of the same volume as the infusion bottles, thus enabling quick, easy measurement and comparison.

UTERINE PERFORATION

This is the one complication that should never occur, as the endoscope is introduced under direct visual control! However, cervical dilatation preceding insertion of the resectoscope does sometimes result in perforation, which, of course, signals immediate termination of the procedure, as a perforated uterus cannot hold the distension medium. Once the resectoscope is inserted into the endometrial cavity, there should be no problem with outright perforation. Incomplete perforation remains a pitfall, however. Although it does not prevent retention of the medium and distension of the uterine cavity, the resultant increased intravasation into the vascular system represents a hazard.

ELECTROSURGICAL ACCIDENTS

Fortunately, electrosurgical accidents rarely occur. Such misadventures are often the result of defective insulation and connectors and, for this reason, electrodes should be considered disposable items. If prolonged contact with any one place on the uterine wall for any extended period of time is avoided, burning through the wall of the uterus will not occur. However, thinner areas (such as the tubal ostia and uterotomy sites) can permit conduction of heat to neighbouring organs, with resulting injury. Particularly where there is direct and continuous contact, as in uterine–bladder or uterine–bowel adhesions, this heat conduction can result in necrosis and

subsequent breakdown of the wall of the bladder or bowel. For this reason, coagulation at the level of the uterotubal junction and at uterotomy scars must be conducted with extreme care.

The most dangerous aspect of accidental electrical burns from large contact electrodes is that no symptoms will be noted until several days following the procedure. For this reason, patients should be instructed to report any unusual symptoms such as haematuria, diarrhoea, fever or pain. Any pain, 24 hours after the procedure, requiring pain medication other than aspirin or panadol, should be carefully investigated. In early reports, mention was made of fistula formation between the uterus and small bowel (treated by expectant management for up to 9 weeks). The large contact electrodes are much less likely to burn through the uterine wall than are the loop electrodes, the latter being designed for precisely that purpose, thus making large contact electrodes the preferred choice for the operator on the learning curve of this technique.

EXCESSIVE UTERINE BLEEDING

Excessive uterine bleeding rarely occurs, and is more likely to be the result of overly energetic cervical dilatation than of electrocoagulation. If electrocoagulation is performed during an episode of heavy bleeding, uterine flow will be reduced significantly postoperatively. Indeed, in the 1930s and 1940s, procedures were performed during ongoing metrorrhagia for the purpose of interrupting (successfully) excessive bleeding. Postoperative bleeding should not exceed that of normal menstrual flow—an annoyingly vague concept, but one the patient understands quite well. Should postoperative bleeding exceed this, a potential problem should be suspected and investigated. Any lacerations of the cervix should be cauterized and repaired. If the bleeding seems to emanate from the uterine cavity itself, an intramuscular injection of methylergometrine (Methergin) (0.2 mg) should be administered. Branches of the uterine vessels can be injured through laceration of the uterine sidewall, whether electrosurgically or mechanically induced. Such injury is rare, however, if only large contact electrodes are used for intrauterine surgery.

Whether antibiotics should be administered prophylactically remains an open question. There have been occasional, unpublished reports indicating that peritonitis can occur in the immediate and late postoperative periods. Baumann reported on three such incidents, out of a series of 387 cases, in 1948. The important thing to remember is that the symptoms of infection did not occur until at least 4 days following the procedure.

PREGNANCY

Pregnancy, either intrauterine or ectopic, can occur as a long-term complication. The estimated risk is approximately 1%. However, there are no reliable statistics for the occurrence of pregnancy, and this figure should be understood to apply only to experienced operators.

Endometrial Suppression

Preoperative endometrial suppression reduces the bulk of the endometrial tissue and makes surgery easier; furthermore, a suppressed endometrium is less likely to recover from a surgical insult, thus enhancing the effectiveness of endometrial electroablation. It is difficult to recommend any one hormonal regimen above another; probably the regimen most familiar to the physician and most convenient for the patient is the one to recommend. We use a single intramuscular injection of LHRH analogue (leuprolide depot (Lupron Depot) 7.5 mg) during the luteal phase of the cycle, and 2–3 weeks prior to the date of surgery. Lupron Depot is effective for approximately 6 weeks, thus a single dose provides both pre- and postoperative endometrial suppression.

Operative Technique

Room Set-up and Positioning of the Patient (Figure 39.1)

The patient should be placed in the dorsal lithotomy position. On one side, the instrument table and scrub technician should be situated; the video monitor and fluid containers should be located on the other. Ideally, a heating blanket should be available.

Anaesthesia

Virtually any form of anaesthesia can be used for endometrial electroablation. Note, however, that heat sensation is not blocked by local anaesthesia and, additionally, patients may experience some pain under local anaesthesia (i.e. paracervical

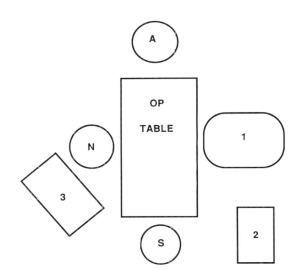

Figure 39.1 Room set-up. This diagram gives a schematic overview of the special arrangement of the operating room. A, anaesthesiologist; N, nurse; S, surgeon; 1, video cart; 2, in and outflow; 3, instrument table.

block) when the surgeon operates in the cornual areas. The anaesthesiologist should be instructed concerning the potential for fluid overload and the need to limit intravenous infusion.

Even when general anaesthesia is used, a paracervical block is useful; its anaesthetic effect will last some hours beyond the actual intervention, reducing the need for postoperative pain medication.

Vasoconstrictive Agents

If one anticipates using the cutting loop, it is helpful to administer a vasoconstrictor (Pitressin) in conjunction with local anaesthesia. In addition, use of such a vasoconstrictive agent permits a virtually bloodless D & C prior to electroablation and, when injected into the cervix, the vasoconstrictor seems to make cervical dilatation easier. We find the use of vasoconstrictive agents extremely helpful, and use them for all hysteroscopic interventions except synechiolysis.

Cervical Dilatation

The operator must take great care in cervical dilatation. First, an obvious laceration or perforation automatically signals termination of the procedure; however, even more importantly, an unnoticed, perhaps incomplete perforation or laceration will almost certainly lead to rapid fluid overload owing to the injury to the large venous sinuses. Many surgeons routinely employ laminaria preoperatively to assist in cervical dilatation. We do not use laminaria, because we find they make it more difficult to distinguish the internal cervical os; furthermore, a cervical dilatation of 10 mm is sufficient, and this can usually be achieved easily with any type of mechanical dilator.

Curettage

Following cervical dilatation, a thorough suction curettage must be carried out to remove as much debris and endometrium as is possible. To encourage thorough curettage, it is helpful for the surgeon to set a time period (e.g. 3 minutes) for this procedure and then have someone actually time him, with a stopwatch, so he does not inadvertently shorten this extremely important step. If no endometrial sampling was performed earlier, a specimen(s) should be obtained at this point for histological evaluation.

Selection of the Electrode

A variety of electrodes are now on the market, presenting the surgeon with the luxury, and burden, of making a choice. What constitutes an ideal electrode? Ideally, it would have no fixed form at all, but would rather adapt itself to whatever contour it encounters. Unfortunately, such an instrument exists only in the imagination at the moment! Given that one must make a very real choice among very real instruments, what factors are important, and what do we know about these factors?

THE SHAPE

My personal favourite is the ball-shaped electrode, because this shape seems best adapted to the irregularities one encounters. However, the effectiveness, electrophysically, of the various shapes of the electrodes has been investigated very little.

THE SIZE

The electrode must permit an adequate field of view for the endoscopist, and thus be relatively small.

TRANSMISSION OF ELECTRICAL ENERGY FROM THE AXIS TO THE ROTATING PART

This is an aspect of configuration that is very important for optimal transmission of the electrical energy from the electrode to the tissue. A loose connection will allow internal sparking between the axis and the bulk of the electrode. This will result in interruption of energy transfer. One example of a good electrode, is one designed by Electroscope (Boulder, CO, USA) where the axis has been eliminated, thus reducing the possibility of uneven energy transfer within the electrode.

BUILD-UP OF CHAR ON THE ELECTRODE DURING SURGERY

The electrode has to allow good cooling within the resectoscope system, thus decreasing the amount of char that builds up on the contact area. Char is an electrical insulator indeed. Ongoing development in the design of electrodes mandates that the surgeon study the underlying principles that determine the effectiveness of each design.

Selection of the Waveform and Power Settings (Figures 39.2–39.5)

When a large electrode makes contact with tissue, coagulation and desiccation occur, because the energy immediately spreads, resulting in a decrease in the power density. Early in this century, studies established that low-power-density electrical energy used over a relatively long period of time will cause deeper tissue destruction than an equivalent amount of energy delivered at a high power density. This is because increased coagulation causes increased tissue impedance and a consequent decrease in current flow. Deep destruction (> 5 mm) would therefore be most effectively accomplished by using power of a continuous low-density waveform ('cutting current' at, e.g. < 20 W). Tissue destruction would be very slow, and therefore extremely difficult for the surgeon to gauge or control. The process is more easily understood, if the reader thinks of it as being divided into two phases: static and dynamic.

FIRST PHASE: INITIATION (Figures 39.2, 39.3)

The operator presses the electrode gently into contact with the tissue and activates the current. A relatively large volume of tissue will be destroyed and the electrode should be held in one spot as long as required until blanching is observed around the electrode (< 1 second).

SECOND PHASE: DYNAMIC (Figures 39.4, 39.5)

When blanching all around the electrode has been observed, the operator can then move the electrode

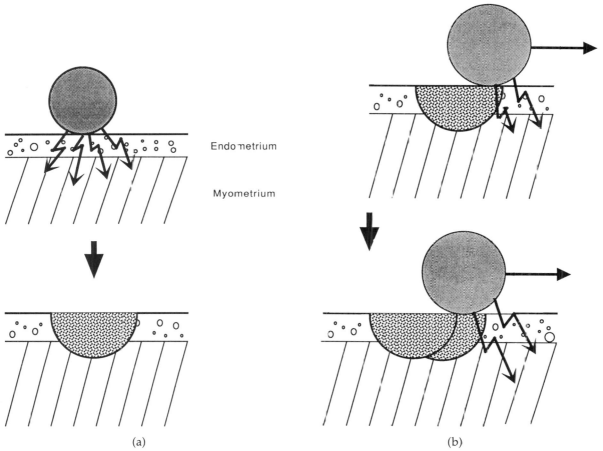

Endometrium

Myometrium

(a) (b)

Figure 39.2 Schematic representation of the bioeffect of electrical current on the endometrium in the initiation phase (a) and dynamic phase (b).

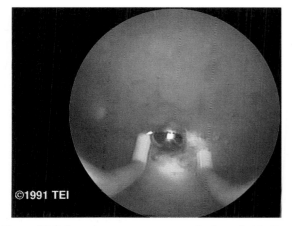

Figure 39.3 *In vivo* appearance of the 'initiation phase'. Courtesy of the Texas Endosurgery Institute.

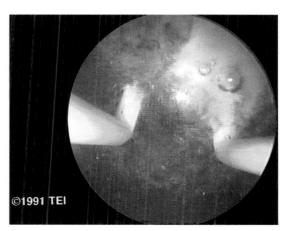

Figure 39.4 *In vivo* appearance of the coagulation effects preceding the electrode. Courtesy of the Texas Endosurgery Institute.

slowly toward the cervical canal. To determine how rapidly the electrode should be moved, the operator must watch the zone of visible tissue destruction preceding the electrode. A relatively high level of power is required to pass through the desiccated tissue and coagulate tissue in front

of it. Low-wattage 'coagulation current' best balances the need for surgical speed and required depth of tissue destruction. Different electrosurgical units vary in the amount of wattage they provide; however, 40–60 W usually will provide

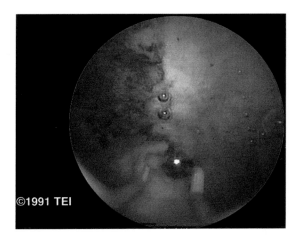

©1991 TEI

Figure 39.5 Aspect of the cavity after a single 'stroke' with the electrode. Courtesy of the Texas Endosurgery Institute.

sufficient energy to cause the desired level of destruction.

After the operator presses the electrode against the uterine wall and presses the control pedal, blanching should be visible around the electrode within one second. If the surgeon observes no visible effect, the connections should be checked and, if found intact, the power setting should be increased. On the other hand, rapid, explosive action indicates that the power setting is too high. When the surgeon is sure the power setting is appropriate, the electrode is rolled slowly toward the optic. The operator should be able to see the coagulation zone preceding the electrode at all times. As the electrode progresses beyond the original, rather wide, area of coagulation, only the advancing edge of the electrode contacts as-yet-uncoagulated tissue—a rather small area, comparatively. The rest of the electrode is passing over already coagulated tissue, where the current is impeded by the previous coagulation. This allows reduction in time of exposure, and therefore forward motion of the electrode. The most important aspect of the surgery is that the operator maintains a steady, but slow pace in moving the electrode over the surface.

The Operation

The point at which coagulation is begun is unimportant, but once begun, coagulation should be pursued in a systematic fashion, and this sequence religiously followed, whether it be clockwise or counterclockwise. During the procedure, the surgeon should inspect both tubal ostia, note any visible uterotomy scars and be on the lookout for any unexpected pathology. The areas where complications are likely to arise are those that are technically most difficult to reach, namely areas of the fundus and tubal ostia. Rolling the electrode is often impossible in these areas; thus, the electrode must be placed in one spot, activated, retrieved, then relocated, activated again, and so on, until the entire fundus and adjacent cornual areas are coagulated. The operator must take care not to force the electrode into the tubal ostia.

It is important to locate the internal cervical os, because this represents the limit of coagulation. The operator should retrieve the resectoscope into the cervical canal, thus temporarily occluding the outflow and permitting visualization of the internal cervical os. It is not all that easy to determine the precise anatomical site and if laminaria have been used for dilatation, this problem is made even more difficult. It is sometimes helpful to stain the mucosa of the uterus with methylene blue (a single drop diluted in 10–20 ml of physiological solution and slowly instilled into the uterine cavity prior to dilatation). The operator can then use a 5 mm endoscope to perform a diagnostic hysteroscopy. The endometrium will be coloured evenly blue, the endosalpinx will appear as dark blue spots, and the endocervix will appear as parallel blue lines.

To wrap up the electrocoagulation, the surgeon inspects the uterine cavity for any areas that appear untouched. Because the coagulation has significantly altered the appearance of the endometrial surface, this is no easy process and emphasizes the need for careful, systematic coagulation in the first place. Evaluation for adenomyosis is aided by the fact that the coagulated interface between endometrium and myometrium presents as transverse grooves (Figure 39.6). This is because the cell-rich tissue of the endometrium conducts electricity better than does the fibrous tissue of the myometrium, and will therefore be more thoroughly destroyed. When the operator rolls the electrode over such an area, he will feel a 'bump', much as the driver of an automobile experiences when he drives over a 'speed bump'. The coagulation of the glandular tissue in such areas may be incomplete, because endometrial glands reach deep into the myometrium, and resection is therefore indicated.

Spontaneous pneumothorax has been treated for several decades by the use of tetracycline hydrochloride as a sclerosing agent. Crystalline tetracycline (500 mg) is suspended in 3 ml of dextran, then slowly and gently injected into the uterine cavity. This drug is extremely caustic and spillage into the peritoneal cavity can lead to

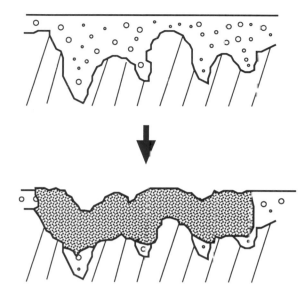

Figure 39.6 Graphic representation of the effect of an irregular interphase between endometrium and myometrium.

chemical peritonitis. Using a viscous distension medium, such as Hyskon, helps avoid this complication. Obviously, some of the instillate will escape into the vagina, and this must be cleansed away prior to concluding the surgery, in order to avoid vaginal irritation.

Follow-up

Vital signs, vaginal bleeding and diuresis must be monitored carefully during the immediate postoperative period. However, it is important to remember that bleeding and infection can arise several days following the surgery. It is therefore vital to keep in close contact with the patient for a period of 10 days or more—an extremely important point, for instance, should one be treating a patient who lives at some distance from the surgical clinic. A postoperative check should be scheduled within 10 days. At that time, any

delayed infection can be diagnosed and therapy begun. Two to three months following surgery, the patient should be checked a second time. Repeat ultrasonography can be performed at this visit, to determine uterine measurements. Many patients will present with an established menogram at this time. No intrauterine manipulation is performed, but pelvic examination should reveal a firm uterus that is slightly smaller than it was preoperatively.

Results

About 80% of patients will be extremely pleased with the results of their operations. Because patient satisfaction is determined to a large extent by patient expectations, adequate preoperative counselling is extremely important. Results should be assessed in terms of reduction in menstrual flow, but, because there is no accurate way to measure this, one must deal in total days per month of vaginal bleeding experienced by the patient. We define bleeding as follows:

- Amenorrhoea: total absence of any cyclic vaginal bleeding;
- Spotting: bleeding lasting less than half a day;
- Hypomenorrhoea: bleeding lasting less than 2 days.

It is often difficult to obtain reliable data concerning bleeding, because patients may not assess their own bleeding patterns reliably, e.g. if bleeding is sporadic, does not occur regularly, is so scant that it requires no protection, etc. In the latter case, the patient may report complete amenorrhoea, when this is not really the case. The difference between scant bleeding for half a day or less and no bleeding at all generally matters very little to the patient, and my initial

Table 39.2 Results of roller-ball electrocoagulation of the endometrium (author's experience: follow-up > 9 months)

Series	0 d	< 1/2 d	< 2 d	> 2 d	Re E.A.	Hyst.
A (n = 15)	*	10 (67)	1 (6)	4 (27)	1	1
B (n = 12)	1 (8)	4 (33)	3 (25)	4 (33)	1	2
C (n = 63)	17 (27)	24 (38)	16 (25)	6 (10)	0	0

Series A starts in June 1986, B in October 1988 and C in October 1989.
Numbers in parentheses are percentages.
Re E.A., repeat ablation; Hyst., hysterectomy; d, average number of days of menstrual bleeding per month.
* In series A the results of '0 d' and '< 1/2 d' are combined.

data also combined these two groups; however, in the interest of precision, I have, in my later data, separated these two groups. In Table 39.2, which shows the results in 90 patients treated between June 1986 and June 1991, series A represents the initial study (Vancaillie, 1989), series B represents the intermediary period, and series C reports the results using the method described in this chapter.

The observer will note that the results obtained in series A are superior to those in series B. This is because I capitulated to every surgeon's instinct to increase the speed of surgery by moving the electrode more rapidly, using an increased wattage. I later learned, through consultation with an electrical engineer, why precisely the reverse—low wattage and 'slow motion' surgery—were more effective in electroablation. The temptation to increase speed is one every surgeon must confront and resist, in the face of everything he has learned previously, if optimal results are to be obtained in electrocoagulation of the endometrium.

The main change made in series C was instillation of tetracycline hydrochloride suspended in dextran 70. The outcome in this series is difficult to assess because of an abundance of variables. For example, many more difficult cases, e.g. larger uterine cavities, were included. However, as yet, no patient in this group, which was larger than the other two, has requested a repeat ablation, nor has hysterectomy had to be performed due to failed treatment. A prospective study is currently under way to obtain more analysable data along the same guidelines.

If one defines monthly bleeding of 2 days or less as an acceptable result, 90% of patients have been cured by electroablation. Of the remaining 10%, three have undergone hysterectomy and two patients requested a second ablation. Both became amenorrhoeic as a result of the second operation. Repeat ablation is performed so seldom that we have no data on outcome following such a procedure. One patient of series B became pregnant. Her postoperative menstrual period lasted an average of 5 days.

Electroablation as a technique for endometrial suppression is still in its evolution. I believe that further investigation and refinement of the three components involved in this technique—hormonal endometrial inhibition, thermal destruction and scar formation—will ultimately produce the optimal technique for endometrial ablation.

References

Baumann A (1948) Ueber die Elektrokoagulation des Endometriums sowie der Zervikalschleimhaut. *Geburtshilfe und Frauenheilkunde* **8**: 221.

Bardenheuer R (1937) Elektrokoagulation der Uterusschleimhaut zur Behandlung klimakterischer Blutungen. *Zentralblatt für Gynäkologie* 209.

Lefler Jr H (1989) Premenstrual syndrome: improvement after laser ablation of the endometrium for menorrhagia. *Journal of Reproductive Medicine* 34: 905.

Lefler, Jr H & Lefler CF (1991) Ablation of the endometrium: a three year follow-up of improvement in perimenstrual symptoms. *Journal of Reproductive Medicine* **36**.

Vancaillie T (1989) Electrocoagulation of the endometrium with the ball-end resectoscope. *Obstetrics and Gynecology* **74**: 425.

40

Nd:YAG Laser Ablation of the Endometrium

MILTON H. GOLDRATH* AND RAY GARRY‡

*Sinai Hospital of Detroit, Michigan, USA
‡Women's Endoscopic Laser Foundation, South Cleveland Hospital, Middlesbrough, Cleveland, UK

Until recently, women with normal uteri who did not respond to pharmacological intervention for the treatment of menorrhagia were limited to one of two options: hysterectomy or continued cycles of heavy menstrual bleeding. With the advent of hysteroscopic laser ablation of the endometrium in 1979 (Goldrath et al., 1981), women with menorrhagia refractory to, or unable to tolerate other methods of therapy were offered an alternative to hysterectomy. Laser ablation has also been employed in recent years to treat menorrhagic patients with moderate-sized fibroids (Goldrath 1990a). Thus, the number of patients for whom this procedure is potentially beneficial is quite sizeable.

The primary objective of laser ablation of the endometrium is to limit uterine bleeding or produce amenorrhoea—in essence, Asherman's syndrome. Asherman (1948), identified uterine synechiae, usually resulting from post-abortal or postpartum uterine curettage, as the cause of the amenorrhoea and infertility in his patients.

It soon became apparent that any technique capable of reproducing Asherman's syndrome might be used to correct excessive uterine bleeding. Subsequently, a variety of chemical and physical methods were used for this purpose, the majority of which proved unsuccessful. While radium and cryocoagulation were both associated with some limited success, radium is no longer used, and the cryocoagulation procedure described by Droegemueller et al. (1971a, b) was abandoned because of the potential for producing painful haematometra. DeCherney and Polan (1983) have successfully destroyed the endometrium and produced amenorrhoea through the use of a high-frequency coagulating current employing a modified urological resectoscope and, more recently, others have done the same using the so-called roller-ball technique (Townsend et al., 1987; Vancaillie, 1989) with electrosurgery.

Photocoagulation of the Endometrium with the Nd:YAG Laser

The neodymium:yttrium–aluminium–garnet (Nd: YAG), is particularly well suited to photocoagulation of the endometrium as a result of its high power and transmission through optical fibres. Its deep-tissue penetration (up to 4 mm beneath the surface) distinguished it from carbon dioxide and argon and KTP lasers.

Because of the danger to the surgeon's eye from backscatter after tissue impact, a protective filter over the eyepiece of the hysteroscope is essential or a video camera can be used.

Surgical Procedure

The human uterus is characterized by a relatively thick myometrium and thin endometrium, thus it is an ideal organ for laser surgery. The fact that only about 5% of the uterine thickness must be ablated in order to destroy the endometrium protects adjacent organs from thermal damage.

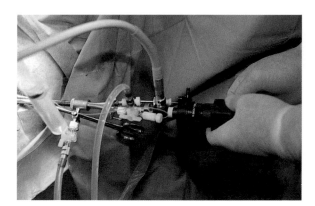

Figure 40.1 A Weck–Baggish hysteroscope with a laser fibre inserted in the left operating channel, a three-way tap with the fluid inflow and a catheter from the uterine cavity to a pressure transducer in the right channel, and a three-way tap for fluid outflow and syringe for channel flushing in the central channel.

Ringer's lactate or physiological saline are currently used to distend the uterus and have both proved to be excellent visualizing media. *Gaseous distending media are useful for diagnostic purposes, but should not be used for extensive therapeutic hysteroscopic surgery because of the risk of fatal gas embolism.*

The procedure is performed with the patient under general or spinal anaesthesia. A continuous-flow hysteroscope is used (Figures 40.1 and 40.2). The fluid flows in by gravity only and is removed by low suction to provide a constant flow of fluid at low pressure. This is important not only for a clear operative field, but also to prevent excessive fluid absorption. Alternatively, a pressure-controlled pump can be used, as described in Chapter 36 (Figure 40.3).

Endometrial photovaporization and photocoagulation are performed under direct visualization using a power output of at least 50 W, continuous

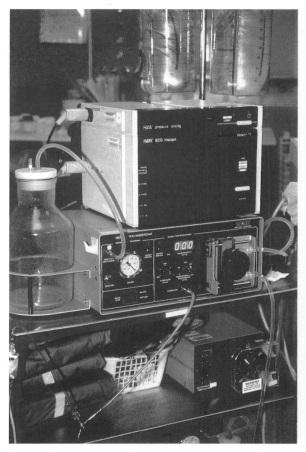

Figure 40.3 A uterine distension system using a Hamou Hysteromat.

wave. The entire endometrial lining is treated, commencing in the cornual area (Figure 40.4) and extending across the fundus and down the anterior and posterior walls to the isthmus (Figure 40.5), terminating 4 cm from the external cervical os. To avoid treating the endocervix, the level of the internal os (4 cm) is marked on the sheath of the hysteroscope. Care is also taken to avoid

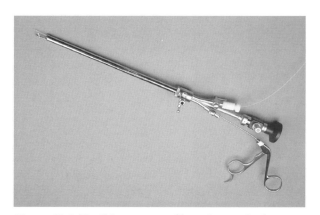

Figure 40.2 Flexible quartz fibre inserted down a channel of an operating hysteroscope.

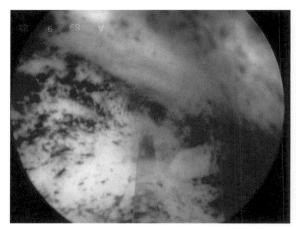

Figure 40.4 Laser quartz fibre applied close to the right tubal ostium prior to ablation.

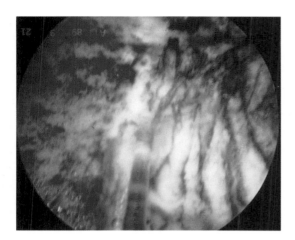

Figure 40.5 Laser quartz fibre 'dragging' a series of parallel furrows across the fundus of the uterine cavity.

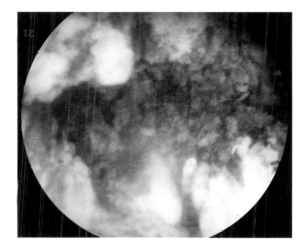

Figure 40.7 A completed ablation. All the endometrium has been removed with the Nd:YAG laser and the He–Ne aiming beam is seen glowing at the tip.

perforation near the tubal ostia, the thinnest portion of the uterus.

The desired end point is coagulation or charring of the entire endometrial surface (Figures 40.6 and 40.7). This procedure takes 30–40 minutes in a normal-sized uterus, longer in a larger uterus. After a long healing period, synechiae develop that are similar to those described by Asherman (Figures 40.8 and 40.9).

The preoperative use of danazol or GnRH agonists greatly facilitates ablation of the endometrium. This pharmacological manipulation decreases the thickness of the endometrial lining (Brooks *et al.*, 1991). Hysteroscopic examination

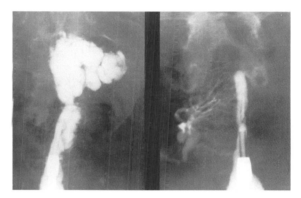

Figure 40.8 Hysterosalpingograms performed 3 months and 1 year post-laser ablation. Note complete obliteration of cavity and intravasation of dye.

reveals a very thin, atrophic endometrium in which telangiectases are prominent. It is interesting to note that this endometrium resembles that of a postmenopausal woman.

Clinical Experience in Detroit (USA) (Milton Goldrath)

To date, over 500 women have been operated upon in my department. The following is an analysis of 407 women aged 12–53 years having undergone 427 hysteroscopic laser procedures for the treatment of menorrhagia in the 11 years ending January 1990. More than 60% of the patients ($n = 274$) had fibroids, most of which

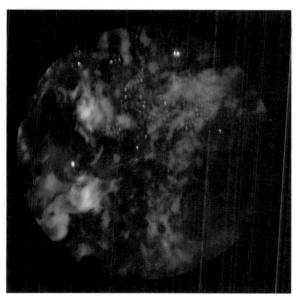

Figure 40.6 Tissue effects of endometrial ablation.

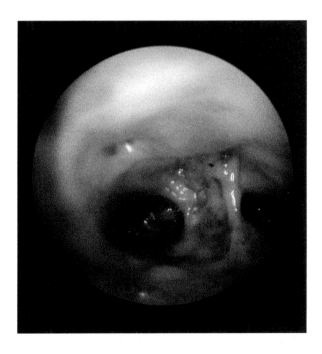

Figure 40.9 Synechiae 10 months post-laser ablation.

were submucous, or adenomyosis. The criteria for patient selection includes:

1. excessive and disabling bleeding;
2. inability or unwillingness to use other therapies;
3. future childbearing not desired; and
4. D & C within 6 months of the surgical procedure to rule out adenocarcinoma of the endometrium or its precursors.

For the past 8 years, patients had preoperative hysteroscopic evaluation as well.

The procedure is usually performed on an outpatient basis, with the patients discharged 2–3 hours later. Although severe cramping typically occurs for the first 2 hours following surgery, it has recently been noted that the use of bupivacaine hydrochloride (Marcaine) 0.25% with epinephrine (adrenalin) 1:200 000 paracervical block upon completion of the procedure greatly reduces the postoperative pain. The other postoperative symptoms resemble those associated with a D & C. All patients have varying degrees of serosanguineous discharge lasting for up to 4 weeks. None of the patients has become febrile.

Results

Table 40.1 summarizes the results of surgery. Overall, the results have been *excellent* in 379 procedures, 60% of which resulted in amenorrhoea and the remainder resulted in a few

days of spotting per cycle. Ten patients reported *good* results, meaning they were satisfied with treatment and experienced what they considered to be normal menstrual flow. Of the 35 procedures which yielded *poor* results, 19 of the 22 which were repeated resulted in amenorrhoea and three failed, necessitating hysterectomy. Of the remaining 13 failed patients, 12 underwent hysterectomy without retreatment and one has decided to put up with her menorrhagia.

Fifty-five of the patients had clotting disorders, all of whom did well following surgery. Twenty-two of the patients were receiving warfarin therapy. It should be noted that patients receiving danazol while on warfarin therapy may have a very marked increase in prothrombin time. This could produce spontaneous retroperitoneal haemorrhage among other complications. It is advisable in these patients to reduce the warfarin by one-half of the maintenance dose. Hysteroscopic laser ablation can be readily performed with the patient fully anticoagulated.

Of a total of 31 hysterectomies, 18 were laser successes (i.e. no excessive bleeding) and 13 laser failures (i.e. excessive bleeding). In two, laser use was abandoned because of the presence of large submucous myomas. In one patient cervical bleeding occurred 10 days postoperative necessitating hysterectomy. The latter complication deserves special comment. At the time, it was our practice to continue administering danazol for 2 weeks after the procedure. The patient was taking warfarin. Ten days following surgery, excessive, uncontrollable bleeding occurred, necessitating hysterectomy. It has since been published that the dose of warfarin must be reduced in patients receiving danazol therapy. The two drugs may be administered concomitantly, but warfarin dosage should be reduced by half. Prothrombin times should be checked every 3 days. However, it should again be restated that the use of GnRH agonists should eliminate the use of danazol in these patients.

Eight of the 13 hysterectomies where laser ablation failed had adenomyosis. Because of the

Table 40.1 Results of hysteroscopic laser surgery (Detroit)

Result		No. procedures
Excellent		379
Good		10
Poor		35
Early failure	17	
Late failure (1.5–8 years)	18	

possibility that adenomyosis was associated with endometrial regeneration, it was decided to administer a single 150 mg dose of medroxyprogesterone acetate to patients with suspected adenomyosis or submucous fibroids on the day of surgery in an attempt to delay regeneration until some scarring occurs. Sixty-nine per cent of the patients treated with medroxyprogesterone acetate became amenorrhoeic, as compared with only 37% of those who did not receive treatment. This difference was highly significant. The remaining patients were hypomenorrhoeic.

Complications

Table 40.2 lists the complications associated with laser ablation of the endometrium. The major complication observed with this procedure has been fluid overload, which led to pulmonary oedema in two cases. It should be noted that this problem occurred early on when a 'push' infusion method was used to distend the uterus. The use of a continuous-flow technique with gravity feed of fluid into the uterus and actively controlled suction out of the uterus, has largely avoided excessive absorption of distending medium.

Following surgery, profuse bleeding developed in 15 patients after release of irrigating pressure. The bleeding was controlled by balloon tamponade using a Foley catheter inserted into the uterus (Goldrath, 1983).

One and three months post-procedure, all patients undergo a suction curettage; if haematometra is found, suction curettage is performed weekly until the condition resolves. Routine suction curettage revealed 11 cases of postoperative haematometra. Experience suggested that if haematometra had not developed within 3 months following laser ablation, it would not develop

Table 40.2 Complications associated with hysteroscopic laser surgery (Detroit)

Complication	No. patients
Fluid overload (2 with pulmonary oedema)	6
Profuse bleeding (tamponade)	15
Urinary tract infection	3
Drug reaction	3
Uterine perforation	1
Cervical bleeding (hysterectomy)	1
Endomyometritis	1
Haematometra	20

subsequently. We have recently discovered nine cases of delayed haematometra. One developed 9 years following laser therapy. Four patients with recurrent haematometra were treated by insertion of an IUD. One had a hysterectomy performed at the time of an operation for stress urinary incontinence. If a patient develops cyclic pain or other symptoms of haematometra, ultrasonic examination should be diagnostic.

Three patients had allergic reactions to danazol. The reaction was mild in two cases, and therapy was continued. One patient had to discontinue treatment because of a severe allergic reaction.

Three patients had postoperative urinary tract infections related to intraoperative catheter drainage.

In one patient purulent endomyometritis developed approximately 1 week postoperatively. Although asymptomatic, she was hospitalized for 2 days and treated with intravenous antibiotics. The purulent discharge immediately stopped. She did not become febrile.

Laser ablation was not completed in one patient due to an instrument-related uterine perforation. The laser was not being used at that time. The patient returned to the hospital 2 months later, at which time the laser procedure was completed.

Clinical Experience in Princeton (USA), Middlesbrough (UK) and Farnborough (UK) (Ray Garry)

Table 40.3 lists the intraoperative and immediate postoperative results of a multicentre study of more than 1000 patients with menorrhagia treated with endometrial laser ablation (ELA) (Garry et al., 1991). After the early learning phase the treatment time fell and the mean time to complete the ablation was 23 minutes (range 11–90). Almost all the patients were discharged home within 24 hours and many went home on the day of surgery. Some complained of menstrual-like cramps for a few hours after ablation but this was almost invariably relieved by simple analgesics and early postoperative pain was not a problem. A variable serosanguineous loss persists for up to 6 weeks after the endometrial ablation and during this time some women experienced a heavy menstrual-like bleed attributed to the shedding of the necrotic endometrium. In those in whom a simple continuous-flow pump was used to distend the cavity the mean volume of normal saline absorbed was 1416 ml. In the 170 patients in whom the fluid was infused with a Hamou Hysteromat the

Table 40.3 Operative details of multicentre study of ELA

	Princeton	Farnborough	Middlesbrough	Total
Number	342	359	318	1019
Operative time (min)	17 (11–27)	27 (17–90)	26 (11–90)	23
Mean fluid deficit (ml)	1500	1500	743 a 1416 b 289	1272

a, 115 cases with continuous-flow non-pressure-controlled pump.
b, 170 cases with pressure-controlled variable flow rate pump.

mean volume absorbed was 289 ml, a reduction of 80%.

More than 500 of these cases have been followed up for more than 6 months and the clinical outcomes are shown in Table 40.4. Of the 514 cases studied 312 (61%) were considered to have an excellent result with either complete amenorrhoea or profound oligomenorrhoea with only vaginal spotting as an outcome. A further 158 (32%) were classified as having a good clinical result associated with continuing menstruation but at a significantly reduced level completely acceptable to the patient as less than 'normal' and much less than pretreatment levels. Thirty-nine (8%) were considered initial treatment failures, but 26 responded to a second ELA and only 13 (3%) required hysterectomy. When the follow-up period was prolonged and those treated more than 12 months previously were studied the apparent success rate fell slightly with 4% of patients who had good early results relapsing. No patient with amenorrhoea at 6 months became worse at 12 months. Overall 470 (97%) women at 6 month review had a satisfactory clinical response to ELA.

These results are similar to those reported by other workers and the clinical outcomes of more than 1000 patients treated by ELA are now in the literature (Table 40.5).

Complications

The principal short-term complications expected following ELA are uterine perforation with damage to bowel, bladder and blood vessels, fluid overload with pulmonary oedema and electrolyte disturbances, intra- and postoperative haemorrhage and infection (Garry, 1990). The incidence of these complications in the 1015 patients reported by Garry et al. (1991) is shown in Table 40.6. The total short-term complication rate was extraordinarily low at only 1%. This was made up as follows. The uterus was perforated on three occasions, a rate of 0.4%. All these occurred during insertion of the rigid hysteroscope. When this happened the procedure was discontinued, the patients allowed home within 24 hours and in each case the treatment was successfully repeated within 4 weeks. No uterine perforation was caused by the laser, nor were there any cases of damage to bowel, bladder or other surrounding structure. None of the women had perioperative bleeding requiring active treatment or blood transfusion and none developed haematometra. Most of these women had uterine distension produced by simple non-pressure controlled pumps. Four women (0.4%) developed symptomatic pulmonary oedema requiring management with postoperative intravenous diuretics. Each

Table 40.4 Clinical results of multicentre trial of ELA

	Princeton	Farnborough	Middlesbrough	Total
Number	198	213	103	514
Excellent	111 (56%)	139 (65%)	62 (58%)	312 (61%)
Good	74 (37%)	55 (26%)	29 (28%)	158 (31%)
First failure	13 (7%)	19 (9%)	18 (17%)	50 (10%)
Successful second laser	10 (5%)	12 (6%)	6 (6%)	28 (5%)
Hysterectomy	3 (2%)	7 (3%)	5 (5%)	15 (3%)

Overall patients satisfaction rate with 1 or 2 ELA 466 (97%).

NdYAG LASER ABLATION OF THE ENDOMETRIUM

Table 40.5 Summary of published results of ELA

Author	Number	Excellent results	Normal results	Failures	Overall success
Goldrath (1990b)	321	292	7	22	93%
Lomano (1988)	62	47	14	1	98%
Loffer (1987)	55	38	11	6	90%
Baggish and Baltoyannis (1988)	14	10	3	1	93%
Daniell et al. (1986)	18	13	1	4	78%
Donnez and Nisolle (1989)	50	47	2	1	98%
Bertrand (1989)	22	16	5	1	95%
Multicentre (Garry et al., 1991)	23	18	3	2	91%
Davis (1989)	25	8	5	12	52%
Gallinatt et al. (1989)	102	95	4	3	97%
Garry et al. (1991)	479	288	178	13	97%
Total	1171	872 (74%)	233 (20%)	66 (6%)	94%

Table 40.6 Complications in multicentre study

Complication	Princeton	Farnborough	Middlesbrough	Total
Pulmonary oedema	2	2	0	4
Perforation with hysteroscope	1	2	0	3
Perforation with laser	0	0	0	0
Haemorrhage	0	0	0	0
Infection	0	2	2	4
Haematometra	0	0	0	0
Total	3	6	2	11 (1%)

responded promptly and all left hospital between 6 and 48 hours. None of these cases required intensive care but in other series severe fluid overload problems have been encountered. Significant postoperative pyrexia was noted in four women but only one of these had proven pelvic inflammatory disease.

In summary, the relative thickness of the myometrium, the ease with which effective uterine tamponade can be produced to arrest haemorrhage, and the fact that endometrial destruction is produced by the Nd:YAG laser energy spreading from the quartz fibre placed superficially on the surface layers of the endometrium minimize the risk of serious complications. The large multicentre study reported above was associated with a very low early complication rate of only 1%. However, ELA, like any surgical procedure, is associated with the risk of severe complications. Three cases of uterine perforation and bowel damage have been reported

(Perry et al., 1990) attributed respectively to an abnormally thin myometrium in a congenitally abnormal uterus, the use of laser power in excess of 90 W, and inexpert use of the laser in an inadequately supervised situation. The inappropriate use of sapphire tips cooled by high-flow CO_2 or air under pressure has caused four deaths and an additional case of severe brain damage due to catastrophic gas embolism has also been reported (Baggish and Daniell, 1989). Significant intraoperative haemorrhage is unlikely but major postoperative haemorrhage remains a possibility. Large amounts of necrotic tissue are produced by ELA and this can provide a focus for infection. The author recommends the use of a preoperative broad-spectrum antibiotic to reduce this risk.

The most common serious complication of ELA remains excessive extravasation of the distending medium into the systemic circulation with the risk of fluid overload, dilutional problems and pulmonary oedema (Leake et al., 1987). This complication, reported in Goldrath's original series, has been noted to a greater or lesser extent in almost every subsequent series. Careful monitoring at frequent intervals of infusion fluid inflow, outflow and deficit is essential. As described in more detail in Chapter 5 the maintenance of a closed circuit, high-flow, low-pressure distension system with a continuously maintained clear outflow channel will minimize this risk. Using a pressure-controlled infusion system has been shown to reduce fluid absorption and directly measuring the intrauterine pressure and adjusting flow rates appropriately has been shown to virtually eliminate the risk of excessive fluid absorption.

Discussion

ELA is a treatment for patients complaining of menorrhagia. Most women suffering from this complaint request relief of the symptom of heavy menstrual loss. They usually do not request amenorrhoea or demand a hysterectomy. In fact, many women are delighted to be relieved of their symptoms and yet still retain their uterus. The distinction between absolute amenorrhoea and profound oligomenorrhoea appears to be of greater consequence to gynaecologists than their patients. Goldrath's original clinical classification of outcome into excellent (which includes both amenorrhoea and oligomenorrhoea), good (with continuing but significantly reduced menstruation) and failure continues to seem relevant. It is the aim of most laser hysteroscopists to produce amenorrhoea in every case and it is not yet clear why this is achieved in some cases and not others. The precise mechanism by which menstrual reduction is produced is not clear. It is certainly not due to the production of a complete Asherman's syndrome and in most cases a much reduced but still patent cavity can be demonstrated at follow-up hysteroscopy. It is of particular interest that in many cases it takes 3–6 months to achieve the maximal reduction in menstrual flow. Many questions remain to be answered about how this technique works and about its long-term safety and effectiveness.

The endometrium is destroyed, the uterotubal junctions damaged and often occluded and considerable myometrial scarring is produced by ELA. These features all combine to reduce the chances of conception. Pregnancy, however, remains possible and one of the author's series of 318 cases has become pregnant. It is important

Table 40.7 Operative details of ELA compared with hysterectomy

	Hysterectomy	ELA
Time in theatre (min)	88	44
Treatment time (min)	60	23
Mean hospital stay (days)	7	1
Mean convalescence (days)	56	10
Proportion with noted post-complication	45%	1%
Postoperative pain (< 24 hours)	94%	0%

to counsel the patients appropriately and to offer those at risk alternative contraceptive protection.

ELA requires a considerable amount of expensive equipment and questions have been raised about the cost effectiveness of the procedure. No meaningful answers can be given until we know the long-term relapse and complication rates. Some facts are, however, already clear. Patients who have had an ELA spend less time in the operating room, less time in hospital, and less time off work or away from their family duties than those who have had a hysterectomy (Table 40.7). These savings in time can also lead to considerable financial savings for the hospital service. The magnitude of these savings will depend much more on the number of cases dealt with than on the capital cost of the equipment. We have calculated that if a laser has a working life of 7 years and 500 patients per year can be treated with it the cost per case of providing the laser is only about £22 (Table 40.8). The cost of theatre consumables such as drapes, swabs and suture materials is 45% less for ELA than for hysterectomy. This saving alone, if continued for the life of the laser, is sufficient to pay for the equipment. We conclude that Nd:YAG lasers when used frequently in large and busy departments are cost effective items and with small cost

Table 40.8 Costs of hysterectomy compared with ELA

	Hysterectomy	ELA
Theatre consumables £ 58.09		£27.77
Laser depreciation		£21.42
Laser fibre costs		£9.60
Staff costs	£107.21	£74.07
Total theatre costs	£165.30	£132.86
Ward costs	£800.00	£50.00
Total procedure costs	£965.30	£182.86

per case the capital costs of buying the equipment are very quickly recovered. If the change from long-term in-patient hospital stay associated with hysterectomy to day-case surgery permits closure of in-patient beds it is estimated that for every 500 patients treated with ELA rather than hysterectomy there could be a saving of £390 000. The financial benefits are even greater, if the savings associated with early return to work and reduced social benefit payments are included. In the short term, endometrial ablation is certainly very popular with the patients and with those who pay for their treatment. With an immediate morbidity of only 1% and a patient satisfaction rate in excess of 90%, it is a technique worthy of further study. From consideration of both the theoretical mode of action and the clinical evidence currently available, Nd:YAG laser ablation seems to be the safest of the ablative techniques now available. Well structured studies are, however, required to determine the long-term relapse rate, the effect of the procedure on various genital tract malignancies and the sustained safety and effectiveness of the procedure.

Conclusion

The data accumulated over the past decade suggest that laser ablation of the endometrium offers an alternative to hysterectomy in patients with menorrhagia who are not good candidates for other forms of conservative treatment. Our current experience in over 900 patients indicates that this procedure is safe and effective and involves minimal postoperative morbidity and discomfort.

References

Asherman JG (1948) Amenorrhea traumatica (atretica). *Journal of Obstetrics and Gynecology* **55**: 23–30.

Baggish MS & Baltoyannis P (1988) New techniques for laser ablation of the endometrium in high risk patients. *American Journal of Obstetrics and Gynecology* **159**: 287–292.

Baggish MS & Daniell JF (1989) Death caused by air embolism associated with neodymium:yttrium–aluminum–garnet laser surgery and artificial sapphire tips. *American Journal of Obstetrics and Gynecology* **161**: 877–878.

Bertrand JD (1989) Endometrial ablation using Nd-YAG laser for menorrhagia. In *Proceedings of the Second*

World Congress of Gynecologic Endoscopy. Clermont-Ferrand, France.

Brooks MD, Philip G, Serden MD, Scott P & Davos I. (1991) Hormonal inhibition of the endometrium for resectoscopic endometrial ablation. *American Journal of Obstetrics and Gynecology* **164**: 1601–1608.

Daniell JF, Tosh R & Meisels S (1986) Photodynamic ablation of the endometrium with the Nd-YAG laser hysteroscopically as a treatment for menorrhagia. *Colposcopy and Gynecologic Laser Surgery* **2**: 43–46.

Davis JA (1989) Hysteroscopic endometrial ablation with the neodymium-YAG laser. *British Journal of Obstetrics and Gynaecology* **96**: 928–932.

DeCherney A & Polan ML (1983) Hysteroscopic management of intrauterine lesions and intractable uterine bleeding. *Obstetrics and Gynecology* **61**: 392–397.

Donnez J & Nisolle M (1989) Laser hysteroscopy in uterine bleeding. Endometrial ablation and polypectomy. In Donnez J (ed) *Laser Operative Laparoscopy and Hysteroscopy.* Leuven: Nauwelaerts Printing.

Droegemueller W, Makowski E & Macsalka R (1971) Destruction of the endometrium by cryosurgery. *American Journal of Obstetrics and Gynecology* **110**: 467–469.

Droegemueller W, Greer B & Makowski E (1971) Cryosurgery in patients with dysfunctional uterine bleeding. *Obstetrics and Gynecology* **33**: 256–258.

Gallinat A, Lueken RR & Moller CP (1989) The use of the Nd:YAG laser in gynecological endoscopy. In MBB-Medizintechnik GmbH (ed) *Laser Brief 14.* Munich.

Garry R (1990) Safety of hysteroscopic surgery. *Lancet* **336**: 1013–1014.

Garry R, Erian J & Grochmal S (1991) A multicentre collaborative study into the treatment of menorrhagia by Nd-YAG laser ablation of the endometrium. *British Journal of Obstetrics and Gynaecology* **98**: 357–362.

Goldrath MH, Fuller TA & Segal S (1981) Laser photovaporization of endometrium for the treatment of menorrhagia. *American Journal of Obstetrics and Gynecology* **140**: 14–19.

Goldrath MH (1983) Uterine tamponade for the control of acute uterine bleeding. *American Journal of Obstetrics and Gynecology* **147**: 869–872.

Goldrath MH (1990a) Use of danazol in hysteroscopic surgery for menorrhagia. *Journal of Reproductive Medicine* **35**: 96.

Goldrath MH (1990b) Intrauterine laser surgery. In Keye WR (ed) *Laser Surgery in Gynecology and Obstetrics,* 2nd edn, pp 151–165. Chicago: Year Book Medical Publishers.

Goulbourne IA & Macleod DAD (1981) Interaction between danazol and warfarin: case report. *British Journal of Obstetrics and Gynaecology* **88**: 950–951.

Leake JF, Murphy AA & Zacur HA (1987) Noncardiogenic pulmonary edema: a complication of operative hysteroscopy. *Fertility and Sterility* **48**: 497–499.

Loffer FD (1987) Hysteroscopic endometrial ablation with the Nd-YAG laser using a non-contact technique. *Obstetrics and Gynecology* **59**: 679–682.

Lomano JM (1988) Photocoagulation of the endometrium with the Nd-YAG laser for the treatment of menorrhagia. *Journal of Reproductive Medicine* **31**: 148–150.

Perry CP, Daniell JF & Gimpelson RJ (1990) Bowel

injury from Nd-YAG endometrial ablation. *Journal of Gynecologic Surgery* **6**: 199–203.

Townsend DE, Richart RM, Paskowitz RA & Woolfork RE (1987) 'Rollerball' coagulation of the endometrium. *Obstetrics and Gynecology* **679**: 679–682.

Vancaillie TG (1989) Electrocoagulation of the endometrium with the ball-end resectoscope ('rollerball'). *Obstetrics and Gynecology* **74**: 425.

41

Electroresection of Fibroids

JACQUES HAMOU

Université Paris XI, Hôpital Antoine Béclére, France

Uterine leiomyomata (fibroids) are usually relatively slow growing and over the course of a decade most submucous fibroids cause progressively heavier menstrual flow, then menometrorrhagia leading to secondary anaemia.

During the reproductive years due to problems with implantation, submucous myomas may impair fertility through inadequate placentation or cornual distortion and it may affect reproductive performance.

Classically the management has been myomectomy by laparotomy or hysterectomy if child bearing is complete. For this reason hysteroscopic operative removal as a non-invasive and safe procedure has been advocated. With recent advances in electrodiathermy, operative hysteroscopy and the use of a resectoscope, such techniques using scissors, or forceps have been abandoned. Hysteroscopy has introduced a more precise diagnostic evaluation and recent advances in electrodiathermy have enabled submucous myomas to be removed by the resectoscope.

Evaluation

Prior to attempting hysteroscopic removal of intracavity myomas, a thorough preoperative work-up should be performed (Hamou and Taylor, 1982; Hamou et al., 1985). Each myoma has its own individual characteristics. The therapeutic approach will depend on the size of the lesion, its position, the importance of the part that is in the interstitial tissues, the degree of vascularity (Figure 41.1), and the presence or absence of any associated lesions. Furthermore, the approach will, to some extent, depend on the indication, be it menorrhagia or infertility (Neuwirth, 1983).

The interstitial and subserous myomas usually remain asymptomatic unless they become extremely large and produce pressure symptoms, at which time they should be removed by formal surgery or even laparoscopic surgery (Chapter 21) (Valle, 1981). It is those intracavity myomas or those submucous tumours, where more than half of the tissue mass resides within the uterine cavity, that, if they are causing symptoms, are

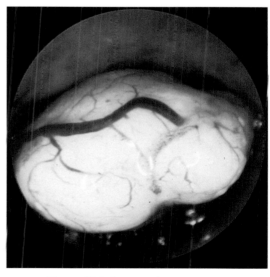

Figure 41.1 Intrauterine myoma.

best dealt with by hysteroscopic electroresection or Nd:YAG laser surgery (Chapter 42).

Preoperative diagnostic hysteroscopy should, at least in principle, provide precise information about the nature of these lesions. At the time of diagnostic hysteroscopy, endometrial biopsy should be performed to determine if there is any degree of associated endometrial hyperplasia. Ultrasonography will identify interstitial or subserous myomata but, unfortunately, the poor electroradiographic gradient between the myoma and the myometrium does not allow this technique to provide reliable information with respect to submucous myomas, particularly those small in size. Similarly, hysterosalpingography does not provide sufficient information to permit the decision to be made as to whether or not the lesion can be resected electrosurgically (Mencaglia *et al.*, 1987).

Preparation

Even with the best technical expertise it is not possible to resect myomas that are greater than 5 cm in diameter or when more than half the fluid lies within the myometrium (Hamou and Salat-Baroux, 1988). Attempts to deal with tumours of this magnitude carry a risk of complications that is prohibitive. GnRH analogues have little effect in the reduction in size of intracavity tumours and their use tends to provoke a fibrous reaction that makes resection more hazardous (Hamou, 1991).

The efficacy of hypo-oestrogenism by GnRH agonists induced to decrease the size of large fibroids may have a useful role in the preoperative management of leiomyomata uteri. Several reports have demonstrated reductions in size up to 50% for large fibroids after 6 months of GnRH. Small submucous fibroids are less responsive to such treatment.

1. Myomas under 2 cm in diameter even if mainly interstitial with only one-third of the surface area protruding in the cavity do not require any particular preparation (Wallach, 1988).
2. Myomas between 2 and 4 cm diameter and with at least 50% protruding into the cavity may benefit from a short preoperative treatment with progestogens or danazol for 3 weeks. Induced endometrial atrophy improves visual control and makes electroresection easier (Mencaglia *et al.*, 1987).
3. For fibroids more than 4 cm with more than

half the volume intra mural, a 2–3 month course of therapy with GnRH agonist will reduce substantially the size and the capillary vascularization with a decreased risk of fluid overload. Longer treatment does produce significant reduction of size but induces a fibrous transformation of the myoma resulting in a more hazardous resection.

Technique

We prefer to use direct hysteroscopic resection of fibroids using a rigid modified urological resectoscope with electrosurgical cutting loops (Figure 41.2). A microhysteroscope No. 2 of 4 mm permits close and magnified vision to differentiate the reticulated structure of the myoma from the fasciculated structure of the myometrium (Figure 41.3). A 7 mm open loop permits morcellation of the fibroid. Two concentric sheaths allow a double flow of distending low-viscosity fluid.

Glycine 1.5% (aminoacetic acid) is widely used. With an osmolarity of 200 mosmol per litre it is a non-haemolytic and non-electrolytic solution. Irrigation is electronically controlled by a Hamou Hysteromat (Figure 41.4) which controls optimal liquid flow and pressure to reduce the risk of intravasation. Liquid used is controlled by negative pressure thus monitoring the amount of liquid used.

A high-frequency current properly blended between cutting and coagulation effect allows precise electroresection without carbonization yet with adequate control of bleeding. A proper understanding of the electrosurgical equipment will avoid the risk of accidents that may include inappropriate stimulation of adjacent muscles and nerves or burns and arcing.

After adequate cervical dilatation the resectoscope is inserted and the myoma clearly identified.

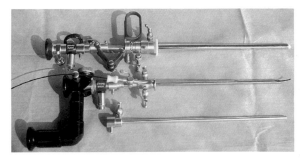

Figure 41.2 Resectoscope.

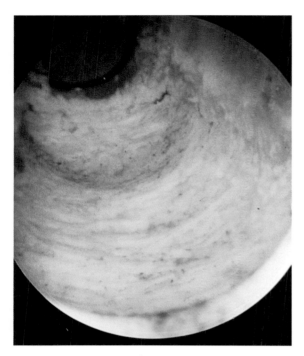

Figure 41.3 Myometrial reticulated structures beneath the fibroid.

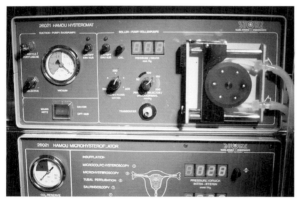

Figure 41.4 Hamou Hysteromat.

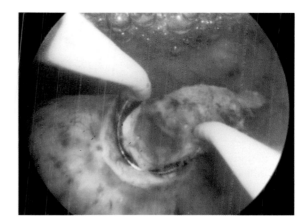

Figure 41.5 More selection of the fibroids.

collected by curettage and sent for pathological examination (Neuwirth, 1985). With adequately controlled irrigation and properly blended high-frequency current, the procedure is generally bloodless and vision is clear throughout. Haemorrhage may occur when resection is too deep and reaches the deep subserous vascular bed.

Results

From 1 March 1985 to 1 June 1987, 103 patients have undergone hysteroscopic resection of fibroids. Intractable uterine bleeding was the indication for 69 patients with a mean age of 42 years, 42 with a myoma of 2–5 cm diameter and 20 with a size up to 2 cm. In the first group five patients required a second resection and two had a hysterectomy for postoperative bleeding. For the second group no other resection was required

Tissue morcellation is started and the loop of the resectoscope is always drawn toward the operator (Figure 41.5). The loop can also be kept at a fixed distance from the resectoscope and drawn back like a curette (Neuwirth, 1983). As the procedure progresses, the slices of tissue are deposited on the side to keep the field clear. Resection of the intramural part of the fibroid should not exceed 8–10 mm below the mucosal level. Progressive enucleation of the deep interstitial part of the myoma may be obtained by massage of the uterus, hydromassage through the hysteromat to obtain a realignment of surrounding myometrium. If such protrusion is not obtained the procedure should be interrupted and a second resection considered 2–3 months later. Chips of tissues are

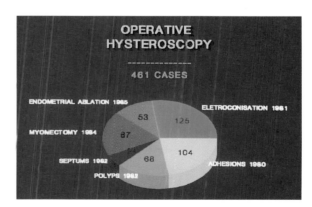

Figure 41.6 Operative hysteroscopy: 461 consecutive cases showing the chronology of the development of operative hysteroscopic procedures.

even when resection was incomplete. Thirty-six patients had an associated hyperplasia and underwent simultaneous partial endometrial ablation.

Thirty-four patients had fibroid resection because of infertility. The mean age was 34 years and in 29 women the myoma was under 2 cm diameter and usually asymptomatic. Particular attention was given to any remaining tissue at the 2 months second look hysteroscopy and in four cases a second resection was performed despite the patient remaining asymptomatic. For 27 of these patients with no other cause of infertility, 19 patients had a pregnancy with term delivery.

Conclusion

Electroresection of fibroids is a very promising procedure as an alternative to conventional abdominal myomectomy of hysterectomy. It is a non-invasive technique requiring a short hospital stay and the patient is usually discharged on the same day as the procedure. Normal activity is resumed within 2–3 days. There is no abdominal scar or fragmentation of the uterus and if the equipment is adequate and the technique mastered, complications are extremely rare.

References

Hamou J & Taylor PJ (1982) Panoramic, contact and microcolpohysteroscopy in gynecologic practice. *Current Problems in Obstetrics and Gynecology*, **4**: 2. Chicago: Year Book.

Hamou J, Salat-Baroux J & Henrion R (1985) Hystéroscopie et microcolpohystéroscopie. *Encyclopédie Méd Chir Gynécologie* **72 (B10)**: 11–14.

Hamou J & Salat-Baroux J (1988) Hystéroscopie et microhystéroscopie opératoires. *Mises à jour en Gynécologie et Obstétrique* **12**: 171.

Hamou J (1991) *Hysteroscopy and Microcolpohysteroscopy, Text and Atlas*, pp 181–185. Norwalk: Appleton and Lange.

Mencaglia L, Perino A & Hamou J (1987) Hysteroscopy in perimenopausal and postmenopausal women with abnormal uterine bleeding. *Journal of Reproductive Medicine* **32**: 577.

Neuwirth RS (1983) Hysteroscopic management of symptomatic submucous fibroids. *Obstetrics and Gynecology* **62**: 509.

Neuwirth RS (1985) Hysteroscopic resection of submucous leiomyoma. *Contemporary Obstetrics and Gynecology* **25**: 103–123.

Valle RF (1981) Hysteroscopic evaluation of patients with abnormal uterine bleeding. *Surgery, Gynecology and Obstetrics* **153**: 521.

Wallach E (1988) Myomectomy: a guide to indications and technique. *Contemporary Obstetrics and Gynecology* **31**: 74.

42

Nd:YAG Laser Hysteroscopic Myomectomy

JACQUES DONNEZ

Infertility Research Unit, Catholic University of Louvain, Brussels, Belgium

Introduction: Nd:YAG Laser or Electrical Current

Both the electrical current of the resectoscope and the energy of the Nd:YAG laser have been effective tools in the destruction of endometrial tissue to sufficient depth to avoid regeneration (Goldrath et al., 1981; Hamou and Salat-Baroux, 1984; Goldrath, 1985; Hallez et al., 1987; Loffer, 1988). The resectoscope has a disadvantage, however, since it is a unipolar electrical instrument. Therefore, there is the potential for damaging the bowel or bladder with a current transmitted through the uterine wall or by actual penetration of the uterine wall with the cutting loop. In addition, there is the risk of bleeding if major uterine vessels are transected by cutting too deeply into the uterine wall. On the other hand, the resectoscope has an advantage over the laser in that the equipment is readily available in most operating rooms: it is virtually the same as that used for urological procedures (Neuwirth, 1983). Use of the resectoscope thus does not require the major capital investment needed for a laser.

On the other hand, laser energy has some advantages in precision of tissue destruction that are not shared by the electrical energy used in resectoscopes. The most popular laser in gynaecology has been the carbon dioxide (CO_2) laser, so it is natural that an effort has been made to adapt this for hysteroscopic use. However, several features of the CO_2 laser make it impractical for hysteroscopic use. There are three reasons making the Nd:YAG laser readily adaptable for hysteroscopic endometrial ablation:

1. its ability to transmit the beam of energy easily into the uterine cavity by means of a flexible quartz fibre;
2. its ability to transmit laser energy to the tissue surface through a liquid distending medium;
3. its ability to penetrate tissue to a controlled depth.

There are other lasers that have some of the same advantages for hysteroscopic work, namely, the argon and the KTP 532. Both can be carried by fibreoptic light guides and can penetrate water. However, neither has the ability to penetrate tissue as deeply as the Nd:YAG laser.

Tissue Effects of the Nd:YAG Laser

The ability of this laser to penetrate the uterine wall and damage the bowel and bladder is limited, since tissue destruction occurs only to a depth of about 5 mm. Although some energy from the laser beam may penetrate more deeply into the uterine musculature and potentially even beyond, it does little more than cause a slight temperature rise in that tissue (Goldrath, 1985). This temperature increase does not denature the enzyme system and therefore does not lead to necrosis. The depth at which tissue destruction will occur can be controlled by varying the power used. The uterine wall averages approximately 1.5 cm in thickness, and deep structures are therefore safe.

Hysteroscopic Equipment

The quartz fibre used to carry the laser light is a 'bare' fibre. It consists of a quartz cylinder surrounded by a thin plastic sheath, beyond which the tip of the fibre extends for several millimetres. The fibre is gas sterilized or wiped with alcohol or Cidex prior to use. The laser power is generally set between 50 and 80 W.

There are several hysteroscopic instruments for endometrial ablation. The disadvantage of the first one used was the inability to suction the interior of the uterine cavity to remove debris during the procedure.

The deflecting arm is not of particular value, since the interior of the uterine cavity is not large enough to allow the fibre to be flexed at right angles to the uterine wall, but allows the fibre to be stabilized. There are now new instruments available. With the hysteroscope, the telescope is inserted into two different sheaths of different diameter, one for inflow and the other one for outflow. This resembles the conventional resectoscope and allows constant irrigation of the uterine cavity, thus ensuring an optimal view.

The technique the author uses to provide constant uterine distension involves attaching two 3000 ml plastic bags of glycine solution to dual blood infusion tubing. Each bag is then wrapped in a pressure infusion cuff similar to that used to infuse blood under pressure. The tubing is connected to the hysteroscope.

In our department, 1.5% glycine solution was chosen for its excellent optical and non-haemolytic properties during endoscopic hysteroscopic surgery. This electrolyte-free solution is widely used by urologists during transurethral resections. The advantages of low-viscosity fluids are numerous. These fluids are less expensive, they are readily available, they cause less pain, and the risks of media intravasation are reduced. However, there is a potential risk of anaphylactic reactions when dextran is used (Van Boven et al., 1989).

Role of Preoperative Therapy with a GnRH Agonist

Two hundred and forty-four women aged between 23 and 40 years (mean 34 years) with symptomatic submucous uterine fibroids were treated with a biodegradable GnRH analogue (Zoladex Implant, ICI Pharmaceuticals, UK). The implant was injected subcutaneously at the end of the luteal phase to curtail the initial gonadotropin stimu-

lation phase always associated with a rise in oestrogen. One implant was systematically injected at weeks 0, 4 and 8.

Endometrial biopsy, hysterography and hysteroscopy were performed before treatment and at 8 weeks. The uterine cavity area and the fibroid area were calculated as previously described (Donnez et al., 1989a, b, 1990) on the hysterography images using the short-line 'multipurpose test system' described by Weibel (Weibel, 1979).

After a well known initial stimulation of E_2 secretion, GnRH analogue administration resulted in a postmenopausal E_2 range (15 ± 6 pg/ml). Throughout the treatment period, LH and FSH concentrations were significantly suppressed by 2 weeks of treatment. Recovery of ovarian secretion occurred on average ± 10 weeks after the last injection (Donnez et al., 1990).

Evaluation of Hormonal Therapy

All patients had a pretreatment uterine cavity area >10 cm². In all patients the uterine cavity was decreased, with an average decrease of 36%. Using the same method, the decrease of very large submucous fibroid areas was also calculated. When more than one fibroid was present, only the largest was evaluated. In all cases except four, the fibroid area was decreased by an average of 38%. However, the response was variable, ranging from 4% to 95%. The fibroid area decreases significantly ($P < 0.01$) from the baseline area (7.2 ± 4.7 cm²) to 4.4 ± 3.5 cm² by 8 weeks of therapy. Figure 42.1 shows the mean fibroid area in patients with a pretreatment fibroid area <5 cm² versus those with an area >5 cm² to <10 cm². In all subgroups, a significant decrease ($P < 0.005$) was noted. There was no significant difference between the different subgroups.

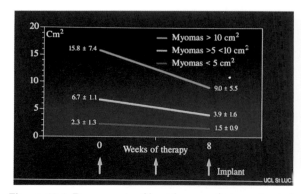

Figure 42.1 Decrease in fibroid area after an 8 week GnRH agonist therapy according to the initial value (<5 cm²; >5 <10 cm²; >10 cm²).

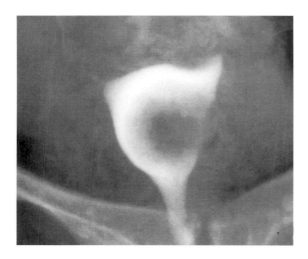

Figure 42.2 Submucosal fibroid of which the greatest diameter was inside the uterine cavity.

Techniques of Hysteroscopic Myomectomy

At 8 weeks, hysteroscopic myomectomy was carried out with the help of the neodymium:YAG (Nd:YAG) laser. A Sharplan 2100 apparatus (Sharplan, Tel-Aviv, Israel) was used for generating the laser. A power output of 80 W was used.

According to hysterosalpingography data, submucosal fibroids were classified as:

1. submucosal fibroid of which the greatest diameter was inside the uterine cavity (Figure 42.2) ($n = 168$);
2. submucosal fibroid of which the largest portion was located in the tubal wall (Figure 42.3). ($n = 44$);
3. multiple (>2) submucosal fibroids (myofibromatous uterus with submucosal fibroids and intramural fibroids diagnosed by hysterography and echography (Figure 42.4) ($n = 32$).

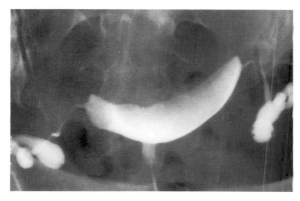

Figure 42.3 Submucosal fibroid of which the largest portion was located in the tubal wall.

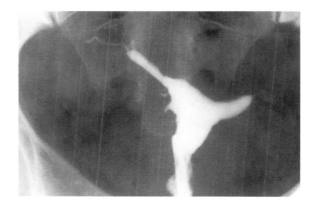

Figure 42.4 Multiple submucosal and intramural fibroids.

Submucosal Fibroid of which the Greatest Diameter was Inside the Uterine Cavity

All patients ($n = 168$) underwent myomectomy by hysteroscopy and Nd:YAG laser. In all cases, except one, the operation was easily performed. The myometrium overlying the myoma was less vascular and the 'shrinkage' of the uterine cavity may have accounted for the relative ease of separating the myomas from the surrounding myometrium (Figure 42.5).

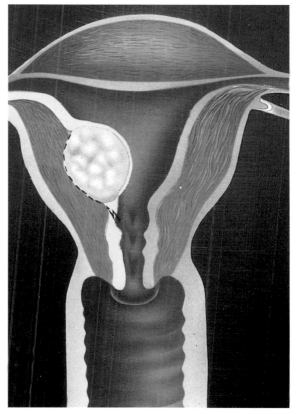

Figure 42.5 Hysteroscopic myomectomy in cases of submucosal fibroids where the greatest diameter was inside the uterine cavity.

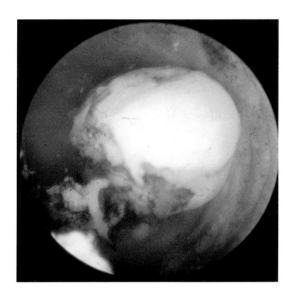

Figure 42.6 Myomectomy: the myoma was left in the uterine cavity.

The myoma was left in the uterine cavity (Figure 42.6). No complications such as infection, bleeding or uterine contractions occurred. Office hysteroscopy done with CO_2 and carried out 2–3 months after myomectomy confirmed the complete disappearance of the myoma, which was probably 'ejected' during the first menstruation occurring after the procedure.

In case of bleeding during the intervention, the pressure infusion was increased so that the intrauterine pressure was above the arterial pressure until the blood vessel provoking the bleeding was coagulated with the help of the Nd:YAG laser. At the end of the procedure, no intrauterine stent was placed in the uterine cavity. No hormonal therapy, such as oestrogens and progesterone, was given. The operating time varied from 10 to 50 minutes (means 24 ± 6 minutes). Blood loss was minimal. Indeed, when blood loss was controlled, the difference between preoperative and postoperative (2 days) haemoglobin concentration was never >1 g/l.

Large Submucosal Fibroid of which the Largest Portion was Located in the Uterine Wall

In cases of very large submucous fibroids of which the largest portion was not inside the uterine cavity but inside the uterine wall ($n = 44$) a *two-step operative hysteroscopy* was proposed (Donnez *et al.*, 1990). After an 8 week preoperative course of GnRH therapy, a partial myomectomy was carried out by resecting the protruding portion of the myoma. Thereafter, the laser fibre

was directed, as perpendicularly as possible, at the remaining (intramural) fibroid portion and was introduced into the fibroid to a length of 5–10 mm (Figure 42.7). During the application of laser energy, the fibre was removed slowly so that the deeper areas were coagulated. The end point of fibroid coagulation with this technique was identified by distinct 'craters' with brown borders on all fibroid areas. The depth of the intramural fibroid portion was already well known due to echographic examination performed the day before surgery. The aim of this procedure was to decrease the size of the remaining myoma by decreasing the vascularity.

GnRH analogue therapy was given for another 8 weeks and a second-look hysteroscopy was then performed. In all cases, the myoma was found to protrude again inside the uterine cavity and appeared very white and without any obvious vessels on the surface. Myomectomy was then carried out as described for myomas in which the largest portion was inside the uterine cavity. The shrinkage of the uterine cavity allowed the residual myoma portion to be easily separated

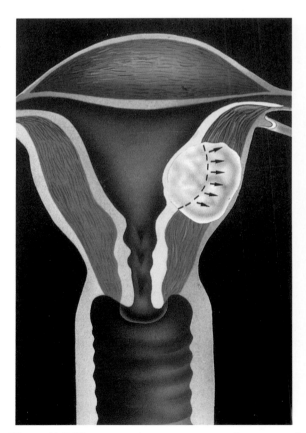

Figure 42.7 Hysteroscopic myomectomy in cases of submucosal fibroids where the largest portion was located in the tubal wall: partial myomectomy and coagulation of the remaining intramural portion.

from the surrounding myometrium and dissected off the myometrium. At the end of the procedure, the myoma was left in the uterine cavity. No concomitant laparoscopy was carried out. In four cases, a third hysteroscopy was carried out because the two-step myomectomy failed. In all cases, hysterography and hysteroscopy, carried out 2–3 months after myomectomy, confirmed the disappearance of the myoma. The uterine cavity was normal.

Fibromatous Uterus

In cases of multiple submucosal fibroids, each myoma was either separated from the surrounding myometrium or totally photocoagulated. When only a small portion of the myoma was visible, the fibre was introduced into the intramural portion to a length depending on the myoma diameter (diagnosed by echography). While firing, the fibre was slowly removed, systematically destroying each myoma. At the end of surgery, endometrial ablation with the Nd:YAG laser was carried out in order to induce uterine shrinkage. Concomitant endometrial ablation was carried out only in women >35 years who did not wish to become pregnant subsequently.

When successfully performed (Table 42.1) the myomectomy permits the restoration of normal flow. Long-term evaluation of the results shows that recurrence of menorrhagia occurred more frequently (22%) in cases of multiple submucosal myomas than in cases of single submucosal myomas. Recurrence of menorrhagia usually resulted from the growth of myomas in other sites, as proved by hysterography and hysteroscopy.

Fertility

A first evaluation in a series of 60 women was published in 1990 (Donnez et al., 1990). Among the 60 women, 24 wished to become pregnant and had no other fertility factors. Sixteen (66%) of them became pregnant during the first 8 months after the return of menstruation. No miscarriage or premature labour was observed in this series; one caesarean section was mandatory because of fetal distress.

Discussion

Because most leiomyomata return to near pretreatment size within 4 months after cessation of

GnRH analogue therapy, these agents cannot be used as definitive medical therapy (Healy et al., 1984; Maheux et al., 1985; Andreyko et al., 1988; Friedman et al., 1988). Several reports have demonstrated reductions in uterine and fibroid volumes by 52–77% after 6 months of GnRH therapy, as assessed by ultrasound imaging. In our study, as documented by hysterographic imaging, an average decrease of 35% in the uterine cavity was found (Donnez et al., 1989a, b).

The current study demonstrated reductions in fibroid volume by 38% after 8 weeks of GnRH analogue therapy. However, the response was variable, ranging from 2 to 9.5%. There was no difference in the extent of decrease according to the pretreatment fibroid area.

In cases of submucosal uterine fibroids, hysteroscopic myomectomy was carried out if the greater diameter of the leiomyoma, as assessed by hysterography, was inside the uterine cavity. A treatment duration of 8 weeks was advised before hysteroscopic myomectomy. Indeed, in a previous study, a significant uterine shrinkage was observed after 8 weeks of therapy.

The preoperative blood loss was minimal, possibly because of decreased vascularity of the myometrium, which was demonstrated by a significant reduction in the uterine arterial blood flow (Doppler) after treatment with a GnRH analogue (Matta et al., 1988). In all cases, the myoma was left in the uterine cavity and there were no complications. Probably after a necrotic phase it was ejected with the menstrual blood.

In cases of very large fibroids where the largest diameter was not inside the uterine cavity, the myomectomy was carried out in two stages. During the first surgical procedure, the protruding portion was removed and the intramural portion was devascularized by introducing the laser fibre into the myoma, to a length of 5–10 mm, depending on the depth of the remaining intramural portion. The distance between the deepest portion of the myoma and the uterine serosa was evaluated by echography. The pelvic structures were protected from injury because the distance between the top of the fibre and the external surface of the uterus was never <1.5 cm. There was no risk of pushing a laser fibre as much as 1 cm into the remaining portion if the diameter of the fibroid was >3–4 cm.

A very interesting finding was that this intramural portion of the myoma became submucosal and protruded again inside the uterine cavity, possibly because of the GnRH analogue-induced uterine shrinkage, which provoked the protrusion of the remaining portion. In all cases, the largest diameter of the remaining portion was inside the

Table 42.1 Surgical procedures and long-term results according to the site of myomas

	Greatest diameter inside the uterine cavity	Largest portion located in the uterine wall	Multiple submucosal myomas (myomectomy and endometrial ablation)
Surgical procedures			
n patients	168	44	32
Successful	167	40	28
Failed	1*	4†	4‡
Long-term results			
1 year follow-up			
n patients	92	21	18
Recurrence¶	1 (%)	1 (1%)	4 (22%)
2 year follow-up			
n patients	34	11	8
Recurrence¶	1 (3%)	1 (9%)	2 (25%)

* Stromal tumour
† A third look hysteroscopy allowed the myoma to be removed.
‡ Myomectomy was not totally successful. (In 2 cases, second-look laser hysteroscopy was successfully performed. In the two other cases, vaginal hysterectomy was proposed and successfully performed.)
¶ Recurrence: recurrence of menorrhagia.

uterine cavity so that myomectomy was easily performed by separating it from the surrounding myometrium with the help of the Nd:YAG laser.

In conclusion, use of GnRH analogue represents an adjunct for preoperative reduction of tumour size so that surgical treatment by hysteroscopy is possible. Even when the largest diameter was in the myometrium, the two-step hysteroscopic therapy combined with GnRH analogue therapy represented an ideal management of large submucous myomas and decreased the chance of myomectomy by laparotomy, which is often accompanied by increased operative blood loss and postoperative adhesion formation.

In cases of numerous submucosal and intramural myomas, a higher risk of recurrence was observed when compared to patients with only one submucosal myoma.

Because of the cessation of uterine bleeding, preoperative therapy resulted in the restoration of a normal haemoglobin concentration, which allows for the possibility of later autologous transfusion (Donnez et al., 1990). The hormonal endometrial status is one of the factors affecting fluid absorption. The endometrial vascularization may account for liquid resorption and it was reduced after a preoperative GnRH analogue therapy. The amount of fluid absorbed was lower if the endometrium was atrophic. By reducing the amount of fluid absorbed, the preoperative GnRH analogue therapy reduced the risk of fluid overload and this represented another major advantage for this combined medical and surgical approach to therapy.

References

Andreyko JL, Blumenfeld Z, Marschall LA *et al.* (1988) Use of an agonistic analog of gonadotropin-releasing hormone (nafarelin) to treat leiomyomas: assessment by magnetic resonance imaging. *American Journal of Obstetrics and Gynecology* **158**: 903.

Donnez J, Schrurs B, Clerckx F & Nisolle M (1989a) Les agonistes de la LH-RH une alternative dans le traitement de la myomatose utérine. *Contraception Fertilité Sexualité* **17**: 47.

Donnez J, Schrurs B, Gillerot S, Sadow J & Clerckx F (1989b) Treatment of uterine fibroids with implants of gonadotropin-releasing hormone agonist: assessment by hysterography. *Fertility and Sterility* **51**: 947.

Donnez J, Gillerot S, Bourgonjon D, Clerckx F & Nisolle M (1990) Neodymium:YAG laser hysteroscopy in large submucous fibroids. *Fertility and Sterility* **54**: 999.

Friedman AJ, Barbieri RL, Doubilet PM, Fine C & Schiff I (1988) A randomized, double-blind trial of gonadotropin releasing-hormone agonist (leuprolide) with or without medroxyprogesterone acetate in the treatment of leiomyomata uteri. *Fertility and Sterility* **49**: 404.

Goldrath MH (1985) Hysteroscopic laser surgery. In Baggish MH (ed) *Basic and Advanced Laser Surgery in Gynecology*, p 357. Norwalk: Appleton-Century-Crofts.

Goldrath MH, Fuller T & Segal S (1981) Laser photovaporization of endometrium for the treatment of menorrhagia. *American Journal of Obstetrics and Gynecology* **140**: 14–19.

Hallez JP, Netter A & Cartier R (1987) Methodical intrauterine resection. *American Journal of Obstetrics and Gynecology* **156**: 1080.

Hamou J & Salat-Baroux J (1984) Advanced hysteroscopy and microhysteroscopy: our experience with 1000 cases. In Siegler AP, Lindermann HJ (eds) *Hysteroscopy: Principles and Practice*, p 63. Philadelphia: JB Lippincott.

Healy DL, Fraser HM & Lawson SL (1984) Shrinkage of a uterine fibroid after subcutaneous infusion of an LH-RH agonist. *British Medical Journal* **209**: 267.

Loffer FD (1988) Laser ablation of the endometrium. *Obstetrics and Gynecology Clinics of North America* **15**: 77.

Maheux R, Guilloteau C, Lemay A, Bastide A & Fazekas ATA (1985) Luteinizing hormone-releasing hormone agonist and uterine leiomyoma: pilot study. *American Journal of Obstetrics and Gynecology* **152**: 1034.

Matta WHM, Stabile I, Shaw RS & Campbell S (1988) Doppler assessment of uterine blood flow changes in patients with fibroids receiving the gonadotropin-releasing hormone agonist Buserelin. *Fertility and Sterility* **49**: 1083.

Neuwirth RS (1983) Hysteroscopic management of symptomatic submucous fibroids. *Obstetrics and Gynecology* **62**: 509.

Van Boven M, Singelyn F, Donnez J & Gribomont BF (1989) Dilutional hyponatremia associated with intrauterine endoscopic laser surgery. *Anesthesiology* **3**: 71.

Weibel ER (1979) Practical methods for biological morphometry. In Weibel ER (ed) *Stereological Methods*, p 101. Bern: Switzerland.

43

Lysis of Intrauterine Adhesions (Asherman's Syndrome)

RAFAEL F. VALLE

Northwestern University Medical School, Chicago, Illinois, USA

Since Asherman (1948) reported 'Amenorrhoea traumatica (atretica)', amenorrhoea following a curettage for postpartum haemorrhage, incomplete abortion or missed abortion, secondary to intrauterine adhesions, the term Asherman's syndrome has been used to describe this entity. Two years after this original description, Asherman (1950) also included in the syndrome the partial occlusion of the uterine cavity secondary to adhesions. Therefore, the term Asherman's syndrome includes both pathological entities.

This condition may result in infertility, menstrual abnormalities, particularly amenorrhoea or hypomenorrhoea, pregnancy complications such as habitual abortions, missed abortions, premature deliveries, and placental insertion abnormalities such as placenta praevia and placenta accreta.

Pathophysiology of intrauterine adhesions

The most important factor in the development of intrauterine adhesions is traumatic curettage or manipulation of the endometrium during the postpartum or post-abortal period, especially at 1–4 weeks following the termination of pregnancy. This is a vulnerable phase when the endometrium seems to be more susceptible to trauma, particularly the denudation of the basalis layer and exposure of the muscularis layer which, by coaptation to the opposing uterine wall, produces adhesions. Although infrequently, infection alone causes intrauterine adhesions, and more often, it follows tuberculous endometritis. Most intrauterine adhesions (over 90%) develop following a pregnancy-related curettage (Klein and Garcia, 1973; Schenker and Margalioth, 1982).

Symptomatology

The presenting symptomatology varies according to the degree of uterine cavity occlusion and the severity of the adhesions, and is represented by infertility, and menstrual abnormalities such as amenorrhoea, hypomenorrhoea, and dysmenorrhoea.

When the occlusion of the uterine cavity includes the proximal portions of the fallopian tubes, infertility follows. Nevertheless, some patients with partial uterine cavity occlusion also develop secondary infertility due, perhaps, to disturbance of sperm migration and interference with the nidation of the blastocyst. Distortions in the symmetry of the uterine cavity may result in habitual abortion, and damage to the basalis layer of the endometrium may predispose to abnormal placental implantation. Polishuk *et al.* (1977) observed, on pelvic arteriography, a decrease of uterine blood vessels in women who develop amenorrhoea or hypomenorrhoea following a postpartum or post-abortal curettage, resulting in uterine fibrosis and poor endometrial development; this decrease of pelvic vascularization may also contribute to the lack of response to oestrogenic stimuli.

Diagnosis

Because of the close association between delayed postpartum, or post-abortal curettage causing menstrual abnormalities, and intrauterine adhesions, a history of these events should alert the clinician to the possibility of intrauterine adhesions. Difficult uterine sounding may suggest adhesions, but sounding should be avoided because of the increased danger of uterine perforation. Dilatation and curettage has not been of diagnostic value for intrauterine adhesions. The progesterone challenge test, resulting in failure of withdrawal bleeding, may be helpful in amenorrhoeic patients with a biphasic basal body temperature curve, showing no evidence of derangement in their hypothalamic–pituitary–ovarian axis, thus suggesting an end organ failure.

Although attempts to diagnose intrauterine adhesions by sonography seemed promising, hysterosalpingography remains the most accurate screening method in the diagnosis of intrauterine adhesions, and when adhesions are suspected by radiographic filling defects, hysteroscopy provides the definite diagnosis.

Intrauterine adhesions are diagnosed on the hysterogram by sharp outlying defects placed at different sites in the uterine cavity which usually persist on sequential films. Routine hysterosalpingography may demonstrate intrauterine adhesions in about 1.5% of infertile patients. Hysterosalpingography performed in patients with habitual abortion show intrauterine adhesions in about 5%, and hysterosalpingograms performed on patients with previous puerperal endometrial curettage demonstrate intrauterine adhesions in about 39% (Klein and Garcia, 1973).

With the renewed interest in hysteroscopy, diagnosis of intrauterine adhesions has been refined and awareness of this condition has increased the number of cases detected, particularly in women with hypomenorrhoea and habitual abortion. Although hysterosalpingography is generally considered the best screening method for diagnosis of this condition, many false-positive findings have been rectified by hysteroscopy. Hysteroscopy confirms the intrauterine adhesions suggested by the hysterogram, delineates them, and allows final surgical treatment.

Treatment of Intrauterine Adhesions

The surgical treatment of intrauterine adhesions consists of dividing the adhesions mechanically or utilizing energy modalities such as electrosurgery and/or fibreoptic lasers.

The blind division of intrauterine adhesions, although somewhat beneficial, does not provide accurate and precise treatment, and may produce damage to the surrounding healthy endometrium. Hysterotomies for the division of adhesions are of only historical interest as are other blind transcervical manipulations. Hysteroscopy is performed in the early follicular phase of the menstrual cycle in menstruating patients. Diagnostic endoscopes (<5 mm outside diameter [o.d.]) can be used to confirm the diagnosis of adhesions; however, for the surgical treatment of adhesions, an operative hysteroscope of 7 ml o.d. and semi-rigid scissors are most beneficial. General anaesthesia is given except to patients with filmy adhesions only partially occluding the uterine cavity. The gynaecological resectoscope with a modified knife electrode has been used to divide the adhesions electrosurgically. Fibreoptic lasers, such as argon, KTP 532, and neodymium:YAG laser with sculptured or extruded fibres, have also been used.

The uterine cavity is distended by fluid as described in Chapter 36.

Care must be exercised to avoid solutions with electrolytes while using electrocoagulation, and to control the volume of fluids not accounted for or collected after infusion, to prevent excessive fluid intravasation, particularly when using fluids without electrolytes.

Low-viscosity fluids are frequently chosen for operative hysteroscopy because of their ability to wash debris and cleanse the uterine cavity, even in the presence of slight uterine bleeding. When mechanical instruments are used to divide intrauterine adhesions, the distending media should contain electrolytes to increase the threshold of tolerance, in case of intravasation of fluid. Normal saline, 5% dextrose in half normal saline (0.45 NaCl), and Ringer's lactate are excellent media to distend the uterine cavity when treating intrauterine adhesions with hysteroscopic scissors.

Fluid delivery methods are also described in Chapter 36. Whatever method is used, the measurement of intrauterine pressure and inflow and outflow volume is important. The differential or non-accounted fluid should be derived by deducting the recovered fluid from the infused volume. This differential will offer an estimate of fluid absorption.

Because intrauterine adhesions, especially those of the moderate and severe type, usually require extensive dissection, the resulting prolonged procedure encourages excessive fluid intravasation. Fluids similar to those used while operating with mechanical instruments can also be used with fibreoptic lasers, because of their lack of conductivity.

Concomitant laparoscopy is performed in those patients with extensive intrauterine adhesions identified at hysterosalpingography, and should be added routinely when tubal blockage is diagnosed by hysterosalpingography, regardless of the degree of uterine cavity occlusion. Hysteroscopic observation of the uterine cavity begins at the internal cervical os, and should adhesions extend to that area, their selective division begins there, preforming a cavity before the hysteroscope is advanced. As the adhesions are divided and the uterine cavity opens, the hysteroscope is advanced to the fundal area, and both uterotubal cones are visualized. The uterine cavity is sculptured systematically until symmetry is achieved. Hysteroscopic semi-rigid scissors are easily inserted through the operative channel and retrieved into the operating channel for better observation (Figures 43.1–43.9).

Rigid scissors fixed in front of the hysteroscope may inadvertently cause perforation of the uterine wall, should panoramic vision be less than adequate. Lasers and/or electrosurgery may damage the uterine wall by obscuring bleeding during hysteroscopic surgery, which usually occurs with mechanical tools when these instruments

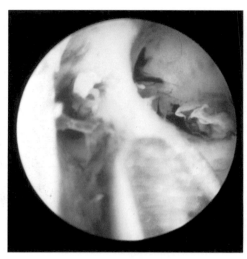

Figure 43.2 Hysteroscopic view of marginal intrauterine adhesion occluding the right cornual region.

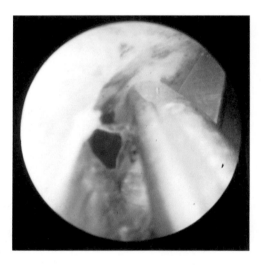

Figure 43.3 Hysteroscopic lysis of marginal intrauterine adhesion.

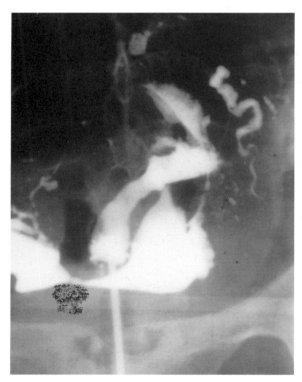

Figure 43.1 Hysterosalpingogram shows right cornual intrauterine filling defect, compatible with intrauterine adhesion.

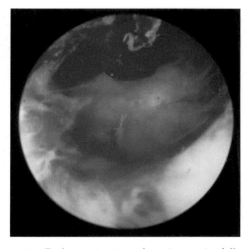

Figure 43.4 Endoscopic view of uterine cavity following division of adhesion.

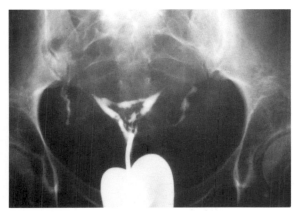

Figure 43.5 Hysterosalpingogram shows extensive uterine cavity occlusion by intrauterine adhesions.

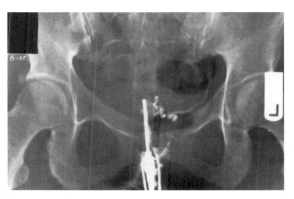

Figure 43.8 Total uterine cavity occlusion on hysterosalpingography. Intravasation of radio-opaque material can be seen.

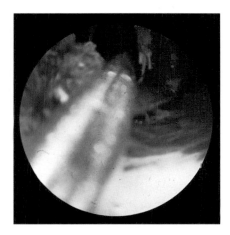

Figure 43.6 Hysteroscopic lysis of intrauterine adhesions with semi-rigid scissors.

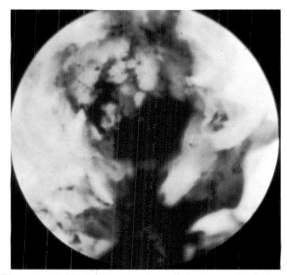

Figure 43.9 Hysteroscopic view of uterine cavity following lysis of severe intrauterine adhesions. Note thick stumps of divided adhesions.

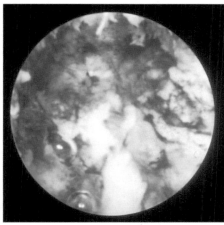

Figure 43.7 Endoscopic view of uterine cavity following lysis of adhesions. Note rugged appearance of uterine cavity.

approach this area. Bleeding is difficult to observe while activating the fibreoptic laser or electrocoagulation devices, due to the coagulation caused by these energies. The lateral, back and front scattering these lasers produce may jeopardize the viability of surrounding healthy endometrium, which is the reservoir for re-epithelialization. When the adhesions are focal and partially occlude the uterine cavity, their division is simple. Removal of the adhesions is not attempted, as the adhesions are divided in the middle, the remaining stumps retract, and the uterine cavity distends, permitting a panoramic view. Both uterotubal junctions should be observed and the tubal openings examined. Once all the adhesions have been divided, chromopertubation with indigo carmine is performed to assess tubal patency under laparoscopic vision.

Marginal or lateral adhesions, particularly if they are extensive and fibromuscular or composed of connective tissue, may be difficult to divide. Utmost care and delicacy are required to avoid uterine perforation. The transillumination of the light provided by the hysteroscope through the uterine walls, as seen by an assistant with a dimmed lighted laparoscope, may alert the hysteroscopist to possible perforation.

To prevent the immediate post-surgical reformation of adhesions, intrauterine splints in the form of intrauterine devices or indwelling catheters are placed in the uterine cavity, particularly in patients with extensive intrauterine adhesions and thick fibromuscular or connective tissue adhesions, which may occlude totally or partially the uterine cavity. Intrauterine contraceptive devices with a large surface area seem to be most suitable for this purpose and are left in place for 1 or 2 months before removal. A paediatric no. 8 indwelling catheter inflated with 3–3.5 ml of saline solution can be used instead, and left in place for a week.

Prophylactic antibiotics are given 1 hour before hysteroscopic treatment and given for 2–3 days postoperatively when a splint is left in the uterine cavity. Cephalosporins such as cefazolin sodium (Kefzol) 1 g i.v. with induction of anaesthesia followed by oral cephalexin (Keflex) 500 mg q.i.d. orally when the patient is able to tolerate fluids for 3–4 additional days. Despite the lack of randomized prospective studies demonstrating the efficacy of prophylactic antibiotics, they are usually administered in cases involving extensive intrauterine manipulations especially if a splint has been left in the uterus. Cyclical oral conjugated oestrogens (Premarin 2.5 mg b.i.d. × 30 days) are administered for two to three cycles with medroxyprogesterone acetate (Provera 10 mg q.d.) added for the last 10 days of each cycle.

To assess the results of the treatment, hysterosalpingography at the completion of the hormonal treatment may be performed in patients with moderate to severe adhesions. If hysterosalpingography demonstrates residual adhesions, a second therapeutic hysteroscopy is performed and the remaining adhesions are divided. Those patients with focal and filmy adhesions may not need post-treatment hysterosalpingography and their follow-up should be individualized (Siegler et al., 1990).

Classification of Intrauterine Adhesions

In order to outline the prognosis and results of the treatment, a classification of intrauterine adhesions is most useful. There are many classifications based on histology, hysterography, symptomatology and hysteroscopy. The important factors that seem to correlate with the final outcome are the extent of uterine cavity occlusion and the type and severity of the adhesions involved. Therefore, a combination of classifications seems more appropriate.

Hysterographic–Hysteroscopic Classification

Valle and Sciarra (1988) utilized a three-stage classification of the extent and severity of intrauterine adhesions (mild, moderate and severe) based on the degree of intrauterine involvement as shown by hysterosalpingography and the extent and type of adhesions found on hysteroscopy. Three stages of intrauterine adhesions are defined: *mild adhesions*, filmy adhesions composed of basalis endometrial tissue producing partial or complete uterine cavity occlusion: *moderate adhesions*, fibromuscular adhesions, characteristically thick, still covered with endometrium that bleeds upon division, and partially or totally occlude the uterine cavity; and *severe adhesions*, composed of connective tissue only; lacking an endometrial lining and not likely to bleed upon division; these adhesions may partially or totally occlude the uterine cavity.

The evaluation of these adhesions by hysteroscopy is not confirmed by histological examination, but by direct hysteroscopic observation of the surface of the adhesions, and their composition is evaluated during division. Histological confirmation has suggested a reasonable correlation between the hysteroscopic evaluation and microscopic examination. The extent of uterine cavity occlusion is best determined by hysterosalpingography.

The American Fertility Society (1988) has proposed a classification of intrauterine adhesions based on the findings at hysterosalpingography and hysteroscopy and the correlation with menstrual patterns. Because this latter classification has not been used uniformly when reporting reproductive outcome following treatment of intrauterine adhesions, assessment and comparisons of the different reports and their outcomes has been difficult. The goals of the treatment, therefore, should be:

1. to treat infertility and pregnancy wastage;
2. to re-establish normal menstruation; and
3. to treat dysmenorrhoea.

The success in establishing normal menstruation in patients treated for intrauterine adhesions has varied, but in collective series, a success rate of 73–92% has been achieved. Successful fertility outcome has not been correlated with conception rates (the latter ranging from 46–55%; and in those patients who carry a pregnancy to term the rate is between 38 and 70%) (Table 43.1; Schenker and Margalioth, 1982).

Conclusions

The hysteroscopic treatment of intrauterine adhesions has resulted in the restoration of normal menstruation in over 80% of the patients treated, and the reproductive outcome has paralleled the severity of the adhesions. The overall rate of term pregnancies in those patients who have become pregnant exceeds 80%. Complications related to placental insertion abnormalities has decreased markedly after hysteroscopic treatment, as compared with the treatment by curettage, hysterotomy, or blind transcervical dissection. Nevertheless, severe obstetric complications have been reported following treatment of intrauterine adhesions utilizing the resectoscope, and/or following the division of adhesions by hysterotomy. With division of the adhesions utilizing hysteroscopic scissors, these complications have not been reported. Of 187 patients with intrauterine adhesions treated hysteroscopically utilizing semi-rigid scissors, only one patient had a serious complication, a partial placenta accreta which failed to separate after birth and required a hysterectomy. Patients treated for moderate or severe adhesions should be considered at risk and their obstetrical surveillance should be closely monitored, particularly in the early stages of pregnancy and following delivery to diagnose early any placental insertion abnormalities such as placenta accreta or percreta (Valle and Sciarra, 1988).

Table 43.1 Hysteroscopic lysis of intrauterine adhesions*

Author	No. patients	Medium	Technique	Menses normal		Reproductive outcome pregnancy		Term	
				no.	%	no.	%	no.	%
Levine and Neuwirth (1973)	10	Hyskon	Flexible scissors	5	(50)	2	(20)		
Edstrom (1974)	9	Hyskon	Biopsy forceps	2	(22)	1	(11)	1	(11)
Siegler and Kontopoulos (1981)	25	CO_2	Target abrasion/ scissors/curettage	13	(52)	11	(44)	12	(44.4)
March and Israel (1981)	38	Hyskon	Flexible scissors	38	(100)	38	(100)	34	(79.1)
Neuwirth et al. (1982)	27	Hyskon	Scissors alongside hysteroscope	20	(74)	14	(51.8)	13	(48.1)
Sanfilippo et al. (1982)	26	CO_2	Curettage	26	(100)	6	(100)	3	(50)
Hamou et al. (1983)	69	CO_2	Target abrasion	59	(85.5)	20	(51.3)	15	(38.4)
Sugimoto et al. (1984)	258	Hyskon/normal saline	Target abrasion/ Kelly forceps	180	(69.7)	143	(76.4)	114	(79.7)
Wamsteker (1984)	36	Hyskon	Scissors/biopsy forceps	34	(94.4)	17	(62.9)	12	(44.4)
Friedman et al. (1986)	30	Hyskon	Resectoscope/scissors	27	(90)	24	(80)	23	(76.6)
Zuanchong and Yulian (1986)	70	Normal saline	Biopsy forceps/ flexible scissors	64	(84.3)	60	(85.7)	17	(48.5)
Valle and Sciarra (1988)	187	D_5W/Hyskon	Flexible/semi-rigid/ rigid scissors	167	(89.3)	143	(76.4)	114	(79.7)
Lancet and Kessler (1988)	93	Hyskon	Flexible scissors/ electrosurgery	98	(100)	86	(87.8)	77	(89.5)
Totals	883			733	(83.0)	535	(60.5)	435	(81.3)

From Siegler AM, Valle RF, Lindemann HJ & Mencaglia L (1990) *Therapeutic Hysteroscopy. Indications and Techniques*, Chapter 6, p 103. St Louis, Baltimore, Philadelphia, Toronto: C.V Mosby.

The hysteroscopic treatment of intrauterine adhesions should be considered the standard treatment for this condition and the adjunctive regimens used postoperatively, such as splints, prophylactic antibiotics, and oestrogen and progesterone hormonal treatments seem to improve the overall treatment of this condition. Nevertheless, in view of the worsening prognosis as the severity of the adhesions increase, early detection followed by early treatment is important, as shown by recent reports correlating the severity of the disease with the final reproductive outcome. Early warning of menstrual abnormalities in patients with a history of delayed postpartum or post-abortal curettage should alert the practitioner of this possibility, assuring evaluation and treatment when the adhesions are mild and filmy and in the early stages of their development.

Therapeutic hysteroscopy for intrauterine adhesions requires experience, dexterity, and understanding of all aspects of operative hysteroscopy, as hysteroscopic treatment of intrauterine adhesions is one of the most difficult therapeutic hysteroscopic procedures. The practitioner embarking in this operation should not only be familiar with diagnostic hysteroscopy but specifically trained in the different methods and techniques of therapeutic hysteroscopy.

References

The American Fertility Society (1988) The American Fertility Society Classifications of adnexal adhesions, distal tubal occlusion, tubal occlusion secondary to tubal ligation, tubal pregnancies, Mullerian anomalies and intrauterine adhesions. *Fertility and Sterility* **49**: 944–955.

Asherman JG (1948) Amenorrhoea traumatica (atretica). *Journal of Obstetrics and Gynaecology of the British Empire* **55**: 23–30.

Asherman JG (1950) Traumatic intrauterine adhesions. *Journal of Obstetrics and Gynaecology of the British Empire* **57**: 892–896.

Edstrom KGB (1974) Intrauterine surgical procedures during hysteroscopy for intrauterine adhesions. *Endoscopy* **6**: 175–181.

Friedman A, DeFazio J & DeCherney A (1986) Severe obstetric complications after aggressive treatment of Asherman's syndrome. *Obstetrics and Gynecology* **67**: 864–867.

Hamou J, Salat-Baroux J & Siegler AM (1983) Diagnosis and treatment of intrauterine adhesions by microhysteroscopy. *Fertility and Sterility* **39**: 321–326.

Klein SM & Garcia CR (1973) Asherman's syndrome: a critique and current review. *Fertility and Sterility* **24**: 722–735.

Lancet M & Kessler I (1988) A review of Asherman's syndrome and results of modern treatment. *International Journal of Fertility* **33**: 14–24.

Levine RU & Neuwirth RS (1973) Simultaneous laparoscopy and hysteroscopy for intrauterine adhesions. *Obstetrics and Gynecology* **42**: 441–445.

March CM & Israel R (1981) Gestational outcome following hysteroscopic lysis of adhesions. *Fertility and Sterility* **36**: 455–459.

Neuwirth RS, Hussein AR, Schiffman BM & Amin HK (1982) Hysteroscopic resection of intrauterine scars using a new technique. *Obstetrics and Gynecology* **60**: 111–113.

Polishuk WZ, Siew FP, Gordon R & Lebenshart P (1977) Vascular changes in traumatic amenorrhea and hypomenorrhea. *International Journal of Fertility* **22**: 189–192.

SanFilippo JS, Fitzgerald MR, Badawy SZA, Nussbaum ML & Yussman MA (1982) Asherman's syndrome. A comparison of therapeutic methods. *journal of Reproductive Medicine* **27**: 328–330.

Schenker JG & Margalioth EJ (1982) Intrauterine adhesions: an updated appraisal. *Fertility and Sterility* **37**: 593–610.

Siegler AM & Kontopoulos VG (1981) Lysis of intrauterine adhesions under hysteroscopic control. A report of 25 operations. *Journal of Reproductive Medicine* **26**: 372–374.

Siegler AM, Valle RF, Lindemann HJ & Mencaglia L (1990) *Therapeutic Hysteroscopy. Indications and Techniques*, pp 82–105. St. Louis, Baltimore, Philadelphia, Toronto: C.V. Mosby.

Sugimoto O, Ushiroyama T & Fukuda Y (1984) Diagnostic and therapeutic hysteroscopy for traumatic intrauterine adhesions. In Siegler AM & Lindemann HJ (eds) *Hysteroscopy. Principles and Practice*, pp 186–192. Philadelphia: J.B. Lippincott.

Valle RF & Sciarra JJ (1988) Intrauterine adhesions: hysteroscopic diagnosis, classification, treatment, and reproductive outcome. *American Journal of Obstetrics and Gynecology* **158**: 1459–1470.

Wamsteker K (1984) Hysteroscopy in Asherman's syndrome. In Siegler AM & Lindemann HJ (eds) *Hysteroscopy. Principles and Practice*, pp 198–203. Philadelphia: J.B. Lippincott.

Zuanchong F & Yulian H (1986) Hysteroscopic diagnosis and treatment of intrauterine adhesions. Clinical analysis of 70 cases. In *Symposium on Hysteroscopy*, p 179. Shanghai: Family Planning Association.

44

Hysteroscopic Tubal Occlusion

FRANKLIN D. LOFFER

Gynecologic Endoscopy, Maricopa Medical Center, Phoenix, AZ, USA

The ease with which the tubal ostium can be seen hysteroscopically has challenged the gynaecological endoscopists to find a transcervical method to occlude the fallopian tube for sterilization. Both blind and hysteroscopically controlled methods have been tried. These methods involve either:

1. the injection of a sclerosing agent into the tube;
2. the destruction of the interstitial portion of the tube; or
3. the occlusion of the tube with a plug.

Although the tubal ostium can be identified in virtually all cases (Loffer, 1984) it is difficult to achieve consistent blockage of the tube at its uterine junction. The primary reason for this difficulty lies in the inability to cause the tube to be occluded by either an induced process of tissue scarring or by tubal occluding devices.

This chapter will review:

1. the practicality of approaching the tube for sterilization procedures;
2. equipment available for this use;
3. the techniques and results of those procedures which have been tried including blind and hysteroscopic approaches involving injection of sclerosing agents, electrical blockage and mechanical plugs;
4. the reason for the difficulty and lack of success in each of these approaches; and
5. the formed *in situ* silicone plug which is the only commercially available hysteroscopic tubal occlusion technique available at this time.

While the number of effective transcervical tubal occlusion techniques are limited it is the author's hope that a review of this chapter will provide historical and clinical information to those who would attempt the currently available methods or develop new ones.

Practicality of Identifying and Approaching the Uterine Tubal Ostia

The tubal ostium can be seen in virtually all patients if certain parameters in patient selection are chosen and appropriate hysteroscopic techniques employed. In the author's 265 hysteroscopic tubal plug occlusion patients who underwent 310 procedures the total ostia were identified in 308 patients (99.3%). One ostium was not identified in two patients. Failure to visualize both ostia occurred in one patient because of inadequate uterine distension related to a very lax cervix. The other patient had a placental polyp from a recent miscarriage which obscured the tubal ostia.

The optimal time for identification of the tubal ostia is in the immediate post-menstrual phase. Identification of the fallopian tube may be difficult if hysteroscopy is done late in the menstrual cycle since the endometrium will bleed easily on contact and the thick endometrium may obscure the tubal opening. It is unnecessary to suppress the endometrium for good visualization with danazol or GnRH analogues.

A 30 degree fore-oblique hysteroscope provides

the easiest optics for viewing the ostia. The hysteroscope can be introduced with the optics directed anteriorly in an anteverted uterus and posteriorly in a retroverted uterus. Once inside the cavity the corresponding tubal ostium will come into full view when the hysteroscope is rotated 45 degrees in that direction.

Visualization of the tubal ostium can be compromised because of blood, mucous and endometrium debris whether carbon dioxide, 32% dextran 70 (Hyskon) or the low-viscosity fluids are used to distend the uterus. Several methods are available for obtaining adequate visualization when the distending media alone is not providing adequate visualization (Loffer, 1990).

When visualization is a problem with CO_2 most authors would probably abandon it and choose one of the other media. Hyskon has the advantage that blood is not miscible with it. A clear view is obtained when the uterine bleeding is pushed aside by the distending media. Although all of the author's tubal occlusion patients were done using Hyskon, the ostium were frequently obscured by mucous, debris and blood (Loffer, 1984). The author found 7 French catheter (No. 104688-7 Karl Storz Endoscopy of America Inc.) with a syringe for suction an indispensable part of visualizing the tubal ostium. When a low-viscosity fluid is used and a continuous flow hysteroscope (Circon ACMI, PO Box 1971, Stamford, CT 06904) is not available, the same catheter described above can be used to 'vacuum' the cavity. The debris obscuring the tubal ostium is forced out of the uterus by the intrauterine pressure of the distending media.

Hysteroscopic Equipment Suitable for Tubal Occlusion Techniques

Both rigid and flexible hysteroscopes can be used to identify and approach the tubal ostium during occlusion procedures. The rigid telescopes have the advantage of easier orientation since the optical view within the uterus has a fixed relationship in all telescopes to the light post. The flexible telescopes allow for variable approaches to the tubal ostium but require greater expertise in intrauterine manipulation and judgment as to its intrauterine location.

When a rigid hysteroscope is used a bridge with a deflecting arm allows the intrauterine position of the surgical instruments which have been passed through the bridge's 7 French operative channel to be varied. A standard operative bridge without the deflecting arm can be used in the majority of cases but limits the surgeon's ability to vary the direction at which the tubal ostium is approached. Equipment and technique for obtaining good visualization has been discussed in the preceding section.

A Review of Techniques Used in Attempting Transcervical Tubal Occlusion Techniques

The appeal of a transcervical tubal occlusion techniques lies in the fact that the tubes can be approached without a surgical incision. A blind method would allow greater application in both developed and developing countries than one which requires hysteroscopic equipment and skills.

Instrumentation for blind methods of injecting into the fallopian tube have been available for many years (Corfman and Taylor, 1966). The Femcet system was developed to inject methyl cyanoacrylate into the fallopian tubes after occluding the uterine cavity with a balloon (Richart et al., 1987). A bilateral tubal occlusion rate was achieved in 71% after one application and 89% after a second application 1 month later. A moderate degree of discomfort existed for the patient during the procedure. In addition there is the inconvenience and expense of a follow-up hysterosalpingogram. Although promising, this procedure is not available to clinicians at the present time.

Ishikawa was reported to have achieved a 98% tubal closure in 136 cases using a blind thermal coagulation technique with the probe at a temperature of 135°C for 30–35 seconds (Rimkus and Semm, 1974). Rimkus and Semm also reported a similar technique but published no statistics. These methods most likely carry the same disadvantage as do the electrical methods and will be discussed later in this chapter.

The injection of quinacrine as a non-specific sclerosing agent has been reported by several authors. Blind injection into the uterine cavity yielded a bilateral closure rate of 88.2% after up to three instillations and a pregnancy rate of 1.2/100 women (Zipper et al., 1970). Direct instillation into the fallopian tube was also tried under hysteroscopic control (Alvarado et al., 1974). This technique is a simple one since it is easy to place catheters at each fallopian tube. A measured amount of quinacrine in saline was injected into each fallopian tube. The small amount of saline used prevented significant intraperitoneal spread in all but one of the 30 patients reported. Bilateral tubal closure rate was evaluated by hysterosalpingogram at 3 months post-application in 16 of the 30 patients. Bilateral closure occurred in six, unilateral obstruction in six and no obstruction in four cases. Failure to occlude the fallopian tube did not appear to be related to the distending media washing the quinacrine out of the fallopian tube since two out of the three unilateral closure failures occurred in the tube that was the second to be injected. Canalization probably occurs since only the tubal epithelium is destroyed, leaving a patent passage which can be re-epithelialized.

Electrical methods using high-frequency unipolar equipment initially appeared to have a great deal of promise as a hysteroscopic tubal occlusion technique. It was assumed it would carry with it a success rate similar to that of laparoscopic tubal coagulation sterilizations. Numerous authors reported their early experience with this technique.

The largest and most successful series of 930 patients (Quinones et al., 1976) had a tubal occlusion rate of 82.7% after the first electrocoagulation. An additional 15.5% of patients could achieve bilateral tubal occlusion for a total of 98.2% if a second electrocoagulation was done. The power used was 25 W for 8 seconds. No pregnancies were reported if bilateral tubal occlusion was demonstrated and the only complication that occurred was a perforation of the uterus with the hysteroscope.

However, further interest in electrical hysteroscopic tubal occlusion techniques essentially ceased after the publication of a collaborative study from 10 institutions involving 773 cases (Darabi and Richart, 1977). Tubal patency demonstrated by hysterosalpingogram or pregnancy occurred in 245 (31.7%) of the cases. Major complications related to the procedure included acute peritonitis in seven patients (0.9%). Bowel damage was documented as to the cause of the peritonitis in three patients. One death occurred as a result of the bowel injury. There were eight ectopic pregnancies (1.0%). Little interest in electrical hysteroscopic methods existed after this collaborative study because of the high failure rate and complications reported. Factors relating to these results were studied in a later publication (Darabi et al, 1978).

The fact that a much higher bilateral closure rate and virtually no complications occurred in an equally as large series performed by one operator (Quinones et al., 1976) further suggests that the experience of the operating surgeon is critical in this procedure.

It is possible that instrumentation could have been developed which would have removed bowel injury as a possible complication. A bipolar probe with markings as to the depth of cornual penetration, as an example, may have been all that was needed. Variations in the length, amount, or type of unipolar current used may also have provided a higher closure rate.

It is not the risk of bowel injury that makes destruction of the fallopian tube at the uterine junction an impractical method of tubal occlusion. What cannot be altered and is, in the author's opinion, the most critical risk is the high ectopic pregnancy rate. All tubal occlusion procedures carry with them a failure rate and a large number are ectopic pregnancies (Loffer and Pent, 1980). However, the risk of an ectopic pregnancy with this technique is higher than acceptable. In addition, interstitial ectopic pregnancy appears to be increased. Half of the six ectopic pregnancies in one series (Quinones et al., 1976) and three-quarters of the ectopic pregnancies in the collaborative study (Darabi and Richart, 1977) were described as cornual. (The term cornual pregnancy denotes an ectopic pregnancy that developed in a rudimentary uterine horn; Hughes, 1977.) Presumably the pregnancies described in these papers were interstitial pregnancies.

The majority of the interstitial pregnancies reported in techniques employing cornual tubal destruction occurs in tubes known not to be closed. However, the risk of interstitial ectopic pregnancies occurring may be even higher with long-term follow-up. The length of follow-up in the collaborative study was less than 1 year in 83.4% of patients. Tubes apparently closed may recanalize or form fistula resulting in pregnancies at long intervals after the sterilization procedure (Loffer and Pent, 1980). The author believes that any method which relies on scarring by necrosing of the interstitial portion of the tube leaves a ready site for re-canalization and subsequent interstitial pregnancy. This problem is especially important because interstitial pregnancies carry a much higher risk to patients than other tubal pregnancies.

There are two reports of using the Nd:YAG laser to occlude the fallopian tubes hysteroscopically. The first series (Donnez et al., 1990) reported 30 patients in whom bilateral tubal occlusion was proven 3 months post-surgery by hysterosalpingography. In this study a touch technique was used in which the laser energy was brought directly to the tissue via the silicone fibre. A power setting of 80 W was used and a total of between 5000 and 8000 J were applied to the tissue. The second series (Brumsted *et al.*, 1991) was discontinued because of a bilateral closure rate of only 4 of 17 (24%) patients. This method differed in that a non-touch technique was used with a power setting of 50–60 W and therefore fewer total joules to tissue. Since the laser method, like the electrical method, depends on the tubes to scar closed and prevent re-canalization the author is concerned that a high interstitial pregnancy rate will also occur with this method.

Numerous mechanical plugs have been designed to occlude the tubal ostium. One only needs to view a picture of some of the many designs (Figure 44.1) to realize that a simple

method does not exist. Retention in the tubal ostium of most plugs is so poor that few underwent any type of clinical trials.

Two tubal plugs have met with some success. One plug (Hamou *et al.*, 1984) is more appropriately defined as an intratubal device since it does not attempt to occlude the fallopian tube. Its expulsion is prevented by a single barb of thread projecting from the device.

The other plug is the formed *in situ* silicone plug (The Ovabloc System®). It avoids the high expulsion rate found with other plugs by virtue of its dumb-bell shape. This plug is formed by the *vivo* hardening of liquid silicone which has been injected into the fallopian tube. This liquid

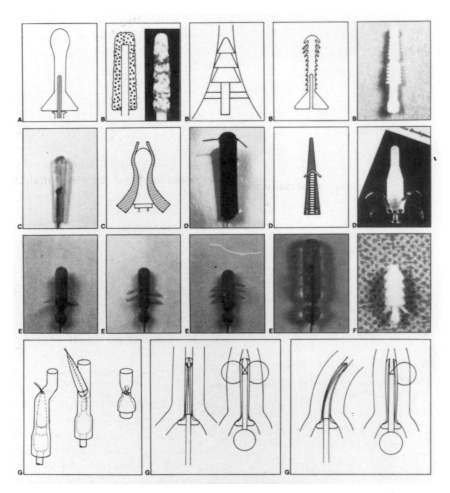

Figure 44.1 Intratubal devices and the principles of their fixation. (A) Insertion without any addition fixation, Bleier. (B) Corrugation of plug surface. (*Left to right*) Craft (porous), Sugimoto (Christmas tree pattern), Bleier, Bleier (fishbone pattern). (C) Swelling after insertion. (*Left to right*) Brundin (hydratization), Popp (inflation). (D) Fixation with spines. (*Left to right*) Chargoy-Vera, Brueschke and colleagues, Hosseinian and colleagues. (E) Combination. Brundin (hydratization plus anchoring protrusions, the far right shows its swollen state). (F) Combination. Bleier (a solid pin is surrounded by a soft and corrugated cover with two spines). (G) Fixation by tubal wall penetration. (*Left*) Cimber (penetration and fixation through ligation; laparotomy is necessary). (*Centre and right*) Popp (the wall penetrating 'claw' fixed the device; a dowel effect and a corrugated surface can also help the fixation). (Reproduced with permission from Siegler AM & Lindemann HJ (eds) (1984) *Hysteroscopy: Principles and Practice*. Philadelphia: J.B. Lippincott.)

silicone welds to a preformed intrauterine tip. The preformed tip and the larger ampullary portion of the plug effectively preclude it from being expelled into either the uterine or peritoneal cavity. This technique is the only transcervical tubal occlusion technique currently commercially available to clinicians.

The Ovabloc System®

Patient selection is important in this procedure since tubal occlusion of 100% of all patients is probably not achievable. The manufacturer (Alphatron, PO Box 12003, 3001 AA, Rotterdam, The Netherlands) lists the following exclusion criteria:

1. acute or chronic cervicitis or vaginal infection— until gonorrhoea and *Chlamydia* are ruled out;
2. a recent history of pelvic inflammatory disease;
3. undiagnosed genital tract bleeding or the presence of a bleeding disorder;
4. congenital malformation of the genital tract or prior tubal surgery;
5. known or suspected genital tract malignancy.

Patients with a retroverted uterus, especially if retroflexed, are more difficult to occlude since the tubal ostia are not readily approached at an angle where silicone instillation can be done. In addition, patients with a history of pelvic inflammatory disease have a high risk of having non-patent fallopian tubes which is necessary for the instillation of the silicone. Finally, the most appropriate time to do these procedures is in the immediate post-menstrual phase when the endometrium is thinnest and less liable to obscure the tubal ostia or to bleed on contact.

This procedure is readily done in an office setting using local anaesthesia. Since these procedures last between 25 and 45 minutes the patients should be placed in a dorsal lithotomy position with their legs cradled in a fashion which will be comfortable for that period of time. The vulva, vagina and cervix are prepped with a povidone-iodine 10% or similar solution. Draping is not necessary although the author placed a sterile drape beneath the buttocks on which to place instrumentation. Anaesthesia is provided by paracervical and intracervical block (Loffer, 1990).

Instruments necessary for this procedure are as follows:

1. paracervical/intracervical block tray;
2. sterile one-sided speculum;
3. tenaculum;
4. cervical dilators (should dilation be required);
5. light source and cable;
6. 4 mm telescope and sheath with a 7 mm operative bridge with deflecting arm; and
7. a method for uterine distension.

The metal instruments are sterilized by autoclaving. Only the hysteroscope and light cables are soaked in activated alkaline 2% glutaraldehyde for 20 minutes. The parts of the Ovabloc system which are purchased for indefinite use include:

1. a mechanical fluid flow actuator (Figure 44.2);
2. a mixing dish;
3. a microsyringe to inject the silicone catalyst; and
4. insulating cup to hold the syringe during mixing.

Those items which are purchased for one time use are:

1. a frozen mixer–dispenser syringe containing raw silicone (Figure 44.3);
2. a vial of catalyst to activate the silicone; and
3. sterile catheters with soft silicone obturator tips (Figure 44.4).

The factors upon which the system depends are standardized by the manufacturer. They include: the amounts of silicone and catalyst used, the time of mixing, injection and the pressures at which the system works. The variable factors which are taken into account by the manufacturer are the rapidity with which the silicone hardens after mixing the catalyst. This depends not only on the silicone temperature but the batch of silicone and the amount of catalyst injected.

When carrying out the procedure, the silicone and catalyst are combined and then mixed by movements of the plunger of the silicone containing syringe. This same syringe can then be converted by a spacer into a dispensing syringe (Figure 44.3). After mixing, the syringe is placed in the fluid flow actuator (Figure 44.2) which begins the injection of the hardening silicone through the catheter into the tube (Figure 44.4). This initial pressure of 300 N is maintained until the silicone is seen by the hysteroscopist to enter the fallopian tube through the catheter. The pressure on the syringe by the fluid flow actuator is then allowed to decrease as the syringe is emptying. The amount of silicone that flows into the fallopian tubes is therefore predetermined by the quickness with which the silicone hardens, the timing of the onset of pressure on the syringe, and the pressure with which it is injected. Final curing of the silicone is determined on a test plate using silicone from the syringe dispenser

Figure 44.2 Fluid flow
actuator system used to drive
the activated and hardening
silicone out of the syringe
and down the coaxial catheter
and into the fallopian tubes.
(Reproduced with permission
from Siegler AM &
Lindemann HJ (eds) (1984)
*Hysteroscopy: Principles and
Practice.* Philadelphia: J.B.
Lippincott.)

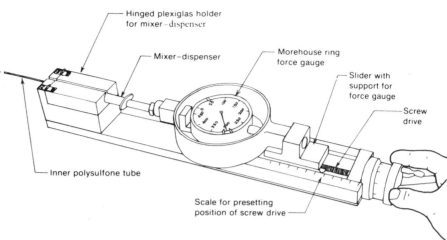

Figure 44.3 Mixer dispenser
syringe allows the catalyst to
be injected with the silicone
and mixed. A spacer converts
it into an injection syringe
which is connected to the
coaxial catheter and placed in
the fluid flow actuator.
(Reproduced with permission
from Siegler AM &
Lindemann HJ (eds) (1984)
*Hysteroscopy: Principles and
Practice.* Philadelphia: J.B.
Lippincott.)

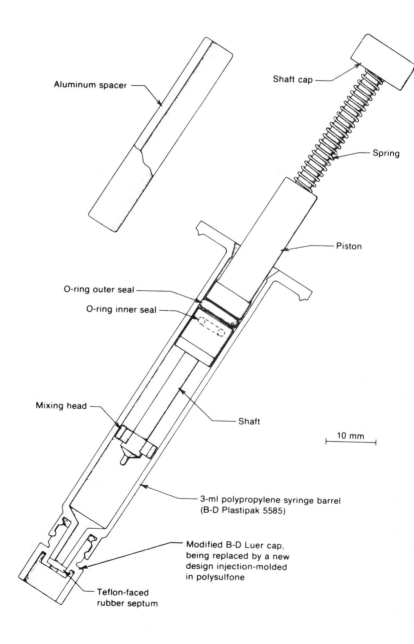

Figure 44.4 Coaxial catheter with pre-formed soft obturator tip.

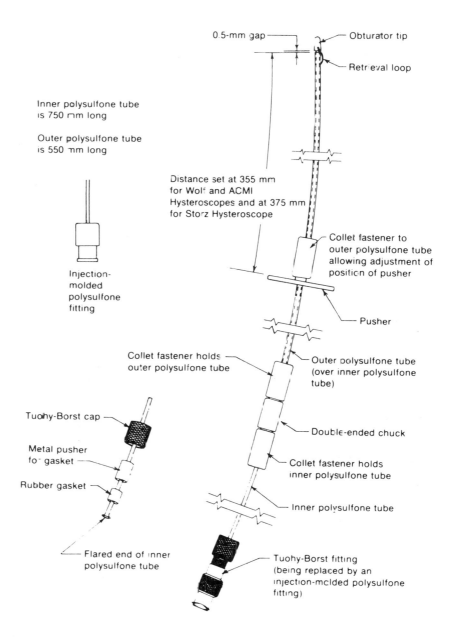

Inner polysulfone tube is 750 mm long

Outer polysulfone tube is 550 mm long

Injection-molded polysulfone fitting

Tuohy-Borst cap

Metal pusher for gasket

Rubber gasket

Flared end of inner polysulfone tube

Collet fastener holds outer polysulfone tube

0.5-mm gap

Obturator tip

Retrieval loop

Distance set at 355 mm for Wolf and ACMI Hysteroscopes and at 375 mm for Storz Hysteroscope

Collet fastener to outer polysulfone tube allowing adjustment of position of pusher

Pusher

Outer polysulfone tube (over inner polysulfone tube)

Double-ended chuck

Collet fastener holds inner polysulfone tube

Inner polysulfone tube

Tuohy-Borst fitting (being replaced by an injection-molded polysulfone fitting)

prior to its being attached to the catheter. Once curing has occurred the interportion of the coaxial catheter is withdrawn which breaks the column of cured silicone at the obturator tip.

The sequential steps in doing this procedure after preparing the patients and administering local anaesthesia are as follows:

1. The operative hysteroscope is inserted. In the author's experience cervical dilatation was necessary in 30% of his patients.
2. The uterine cavity is distended. Carbon dioxide, Hyskon and low viscosity fluid can be used.
3. The cavity is cleaned of blood, debris and other tissue so the fallopian tubes can be identified.
4. The prepackaged sterile coaxial catheter with a preformed silicone obturator tip at the end is introduced through the hysteroscope operative channel into the uterine cavity. It is brought

into contact with the tubal ostium. When Hyskon is used debris can be seen to pass with the Hyskon out through the fallopian tubes. This alerts the hysteroscopist to the direction the intramural portion of the tube is coursing.

5. Once the hysteroscopist feels that appropriate application of the obturator tip to the ostium has taken place, the assistant is asked to inject a methylene blue dye solution through the coaxial catheter into the fallopian tube. This is done to demonstrate tubal patency and proper alignment of the obturator tip. The assistant should feel a free flow of the methylene blue solution. If the solution refluxes back into the uterine cavity a tight application has not been made to the ostium. If a free flow is not determined it may be due to spasm of the fallopian tube, a blocked fallopian tube or the

obturator tip may be inappropriately applied and thus occluded. Tubal spasm is a frustrating problem for which no method of relaxing is available. Time will occasionally provide relaxation and the silicone can be injected.

6. The procedure cannot be carried forward until there is a free flow of the methylene blue test. Once this has been determined the hysteroscopist holds the catheter in place without movement while the assistant removes the silicone syringe from the freezer and places it in the insulated holder. An insulator is necessary in order not to raise the silicone temperature and alter its curing properties.

7. A predetermined amount of catalyst is then injected into the silicone syringe and the mixer

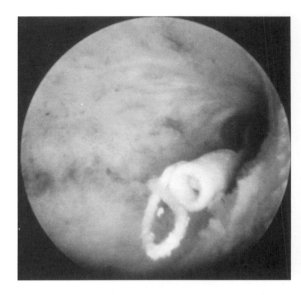

Figure 44.6 The larger pre-formed tip is seen lying in the uterine cavity attached to the thinner isthmic portion. Beyond and out of sight, in the isthmic part of the fallopian tube, is a large distal portion.

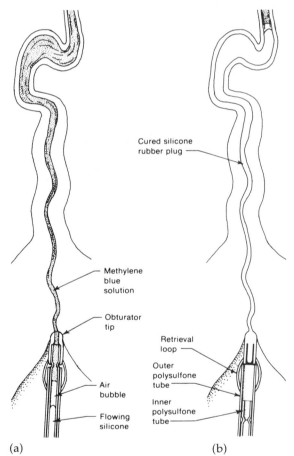

Cured silicone rubber plug

Methylene blue solution

Obturator tip

Retrieval loop

Outer polysulfone tube

Air bubble

Inner polysulfone tube

Flowing silicone

(a)   (b)

Figure 44.5 When methylene blue and silicone are injected into the fallopian tube the obturator tip is held in place by the outer catheter (a). When the silicone has hardened the inner part of the coaxial catheter is then withdrawn and breaks the silicone column (which had extended from the syringe to the ampullary part of the plug) at the junction of the pre-formed obturator tip (b). (Reproduced with permission from Siegler AM and Lindemann HJ (eds) (1984) *Hysteroscopy: Principles and Practice.* Philadelphia: J.B. Lippincott.)

syringe handle is then pumped to mix the silicone and catalyst. Once a predetermined number of mixing strokes have been done, a spacer converts the mixing syringe into a dispensing syringe. A small portion is injected onto a test plate before the syringe is attached to the coaxial catheter.

8. At a predetermined time the fluid flow actuator is brought up to 300 N and the silicone is injected down the catheter. If curing is taking place in an appropriate fashion the hysteroscopist will see the silicone appear at the end of the coaxial catheter and proceed on into the tube in a predetermined time span (Figure 44.5a).

9. The surgeon will see when the silicone has become so hardened that the pressure of the fluid flow actuator is insufficient to cause further infusion into the fallopian tube.

10. Once the flow has stopped the assistant begins checking the curing of the silicone on the test plate.

11. If curing occurs in an appropriate period of time the interportion of the coaxial catheter is pulled back breaking the bond (Figure 44.5b). Then the whole catheter can be removed leaving an intact plug (Figure 44.6).

12. The procedure is carried out on the opposite side in this same fashion.

13. Bilateral normal plugs can be determined by X-ray. They appear as a tip with a narrow isthmic portion and enlarged ampullary portion (Figure 44.7a).

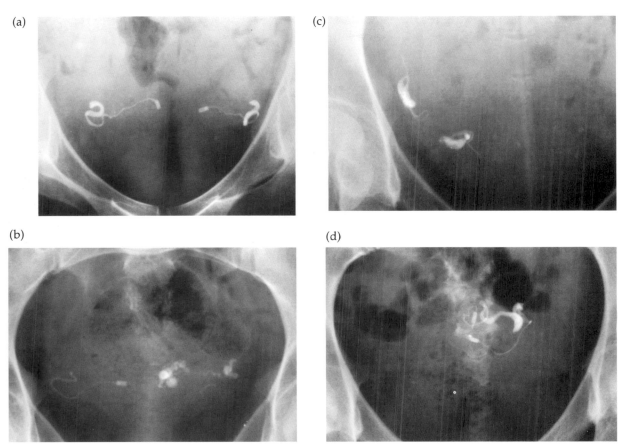

Figure 44.7 Types of formed, *in situ* plugs as seen on X-ray; (a) bilateral normal dumb-bell shaped plugs; (b) *left*, an inadequate distal tip occurring from premature hardening of the silicone may also occur resulting in reflux of the plug into the uterine cavity; *right*, intravasation of silicone into myometrium; (c) bilateral tip separation resulting from inadequate bonding of the tip to the formed *in situ* portion of the plug. Both distal portions lie intraperitoneally; (d) *left*, migrated intact plug lying free in the peritoneal cavity above a normal plug.

One of the problems that can occur during the instillation of silicone into the fallopian tube is reflux of silicone back into the uterine cavity. Slight additional pressure of the catheter against the tubal opening will usually solve this problem. If it does not, the procedure must be aborted since an undetermined amount of silicone will enter the fallopian tube and may result in a small distal enlargement (Figure 44.7b). In these cases the plug will eventually be lost into the uterus. Inadequate silicone may also enter the fallopian tube if the curing time has occurred too rapidly.

When an inadequate plug is to be removed the preformed tip can be grasped and removed from the uterus. During this process the whole plug may be removed but more likely it will break its connection with the formed *in situ* portion of the plug. The remaining part of the plug can then be flushed with the methylene blue test into the peritoneal cavity and another plug attempted.

When the pre-formed obturator tip is not appropriately bonded to the formed *in situ* plug it will migrate into the peritoneal cavity (Figure

44.7c). A small number of patients will have plugs that migrate intact into the peritoneal cavity by virtue of anatomically larger than normal interstitial portions of the tube (Figure 44.7d).

The author enrolled 265 patients in his part of the formed *in situ* silicone plug study. Thirty-seven patients had two procedures and four patients had three procedures for a total of 310 procedures. Six patients were unable to have silicone injected and were dropped from the study. A successful procedure was defined as the formation of bilaterally normal devices. Tip separation and tubal spasm were the primary reason the initial procedure had to be repeated. Of the 259 patients who had silicone installed and were included in the study, 248 (96%) had normal devices and were felt to be occluded immediately following the final procedure. Before allowing a patient to rely on the Ovabloc device for contraception an X-ray was obtained at 3 months. At that time 225 (88%) of the 255 women who were seen had continuing normal devices. They were then allowed to rely on the Ovabloc method as their only method of contraception. Improved techniques and product modifications should significantly increase the number of plugs that remain normal from the immediate postoperative period to the 3 month follow-up.

There are currently 208 patients in the author's series who are being followed and 190 rely on the formed *in situ* plugs as their only form of birth control. The remaining 18 patients are not considered sterilized because their plugs were inadvertently damaged by a D & C or removed at the patient's request. Fifty-one patients who had silicone instilled have been dropped from the study. Failure to achieve bilateral devices were the reason 31 patients are no longer being followed. In addition, 19 patients were lost to follow-up. One patient became pregnant while presumed sterilized.

The efficacy of the procedure is shown by the fact that only one patient became pregnant while presumed protected by the Ovabloc procedure. She had an ectopic pregnancy. Another patient had an ectopic pregnancy while never being presumed protected by the device and another patient had the devices removed in order to become pregnant. She became pregnant but only after a tuboplasty. Removal of plugs will not result in pregnancies. The tubes appear to scar closed in essentially all patients.

The Ovabloc procedure is an effective, safe method of permanent contraception. Follow-up of the author's series in 12 022 months of use have shown no serious side-effects other than the one ectopic pregnancy. In 9950 women-months of use the failure rate has shown a Pearl index of 0.12 and a life table pregnancy rate at 5 years per 100 women of 0.0067. Other series have found similar results. The oldest series which is based on 14 300 women-months exposure had a Pearl index of 0.84 a life table pregnancy rate of 0.0093 per 100 women (T Reed, 1991, personal communication). Similar results based on 8040 women-months exposure gave a life table rate exactly the same as the authors (0.0067) and a Pearl index of 0.30 (J DeMaeyer, 1991, personal communication).

This method is well received by patients and provides an excellent office-based tubal occlusion procedure. It is commercially available in many areas of Europe. It has not yet completed the regulatory requirements of the FDA in the United States.

References

Alvarado A, Quinones R & Aznar R (1974) Tubal instillation of quinacrine under hysteroscopic control. In Sciarra JJ, Butler JC & Speidel JJ (eds) *Hysteroscopic Sterilization*, pp 85–94. New York: Intercontinental Medical Book Corporation.

Brumsted JR, Shirk G, Soderling MJ & Reed T (1991) Attempted transcervical occlusion of the fallopian tube with the Nd:YAG laser. *Obstetrics and Gynecology* **77**: 327–328.

Corfman PA & Taylor HC (1966) An instrument for transcervical treatment of the oviduct and uterine cornua. *Obstetrics and Gynecology* **27**: 880–883.

Darabi KF & Richart RM (1977) Collaborative study on hysteroscopic sterilization procedures. A preliminary report. *Obstetrics and Gynecology* **49**: 48–54.

Darabi KF, Roy K & Richart RM (1978) Collaborative study on hysteroscopic sterilization procedures: final report. In Sciarra JJ, Zatacuni GI & Speidel JJ (eds) *Risks, Benefits and Controversies in Fertility Control*, pp 81–101. Hagerstown: Harper and Row.

Donnez J, Malvaux V, Nisolle M & Casanas F (1990) Hysteroscopic sterilization with the Nd:YAG laser. *Journal of Gynecologic Surgery* **6**: 149–153.

Hamou J, Gasparri F, Scarselli GF et al. (1984) Hysteroscopic reversible tubal sterilization. *Acta Europaea Fertilitatis* **15**: 123–129.

Hughes EC (ed) (1977) *Obstetric-Gynecologic Terminology* pp 418–419. Philadelphia: F.A. Davis Co.

Loffer FD (1984) Hysteroscopic sterilization with the use of the formed in-place silicone plugs. *American Journal of Obstetrics and Gynecology* **149**: 261–270.

Loffer FD (1990) Hysteroscopy. In Stangel JJ (ed) *Infertility Surgery: A Multi Method Approach to Female Reproductive Surgery*, pp 72–85. Norwalk: Appleton and Lange.

Loffer FD & Pent D (1980) Pregnancy after laparoscopic sterilizations. *Obstetrics and Gynecology* **55**: 643–648.

Quinones R, Alvarado A & Ley E (1976) Hysteroscopic sterilization. *International Journal of Gynecology and Obstetrics* **14**: 27–34.

Richart RM, Neuwirth RS, Goldsmith A & Edelman DA (1987) Intrauterine administration of methyl cyanoacrylate as an outpatient method of permanent female sterilization. *American Journal of Obstetrics and Gynecology* **155**: 981–987.

Rimkus V & Semm K (1974) Sterilization by carbon dioxide hysteroscopy. In Sciarra JJ, Butler JC & Speidel JJ (eds) *Hysteroscopic Sterilization*, pp 75–84. New York: Intercontinental Medical Book Corporation.

Zipper JA, Stachetti E & Medal M (1970) Human fertility control by transcervical application of quinacrine on the fallopian tube. *Fertility and Sterility* **21**: 581–589.

45

Hazards and Dangers of Operative Hysteroscopy

BRUNO van HERENDAEL

Algemeen Ziekenhuis Jan Palfijn, Antwerp, Belgium

Operative hysteroscopy is a new and valuable technique in the treatment of non-malignant conditions of the uterine cavity. As the indications for endoscopic surgery become wider (Siegler and Valle, 1988) safety protocols become more important in the prevention of complications. This is particularly important since most complications tend to occur in the hands of inexperienced surgeons (Lindemann, 1975).

As with any other surgical technique, operative hysteroscopy requires an intensive training period. The operative field is new to gynaecologists and requires a different approach when compared with classical surgery (Slangen, 1991; Martens, 1991). It is therefore advisable that a surgeon starting hysteroscopic surgery should have performed at least 250 diagnostic procedures before embarking on operative work.

A further recommendation is that there should be a gradation of difficulties tackled and that the beginner should begin with minor surgery and do some 50 procedures, then do 50 intermediate procedures and only after about 350 hysteroscopies start doing major hysteroscopic surgery.

The safety committee of the European Society of Hysteroscopy has issued a classification of hysteroscopic operative procedures. It seems reasonable to use such a classification to assess the progress of any trainee (Table 45.1).

Every uterine septum operation performed with the hysteroscope should have a full investigation including a laparoscopy prior to surgery to ascertain that the uterus is not bicornuate (Valle and Sciarra, 1986).

Table 45.1 Classification of operative difficulty

Minor hysteroscopic surgery
 Endometrial biopsy
 Small polyps
 Non-embedded IUCD (non-pregnant)
 Simple adhesions

Intermediate hysteroscopic surgery
 Cannulation of the fallopian tube
 Sterilization

Advanced hysteroscopic surgery
 Myomectomy*
 Large polyps
 Endometrial resection or ablation
 Resection of uterine septum*
 IUCD removal in pregnancy
 Extensive adhesiolysis*

---

* These procedures should probably be combined with either a laparoscopy or an ultrasound examination (Sugimoto *et al.*, 1984; Taylor *et al.*, 1984; van Herendael, 1988).

Complications of Hysteroscopic Surgery

Dilation of the Cervix

The use of rigid instruments may cause damage to the cervical canal if appropriate care is not taken. The cervix can be lacerated by the tenaculum due to excessive traction whilst dilating (Siegler, 1983). Dilation itself can provoke bleeding. A certain amount of force is often necessary to dilate a cervical canal up to Hegar 9. Therefore the position taken with the direction of the force as well as a certain amount of patience. The use of Hegar dilators increasing by half a size at a time is less traumatic. Some instruments such as the Pratt dilator seem to cause less trauma.

Pharmacological cervical dilatation is useful in overcoming these problems. Laminaria stents are hygroscopic and distend by absorption of fluid over the course of a few hours. However, the laminaria tends to swell beyond the confines of the cervical canal and can therefore be difficult to remove and can introduce infection. Synthetic laminaria such as Lamicel® overcome this problem. The dilator consists of a polyvinyl core impregnated with less than 500 mg of sodium phosphate.

A better method of pharmacological dilatation is the use of prostaglandins. The synthetic derivative of prostaglandin E_2 (Sulprostone) is more effective at a lower dosage than prostaglandin $F_{2\alpha}$ and its maximum effect is reached within the hour. The route of administration is local by vaginal suppositories. The action is due to softening of the cervical stroma resulting in dilatation of the canal. This is enhanced by contractions of the myometrium induced by the drug. Doses of 125–250 mg given 1–2 hours prior to surgery produce sufficient cervical dilatation in 80% of women. Side-effects reported include nausea, vomiting, hypertension, hypotension and occasionally a cutaneous rash.

Hazards of Distension Media

Both CO_2 and liquid distension media are used in hysteroscopic surgery (Lindemann, 1983) and are comprehensively covered in Chapter 36 by Ray Garry.

Minor and intermediate hysteroscopic surgery can be performed using CO_2 gas with a specially adapted insufflator for hysteroscopy. Advanced hysteroscopic surgery is always performed using liquid distension with the one exception being the removal of an IUCD in the gravid uterus where the distension medium of choice is still CO_2 under carefully controlled pressure.

Complications of CO_2 and other Gases

CO_2 is a soluble gas at body temperature since 57 ml of CO_2 per minute are absorbed in 100 ml of blood (Lindemann, 1972). There are no changes in Po_2, Pco_2 or pH if 100 ml of CO_2 are infused into the bloodstream per minute but changes start to occur when more than 400 ml of CO_2 per minute are used. If 1000 ml are infused per minute an irreversible cardiac shock occurs due to acute CO_2 intoxication of the heart muscle.

This means that for operative hysteroscopy where the time used for the procedure is longer than for a classical diagnostic hysteroscopy it is mandatory to have a reliable and calibrated hysteroflator. The flow should not exceed 80 ml/min. The insufflation pressure should not exceed 200 mgHg. The use of cervical cups is contraindicated as it prevents the outflow of gas through the cervical canal.

The use of hysteroflators equipped with the possibility of giving a boost of gas is dangerous and should not be used for hysteroscopy. These deliver a bolus of gas of 120 ml in ten (10) seconds with the ability to repeat the bolus every minute; in doing so the blood buffer system could be overloaded. These hysteroflators should therefore *not* be used for operative procedures (Gallinat, 1978). Gas embolism is probably underdiagnosed due to this very high solubility of CO_2. It must, however, be assumed that because of the fact that the intrauterine pressure rises above the diastolic blood pressure there must be frequent entry of gas into venous circulation.

The physical properties of CO_2 are such that the mixing with the blood and the mucus of the endocervix and the endometrium creates bubbles. Bubbles impair the vision but invariably disappear when the physical reaction of mixing ends. However, this can take a long time and CO_2 is less appropriate for hysteroscopic surgery since liquid distension media are safer and afford good visibility for the surgeon.

Air and other gases must never be used for uterine distension. Fatal air embolism has been recorded with both tubal persufflation and with hysteroscopy. Baggish and Daniell (1989) reported five fatal cases where air had accidentally been used to cool the sapphire tips of Nd:YAG laser fibres. Several other deaths have been reported throughout the world. All these women had sudden irreversible circulatory failure due to massive air embolism.

Complications of Liquid Distension Media

High-viscosity Fluids

Thirty-two per cent dextran 70 in 10% dextrose (Hyskon) is colourless, has excellent optical properties and does not conduct electricity.

The risks are the same in hysteroscopy as in intravenous infusion and in intraperitoneal instillation. Blood coagulation can be impaired and sensitivity has been associated with allergic reactions including anaphylaxis based on a direct toxic effect on the pulmonary vessels—the so-called dextran-induced anaphylactic reaction (DIAR). This results in extravasation and interstitial oedema. The incidence is of 1 in 10 000 cases (Leake *et al.*, 1987; McLucas, 1991) and can be fatal. Treatment consists of administration of adrenaline, vasopressin and corticosteroids.

Low-viscosity Fluids

GLYCINE 1.5%

Glycine is a non-essential amino acid which is normally present in the circulation and in solution gives poor electrical conductivity and good visibility (Baumann *et al.*, 1990). Intravascular absorption of large volumes of glycine causes hyperammonaemia due to rapid metabolism. High ammonia concentrations in the central nervous system alter neural amino acid metabolism, resulting in the production of false neurotransmitters causing encephalopathy.

Oxalate, the metabolic end product, is contraindicated in renal failure. Glycine in iso-osmotic concentration can lead to haemodilution and extracellular volume expansion with consequent decrease of serum sodium.

From the experiments of Donnez we know that it is possible to lose up to 1300 ml (Pers. commun.) into the circulation without any adverse effect. It is therefore mandatory to monitor very carefully the fluid input and output and to stop surgery when the deficit is more than 1300 ml.

Mannitol Sorbitol

Mannitol is an isomer of sorbitol and is soluble in water and is iso-osmotic with serum in a 5.07% solution. Intravasation of large amounts may cause nausea, vomiting, headache and hyponatraemia. It should not be used in patients with renal failure. The only severe complication known is fluid overload due to prolonged surgical procedures which result in pulmonary oedema (Wamsteker, 1991).

Mechanical Complications

Perforation

It is an accepted fact that perforations do occur when using dilators to dilate the cervix or when inserting the hysteroscope. Subsequently therapy is seldom necessary but the patient should be carefully observed for several hours. A rising pulse and falling blood pressure usually indicates ongoing haemorrhage in which case a laparoscopy should be performed to assess the bleeding. Usually the haemorrhage can be stopped by laparoscopic endocoagulation, diathermy or sutures but occasionally it is necessary to perform a laparotomy or even a hysterectomy.

Instrumental Injuries

The more sophisticated the instrument the more essential it is that the surgeon must know the physical properties of the instruments that he is using. Electric instruments have quite different physical properties than mechanical and laser instruments.

If the instrument or the heat generated by the instrument diffuses beyond the myometrium adherent bowel loops may be damaged. For this reason if a patient complains of increasing abdominal pain after surgery, a laparoscopy should be performed to check for bowel damage. A pelvic drain should be inserted and the patient kept under careful observation for signs of peritonitis.

Mechanical injury is circumscribed and mostly easy to detect with the laparoscope. If a perforation occurs during instrumentation, the operation must be terminated immediately. On no account must a laser or electric current be activated if perforation is suspected. The surgeon has to ascertain that there has been no major vessel injury and has to withdraw the hysteroscope only after removing the ancillary instruments (Haning *et al.*, 1980).

A possible complication is fluid overload due to the massive absorption of the distension medium at the time of the perforation. The rate of fluid absorption is increased 20-fold. Sometimes collections of distension medium have been reported in the broad ligament, especially after perforations at the time of extensive adhesiolysis. These should be left undisturbed and will disappear over a period of time. Only if the patient complains of pressure in the iliac fossa or persistent fever should laparoscopic drainage be performed.

Injuries to the bowel, mostly colon or rectum (and very seldom the small bowel) due to electric current are often not so obvious and require some expertise to be detected. If the perforation is performed by an experienced surgeon the current will not be activated at the time of the perforation in most cases. The injury will therefore be a thermal injury and sometimes it will take as long as 5 days before the bowel perforates and the patient will present with a septic peritonitis. For this reason if perforation is suspected the patient should be kept under close observation in hospital for several days.

If, however, the current is activated during the perforation the results are more spectacular and require immediate intervention. There have been case reports of the aorta, the external and internal iliac vessels, mesenteric and sacral vessels being damaged in these circumstances. Prompt intervention using emergency laparotomy and preferably the assistance of a vascular surgeon is necessary to save the life and limb of the patient.

PREOPERATIVE PREPARATION

Patients should have received some kind of bowel preparation. The easiest to perform is the one used by the radiologists to prepare the bowels for contrast X-ray studies. The least expensive is a combination of an oral laxative the morning and the evening of the day preceding the hysteroscopy and an enema some 2 hours prior to the procedure.

ACTIVE AND PASSIVE RESECTOSCOPE

The procedure is best performed with a passive resectoscope (DeCherney et al., 1987). The active resectoscope features a loop, a ball or a knife that protrudes in front of the instrument. This is useful for the urologist but offers no advantage whatsoever to the gynaecologist. The automatic advancement of the loop can cause a perforation if the resectoscope is held too close to the uterine wall. The passive resectoscope automatically retracts the loop towards the end of the hysteroscope and requires an active movement from the fingers of the surgeon to move it outwards, thus reducing the danger of perforation.

When using a resectoscope the active phase should always be towards the lens so that the surgeon is able to control the section at all times. As long as the loop, the ball or the knife are not completely visible the current should not be activated.

HAZARDS OF ELECTROCAUTERY AND LASERS

Electricity has an effect beyond the visual field of the surgeon. Coagulation and devitalization occur up to 6 mm into the tissues. This has serious implications in the region of the uterine cornu where the safety margin before reaching the serosa is only some 8 mm (Neuwirth and Amin, 1976).

Inside the cavity the zona compacta of the myometrium, situated directly under the endometrium is some 6–8 mm thick, and beneath this lies the vascular bed. Perforation of this layer causes intensive bleeding. Secondary bleeding a week or more after surgery has been reported due to the deep devitalization of the tissues after overzealous coagulation (DeCherney and Polan, 1983).

The most widely used laser for intrauterine surgery is the Nd:YAG laser (Goldrath et al., 1981). All lasers used at hysteroscopy are fibre lasers. Some incidents have occurred where the fibre has perforated the uterus and the laser has been activated. As the fibre is then in the abdominal cavity out of the visual field of the surgeon trauma to bowel and major vessels is possible. The power setting needed for intrauterine laser surgery is high so damage could be extensive. If the surgeon recognizes the problem a laparotomy should be performed to assess the damage as laparoscopy is not sufficient or reliable in these cases.

The Nd:YAG laser has a penetration of 6 mm into the tissues and therefore the surgeon needs to take the same precautions as when using electricity.

The argon or KTP 532 lasers have a penetration of some 3 mm and require fewer precautions. The holmium:YAG laser seems to have even less penetration, some 1–2 mm, and this could be an advantage in some cases.

Laser procedures take much longer than electrosurgery; hence they increase the risk of fluid overload and should therefore only be used with continuous-flow hysteroscopes or flexible hysteroscopes which require less fluid. Flexible hysteroscopes, however, are more difficult for the beginner to use (Baggish and Baltoyannis, 1988).

There is one more pitfall in the tissue penetration. The endometrium is not a homogeneous layer and in the case of adenomyosis crypts of endometrial tissue infiltrate the myometrium and facilitate conduct in both electricity and laser energy far deeper than would be expected in myometrium.

In an unpublished study on the follow-up of

70 patients after endometrial resection after 3, 6, 9 and 12 months both with hysteroscopy and vaginal endosonography, we found in 5% of patients lesions up to 3 mm from the serosa as measured by vaginal ultrasound. The healing of the endometrial wound takes many months and hysteroscopically stabilization of scar tissue occurs only after 9 months, thus explaining some of the delayed complications.

There is no evidence that hysteroscopic surgery causes displaced fragments of endometrium to seed and to produce endometriosis or encourage metastasis of endometrial carcinoma cells (Labastida *et al.*, 1991).

Table 45.2 Recommended doses of commonly used anaesthetics

Local anaesthetic	Maximum doses – vasoconstrictor	Maximum doses + vasoconstrictor
Lignocaine (1–2%) (Xylocaine)	200 mg	500 mg
Mepivacaine (1–2%) (Scandicaine, Carbocaine)	300 mg	500 mg
Prilocaine (1–2%) (Citanest)	400 mg	600 mg

Anaesthesia

Local Anaesthesia

The main problems which may be encountered are anxiety, vasovagal reaction and pain. Most patients are understandably anxious when entering the hysteroscopy room. Not all patients are suitable for outpatient hysteroscopy and hysteroscopic surgery (Magos *et al.*, 1989). It is important to create a relaxed setting which includes a gynaecological examination chair or couch and, above all, good communication between the surgeon and the patient.

Traction on the cervix itself and dilatation may cause a vasovagal reaction. The patient may feel unwell, have a slow pulse rate and a fall in blood pressure. Vagal reactions can be prevented by giving atropine 0.6 mg by intramuscular injection some 20 minutes before the procedure. Glaucoma is uncommon but should be excluded before this drug is given. The patient has to be warned about blurred vision afterwards and it is advisable to ask patients to provide transport and an escort to take them home.

Pain results from dilatation of the cervix beyond Hegar 5–6 and also from overdilatation of the uterine cavity with carbon dioxide. Pain can be diminished by preoperative administration of naproxen sodium 500 mg by rectal suppository 2 hours prior to the operation and/or by using a local anaesthetic in a paracervical block.

The recommended doses of the commonly used anaesthetics are shown in Table 45.2. The preparations are effective in 2–3 minutes and provide good pain relief for up to 30 minutes. The effect is prolonged threefold by combination with vasoconstrictive agents but these are rarely necessary in office hysteroscopy where most procedures are of short duration.

COMPLICATIONS OF LOCAL ANAESTHETICS

Provided the dosage is within accepted limits and care is taken to avoid an intravascular injection, complications are rare although toxic reactions can occur. It is therefore imperative for the hysteroscopist to recognize and deal with them.

1. An inhibiting effect on the conduction system of the heart may be caused by rapid absorption from the injection site, accidental intravascular injection or exceeding the maximum dose. The cardiac effect is evidenced by bradycardia, cardiac arrest, shock or convulsions. The emergency treatment is:
    atropine 0.5 mg i.v.i.;
    intubation and oxygen at a rate of 4–6 l/min;
    adrenaline 0.5–1.0 ml i.v. of 1:1000 solution;
    respiratory and cardiac resuscitation.
2. An excitatory effect on the central nervous system may be caused by the same factors. The signs are drowsiness, tremor or convulsions and above all paraesthesia of the tongue and the perioral area. The treatment is:
    diazepam 10–20 mg i.v.i.;
    respiratory support.
3. Allergic reactions are mainly caused by hypersensitivity to the distension medium used. Agitation, palpitations, pruritis, urticaria, coughing, bronchospasm, shock and possibly convulsions occur after a very short period of time—usually within minutes. The emergency treatment is:
    adrenaline 0.5 ml (1:1000) s.c. or i.m.;
    clemastine (Tavegyl) 2 mg (2 ml) i.v.;
    prednisolone 25 i.v.;

aminophylline 240 mg (10 ml) slowly i.v. over several minutes;
supportive measures including i.v. fluids and oxygen.

General Anaesthesia

General anaesthesia should be administered with controlled positive pressure respiration and an endotracheal tube for all diagnostic and operative hysteroscopies and for combined laparoscopy and hysteroscopy. This is especially the case when carbon dioxide is used as the distension medium. Carbon dioxide absorption leads to a raised plasma level of CO_2 especially if there is an associated hypoxia, as is often the case during the induction of the anaesthesia. The blood pH falls and there is release of catecholamines which, in turn, leads to vasoconstriction, raised central venous pressure and cardiac arrhythmia. The side-effects of CO_2 absorption can usually be prevented by hyperventilation with 30% oxygen although complications can occur if the patient has a metabolic acidaemia, even if there has been compensation.

CONTRAINDICATIONS

Absolute Contraindications
The one and only absolute contraindication is an inexperienced endoscopist. There is no area of gynaecological surgery that can result in such sudden and catastrophic disasters as a result of lack of adequate supervised training.

Relative Contraindications

1. Infection
2. Cardiorespiratory disease
3. Metabolic acidosis
4. Pregnancy
5. Uterine bleeding
6. Occult cervical malignancy

1. *Infection.* Sometimes we have to perform an operation with an IUCD *in situ* in the non-gravid uterus when we become aware that endometritis is present. It is then necessary to treat the patient for 48 hours with broad spectrum antibiotics (Salat-Baroux, 1984).
2. *Cardiorespiratory disease.* As most of the operations are performed under general anaesthesia there should be adequately controlled respiration with an endotracheal tube or a laryngeal mask. This should limit the risks. If CO_2 is used under local anaesthesia or without anaesthesia, cardiopulmonary disease is an absolute contraindication.
3. *Metabolic acidosis.* This condition should be corrected prior to any surgery.
4. *Pregnancy.* If operative hysteroscopy must be performed in pregnancy it should be before the tenth week of gestation with a flow of 50 ml/min and a maximum pressure of 100 mmHg. As the gestational sac does not adhere completely to the uterine cavity there should be no mechanical trauma and as the nervus opticus does not function before the tenth week there should be no risk of damage to that nerve (Lindemann and Lueken, 1978).
5. *Uterine bleeding.* This condition requires more experience but is not a contraindication to surgery. The continuous-flow hysteroscope allows good visibility, even in the presence of active bleeding.
6. *Occult cervical malignancy.* Operative hysteroscopy should not be performed in the presence of cervical or endometrial malignancy and if recognized during the procedure, the appropriate biopsies should be taken, the neoplasm should be staged according to the FIGO criteria, the operative procedure discontinued and the patient's future treatment planned in the conventional manner.

References

Baggish MS & Baltoyannis P (1988) New techniques for laser ablation of the endometrium in high risk patients. *American Journal of Obstetrics and Gynecology* **159**: 287–292.

Baggish MS & Daniell JF (1989) Death caused by air embolism associated with Nd:YAG laser surgery and artificial sapphire tips. *American Journal of Obstetrics and Gynecology* **161**: 877–878.

Baumann R, Magos A, Kay JDS & Turnbull AC (1990) Absorption of glycine irrigating solution during transcervical resection of the endometrium. *British Medical Journal* **300**: 304–305.

DeCherney A & Polan MH (1983) Hysteroscopic management of intrauterine lesions and intractable uterine bleeding. *Obstetrics and Gynecology* **61**: 392–397.

DeCherney AH, Diamond MP, Lavy G & Polan ML (1987) Endometrial ablation for intractable uterine bleeding: hysteroscopic resection. *Obstetrics and Gynecology* **70**: 668–670.

Gallinat A (1978) Metromat—a new insufflation apparatus for hysteroscopy. *Endoscopy* **3**: 234.

Goldrath MH, Fuller T & Segal S (1981) Laser photovaporization of endometrium for treatment of menorrhagia. *American Journal of Obstetrics and Gynecology* **140**: 14–19.

Haning RV *et al.* (1980) Preservation of fertility by transcervical resection of a benign mesodermal uterine tumor with a resectoscope and glycine distension medium. *Fertility and Sterility* **39**: 209.

Labastida R, Montesinos M, Cararach M *et al.* (1991) Endometrial carcinoma and hysteroscopy. In van Herendael B, Slangen T & Martens P (eds) *Operative Endoscopy, Practical Aspects*, pp 52–58. Antwerp: Gyntech.

Leake JF, Murphy AA & Zacur HA (1987) Non-cardiogenic pulmonary oedema: a complication of operative hysteroscopy. *Obstetrics and Gynecology* **48**: 497.

Lindemann HJ (1972) The use of CO_2 in the uterine cavity for the hysteroscopy. *International Journal of Fertility* **17**: 221.

Lindemann HJ (1975) Komplikationen bei der CO_2 Hysteroskopie. *Archiv für Gynäkologie* **219**.

Lindemann HJ (1983) The choice of distension medium in hysteroscopy. In Van der Pas H, van Herendael B, Van Lith D & Keith L (eds) *Hysteroscopy*, p 83. Lancaster: MTP Press.

Lindemann HJ & Lueken RP (1978) Transcervical amniocentesis via hysteroscopy within the first three months of pregnancy. In Philips J (ed) *Endoscopy in Gynecology*. Downey, CA: American Association of Gynecologic Laparoscopists.

Magos A, Baumann R, Cheung K & Turnbull AC (1989) Intrauterine surgery under intravenous sedation as an out-patient alternative to hysterectomy (letter). *Lancet* **ii**: 925–926.

Martens P (1991) Basic notions for the endoscopic nurse. In van Herendael B, Slangen T & Martens P (eds) *Operative Endoscopy, Practical Aspects*, pp 6–9. Antwerp: Gyntech.

McLucas B (1991) Hyskon complications in hysteroscopic surgery. *Obstetrical and Gynecological Survey* **46**: 196–200.

Neuwirth RS & Amin HK (1976) Excision of submucous fibroids with hysteroscopic control. *American Journal of Obstetrics and Gynecology* **126**: 95–97.

Salat-Baroux J (1984) Complications. In Hamou J (ed) *Hysteroscopie et Microcolpohysteroscopie Atlas et Traité*, pp 79–84. Palermo: COFESE.

Siegler AM (1983) Risks and complications of hysteroscopy. In Van der Pas H, van Herendael B, Van Lith D & Keith L (eds) *Hysteroscopy*, pp 75–80. Lancaster: MTP Press.

Siegler AM & Valle RF (1988) Therapeutic hysteroscopic procedures. *Fertility and Sterility* **80**: 685.

Slangen T (1991) Adaption of a conventional operating theatre to a practical set-up for endoscopic surgery. In van Herendael B, Slangen T & Martens P (eds) *Operative Endoscopy, Practical Aspects*, pp 19–21. Antwerp: Gyntech.

Sugimoto O, Ushiroyama T & Fukuda Y (1984) Diagnostic and therapeutic hysteroscopy for traumatic intrauterine adhesions. In Siegler AM & Lindemann HJ (eds) *Hysteroscopy, Principles and Practice*, pp 58–62. Philadelphia: J.B. Lippincott.

Taylor PJ, Leader A & George RE (1984) Combined laparoscopy and hysteroscopy in the investigation of infertility. In Siegler AM & Lindemann J (eds) *Hysteroscopy, Principles and Practice*, pp 207–210. Philadelphia: J.B. Lippincott.

Valle RF & Sciarra JJ (1986) Hysteroscopic treatment of the septate uterus. *Obstetrics and Gynecology* **67**: 253.

van Herendael BJ (1988) Hysteroscopy in infertility. *Pakistan Journal of Obstetrics and Gynaecology* **1**: 136–147.

Wamsteker K (1991) Fluid intravasation: risk and management. In van Herendael, Slangen T & Martens P (eds) *Operative Endoscopy, Practical Aspects*, pp 81–83. Antwerp: Gyntech.

The Future

46

Radiofrequency Endometrial Ablation (RaFEA)

JEFFREY H. PHIPPS* AND B. VICTOR LEWIS‡

*George Eliot Hospital, Nuneaton, Warwickshire, UK
‡Watford General Hospital, Watford, Hertfordshire, UK

Introduction

An alternative method of ablating the endometrial cavity in the management of dysfunctional uterine bleeding (DUB) to the hysteroscopic methods is the use of radiofrequency (RF) heating to induce irreversible damage to the basalis layer.

The potential advantages of such an approach are that the toxic effects of flushing media—fluid overload and glycine toxicity—are avoided, there is no long learning curve as is the case for hysteroscopic surgery, and the necessary equipment is cheaper than laser systems.

Attempts in the past to use toxic chemicals or physical agents have been universally disappointing. Silver nitrate or fuming nitric acid infused into the uterine cavity was recommended by Tilt (1881), but by the turn of the century were no longer used. Quinacrine or urea instillation, cyanoacrylate ester ('superglue') injection, super-heated steam and radium packing have all been tried but abandoned (Goldrath, 1987). Cahan and Brockunier (1971) and Droegemueller et al. (1971) studied the use of an intracavity cryoprobe, but only partial success was achieved, and the technique has now been abandoned. Hot water has been used to irrigate the uterine cavity either in direct contact with the endometrium or contained within balloons, but recent use of these techniques has led to two consecutive cases of severe intraperitoneal burns, where one patient died (Hardt and Genz, 1989).

This chapter describes the investigation and development of the use of RF electromagnetic energy to ablate the endometrial cavity.

Physical Principle

Heating tissue above 43°C is referred to as 'hyperthermia', and has been used in the treatment of malignant disease, either alone or as an adjunct to radiotherapy, for many years (Streffer, 1977). More recently, Yerushalmi (1985) reported the use of microwave energy induced hyperthermia in the treatment of both malignant and benign prostatic disease as an alternative to resection. We reported the first use of RF-induced hyperthermia for treating DUB in 1990 (Phipps et al., 1990).

Human tissues suffer irreversible damage after exposure to temperatures above 42°C in a manner which is both time- and temperature-dependent. Cells appear to survive thermal exposure up to approximately 42°C, but exposure to 43°C for 60 minutes or more causes cell death. For each degree rise, this 'thermotolerance' time is approximately halved. Cell damage occurs because of critical changes in cytoskeletal protein structure, and at higher temperatures because of enzyme denaturation and nuclear damage (Hahn, 1982). Thus heating of the endometrium, including the basalis layer, to a sufficiently high degree for sufficient time, results in endometrial ablation.

The use of simple conductive thermal devices has been tried (heated rods or water-filled balloons), but has proved unsuccessful in the past for a number of reasons. Any conductive intrauterine thermal device would have to be of sufficient temperature to drive a thermal gradient such that the basalis layer is heated to histotoxic levels. Blood and protein coagulate above 60°C and this coagulum within the cavity rapidly forms a progressively insulating layer between the device and the endometrium, preventing thermal penetration. Secondly, tissue heating will depend upon the volume of local blood flow, since those areas where blood flow is high will be spared due to the cooling effect of perfusing blood. Penetration is therefore erratic. After initial experimentation with simple conductive techniques, we therefore explored the use of RF energy.

In RF endometrial heating, a conductive angulated probe (Figure 46.1) is placed within the endometrial cavity, and an insulated 'belt' is placed around the patient's waist which acts as a ground-plane earth electrode to complete the circuit. A 27.12 MHz signal is applied to the RF thermal probe, and the endometrial surface is heated to between 62 and 65°C for approximately 15 minutes. Applied power is varied during treatment to maintain therapeutic temperatures. Such temperatures have been experimentally determined (see below).

The electrical load presented by the RF thermal probe, patient and external ground-plane electrode is impedance-matched to the output of a linear-amplified 27.12 MHz signal generator, such that maximum power is deposited as heat within the target tissues (Figure 46.2).

At this frequency, current flows primarily capacitatively. The tissues act as a 'lossy' capacitor,

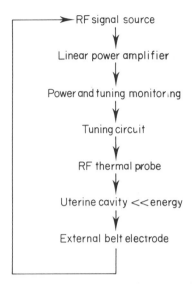

RF signal source

↓

Linear power amplifier

↓

Power and tuning monitoring

↓

Tuning circuit

↓

RF thermal probe

↓

Uterine cavity << energy

↓

External belt electrode

Figure 46.2 Block circuit diagram of the radiofrequency generating apparatus.

that is, a proportion of the energy transfer across the capacitor is 'lost' as heat. An electric field is set up around the active tip of the probe, and tissue lying within the boundaries of the field becomes heated. The density of the electric field, and therefore the heating effect, fall off geometrically with distance from the probe surface in an 'inverse square' fashion (although the precise mathematical relationship is more complex than $1/r^2$). Heating beyond the confines of the endometrial cavity at the powers used clinically is prevented by three major factors. First, the physical attributes of an electric field at this frequency and applied power mean that penetration beyond approximately 5–7 mm is negligible. Secondly, the uterine blood flow acts as a highly effective heat sink to cool the outer myometrium, and thirdly, the myometrium itself, like all biological tissues, is a poor conductor of heat.

Equipment

The RF generator is combined with the temperature monitoring apparatus, and is now purpose-built ('Menostat', Rocket of London Limited, UK). The machine is capable of generating up to 400 W of power at 27.12 MHz, although clinically between 150 and 300 W are generally used. The unit also measures applied power, duration of treatment and intrauterine temperature (Figure 46.3). The patient application apparatus consists of the thermal probe and vaginal guard, which is a tapered plastic tube inserted into the vagina.

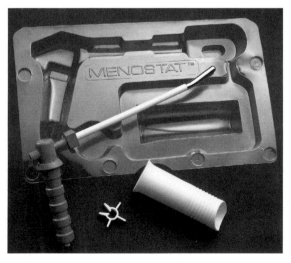

Figure 46.1 The radiofrequency thermal probe and vaginal guard.

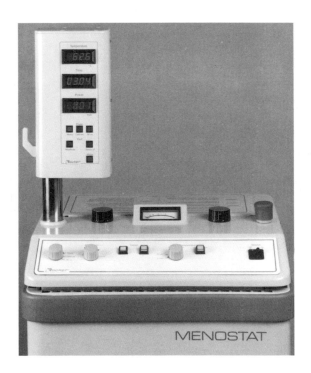

Figure 46.3 The 'Menostat' radiofrequency endometrial ablation unit (courtesy of Rocket of London Limited).

The thermal guard is necessary to retract the vagina, particularly the anterior vaginal wall, to protect the bladder from heating. Inadequate retraction of the anterior vaginal wall may result in fistula formation (Phipps *et al.*, 1990, Figures 46.1 and 46.4). The external ground-plane electrode is an insulated conductive wire mesh 'belt', which is wrapped around the patient's waist before treatment, and is connected to the generator machine to provide the 'return' arm of the circuit.

Experimental Studies

All studies were carried out with Ethical Committee approval.

Temperatures achieved during treatment were measured in ten volunteers undergoing abdominal hysterectomy. Electronic thermometry was used to measure the temperatures during treatment within the uterine cavity, at various distances from the probe within the myometrium, on the surface of the uterus and bowel, and at the base of the bladder. These studies showed that with an intracavity temperature of around 63°C the surface of the uterus was between 37

and 39°C and all other tissues remained at normal body temperature (Figure 46.5).

The heat sink effect of uterine blood flow was demonstrated when RF endometrial heating was performed before and after clamping the uterine arteries on two abdominal hysterectomy patients. The intracavity temperature rose much faster when the uterine vessels were clamped, showing that blood flow has a profound cooling effect (Figure 46.6).

Systemic venous blood samples were collected before surgery, immediately afterwards, and at 1 and 6 weeks. Free haemoglobin, coagulation profiles, and bilirubin levels were all normal and unchanged before and after surgery. Uterine venous blood was sampled from an isolated uterine vein during RF endometrial heating, and examined microscopically. No blood sample showed any red cell crenellation, a sensitive indicator of thermal damage to blood (Coakley, 1987).

Patient Selection

Patients with dysfunctional uterine bleeding were fully informed of the experimental nature of the surgery, and volunteered to undergo the procedure. They had all completed their families, since the effects of endometrial ablation on fertility are unknown. Permanent sterility after the procedure cannot be guaranteed, and so simultaneous laparoscopic sterilization was offered. Organic disease is excluded by hysteroscopy, ultrasound scan, and endometrial biopsy. The distance across the cornua (measured ultrasonically) must not exceed 35 mm, because thermal probes currently available are unable to reach the cornual regions in abnormally large uteri.

The uterus must be clinically of normal size and shape, and freely mobile. There must be no suspicion of endometriosis. Patients complaining of cyclic pain or dyspareunia are advised against treatment because of the likelihood of adenomyosis. A history suggestive of significantly heavy menstruation was elicited as follows: changing pads or towels every one and a half hours or more frequently because of saturation or near-saturation, and bleeding heavily for three or more consecutive days.

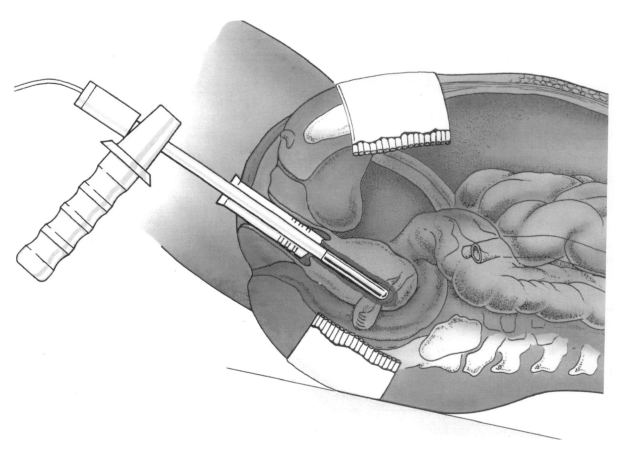

Figure 46.4 Sagittal view of the radiofrequency thermal probe and vaginal guard *in situ*.

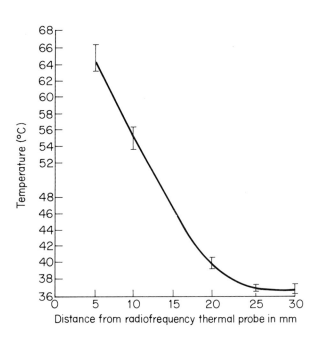

Figure 46.5 Temperature as a function of distance from the radiofrequency thermal probe (*n* = 10, maximum variation between patients 1.2°C).

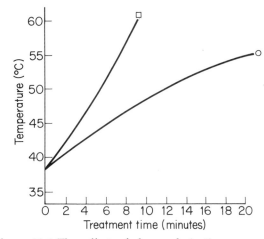

Figure 46.6 The effect of devascularization on endo-metrial cavity temperature rise (*n* = 2) ○, vascular supply intact; □, devascularized.

Treatment Technique

The patient may be treated under general or regional anaesthesia. We have found that a 'single shot' epidural anaesthetic is ideal for both intra- and postoperative pain relief.

The external electrode is placed around the patient's waist, and she is positioned in the lithotomy position. No part of the patient should touch earthed metal such as the operating table or metal stirrups frames, because of the risk of skin burns (as is the case with standard electrosurgery). The cervix is dilated to size 10 Hegar, and the length of the cavity is measured using a sound. The length of the cervical canal is estimated using a special angulated fine probe to detect the internal os. The estimated length of the cervical canal is subtracted from the total length, and the appropriate probe size selected. This is necessary so that the cervical canal is not heated, which would place the base of the bladder at risk of damage.

The thermal guard is inserted into the vagina until the leading edge is in the fornices with the cervix 'captured' centrally. No vaginal skin should be visible in order that the bladder and rectum are protected. The cervix is held in position using two stay sutures placed through the anterior and posterior lips, and passed through the aperture of the guard where they are anchored. The probe is then inserted fully into the cavity of the uterus. If difficulty is encountered in dilating the cervix, if there is any suspicion of perforation or if rotation is not free, it is essential that the procedure be abandoned because of the risk of probe insertion elsewhere other than the endometrial cavity. If the probe is placed inappropriately, and the surgeon is unaware, the equipment is capable of detecting the error because circuit tuning occurs outside the normal range for the uterine cavity. If difficulty is experienced in tuning, perforation should be excluded.

A safety check is carried out by the surgeon and the anaesthetist before the generator is switched on. There must be no contact by the patient with any metal, and ECG and pulse oximeter must be filtered and compatible with the RF equipment. Most older monitoring equipment is unstable in the presence of RF energy, and may cause burns at the site of ECG electrodes or pulse oximeter sensors if used without adequate filtering and screening because a pathway to earth may form. If monitoring equipment is left connected to the patient but switched off, burns may also occur.

The probe and belt electrode are connected to the RF generator/monitor unit, which is switched on and set to the calibration mode. Tuning is achieved by manipulation of the two calibration controls. After tuning, the machine is switched to treat mode, and the power increased to 200 W. Recent advances in equipment efficiency mean that much lower power levels may be used for the same therapeutic effect. Probe temperature is measured every 3 minutes via a built-in thermistor

in the probe tip, and power levels are varied so that a probe temperature of 62–65°C is maintained. The uterus is treated for a total of 15 minutes, during which time the probe is rotated through 360 degrees. At the end of the procedure, the probe, guard, clip and external belt are removed.

Postoperative analgesia requirements are very variable. Approximately half of patients treated require narcotics for the first 3–4 hours, but the pain quickly settles thereafter. It may be the case that the pain experienced is mediated by prostaglandin synthesis (many patients complain of 'labour pains'). We have yet to study the use of anti-inflammatory agents, but it may well be that these may be the drugs of choice.

Results

To date, 347 patients have been treated. Of these, 203 have been treated according to the definitive protocol (62–65°C at the endometrial surface for 15 minutes) and have been followed up for between 7 and 18 months. Results are shown in Figure 46.7, and show that using the definitive treatment regimen in patients where the endometrial cavity is ultrasonically and hysteroscopically normal, either amenorrhoea or significantly reduced flow was achieved in almost 87% of cases. A 'cure' was judged when patients did not want further treatment, and considered their periods (or absence of bleeding) acceptable.

In 15 patients menstrual loss was recorded over two cycles before and after RaFEA. The radioactive ^{59}Fe iron/whole body gamma counting method was used which is more accurate than, and does not suffer the practical disadvantages of, pad-saving studies. Patients were given radioactive

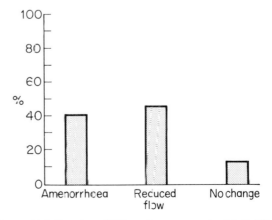

Figure 46.7 Results of 203 patients treated with RaFEA, normal uterine cavity.

iron before a menstrual period, and whole-body radioactivity measured before and after two cycles. The deficit between the two measurements is directly proportional to blood loss (Holt *et al.*, 1967). The pretreatment loss was 97–1330 ml, and after RaFEA was 0–266 ml, with a mean reduction of 195 ml per cycle (74% reduction in loss, see Figure 46.8). It is a feature of the technique that several cycles may elapse before the patient achieves her definitive result. Many patients experience several heavy periods after treatment, which subsequently diminish, presumably because of cavity fibrosis. We have yet to obtain long-term follow-up data.

The majority of patients were treated as day cases, and in a series of 140 patients treated, only three have required overnight admission for pain relief. All were able to go home the following day. Fifty per cent of women are able to resume work within 10 days, and the majority of the rest within 2 weeks. Approximately 10% of patients need between 2 and 4 weeks of recovery. The principal complaint that prevents return to work seems to be a feeling of general malaise and tiredness. This may be because some patients are susceptible to a form of 'burn syndrome', seen in some cases of severe burns, which is presumed to be due to absorption of toxic products from damaged tissue. Patients are told that they should refrain from sexual intercourse and take cephradine 250 mg four times a day for a week as prophylaxis against possible infection. We have

yet to ascertain whether or not this precaution is necessary.

Postoperative hysteroscopy at 6 months after surgery has shown a variable appearance within the uterus. In some cases the cavity is completely stenosed. In others, the endometrium appears to be replaced by fibrous tissue.

Complications

Most patients complain of a varying degree of abdominal pain after RaFEA, which disappears or becomes a dull ache after 4–6 hours. All patients report a blood stained vaginal discharge lasting 1–4 weeks.

Of the patients treated in the recent series using the vaginal guard, one patient developed a vesicovaginal fistula, which was subsequently repaired without further complication. The cause of this was a fold of anterior vaginal wall (and therefore bladder) was trapped by the thermal guard and was in contact with the thermal probe shaft.

Four patients from the series have complained of cyclical pain. One of these has settled spontaneously, but the other three continue. Ultrasound scans are unremarkable, but the possibility of small haematometra remains. Two patients have required hysterectomy for recurrence of their heavy bleeding, and one for pain, between 8 and 14 months after treatment. Histology failed to reveal any significant features to account for their symptoms.

ECG electrode and a pulse oximeter sensor burn have occurred due to the use of non-compatible equipment. It is vital that only approved monitoring equipment is used. Standard ECG machines are suitable *provided* a special filter is interposed between the monitor and the patient. Self-powered battery operated pulse oximeter units are also suitable for use *provided* they have been examined and approved, but a purpose-built combined monitoring unit may also be used. Built-in fuses in the latest monitoring equipment (which may also be used for general theatre purposes) mean that even if a fault develops, burns are prevented by stopping current flow.

Studies have shown that environmental radiofrequency electromagnetic energy levels are below the government recommended maximum levels with the equipment operating at power levels in excess of those used clinically. Therefore hazards to theatre staff and patient due to excessive

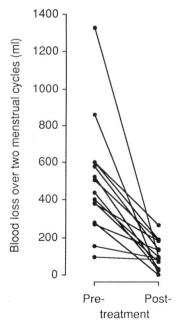

Figure 46.8 Effect of RaFEA on measured menstrual blood loss over two menstrual cycles before and after ablation.

radiofrequency exposure are not a problem. The prevention of complications depends upon the surgeon, the anaesthetist and the theatre staff who should be familiar with the safety protocol, with the patient under constant vigilance during treatment. Theatre doors should be labelled with appropriate signs stating that radiofrequency energy is in use, and entry forbidden by non-authorised staff during surgery.

Future Development

Currently, a multicentre trial is underway in six centres in the UK and Europe. The equipment is under constant development to improve safety and efficiency.

RaFEA is particularly suitable for patients with severe cardio-pulmonary disease, where the possibility of even a minor degree of fluid intravasation with the hysteroscopic methods might be dangerous. It may be the case that RaFEA has a unique role under these circumstances.

The absence of any need for high technology operating facilities or special training may mean that RaFEA is especially suitable for developing countries, particularly in Moslem communities where hysterectomy is considered culturally unacceptable.

In conclusion, RaFEA may offer another alternative to hysterectomy that is simple, effective and relatively inexpensive, and may offer specific advantages over the hysteroscopic methods in certain groups of patients.

References

Cahan WG & Brockunier A (1971) Cryosurgery of the uterine cavity. *Obstetrics and Gynecology* **38 (2)**: 256–258.

Coakley WT (1987) Hyperthermia effects on the cytoskeleton and on cell morphology. *Symposia of the Society for Experimental Biology* **41**: 187–211.

Droegemueller W, Greer B & Makowski E (1971) Cryosurgery in patients with dysfunctional uterine bleeding. *Obstetrics and Gynecology* **38**: 256–258.

Goldrath MH (1987) Hysteroscopic laser ablation of the endometrium. In Sharp F and Jordan JA (eds) *Gynaecological Laser Surgery*, pp 253–255. New York: Publishers Perinatology Press.

Hahn GM (1982) *Hyperthermia and Cancer*. New York: Springer-Verlag.

Hardt W & Genz T (1989) Atmocausis vaporisation. Most severe internal burns following intrauterine use of steam, *Geburtshilfe und Frauenheilkunde* **49 (3)**: 293–295.

Holt JM, Mayet FGH, Warner GT & Callender ST (1967) Measurement of blood loss by means of a whole body counter. *British Medical Journal* **4**: 86–88.

Phipps JH, Lewis BV, Roberts T et al. (1990) Treatment of functional menorrhagia with radiofrequency endometrial ablation. *Lancet* **335**: 374–376.

Streffer C (ed) (1977) *Cancer Therapy by Hyperthermia and Radiation*, pp 122–124. New York: American Institute of Physics.

Tilt EJ (1881) Caustic medication. In *A Handbook of Uterine Therapeutics*, 4th edn, pp 137–148. New York: William Wood and Company.

Yerushalmi V (1985) Localised deep microwave heat treatment of poor operative risk patients with benign prostatic hyperplasia. *Journal of Urology* **133**: 873–879.

47

Circumferential Nd:YAG Endometrial Destruction

M.D. JUDD AND S.G. BOWN

National Medical Laser Centre, University College, London, UK

Introduction

Hysterectomy still remains the commonest surgical procedure for women whose menorrhagia has failed to respond to medical treatment for, until recently, most methods of local endometrial destruction had met with limited success.

The endometrium is well known for its regenerative capacity: in menstruating women complete endometrial regrowth has occurred within 48 hours (Ferenczy, 1976) and in rabbits following curettage the first regenerated epithelial cells can be seen after 3 hours (Schenker et al., 1971). Uterine occlusion and resultant amenorrhoea rarely occur except in the case of Asherman's syndrome which seems to be solely related to postpartum and post-abortal curettage. Intrauterine adhesions are occasionally found following myomectomy or in cases of endometrial tuberculosis (Polishuk, 1975). However, the fact that Asherman's syndrome (Asherman, 1948) does occur, in which the endometrium is almost completely obliterated and the uterine cavity occluded with extensive fibrosis, has led gynaecologists to seek a way of inducing this situation as a treatment for menorrhagia.

Local destruction has been tried using a variety of physical and chemical methods and have included methylcyanoacrylate, oxalic acid, paraformaldehyde, silicone rubber, superheated steam (Droegemueller et al., 1978), intracavitary radium (Crossen and Crossen, 1947; Rongy, 1947), quinacrine (Schenker and Polishuk, 1973), cryocoagulation (Cahan and Brockunier, 1967; Droege-

mueller et al., 1971a, b) and autologous (Polishuk and Schenker, 1973; Schenker et al., 1975) and homologous (Polishuk and Sadovsky, 1975) fibroblast implants. However, most met with little success and until Goldrath ablated the endometrium using a high power (55–60 W) Nd:YAG laser under hysteroscopic control (Goldrath et al., 1981). This procedure had a 93% success rate after one application and a minimal morbidity. Since then Loffer (1987) and Lomano (1986) have treated women in a similar way with equally good results.

Neuwirth first described the use of the urological resectoscope in the treatment of menorrhagia resulting from submucosal fibroids (Neuwirth and Amin, 1976). This technique has since been used to perform endometrial ablation and has been shown to have an 80% success rate after one treatment (Magos et al., 1989). More recently radiofrequency-induced thermal endometrial ablation has been described (Phipps et al., 1990).

Both the laser and the resectoscope are associated with well recognized complications; major ones are uterine perforation, haemorrhage and fluid overload (Goldrath, 1986; Morrison et al., 1989). Minor problems after these techniques include vaginal discharge, cervical stenosis, haematometria and pelvic or urinary tract infections. Unfortunately each technique has produced fatalities which need to be considered against the mortality rate for hysterectomy which is 0.6 deaths per 1000 procedures (Wingo et al., 1985). In the USA, two young medically fit women have died from air embolism when using the Nd:YAG laser with artificial sapphire tips which are cooled by carbon dioxide gas (Baggish and Daniell, 1989).

There is little evidence for the usefulness of sapphire tips in intrauterine surgery, as endometrial ablation with a bare quartz fibre is faster and more effective than these (Zumwalt *et al.*, 1986). In the UK and Europe, five women have died while undergoing endometrial resection (Hamou, 1989; Irwin, 1991).

There is also a risk of damage to adjacent organs if uterine perforation occurs. Goldrath describes perforating a uterus during manipulation of the hysteroscope but there are no reports of the laser causing thermal damage to any pelvic or intra-abdominal structures (Goldrath *et al.*, 1981; Goldrath, 1986). The resectoscope and extrauterine damage are now receiving much publicity: this includes trauma to major blood vessels (aorta, inferior vena cava, mesenteric and sacral vessels), the bowel, ureter and even the loss of a lower limb (Irwin, 1991; Pittroff *et al.*, 1991).

Various liquid media are used to distend the uterus including dextran 70 (Hyskon), 5% dextrose, physiological saline and 1.5% glycine and another major complication of intrauterine surgery is fluid overload (Macdonald and Singer, 1989; West and Robinson, 1989). This can cause dilutional hyponatraemia (Morrison *et al.*, 1989; Van Boven *et al.*, 1989) with resultant hypovolaemia, pulmonary oedema, confusion, coma and even death (Rao, 1987). Therefore careful measurement of fluid balance is mandatory, although the exact volume at which complications occur is unknown. There have been reports of more than 2 litres being absorbed without ill effect (Lomano, 1986). Measured average fluid absorption ranges from approximately 300 to 650 ml (West and Robinson, 1989; Baumann *et al.*, 1990). The patency of the fallopian tubes on fluid absorption either has no effect (Lomano, 1986) or when occluded reduce absorption (Baumann *et al.*, 1990). Excessive absorption of glycine when metabolized causes hyperammonaemia which results in delayed recovery from general anaesthesia (Sturdle and Hoggart, 1991). Also, recent reports suggest that glycine as an irrigation fluid is cardiotoxic (Coppinger and Hudd, 1989) and Hyskon can cause coagulation defects and anaphylaxis (McLucas, 1991).

Haemorrhage is the final problem of these techniques; intractable uterine bleeding at the end of the procedure can usually be stopped by applying uterine tamponade via a Foley catheter (Goldrath, 1983). The commonest cause of delayed haemorrhage is from coagulation necrosis of the cervical artery and can be prevented by avoiding treating the lower part of the cervical canal.

Obviously the main advantages of the radio-frequency-induced endometrial destruction is the simplicity of the technique which requires no hysteroscopic manipulation and no irrigating fluids. This technique may prove to have the best safety record though two vesicovaginal fistulae occurred in the first preliminary study (Phipps *et al.*, 1990). The relative effectiveness, safety and true cost of each procedure for intrauterine destruction are not yet established. It is important that each technique is fully assessed in correctly structured, collaborative prospective clinical studies.

Hyperthermia

Hyperthermia has been used to treat a variety of diseases. Since the last century fever-inducing infections were used to kill tumours, while whole-body heating was used in patients with resistant gonococcal and non-specific urethritis (King *et al.*, 1943; Macdonald, 1944). Generalized hyperthermia was not very specific and had a high morbidity and mortality; these techniques produced jaundice, deranged liver function and irreversible liver and cardiac failure. Therefore localized hyperthermia has been directed at specific organs and has attempted to produce uniform heating of tissue to temperatures in the range of 42.5–50°C for extended periods of time (often over 1 hour). There is a relationship between temperature and cell death, such that at 42°C and above the temperature required to cause cell death by heating is halved with every increase of 1°C. Canine bladder can be completely destroyed at temperatures ranging from 59 to 69°C and replaced by a fibrous nodule (Linke *et al.*, 1972). A number of methods of inducing hyperthermia have been tried including radiofrequency, microwave and ultrasound (Hand and Ter-Haar, 1981) but they all produce irregular tissue heating with damage to surrounding structures.

Interstitial Laser Hyperthermia

Laser light can interact with biological tissue in four ways: it can be absorbed, reflected, transmitted or scattered. Transmitted and reflected laser light will produce no biological effect. Scattering of laser light causes it to be absorbed by a larger volume of tissue. Nd:YAG laser light which has a wavelength of 1064 nm is poorly absorbed but considerably scattered by biological tissue; therefore light distribution within irradiated tissue is relatively uniform. Absorbed laser energy is converted to heat and at low powers local tissue necrosis is produced.

Interstitial laser hyperthermia (ILH) has been shown to be a safe and predictable technique when used to treat solid structures. The necrosis produced is well defined and reproducible and resolves by healing with fibrosis or regeneration. ILH has been used in many experimental models including rat (Matthewson *et al.*, 1987) and canine liver (Steger *et al.*, 1987b), canine pancreas (Steger *et al.*, 1987a), chemically induced rat colon tumour (Matthewson *et al.*, 1988) and in an implanted flank fibrosarcoma (Matthewson *et al.*, 1989). Single bare quartz fibres placed into a solid structure or organ using low powers (1–2 W) produced areas of thermal necrosis up to 16 mm in diameter. These healed by resolution and fibrosis. There was a clear 'dose-response' between energy delivered to the tissue and the final lesion size. A clear border between normal and necrotic tissue existed and there was evidence of a reduction in blood flow.

ILH has also been used in small clinical studies to treat solitary liver metastases, inoperable pancreatic carcinoma and metastatic breast tissue (Steger *et al.*, 1989, Masters and Brown, 1990) using either single or multiple fibres.

Hollow organs like the uterus are not particularly suited to interstitial therapy; obviously a single bare fibre placed in the endometrium at low powers would not be a practical treatment for menorrhagia. However, using a modified fibre tip in which the light is reflected in a suitable distribution has the potential to treat the entire endometrium in a safe and predictable manner. Thermal damage to the entire endometrium would potentially result in safe healing with the structural integrity of the surrounding tissue maintained.

Experimental Work

An animal model was used to assess the feasibility of destroying and preventing the regrowth of the endometrium using a low-power laser hyperthermia technique (Judd *et al.*, 1991). The fibre tip was passed into the uterine horn at laparotomy (Figure 47.1). The endometrium was exposed to laser light using 1–3 W either to produce single lesions or to destroy the entire endometrium by treating a series of adjacent sites.

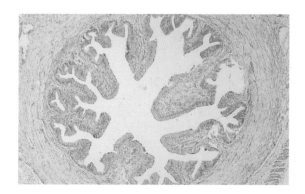

Figure 47.1 Cross-section of a normal uterine horn showing the stellate-shaped endometrial cavity (H & E, magnification ×8, reproduced at 215% of original).

A continuous wave Nd:YAG laser was used at powers of 1–3 W. A modified fibre tip (Figure 47.2) was used in which the light was incident upon a gold cone and reflected in a disc-shaped distribution. This arrangement produced circumferential lesions. Gold was used for the tip because it is durable and has a high reflectivity. The tip was securely fixed to a plastic clad silicone fibre (core diameter 400 μm) which was polished at both ends. The length of the tip was 20 mm and the diameter 3 mm which allowed it to be passed easily through the cervix into the uterine horn. Its output was measured at the start and finish of each procedure using an integrating sphere power meter. A copper–constantan thermocouple was used in conjunction with a display unit to monitor serosal temperature changes.

Single Lesion Procedure

In this part of the study three to four separated lesions were produced in each uterine horn. The powers used were 1–3 W with maximum exposure times of 100 seconds. All specimens were exam-

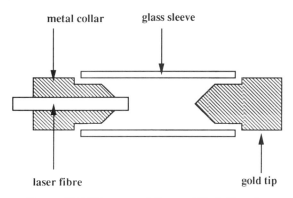

Figure 47.2 Diagram of the modified fibre tip.

ined 6–8 days following treatment when the maximum amount of damage had occurred.

These results are summarised in Table 47.1. Lesions produced using 2 W at exposure times of 100 seconds were symmetrical in 89% of cases. They had a mean serosal length of 6.3 mm (range 5–9 mm) and were easily identifiable being paler in colour than the untreated tissue. Symmetrical endometrial destruction occurred causing loss of all villi. Myometrial and serosal damage was seen in some specimens. When using 3 W at exposure times of 50–100 seconds, 69% of the lesions showed asymmetrical endometrial damage. The most suitable lesions were produced at 2 W × 100 seconds and these parameters were used to treat the entire endometrium.

Overlapping Lesions Procedure

When destroying the whole endometrium the tip was passed to the cornual end of the horn and positioned to ensure that it was pressed equally against all parts of the uterine cavity. After each delivery of laser light (2 W × 100 seconds) the fibre was withdrawn approximately 5 mm before the next site was treated. A 5 mm gap would ensure overlap of treated areas because single lesions produced at 2 W × 100 seconds were approximately 6 mm in length.

However, early on in the work it was discovered that areas of endometrium were consistently difficult to treat. First, the upper 5 mm of each horn remained undamaged because its diameter was too narrow to allow the passage of the fibre tip. Secondly, the lowest part of the cervix which had the most complex villi was often only partially destroyed. Therefore, in subsequent animals the

upper quarter of each uterine horn was tied off with sutures and only the lower part and the cervix were treated with maximum exposure times of 200 seconds. The sutures occluded the uterine cavity along 2–3 mm of its length but the horn above and below remained intact. Animals were killed at intervals from 24 hours to 14 weeks after treatment.

The results are summarized in Table 47.2. From 28 days post-treatment macroscopically the horn was either completely absent except for a thin fibrous strand (Figure 47.3) or present and distorted by adhesions. In the intact horns endometrial regeneration had occurred but with reduced numbers of glands and abnormal regrowth of villi (Figure 47.4). There were areas of fibrosis within the myometrium. Histology performed at 2 months post-treatment showed intermittent fibrous occlusion of the uterine cavity and areas completely denuded of glands.

The technique was safe with other pelvic organs suffering no thermal damage. Animals remained well even when an entire uterine horn was destroyed and replaced by a fibrous strand. At post-mortem examination in this group there was no evidence of peritonitis, bowel or bladder damage and adhesion formation was minimal. These animals were possibly able to reabsorb the

Table 47.1 Single lesions produced using 1–3 W, all specimens were examined 6–8 days after laser treatment

Power (W)	Exposure time (s)	Number of lesions	Result
1	50	13	Little effect
	100	9	Little effect
2	50	10	Little effect; few lesions symmetrical
	100	36	Symmetrical lesions
3	50	14	Asymmetrical lesions
	100	7	Asymmetrical lesions

Table 47.2 Results of the horns treated with overlapping lesions

Survival (days)	Uterine horns	Macroscopic appearance	Microscopic appearance
4–8	Non-ligated (4) Ligated (4)	Haemorrhagic	Full thickness lesions except upper 5 mm and cervix
14–21	Non-ligated (1)	Normal	Intact endometrium
	Ligated (10)	Thinned, necrotic and haemorrhagic	Incomplete surface epithelium. Few villi and glands
28–34	Non-ligated (5)	Horn absent (1) Distorted (4)	Intact surface epithelium Few villi and glands
	Ligated (2)	Distorted	
63–98	Non-ligated (5)	Horn absent (4) Normal (1)	Intact surface epithelium Few glands and villi
	Ligated (4)	Horn absent	

The upper end of each ligated horn was tied off with sutures and only the endometrium below this treated.

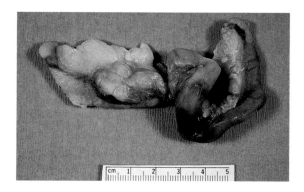

Figure 47.3 At 32 days the rabbit uterine horn treated with overlapping lesions has been replaced by a fibrous strand. The untreated left horn has a normal appearance.

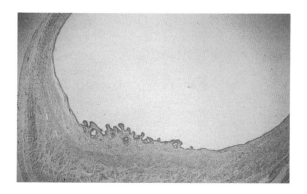

Figure 47.4 Histological section of a uterine horn which was treated with overlapping lesions 30 days after treatment. There is abnormal regrowth of villi but re-epithelialization of the endometrial surface is complete (H & E, magnification ×8, reproduced at 215% of original).

necrotic uterine tissue over many weeks and this process appeared to be well tolerated. The absence of a horn was first noted at 32 days post-treatment. A similar phenomenon was described when canine bladder was completely destroyed at temperatures ranging from 59 to 69°C and replaced by a fibrous nodule (Linke *et al.*, 1972).

Discussion

This study confirms that the endometrium regenerates if any undamaged epithelial cells or glands remain intact. In both menstruating women and rabbit endometrium subjected to mechanical or chemical trauma, the regrowth of the surface epithelium is derived from the proliferation of

two areas: the exposed ends of basal glands and the persistent and intact lining of cornual and cervical regions bordering the denuded areas. This regrowth is initiated in response to tissue loss and is not hormonally dependent (Ferenczy, 1976). Even when there is extensive endometrial and myometrial damage, for instance after cryosurgery, the epithelial surface has regenerated within 7–10 days and after a month the endometrium and its components appear the same as an untreated horn except for patches of fibrosis within the myometrium (Schenker and Polishuk, 1972).

These results show that in this animal model if there is inadequate endometrial destruction glandular regrowth occurs. However, because of the extreme thinness of rabbit myometrium (approximately 1–3 mm) the depth of destruction needed was a fine balance between either too much, causing entire horn loss, or too little, leaving undamaged areas which subsequently regenerated to replace all endometrial components.

The fibre tip used produced cylindrically shaped lesions which were ideal for treating the tube-like uterine horns. These diffuse lesions were produced at irradiances of approximately $0.1/mm^2$ and could not have been achieved with a bare fibre. Rabbit endometrium was successfully destroyed using this low-powered method and with a suitably designed fibre tip similar biological effects should be produced in the human uterus which might prove useful in treating women suffering from menorrhagia.

In Goldrath's technique a contact (Goldrath *et al.*, 1981) or non-contact (Lomano, 1987b; Loffer, 1987) bare fibre was used to produce small lesions by vaporization and charring. Our technique is to use a modified fibre tip to produce large diffuse lesions at temperatures around 60°C. It is a simple technique and lasted 25–30 minutes when treating 10–15 sites within each uterine horn.

The aim of this work was to assess the suitability of using a similar method to treat menorrhagia. Our proposed technique would be to place a suitable fibre tip (diameter 3 mm) into the uterine cavity without cervical dilatation under ultrasonic control. Three to four sites would be treated within the uterus to produce one converging lesion.

Destruction of the entire endometrium would be most unlikely and is frequently unnecessary when using Goldrath's technique. A subjectively successful response was not dependent on producing amenorrhoea but on reducing heavy menstrual loss. This procedure could potentially be repeated at intervals until the menopause occurred. If treatment failed it would not affect a subsequent hysterectomy which remains the treatment for intractable menorrhagia.

This low powered technique is shown to be effective, simple and safe and early clinical studies have begun.

References

Asherman JG (1948) Amenorrhoea traumatica (atretica). *Journal of Obstetrics and Gynaecology of the British Empire* 55: 23–30.

Baggish MS & Daniell JF (1989) Death caused by air embolism associated with neodymium; yttrium–aluminium–garnet laser surgery and artificial sapphire tips. *American Journal of Obstetrics and Gynecology* 161: 377–878.

Baumann R, Magos AL, Kay JD & Turnball A (1990) Absorption of glycine irrigating solution during transcervical resection of endometrium. *British Medical Journal* 300: 304–305.

Cahan WG & Brockunier A (1967) Cryosurgery of the uterine cavity. *American Journal of Obstetrics and Gynecology* 99: 138–153.

Coppinger SW & Hudd C (1989) Risk factor for myocardial infarction in transurethral resection of prostate. *Lancet* ii: 895.

Crossen RJ & Crossen HS (1947) Radiation therapy of uterine myoma. *Journal of the American Medical Association* 133: 593–599.

Droegemueller W, Greer BE & Makowski E (1971a) Cryosurgery in patients with dysfunctional uterine bleeding. *Obstetrics and Gynecology* 38: 256–258.

Droegemueller W, Malowski, E & Macsulka R (1971b) Destruction of the endometrium by cryosurgery. *American Journal of Obstetrics and Gynecology* 110: 467–469.

Droegemueller W, Greer BE, Davis JR et al. (1978) Cryocoagulation of the endometrium at the uterine cornua. *American Journal of Obstetrics and Gynecology* 131: 1–7.

Ferenczy A (1976) Studies on the cytodynamics of human endometrial regeneration. I. Scanning electron microscopy. *American Journal of Obstetrics and Gynecology* 124: 64–74.

Goldrath MH (1983) Uterine tamponade for the control of acute uterine bleeding. *American Journal of Obstetrics and Gynecology* 147: 869–872.

Goldrath MH (1986) Gynaecological laser surgery. In Sharp F & Jordan JA (eds) *Proceedings of the 18th Study Group of the Royal College of Obstetricians and Gynaecologists*, pp 253–265. New York: Perinatology Press.

Goldrath MH, Fuller TA & Segal S (1981) Laser photovaporization of endometrium for the treatment of menorrhagia. *American Journal of Obstetrics and Gynecology* 140: 14–19.

Hamou J (1989) Partial endometrial resection. *Proceedings of Second World Congress of Gynecologic Endoscopy.* Clermont-Ferrand, France, p 53.

Hand JW & Ter-Haar G (1981) Heating techniques in hyperthermia. *British Journal of Radiology* 54: 443–466.

Irwin A (1991) New gynaecology technique 'risky'. *Pulse* July: 23.

Judd MD, Hill PD, Potter LA, Bown SG & McColl I (1991) Destruction of the rabbit endometrium using a low-powered neodymium-YAG laser. *Lasers in Medical Science* 6: 133–140.

King AJ, Williams DI & Nicol CS (1943) Hyperthermia in the treatment of resistant gonococcal and non-specific urethritis. *British Journal of Venereal Diseases* 19: 141–154.

Linke C, Elbadawi A, Netto V et al. (1972) Effect of marked hyperthermia upon the canine bladder. *Journal of Urology* 107: 599–602.

Loffer FD (1987) Hysteroscopic endometrial ablation with the Nd-YAG laser using a non-touch technique. *Obstetrics and Gynecology* 69: 679–682.

Lomano JM (1986) Photocoagulation of the endometrium with the Nd-YAG laser for the treatment of menorrhagia. *Journal of Reproductive Medicine* 31: 148–150.

Macdonald RM (1944) Toxic hepatitis in fever therapy. *Canadian Medical Association Journal* 51: 445–449.

Macdonald R & Singer A (1989) Endometrial resection and fluid absorption. *Lancet* ii: 1387.

Magos AL, Baumann R & Turnball AC (1989) Transcervical resection of endometrium in women with menorrhagia. *British Medical Journal* 298: 1209–1212.

Masters A & Bown SG (1990) Interstitial laser hyperthermia in the treatment of tumours. *Lasers in Medical Science* 5: 129–135.

Matthewson K, Coleridge-Smith P, O'Sullivan JP, Northfield TC & Bown SG (1987) Biological effects of intrahepatic Nd:YAG photocoagulation in rats. *Gastroenterology* 93: 550–557.

Matthewson K, Barton T, Lewin MR et al. (1988) Lower power interstitial Nd-YAG laser photocoagulation in normal and neoplastic rat colon. *Gut* 29: 27–34.

Matthewson K, Barr H, Traulau C & Bown SG (1989) Low power interstitial Nd-YAG laser photocoagulation: studies in a transplanted fibrosarcoma. *British Journal of Surgery* 76: 378–381.

McLucas B (1991) Hyskon complications in hysteroscopic surgery. *Obstetrical and Gynecological Survey* 46: 196–200.

Morrison LMM, Davis J & Sumner D (1989) Absorption of irrigating fluid during laser photocoagulation of the endometrium in the treatment of menorrhagia. *British Journal of Obstetrics and Gynaecology* 96: 346–352.

Neuwirth RS & Amin HK (1976) Excision of submucous fibroids with hysteroscopic control. *American Journal of Obstetrics and Gynecology* 126: 95–97.

Phipps JH, Lewis BV, Roberts T et al. (1990) Treatment of functional menorrhagia by radiofrequency-induced thermal endometrial ablation. *Lancet* 335: 374–376.

Pittroff R, Darwish DH & Shabib G (1991) Near fatal uterine perforation during transcervical endometrial resection. *Lancet* 338: 197–198.

Polishuk WZ (1975) Endometrial regeneration and adhesion formation. *South African Medical Journal* 49: 440–442.

Polishuk WZ & Sadovsky E (1975) A syndrome of recurrent intrauterine adhesions. *American Journal of Obstetrics and Gynecology* 123: 151–158.

Polishuk WZ & Schenker JG (1973) Induction of intrauterine adhesions in the rabbit with autologous fibroblast implants. *American Journal of Obstetrics and Gynecology* **115**: 789–794.

Rao PN (1987) Fluid absorption during urological endoscopy. *British Journal of Urology* **60**: 93–99.

Rongy AJ (1947) Radium therapy in benign uterine bleeding. *Journal of the Mount Sinai Hospital* **14**: 569–575.

Schenker JG & Polishuk WZ (1972) Regeneration of rabbit endometrium after cryosurgery. *Obstetrics and Gynecology* **40**: 638–645.

Schenker JG & Polishuk WZ (1973) Regeneration of rabbit endometrium following intrauterine instillation of chemical agents. *Gynecological Investigation* **4**: 1–13.

Schenker JG, Sacks MI & Polishuk WZ (1971) Regeneration of rabbit endometrium following curettage. *American Journal of Obstetrics and Gynecology* **111**: 970–978.

Schenker JG, Nicosia SV, Polishuk WZ & Garcia CR (1975) An in vitro fibroblast-enriched sponge preparation for induction of intrauterine adhesions. *Israel Journal of Medical Sciences* **11**: 849–851.

Steger AC, Barr H, Hawes R, Bown SG & Clarke CG (1987a) Experimental studies on interstitial hyperthermia for treating pancreatic cancer. *Gut* **28**: A1382.

Steger AC, Matthewson K, Bown SG & Clark CG (1987b) Interstitial hyperthermia: a new technique for intrahepatic neoplasms. *Gut* **28**: A1350.

Steger AC, Lees WR, Walmsley K & Bown SG (1989) Interstitial laser hyperthermia: a new approach to local destruction of tumours. *British Medical Journal* **299**: 362–365.

Sturdle D & Hoggart B (1991) Problems with endometrial resection. *Lancet* **337**: 1474.

Van Boven MJ, Singelyn F, Donnez J & Gribomont BF (1989) Dilutional hyponatraemia associated with intrauterine endoscopic laser surgery. *Anaesthesiology* **71**: 449–450.

West JH & Robinson DA (1989) Endometrial resection and fluid absorption. *Lancet* **ii**: 1387–1388.

Wingo PA, Huezo CM, Rubin GL, Ory HW & Peterson HB (1985) The mortality risk associated with hysterectomy. *American Journal of Obstetrics and Gynecology* **152**: 803–808.

Zumwalt T, Wesseler T & Joffe SN (1986) A comparison of artificial sapphire tip with the quartz; in in vitro endometrial ablation. *Colposcopy and Gynecological Laser Surgery* **2**: 47–51.

48

Laser Microsurgery and Manipulations of Single Cells

Y. TADIR*‡, J. NEEV* AND M.W. BERNS*

*Beckman Laser Institute and Medical Clinic, Department of Surgery
‡Department of Obstetrics and Gynecology, University of California, Irvine, CA, USA

From Pelvic Organ Laser Surgery to Cellular Laser 'Microsurgery'

Laser energy was first applied to reproductive organs by Kaplan et al. in 1973 for the treatment of uterine cervix erosion, and intra-abdominally by Bellina in 1974. In the time span since this initial work advances in endoscopic technology enabled detailed visualization of almost every cavity in the human body. It was soon after realized that the same optical technology used for imaging could also be used to couple laser light sources into the endoscopic system. In turn, this natural marriage between optical imaging devices and optical fibre delivery systems stimulated adaptation of additional laser sources with suitable delivery systems for reconstructive pelvic surgery (Bruhat et al., 1979; Tadir et al., 1981).

In surgery the effect of the laser beam on tissue is mainly of thermal origin since wavelengths normally used correspond to photon energies which are insufficient for direct bond breaking or photochemical processes. The weaker visible and infrared photons used in endoscopic surgery are thus converted into heat. This conversion allows it to be used for treating a wide variety of lesions, by changing laser parameters such as power, wavelength and spot size. The most commonly used lasers in reproductive surgery are the carbon dioxide (10 600 nm) (Daniell, 1984; Bellina et al., 1985; Baggish, 1986; Sutton, 1986), the neodymium:yttrium–aluminium–garnet (Nd: YAG 1064 nm) (Lomano, 1985) the argon-ion laser (515 nm) (Keye and Dixon, 1983) and the frequency

doubled Nd:YAG operating at 532 nm (typically a 1064 nm Nd:YAG used in conjunction with a potassium–titanyl–phosphate (KTP) frequency-doubling crystal) (Daniell et al., 1986).

The application of lasers to treatment and research in biology and medicine crossed an additional threshold with the coupling of laser radiation through microscopes to cellular and subcellular organelles (Berns et al., 1969). The use of microscopes allows the beam's spot sizes to be focused down to a diameter as small as 1 μm. These capabilities, along with the development of tunable dye lasers (the wavelength of which can be tuned, depending on the type of dye and optics used, from the UV at 217 nm to the near IR 800 nm) permitted selective interaction with and alteration of subcellular organelles in a single living cell (Berns et al., 1981). Finally, additional opportunities for cell micromanipulation were made possible by the development of the gradient force optical trap using a single laser beam (Ashkin and Dziedzic, 1987).

At the same time, we have witnessed the rapid proliferation of infertility investigations and treatments which incorporate a wide variety of new technologies. These, in turn, call for the application of micromanipulation procedures and the refinement of new tools. In a series of experiments, human sperm, various species of oocytes and other living cells were exposed to laser microbeams in order to evaluate their potential contribution to reproductive technologies.

To summarize the above, Figure 48.1 lists the parameters used in the application of lasers for reconstructive pelvic surgery and the newly developed cellular micromanipulation.

Micromanipulation of Human Sperm with Laser Optical Trap

The zona pellucida of the mammalian egg is a barrier which sperm must penetrate if fertilization is to proceed. Flagellar movement is a fundamental expression of the viability of sperm and is essential for its reproductive capabilities. In order to combine these observations and develop a micromanipulating device for testing sperm force or assisting sperm penetration potential, we applied the recoil forces generated by the scattering of low power laser light to induce optical traps which are capable of manipulating microscopic particles (Tadir *et al.*, 1989).

A single beam gradient force trap consists of a Gaussian laser beam focused to a very small spot of the same order as the light wavelength in diameter. This trap confines the particle to a fixed position just below the focal point of the laser beam in the axial direction, and at the centre of the beam in the transverse direction. The magnitude and direction of the net force on the particle is dominated by the refraction of the laser light by the object. As the photons in the beam are refracted in opposite directions, their momentum is changed. Momentum conservation requires that equal and opposite forces will be exerted by these photons on the refracting object— the trapped cell. These forces are distributed symmetrically about the axis which defines the beam's direction of propagation. Analysis of the refraction geometry (Ashkin, 1980) shows that when the trapped particle is displaced from a

symmetrical position with respect to the beam's axis of propagation, the refraction force in the direction which opposes the change increases, while the opposite force decreases. A net force in the direction opposing the displacement is generated, thus restoring the particle to its original position. This restorative force is power dependent and, for even low power levels, is considerably larger than all other forces (such as liquid viscosity) normally acting on the particle (Ashkin and Dziedzic, 1986). As already mentioned, this was used to trap and micromanipulate sperm, for assessment of its potential effects on motility during and following exposure to the laser light.

In our optical trapping experiments, a continuous-wave (CW) Nd:YAG laser beam (1064 nm) was directed into a Zeiss photo microscope and focused into the field of view. A second beam was added to the unit in order to allow for combined procedures such as cell fusion or chromosomal manipulations (later in text). The power of the laser beam on the target was measured to be 0.1–1 W. The estimated beam's diameter at the focused spot was 2–3 μm. Sperms were placed on a joystick coupled to a motorized X–Y stage that allows positioning in the optical trap. Remote real time viewing of the sperm in the trap was performed using a video camera collinear with the path of the trapping beam (Figure 48.2). A dichoric mirror was used to separate the trapping beam from the image projected onto the video camera. All experiments were recorded on a videotape for later analysis. The recorded images were analysed using a computer and an image processor. This image processor allowed us to analyse the video tape on a frame-by-frame basis, thus allowing measurements of position velocities and other characteristics of sperm movement before and after

Figure 48.1 Comparative parameters for the application of lasers in reconstructive pelvic surgery and cellular micromanipulation.

Spot Size ⌀ Micrometer	Reconstructive Pelvic Surgery and Laparoscopy	Cell Microsurgery and Optical Trap
	300-1000 μm	1-5 μm
Wavelength Nanometer	CO2 ∿∿∿ 10.600 nm Nd:YAG ∿∿ 1.064 nm Frequency doubled Nd:YAG (KTP) 532 nm Argon ·∿∿∿ 515 nm	1064 nm^ 532 nm^^ 366 nm^^ 355 nm^^ * 308 nm^^^^ 266 nm^^ 193 nm^^^
Power ⚡ Watt & Milliwatt	5-30 W Continuous Wave	10^2-10^6 W** @532nm Pulse width 10-14 ns 10-1000 mW***

Figure 48.2 Schematic diagram of the optical trap. The microscope is represented by the objective lens and the focusing lens was mounted above the microscope. An attenuator was used to control the laser power at the optical trap. The power meter indicates the laser power when the sperm is released from the trap.

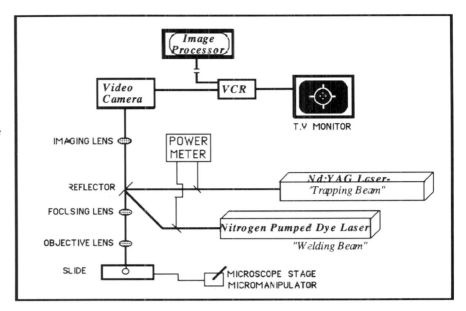

exposure to the optical trap. Sperm exposure times in the trap were 15, 30, 45, 60, 90, and 120 seconds. In the first experiment (Tadir *et al.*, 1989), a total of 514 sperm from 11 donors were trapped. Following the different laser exposure time periods, motility characteristics such as linear velocity, actual distance travelled, maximum lateral head displacement and motility patterns (before, during and after exposure) were recorded and analysed. No significant change in the mean velocity was found when the sperms were exposed to trapping light for 15 and 30 seconds (33.4 μm/s and 34 μm/s before as compared with 32 μm/s and 31.8 μm/s after release, respectively). Sperm exposed to the trap beam for 45 seconds or longer had a statistically significant decrease in velocity when released (36.4 μm/s before compared with 29.2 μm/s after exposure; $P < 0.0116$).

The sperm population was subdivided into two groups based on their initial velocity: slow (1–30 μm/s) and rapid (31–60 μm/s). In the slow motility group, sperm exposed to trapping radiation for 15 seconds showed a 20% *increase* in linear velocity (from 19.6 μm/s before to 23.5 μm/s after exposure). Following 30 and 45 seconds of exposure there was no significant additional change of mean velocity in this group. A gradual *decrease* in sperm velocity was observed in the entire sperm population following 60, 90 and 120 seconds in the trap. The mechanism that may explain the increased linear velocity of the slow motile sperm is not clearly understood. Heat generation or direct light activation may contribute to these changes. In addition, we suspect that trapping-induced motility pattern changes (from zig-zag to straight motion) may also be a contributing factor.

The final decrease in sperm velocity following

longer exposure duration is probably related to gradual localized heating of the trapped sperm. Since the small size of the sperm (or any other trapped particle) prevented direct measurement of the temperature (using the instrumentation at our disposal), it was not possible for us to determine at this stage the localized temperature. However, comparing our observed sperm motility pattern with 'normal' patterns observed in most circumstances, we believe that temperature changes are not significant within the first 30 seconds. Capturing and manipulating up to three sperm at the same time in the trap is possible. Gradual reduction of the laser power in the range of 50–95% from the highest setting lowered the number of sperm that could be manipulated in the trap. Our observation clearly showed a power threshold that allowed the sperm to be spontaneously released. Since the trapping force is proportional to laser power, it was possible to measure the relative force generated by trapped sperms (Tadir *et al.*, 1990). Tabulation of the threshold power level at which each spermatozoan was released enabled the determination of the relative force required to hold the sperm. Conversion of the relative force measurements into absolute units of force (e.g. dynes) requires calibration of the optical trap. This procedure is very difficult given that the force exerted on a cell depends on its optical and physical properties.

A total of 705 morphologically normal human sperm from six donors were trapped at room temperature. In order to evaluate the possible influence of time on sperm power, measurements were also recorded for two specimens 24 hours following the initial observations. The length of exposure to the trap prior to spontaneous release was kept to a minimum (less than 10 seconds).

Sperm head size was measured using the image processor. The sperm patterns were classified as straight and zig-zag motile, and linear velocities were subdivided into three groups: (a) slow (≤ 20 μm/s); (b) medium (21–40 μm/s); and (c) fast (≥ 41 μm/s) motile. The power measurements were compared to the linear velocity and the motility pattern. A direct correlation was found between velocity and trapping power in the entire sperm population. The mean power readings for these groups were 57 mW; 73 mW; and 84 mW, respectively. The analysis of power in the total population demonstrated that zig-zag motile sperm had significantly higher mean power readings, when compared to straight motile sperm with similar mean linear velocities. The measurement of the power threshold that was repeated 24 hours later revealed significantly lower power thresholds for trapping. In the slow motile group, the mean velocity decreased along with the power. The mean release laser power for the slow motile group 4 hours following ejaculation was 55 mW (± 9 mW). This value decreased to 25 mW (± 3 mW) 24 hours later ($P < 0.0001$). However, for the medium motile sperm, the power dropped from an initial reading of 99 mW to 50 mW one day later ($P < 0.016$) despite the similarity in the mean velocity.

These studies demonstrated that optical trapping and micromanipulation of sperm using a low-power laser beam is technically feasible. The optical trap may thus be used as a micromanipulator, allowing sperm traction *in vitro* and may also be used in combination with other micromanipulating techniques described below. Measurements of sperm relative force may also contribute to better understanding of sperm physiology. Such measurements, before and after the introduction of various drugs that are known to affect sperm motility, may provide a more qualitative measure of the possible effects of such chemicals.

Intracellular Application of Laser Beams

One of the key questions in cell biology centres on the forces involved in the movement of chromosomes during mitosis. Various models have been proposed to explain how forces are exerted on chromosomes but have not been adequately tested due to the difficulty involved in the measurement of forces within a cell. An optical trap provides a new approach to the measurement of intracellular forces without physical contact with the cell. Some of the methods

and procedures described below may highlight the potential use of lasers in gamete research. Berns *et al.* (1989) used an optical trap similar to the one described earlier to alter (*in vitro*) the movement of chromosomes in prometaphase and metaphase of *Potorus tridactylis* kidney (Pt K2) cells. Two experiments were conducted by using the optical trap to exert transverse forces on chromosomes. In the first case, the optical trap was applied adjacent to centrophilic chromosomes that were off the mitotic spindle. The second experiment involved late moving chromosomes between a mitotic pole and the metaphase plate. In both experiments, the movement of chromosomes away from the laser beam was initiated by the optical trap with resulting velocities that were higher than previously reported (McNeill and Berns, 1981). Control experiments were performed by applying the optical trap to other regions of the cell with no effect on mitosis. These observations suggest that the chromosome has an ability to sense and respond to external forces exerted on it. When a pulling optical force was applied to one side of the chromosome, the spindle attached to the other side responded by pulling the chromosome in the other direction.

Microdissection of selected nucleolar genetic regions of mitotic chromosomes and cytoplasmic organelles is also possible (Berns *et al.*, 1981). Living cells were exposed to a tunable dye laser microbeam at very short (a few nanoseconds) pulses. The damage was confined to specific cellular or subcellular targets. For better understanding of the feasibility of these delicate manipulations it is important to highlight some theoretical and practical determinants. The diameter of the focused laser spot is directly proportional to the wavelength and inversely related to the numerical aperture of the objective. However, the actual diameter of the effective lesion may be smaller than the theoretical limit of the focused laser beam. The tissue may have a damage threshold that is exceeded only by the centre region of the Gaussian laser beam. Another explanation for the smaller effects is the selective disruption of the molecules at the target zone. In these studies the authors demonstrated that cells with destroyed centrioles, but intact pericentriolar material, were capable of proceeding through mitosis in a normal fashion. Presumably, the laser was able to destroy selectively the molecules in either the centrioles or the pericentriolar material, and then follow the cells to determine if they could continue cell division.

Laser Zona Drilling (LZD)

Mammalian fertilization is an inefficient process in which only one sperm, of millions initially deposited in the female reproductive tract, penetrates the egg. *In vitro* fertilization may provide an approach for correction of infertility in oligospermic males. However, the ratio of sperm to eggs needed for successful fertilization is several thousands to one. By drilling a small hole through the zona pellucida of the mouse oocytes with acidified Tyrode solution, Gordon and Talansky (1986) were able to achieve *in vitro* fertilization with only 1% of the sperm concentration that would otherwise be required. An increased fertilization rate of human oocytes in cases of male infertility after partial zona dissection (PZD) has also been observed by Malter and Cohen (1989a, b).

In order to assess the potential use of laser microbeams for controlled, 'non-contact' zona drilling, a different approach was used on 420 oocytes (231 hamster, 148 mouse and 41 human oocytes; Tadir *et al.*, 1991). Laser pulses (15 ns in duration) at 532 nm, 366 nm, 355 nm and 266 nm wavelengths with the energy range of 5–9 mJ were applied through an inverted microscope (Zeiss-Axiomat, Thornwood, NY) with a 25 × objective. The oocytes, incubated in Ham's-F 10 medium, were placed in a specially designed glass container, on the motorized X–Y microscope stage. The laser beam was directed towards the oocyte. Better control on the depth of zonal damage is obtained when the beam is directed tangent to the egg sphere rather than oriented towards the lower pole (Figure 48.3). Following exposure to the laser light, oocytes were fixed in 4% glutaraldehyde solution and stored in cocodylate buffer. Light and scanning electron microscopy confirmed the laser effects. These results indicated that the optimal configuration incorporates the use of 366 nm laser light at spot diameters of 2–4 μm (unpublished data). A well shaped controlled crater in the zona pellucida was produced. The accuracy of this method enables drilling several neighbouring apertures, without causing damage to the vitelline membrane and the ooplasm content.

More recently, Neev *et al.* (1992) used a short pulse (15 ns) excimer laser as well as ultra-short pulses from an Nd:YAG laser, in order to drill human zone pellucidae in eggs which failed to fertilize in clinical IVF cycles. They demonstrated that the excimer laser with xenon chloride (XeCl) gas fill, emitting at 308 nm, produced superior results in several categories, including precise

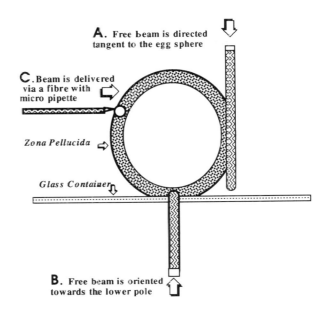

Figure 48.3 Laser beam directed towards the zona pellucida in three modes. Better control on the depth of zonal damage is obtained when the beam is directed tangent to the egg sphere (B) rather than oriented towards the lower pole (A). The ArF laser (Palanker *et al.*, 1991) is delivered through a micropipette located in contact with the drilling site on the zona pellucida.

control of the amount of material removed, and the ease of energy delivery to the drilling site (Figure 48.4). At the same time, these XeCl excimer lasers were virtually free of thermal damage to adjacent areas. It was also noticed that radiation from the shorter pulse (70 ps) Nd:YAG (here, again, a non-linear crystal was used to generate higher harmonics at 532 nm and 266 nm) failed to cause sufficient damage to the drilled site (probably due to the pulse's lower absorption or lower energy), while the argon fluoride (ArF) excimer laser was very difficult to work with because of its extremely high absorption by water, which prevents it from being delivered through the liquid interfaces or through optical fibres. Palanker *et al.* (1991), however, found a way to circumvent this shortcoming of the ArF laser by delivering the 193 nm radiation through a micropipette filled with a positive pressure gas, which is in contact with the drilling site on the zona (Figure 48.3). Their methods produced a highly localized (< 5 μm) hole in the zona with minimal damage to the surrounding area. The main disadvantage of this method, however, is the necessity to use a micropipette and maintain manual contact with the drilled site. It is believed that using the XeCl with its less absorptive 308 nm radiation will allow the same high precision and control, with minimal collateral

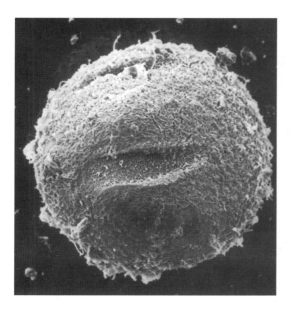

Figure 48.4 Superficial crater in the zona pellucida of human oocyte exposed to 308 nm wavelength laser light, at an energy level of 10 mJ. The beam was directed tangent to the egg sphere. (SEM magnification × 710, reproduced at 81% of original.)

damage and permitting the user to take advantage of the ability to deliver this wavelength (308 nm) through optical fibres and liquid media. The fact that the short pulse XeCl interaction with the oocyte is threshold dependent (i.e. the light will pass through the liquid medium without interaction if the pulse's energy per time per unit area is below a threshold level) can be used, by focusing the beam onto the desired target area, to interact with highly selective targets, and even with a selected site within the zona or within the ooplasm. This can be applied, for example, to selectively destroy excess pronuclei in cases of polyspermic fertilization. Currently, research is being conducted on the potential advantages, possible adverse effects, improving laser performance and ease of use, in order to evaluate the need and allow introduction of these techniques to IVF clinics in the future. If this research is proved successful, the highly reproducible, accurate (and perhaps even partly automated) use of lasers like the XeCl excimer could make this method accessible to clinical application on a large scale and with relative ease.

Laser-induced Inactivation of Extra Pronucleus Following Polyspermic Fertilization

Polyspermy is a potential complication of human *in vitro* fertilization with a reported incidence of between 4 and 5%, depending on the hormonal stimulation used for super ovulation (Wentz *et al.*, 1983; Kola *et al.*, 1987). Rawlins *et al.* (1988) reported identification of the supernumerary male pronucleus in tripronuclear (3 PN) human zygotes, removal of one male pronucleus, and syngamy without subsequent cleavage of the resultant diploidized zygotes. Malter and Cohen (1989a) described the correction of polyspermy through pronucleus extraction in the absence of membrane relaxants in 25 polyspermic zygotes. We were able to inactivate extra pronuclei using a different 'non-invasive' method.

Nine 3 PN human oocytes were exposed to lasers at 532 nm and 355 nm wavelength, with the power setting of 5 mJ, through the inverted microscope with a 100 × objective. A specially designed glass dish was placed on an X–Y motorized stage and the beam was directed towards one of the extra pronuclei. The high magnification and the marked changes in power density within short distances allowed non-traumatic penetration through the zona pellucida, and selective destruction of the pronucleus. Two out of the nine fertilized ova exposed to the laser light were cleaved to the 6–8 cell stage and further processed for chromosomal analysis. Unfortunately, the processing could not be successfully completed. It is important to emphasize that it is difficult to distinguish between male and female pronuclei although several authors described criteria to identify the male pronuclei (Malter and Cohen, 1989b). Our experiment demonstrated that this selective, non-touch procedure is technically feasible. More experience is needed to assess its effectiveness and necessity.

Cell Fusion

A single-beam gradient force optical trap was combined with a pulsed UV laser microbeam in order to perform laser-induced cell fusion (Wiegand-Steubing *et al.*, 1991). This combination offers the possibility to selectively fuse two single cells without critical chemical or electrical treatment. The optical trap was created by directing a Nd:YAG laser into a microscope and focusing the beam with a high numerical aperture

Figure 48.5 Laser microbeam facility. The laser beam is delivered through the laser cavity (upper right) into an inverted microscope and reduced to 1–5 μm spot size. The image of the oocyte is monitored on the television screen.

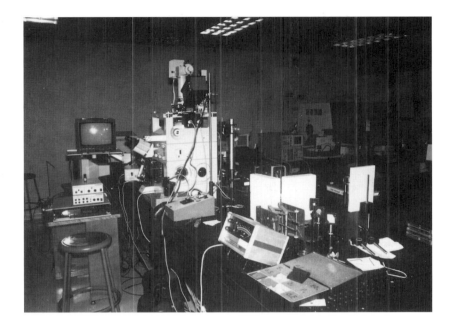

objective. The UV laser microbeam, produced by a nitrogen pumped dye laser (366 nm), was collinear with the trapping beam. Once inside the trap, two cells could be fused with several pulses of the UV laser, attenuated to an energy of ~1 μJ/pulse in the object plane. This method of laser-induced cell fusion should provide increased selectivity and efficiency in generating hybrid cells.

Conclusion

The field of reproductive technologies is being rapidly developed since the introduction of *in vitro* fertilization as a clinical service in the early 1980s. Many questions and potential solutions are being suggested as a result of exposure to new technologies. Various procedures, especially in the field of male infertility, may require micromanipulating manoeuvres. It appears that laser microbeams, optical microscopy and high resolution television systems integrated with computerized image processing may greatly contribute to this area.

Acknowledgement

This research was supported by the following grants and contracts: US NIH RR01 102, US Department of Energy DE-FG03-91ER61227, and the US Department of the Navy contract N000 14-91-0134.

References

Ashkin A (1980) Application of laser radiation pressure. *Science* **210**: 1081–1088.

Ashkin A & Dziedzic JM (1987) Optical trapping and manipulation of viruses and bacteria. *Science* **235**: 1517–1520.

Ashkin A, Dziedzic JM, Bjorkholm JE & Chu S (1986) Observation of a single beam gradient force optical trap for dielectric particles. *Optics Letters* **11**: 288–290.

Baggish MS (1986) The state of the art of laser surgery in gynecology. *Lasers in Surgery and Medicine* **6**: 390–395.

Bellina JH (1974) Gynecology and the laser. *Contemporary Obstetrics and Gynecology* **4**: 24–29.

Bellina JH, Fick AC & Jackson JD (1985) Lasers in gynecology: an historical/developmental overview. *Lasers in Surgery and Medicine* **5**: 1–22.

Berns MW, Rounds DE & Olson RS (1969) Effects of laser microirradiation on chromosomes. *Experimental Cell Research* **56**: 292–298.

Berns MW, Aist J, Edwards J *et al.* (1981) Laser microsurgery in cell and development biology. *Science* **213**: 505–513.

Berns MW, Wright WH, Tromberg BJ *et al.* (1989) Use of a laser-induced optical force trap to study chromosome movement on the mitotic spindle. *Proceedings of the National Academy of Sciences (USA)* **86**: 4539–4543.

Bruhat M, Mage C & Manhes M (1979) Use of the CO_2 laser via laparoscopy. In Kaplan I (ed) *Laser Surgery III, Proceedings of the Third International Society for Laser Surgery*, pp 274–276. Tel-Aviv: Ot-Paz.

Daniell JF (1984) The role of lasers in infertility surgery. *Fertility and Sterility* **42**: 815–823.

Daniell JF, Miller W & Tosh R (1986) Initial evaluation of the use of potassium–titanyl–phosphate (KTP 532) laser in gynecologic laparoscopy. *Fertility and Sterility* **46**: 373–377.

Gordon JW & Talansky BE (1986) Assisted fertilization

by zona drilling: a mouse model for correction of oligospermia. *Journal of Experimental Zoology* **239**: 347–354.

Kaplan I, Goldman J & Ger R (1973) The treatment of erosions of the uterine cervix by means of the CO_2 laser. *Obstetrics and Gynecology* **41**: 795–796.

Keye WR & Dixon J (1983) Photocoagulation of endometriosis by the argon laser through the laparoscope. *Obstetrics and Gynecology* **62**: 383–386.

Kola I, Trounson A, Dawason G & Rogers P (1987) Tripronuclear human oocytes altered cleavage patterns and subsequent karyotype analysis of embryos. *Biology of Reproduction* **37**: 395–399.

Lomano JM (1985) Nd:YAG laser applications in gynecology. In Joffe SN & Ogurs Y (eds) *Advances of Nd:YAG Laser Surgery*, pp 201–207. Berlin: Springer Verlag.

Malter EH & Cohen J (1989a) Partial zona dissection of the human oocyte: a non-traumatic method using micromanipulation to assist zona pellucida penetration. *Fertility and Sterility* **51** 139–148.

Malter HM & Cohen J (1989b) Embryonic development after microsurgical repair of polyspermic human zygotes. *Fertility and Sterility* **52**: 373–380.

McNeill PA & Berns MW (1981) Chromosome behavior after laser microirradiation of a single kinetochore in mitotic PTK2 cells. *Journal of Cell Biology* **88**: 543–553.

Neev Y, Tadir T, Asch R *et al.* (1992) Laser zona drilling and partial zona dissection: a comparative study. *Proceedings of the International Society for Photo-Optical Instrumentation Engineers (SPIE)*, no. 1650 (in press).

Palanker D, Ohad S, Lewis A *et al.* (1991) Technique for cellular microsurgery using the 193 nm excimer laser. *Lasers in Surgery and Medicine* **11**: 580–586.

Rawlins RG, Binor Z, Radwanska E & Dmowski WP (1988) Microsurgical enucleation of tripronuclear human zygotes. *Fertility and Sterility* **50**: 266–272.

Sutton CJG (1986) Initial experience with carbon dioxide laser laparoscopy. *Lasers in Medical Science* **1**: 25–31.

Tadir Y, Kaplan I, Zukerman Z & Ovadia J (1981) Laparoscopic CO_2 laser sterilization. In Semm K & Mettler L (eds) *Human Reproduction*, pp 429–431. Amsterdam: Excerpta Medica.

Tadir Y, Wright WH, Vafa O *et al.* (1989) Micromanipulation of sperm by a laser generated optical trap. *Fertility and Sterility* **52**: 870–873.

Tadir Y, Wright WH, Vafa O *et al.* (1990) Force generated by human sperm correlated to velocity and determined using a laser trap. *Fertility and Sterility* **53**: 944–947.

Tadir Y, Wright WH, Vafa O *et al.* (1991) Micromanipulation of gametes using laser microbeams. *Human Reproduction* **6**: 1011–1016.

Wentz AC, Repp RE, Maxson WS, Pittaway DE & Torbit CA (1983) The problem of polyspermy in *in vitro* fertilization. *Fertility and Sterility* **40**: 748–754.

Wiegand-Steubing R, Cheng S, Wright WH, Numajiri Y & Berns MW (1991) Laser induced cell fusion in combination with optical tweezers: the laser cell fusion trap. *Cytometry* **12**: 505–510.

49

Photodynamic Therapy

WILLIAM R. KEYE

Division of Reproductive Endocrinology, William Beaumont Hospital, Royal Oak, Michigan, USA

Introduction

During the 1980s the use of lasers in gynaecology grew rapidly both in terms of the number and types of procedures as well as the percentage of gynaecologists using lasers. In addition, there was development of an increasing number of different wavelengths as well as the development and application of new delivery systems. Each of these lasers and delivery systems has been developed for the purpose of ablating abnormal tissues through the conversion of light energy to heat (photothermal effect).

While the use of this photothermal effect of lasers has simplified operative laparoscopy and hysteroscopy, lasers have not yet been shown to significantly improve the clinical results in the treatment of any gynaecological disease. In addition, the final clinical effect of currently available lasers is determined more by the skill and dexterity of the surgeon than by the type of laser or delivery system used. However, the 1990s may see the emergence of a different type of laser and a different principle of laser tissue interaction in the treatment of benign gynaecological disease. Instead of using the photothermal effect of lasers, gynaecologists of the next decade may utilize the photochemical effect of lasers. The use of this photochemical effect has been termed photodynamic therapy.

Principles of Photodynamic Therapy

'Photodynamic therapy', which is based on a phenomenon known as photodynamic action, was developed in the first part of this century by Niels Finsen and others when they used natural and artificial sources of ultraviolet radiation for the treatment of lupus vulgaris (Bloom, 1964). Photodynamic therapy involves the interaction of light or other forms of electromagnetic radiation with dyes or pigments within tissues. In contradistinction to 'phototherapy' which involves the interaction of light with endogenous pigments within tissues, photodynamic therapy (PDT) involves the excitation of exogenously administered drugs by various forms of light or electromagnetic radiation. Typically, photodynamic therapy utilizes visible laser light in the 400–800 nm wavelength range and exogenously administered photosensitive dyes such as the haematoporphyrin derivative (HPD). The haematoporphyrin derivative absorbs photons of light energy and in the process photophysical and photochemical reactions are initiated that lead to the destruction of target tissues which have concentrated the dye.

The exact nature of the photochemical reaction involved in photodynamic therapy has been studied intensively and in the case of haematoporphyrin derivatives involves the generation of reactive oxygen, primarily singlet oxygen, and perhaps the development of free radical reactions and radical oxygen species (Straight and Spikes, 1985). Singlet oxygen then reacts with a variety of biological molecules including amino acids, nucleic acids, unsaturated lipids, proteins and other compounds sensitive to oxidation (Straight and Spikes, 1985). This interaction of singlet oxygen with biological molecules results in irreversible oxidation of these molecules and irreversible damage to cellular macromolecules in structures such as nucleic acids, enzymes and cell membranes. Singlet oxygen may also interact with multiple targets within cells and thus destroy target tissues in a variety of ways. The principle of selective tissue destruction using photodynamic therapy requires the localization of exogenously administered dye such as haematoporphyrin derivatives (HPD) within target tissues. In general this takes place as the result of delayed clearance and extended retention of the exogenous dyes within the target tissue. For example, the treatment of malignancies by photodynamic therapy requires the retention of photosensitive dyes within the tumour or its stroma and vessels and the subsequent exposure of the tumours to laser light of such a wavelength that will activate the dye. The retention of the photosensitivity dyes may occur within one or more compartments of the tumour tissue, such as blood vessels, intercellular stroma, connective tissue or the malignant cell itself. In some cases the process of tumour destruction following photodynamic therapy is the result of damage to the vascular system within the tumour which in turn causes coagulation necrosis. This indirect effect may be superimposed upon a direct effect of the light and dye within the malignant cells themselves.

The localization and retention of haematoporphyrin derivative (HPD) occurs as a result of the competitive binding of this dye to plasma proteins such as albumin, haemopexin, lipoproteins or tumour tissue proteins. The haematoporphyrin derivative, which is composed of monomers, dimers and tetramers, aggregate within the tumour cells and the vascular network within tumours. They may be selectively retained within the tumour as a result of altered capillary permeability in the vessel supplying the tumour. When the haematoporphyrin aggregates leak out of the capillaries, they may then localize within tumour cells by binding to extracellular and cellular components of the tumour.

The toxic effects of singlet oxygen manifest themselves at the cell surface as membrane blebbing or lysis, the inactivation of enzyme and the destruction of protein cross-linking. There may also be damage at the mitochondrial, microsomal, lysosomal membrane and nuclear membrane levels. Damage to the DNA appears to be minimal. As a result of destruction of membranes of the lysosome, lysosomal enzymes are released and

ultimately photoinactivated. In *in vivo* models this initial sequence of events often occurs first at the site of the capillary endothelial cell.

In order to be effective, laser light must be chosen so that its wavelength falls within the absorption band of the photosensitive dye and must reach the dye and the tissues that contain the dye with enough intensity to initiate the photo-oxidation reactions described above. It appears that the window of electromagnetic energy that is most effective ranges between 600 nm and 1200 nm. In addition, the wavelength must be chosen so that absorption of the light by endogenous tissue pigments such as haem, bilirubin and melanin is minimal so the activating light energy will be able to penetrate through normal tissues and reach the sensitized tissues containing the dye. Above 600 nm the absorption of light by endogenous pigments is at its lowest, thus permitting the maximum depth of tissue penetration by the activating light energy. Some superficial lesions may be treated by shorter wavelengths ranging between 410 and 580 nm. Thus the impact of the laser energy is determined by the absorption characteristics of the dye, the geometry of the target tissue that contains the dye, the type of tissue that composes the target tissue and the type of tissue that surrounds the target. In addition, the efficacy and efficiency of photodynamic therapy can be enhanced by the selection of an appropriate dye as well as the selection of specific wavelengths and intensities of laser to match the wavelengths of the sensitizer. Finally, the selection of optimal pulse parameters such as pulse duration and pulse frequency may be useful in photodynamic therapy. Appropriate studies evaluating these pulse parameters are now being performed. Fortunately the efficiency of this system requires only very low oxygen concentrations (10^{-6}–10^{-8} M).

There are four classes of photosensitizers or light-activated drugs that may be useful in photodynamic therapy in the 1990s. The first are porphyrin derivatives which include the aforementioned haematoporphyrin derivative as well as other porphyrins such as benzoporphyrin. The second category are chlorin derivatives including chlorin, E^6, monoaspartic acid and monoethylene diamine chlorin derivatives. The third class of photodynamic dyes include synthetic dyes such as purpurins, zanthine dyes, thiazine dyes and phthalocyanines. Finally, the last group of dyes are light absorbing drugs and precursors of photosensitizers such as alpha-aminolaevulinic acid. Many of these agents can be administered either systemically or topically. Topical application often results in maximum uptake by the target tissue with limited uptake by other non-specific and normal tissues. In addition to using these photodynamic agents for the therapy of target tissues, the fact that these agents and dyes fluoresce may make it possible for the early diagnosis of subclinical lesions and their treatment before they become invasive or otherwise destructive.

Unfortunately these aggregates of haematoporphyrin derivative may also accumulate in normal tissues whose structure is readily accessible to proteins and colloids and in pathological but non-tumorous tissues that have altered or increased vascularity. Thus haematoporphyrin derivatives have been observed in significant concentrations in liver, kidney, spleen, skin, lung, muscles and fat. As a result when there is inflammation or wound healing within normal tissues, there may be excessive uptake or retention of the dye within these tissues. This has posed a major problem in the use of haematoporphyrin derivative as a photosensitizer, i.e. the unwanted and inadvertent damage to normal tissues. While there is a selective retention of haematoporphyrin tissue within tumour cells and the tumour itself, the low level presence of dye within other tissues renders them photosensitive and, as a result, patients must avoid direct sunlight for as long as 4 or 5 weeks after the administration of dye. This has thus far almost completely limited the use of haematoporphyrin derivative to the treatment of malignancies where the potential benefit far outweighs the inconvenience and potential toxic effect of the dyes. As a result, the use of photodynamic therapy in the treatment of benign diseases such as endometriosis or the endometrium of women with menorrhagia will depend on the development of new dyes which are more rapidly and fully cleared from normal tissue or on the development of techniques of local application which would avoid the systemic distribution of the drug and thus the sensitization of normal tissue.

Treatment of Endometriosis with Photodynamic Therapy

The detection of endometriosis currently depends on the visual identification of peritoneal lesions at the time of pelvic laparoscopy. However, it is often very difficult to detect all the lesions of endometriosis that may be present in the pelvis and, as a result, our inability to detect occult lesions limits our ability to completely eradicate the disease. In addition, the destruction of lesions depends upon our ability to direct the laser energy at each lesion and vaporize the entire lesion as well as our ability to identify each lesion. Preliminary studies utilizing animal models of endometriosis suggest a possible role for photodynamic therapy in the treatment of endometriosis. This laser light-induced luminescence of endometriotic lesions may be useful in the early detection and diagnosis of the disease.

The work of Vancaillie and his colleagues suggests that endometriosis may be amenable to light-induced luminescence for its diagnosis (Vancaillie et al., 1989). This light-induced fluorescence using differentially retained photosensitizers for the detection of occult lesions of many types is not new. Research is currently under way to develop techniques for the early detection of occult tumours as well as atherosclerotic lesions. Vancaillie has demonstrated laser-induced fluorescence of ectopic endometrium in rabbits and has suggested a role for this technique in the early diagnosis of endometriosis (Vancaillie et al., 1989). Manyak and his colleagues have also recently demonstrated the feasibility of the detection of endometriotic implants using fluorescent porphyrins and a rabbit model of the disease (Manyak et al., 1990).

The use of both exogenous and endogenous porphyrins for the fluorescent diagnosis of tumours was founded on the early work of Policard (1924) who observed reddish fluorescence of endogenous porphyrins in human and animal tumours. Early studies utilizing fluorescence for the diagnosis of occult tumours relied upon photographic methods utilizing either standard film or digital charge-coupled devices (CCD). While standard film photography is capable of detecting and recording the presence of fluorescences, recently videocons and digital CCD-based camera systems can enhance the sensitivity of detection by their ability to detect and record low-intensity light signals and by their ability to subtract interfering autofluorescence background from the fluorescence of the tumour.

One can envisage in the future that hours before laparoscopy a patient with suspected endometriosis will receive a drug designed to be retained within endometriotic implants within the pelvis. At the time of laparoscopy the pelvis will be illuminated with light of specific wavelengths designed to excite the dye and, subsequently, fluorescence from the dye will then be observed and recorded. In this way not only gross but microscopic areas of endometriosis may be detected. Following the recording of the areas of endometriosis, the pelvis will be exposed to a longer pulse of laser light energy which will activate the dye within the implants of endometriosis. As described above, singlet oxygen will then trigger a series of irreversible, biochemical events within the endometriosis which will ultimately lead to its destruction.

Utilizing a rabbit model of endometriosis, Petrucco *et al.* (1990) have established the differential uptake and retention of haematoporphyrin derivatives in explants of endometrium in the peritoneal cavity of New Zealand white rabbits. Following the systemic and topical application of haematoporphyrin derivatives, they were able to demonstrate the specific and selective destruction of these implants following exposure to the gold vapour laser. In their experiments they determined that following the pretreatment with haematoporphyrin derivative and exposure to gold vapour laser 24 hours later, that the endometriotic implants were totally destroyed. However, normal surrounding tissue that had also been exposed to the dye and to the laser light was unaffected. In addition, exposure to either the dye or the laser light was not sufficient to destroy the areas of endometriosis. Similar findings were observed by Keye *et al.*, utilizing the Rhesus monkey and subcutaneous experimentally induced lesions of endometriosis haematoporphyrin derivative and an argon laser (unpublished data).

It is hoped that this approach to the treatment of endometriosis will not only lead to the more reliable diagnosis of the disease and a more reliable means of determining the extent of the disease but also to more thorough destruction of the lesions. This would be achieved in the hope of reducing the chance of recurrence and improving the clinical result following the surgical treatment of the disease.

The Destruction of the Endometrium

The treatment of idiopathic menorrhagia currently relies upon a number of medications, hysterectomy or in some cases the hysteroscopic destruction of the endometrium using the photothermal effect of the Nd:YAG laser, KTP laser or argon laser. In addition, the endometrium may be destroyed by radiofrequency or by electrocautery. Unfortunately each of these techniques relies upon extensive experience of the operator and mastery of the difficulties of operative hysteroscopy. As a result, the techniques of endometrial ablation are not widely available and will never be practical for all gynaecologists. Preliminary

studies in experimental animals have demonstrated that haematoporphyrin derivative is present in the endometrium after the systemic administration to ovariectomized Sprague–Dawley rats (Schneider *et al.*, 1988a–c). In a series of studies, Schneider *et al.* (1988a–c) observed the uptake of haematoporphyrin derivative in the uterus with levels that were constant between 3 and 72 hours after its administration. They also observed that there was initial concentration of the dye within the endometrium followed by a shift in the concentration of the dye to the myometrium and finally to the serosa. Using iodine-125 labelled haematoporphyrin derivative and fluorescence microscopy they were able to demonstrate the dye in the temporal sequence noted above. The dye was noted to be concentrated in the endometrium within 3 hours after the injection of the haematoporphyrin derivative. By 6 hours the haematoporphyrin derivative had disappeared from the endometrium, was found in the myometrium and finally the serosa. By 24 hours it was seen only in the serosa. Similarly Keye and colleagues demonstrated in New Zealand white rabbits the concentration of dye within the uterus following either systemic or topical application of haematoporphyrin derivative (unpublished data). Following the administration of very small amounts of haematoporphyrin derivative, this dye was present within several hours within the uterus. Using laser energy from an argon pumped dye laser with a wavelength of 630 nm, destruction of the endometrium as well as the superficial myometrium was demonstrated (Figures 49.1–49.4).

It is envisaged that in the future women with idiopathic menorrhagia may be treated using photodynamic therapy. Several hours before the photodynamic therapy haematoporphyrin derivative or some other photosensitizer would be administered either systemically or topically into

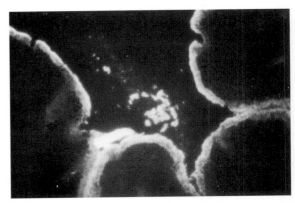

Figure 49.1 Fluorescence of haematoporphyrin derivative in the rabbit endometrium.

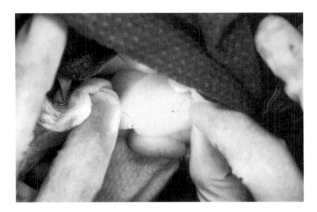

Figure 49.2 Illumination of the rabbit uterus with the argon pumped dye laser.

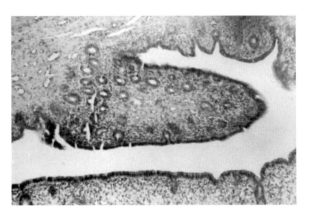

Figure 49.3 Control endometrium which had been exposed to the laser but not the HPD rabbit.

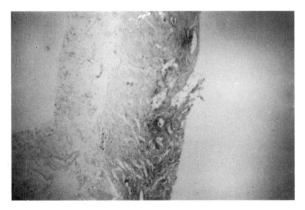

Figure 49.4 Ablated rabbit endometrium after exposure to HPD and the argon pumped dye laser.

the uterus. Ideally a small catheter would be placed through the cervix and into the endometrial cavity. The endometrial cavity would then be flushed with a solution containing the photosensitizer. Within minutes to hours an optical fibre would be placed into the uterus. The fibre would be modified in such a way to enhance the illumination of the endometrial surfaces. Over

the course of several minutes the endometrium would be exposed to laser light energy of a wavelength chosen to excite the photosensitizer. The patient would then return to her normal activities and over the course of the next several weeks the endometrium would be totally destroyed by photodynamic therapy. This technique could also possibly be of some use as an non-operative approach to sterilization.

Conclusions

While photodynamic therapy is currently limited to the treatment of malignant diseases, the development of new and more specific dyes may make it possible to treat benign conditions such as menorrhagia or endometriosis using photodynamic therapy. The dyes of the future will not only be more specific but also will have the ability to be cleared more rapidly from normal tissues. In addition, the dyes may be of such a nature that the light energy required will not be laser light but will simply be a range of wavelengths of light which includes the wavelengths that are known to excite the dye. The treatment of such benign conditions such as endometriosis by this method may make the treatment more successful and less invasive than the techniques commonly available.

References

Bloom HF (1964) *Photodynamic Action and Diseases Caused by Light.* New York: Hafner Publishing Co.

Manyak MJ, Nelson LM, Solomon D et al. (1990) Fluorescent detection of rabbit endometrial implants resulting from monodispersed viable cell suspensions. *Fertility and Sterility* **54**: 356–359.

Policard A (1924) Etudes furles. Aspects offerts par des tumeurs expérimentales examinées à la lumière de Woods. *Comptes Rendus des Séances de la Société de Biologie et de ses Filiales* **91**: 1423–1424.

Petrucco DM, Sathanandan N, Knowles S et al. (1990) Ablation of endometriosis in rabbits by haematoporphyrin derivative (HPD)—photoradiation therapy using the gold vapor laser. *Lasers in Surgery and Medicine* **10(4)**: 344–348.

Schneider DF, Schelthas HF, Wesseler TA, Chen I-W & Moulton BC (1988a) Hematoporphyrin derivative uptake in uteri of estrogen-treated ovariectomized rats. *Colposcopy and Gynecologic Laser Surgery* **4**: 67.

Schneider DF, Schelthas HF, Wesseler TA, Chen I-W & Moulton BC (1988b) Endometrial ablation by

DHE photoradiation therapy in estrogen-treated ovariectomized rats. *Colposcopy and Gynecologic Laser Surgery* **4**: 73.

Schneider DF, Schelthas HF, Wesseler TA, Chen I-W & Moulton BC (1988c) Fertility in rats following endometrial ablation by DHE photodynamic therapy. *Colposcopy and Gynecologic Laser Surgery* **4**: 79.

Straight RC & Spikes JD (1985) Photosensitized oxi-

dation of biological molecules. In Frimer A (ed) *Singlet Oxygen*, Vol. 4, pp 91–143. Boca Raton: CRC Press.

Vancaillie TG, Hill RH, Riehl RM, Gilstad D & Schenken RS (1989) Laser-induced fluorescence of ectopic endometrium in rabbits. *Obstetrics and Gynecology* **74**: 225–230.

Directory of Manufacturers

Acufex

Acufex UK, Cyanamid of Great Britain Ltd, Fareham Road, Gosport, Hants PO13 0AS, UK, Tel: +44 (0)329 224 116, Fax: +44 (0)329 220 213;

Acufex Europe, Acufex Microsurgical Inc, Crown House, Hornbeam Square North, Harrogate, HG2 8PB, UK, Tel: +44 (0)423 879 379, Fax: +44 (0)423 873 202;

Acufex Microsurgical Inc, 130 Forbes Boulevard, Mansfield, MA 02048, USA, Tel: +1 (508) 339 9700, Fax: +1 (508) 339 8853

Endoscopic video equipment

Aesculap Ltd

Parkway Close, Parkway Industrial Estate, Sheffield S9 4WJ, UK, Tel: +44 (0)742 730346, Fax: +44 (0)742 701 840

Surgical instruments

Albert Waeschle Co

123/125 Old Christchurch Road, Bournemouth, BH1 1EX, UK, Tel: +44 (0)202 557 513/290 502, Fax: +44 (0)202 299 683;

Martin Medizin-Technik, Ludwigstaler Str 132, Postfach 60, 7200 Tuttlingen, Germany, Tel: +49 (0 74 61) 706 233, Fax: +49 (0 74 61) 706 193;

Medline Industries Inc, One Medline Place, Mundelein, IL 60060, USA, Tel: +1 (800) 323 5886, Fax: +1 (708) 949 2686

Martin – Minimal invasive surgery system
Surgical diathermy units
Arm system to hold endoscopes
Surgical and endoscopic instruments
Electrosurgical units
Lights, insufflators, suction pumps, optics

Apple Medical Corporation

Distributor: Sinergy SA, 38 Ave Croix, St Martin, 03200 Vichy, France, Tel: +33 117097 8804, Fax: +33 7059 8377;

93 Nashaway Road, Bolton, MA 01740, USA, Tel: +1 (508) 779 2926, Fax: +1 (508) 779 6927

Trocar/Cannula 5 mm, 10 mm, 12 mm
Lehrer open lap cannula 10 mm, 105 mm length
Pneumo-matic insufflation needles, 120 mm, 150 mm
Bi-polar insert

Aspen Lab

(see CONMED)

Auto Suture Company UK

2 King's Ride Park, King's Ride, Ascot, Berks SL5 8BF, UK, Tel: +44 (0)344 277 21, Fax: +44 (0)344 275 12;

Auto Suture Europe SA, 22 Rue Berlioz, Brive 19100, France, Tel: +33 5524 5656, Fax: +33 5574 4702;

United States Surgical Corporation, 150 Glover Avenue, Norwalk, CT 06856, USA, Tel: +1 (203) 866 5050

Various disposable laparoscopic stapling, clipping, cutting, grasping and manipulation instruments and devices

Baxter Healthcare Ltd

Baxter Healthcare Ltd UK, Wallingford Road, Compton, Newbury, Berks RG16 0QW, UK, Tel: +44 (0)635 200 020, Fax: +44 (0)635 578 800;

Multiple subsidiaries/agents across Europe;

Baxter Healthcare Corp, V Mueller Division, 1500 Waukegan Road, Mcgaw Park, IL 60085, USA, Tel: +1 (708) 473 1500, Fax: +1 (708) 473 0879

Laparoscopes
Camera systems
Light source
Insufflators
Instruments

Beacon Lab

European Consultant: Harvey Grossman, Tel: +44 (0)532 689 579; 2150 W 6th Avenue, Unit P, Broomfield, CO 80020–7116, USA, Tel: +1 (303) 466 3042, Fax: +1 (303) 466 0662

Argon Beam Coagulator (for general purpose, laparoscopic units, open procedures)
Hand pieces

Berchtold GmbH & Co

Arthrodax Surgical Ltd, Great Western Court, Ross-on-Wye, Herefordshire HR9 7DW, UK, Tel: +44 (0)989 66669, Fax: +44 (0)989 768140;

Berchtold GmbH & Co – Medizin Elektronik, POB 4052, Ludwigstaler Str 28, D-7200 Tuttlingen, Germany, Tel: +49 7461 1810, Fax: +49 7461 181 200;

Berchtold Corporation, 2050 Mabeline Road, Suite C, North Charleston, SC 29418, USA, Tel: +1 (803) 569 6100, Fax: +1 (803) 569 6133

ELEKTROTOM BICUT II – New bipolar technology for cutting and coagulation with HP current
Bipolar instruments for laparoscopic surgery

Bioplasty Ltd

Unit 3, Woodside Business Park, Whitley Wood Lane, Reading, Berks RG2 8LW, UK, Tel: +44 (0) 734 755 180, Fax: +44 (0) 734 312 120;

Bioplasty BV, International Headquarters, Zinkstraat 70, 4823 AC, Breda, The Netherlands, Tel: +33 76 423 770, Fax: +33 76 423 737;

Bioplasty Incorporated, 1385 Centennial Drive, Saint Paul 55113, MN, USA, Tel: +1 (612) 636 4112, Fax: +1 (612) 633 3204

Minimally invasive, endoscopic, incontinence products

Birtcher Medical Systems

Huizer Maatweg, 1273 NA Huzen, The Netherlands, Tel: +31 2152 68344, Fax: +31 2152 63065;

SOLOS Endoscopy, 50 Technology Drive, Irvine, CA 92718, USA, Tel: +1 (714) 753 9400, Fax: +1 (714) 753 9171

ENDOTYER − suturing for advanced laparoscopic technique

Cabot Medical Corporation

Distributor: Cory Bros (Hospital Contracts) Co Ltd, 4 Dollis Park, Finchley, London N3 1HG, UK, Tel: +44 (0)81 349 1081, Fax: +44 (0)81 349 1962;

2021 Cabot Boulevard West, Langhorne, PA 19047, USA, Tel: +1 (215) 752 3834, Fax: +1 (215) 752 0161

Hysteroscopic instrumentation e.g. DeCherney Hysteroscopy Pump
Laparoscopic equipment e.g. Nanticoke advanced laparoscopic/thoracoscopic instruments
Video equipment e.g. High performance video endoscopy system and equipment
Insufflators – KLI electronic insufflator 2001
Instrumentation e.g.
  5 mm Diagnostic sheath with obturator
  Semi rigid operating instruments
  Cervical dilators
  Biopsy instruments
Colposcopes and accessories
Niagara High Flow irrigator system
Zinnanti uterine manipulator injector 4.5 and 4.0
Electrosurgery Units – Models: 110G, 91A
Cryosurgical systems
Re-section equipment for endometrial ablation

Carl Zeiss (Oberkochen) Ltd

PO Box 78, Woodfield Road, Welwyn Garden City, Herts AL7 1LU, UK, Tel: +44 (0)707 331144, Fax: +44 (0)707 373210;

Carl Zeiss Strasse, P O Box 1380, D-7082 Oberkochen, Germany, Tel: +49 (0)736 4200, Fax: +49 (0) 736 46808;

Carl Zeiss Inc, One Zeiss Drive, Thornwood, NY 10594, USA, Tel: +1 (914) 747 1800

OPMILAS CO-2 25 watt laser

OPMILAS CO-2 50 watt laser
OPMILAS YAG M CW Nd:YAG 60 watt laser
OPMILAS 144 pulsed Nd:YAG 1.4 μm 30 watt laser
OPMILAS 144 Plus pulsed Nd:YAG 1.44 μm 30 watt, plus CW Nd:YAG
1.06 μm 100 watt laser (dual wavelength)

Circon ACMI
Distributor: Cory Bros (Hospital Contracts) Ltd, 4 Dollis Park, Finchley, London N3 1HG, UK, Tel: +44 (0)81 349 1081, Fax: +44 (0)81 349 1962;
Circon GmbH, Mehlbeerenstrasse 2, 8028 Taufkirchen, Germany, Tel: +49 89 612 9070, Fax: +49 89 612 90766;
300 Stillwater Avenue, PO Box 1971, Stamford, CT 06904-1791, USA, Tel: +1 (203) 357 8300

Laparoscopy and thoracoscopy instrumentation
HYDROLAPAROSCOPE system
ENDOVIDEO beamsplitter camera with DOCUTROL II
OFFICE CAM office video system

Coherent Inc
Coherent (UK) Ltd, Cambridge Science Park, Milton Road, Cambridge CB4 4RF, UK, Tel: +44 (0)223 424048, Fax: +44 (0)223 425902;
Coherent GmbH, Senefelder Str 10, 6074 Rodermark 2, Ober Roden, Germany, Tel: +49 6074 9140, Fax: +49 6074 95654;
Coherent Medical Division, 3270 West Bayshore Road, Box 10321, Palo Alto, CA, USA, Tel: +1 (415) 858 2250, Fax: +1 (415) 857 0146

Ultrapulse laser system
CO$_2$ laser systems
Coherent/Nezhat laser laparoscope coupler

Conkin Surgical Instruments
PO Box 6707, Station A, Toronto, Ontario, Canada M5W 1X5, Tel: +1 (416) 922 9496, Fax: +1(416) 922 3501

Valtchev uterine mobilizer, VUM-4

CONMED Corporation/Aspen Labs Surgical Systems
Distributor: Cory Bros, 4 Dollis Park, London N3 1HG, UK, Tel: +44 (0)81 349 1081, Fax: +44 (0)81 349 1962;
Intraveno Ltd, 55 Broomhill Drive, Tallaght, Dublin 24, Ireland, Tel: +353 (1) 520 388, Fax: +353 (1) 520 864;
CONMED Corporation, 310 Broad Street, Utica, NY 13501, USA, Tel: +1 (315) 797 8375, Fax: +1 (315) 797 0321

SABRE 180 patient monitoring diathermy machine
ASPEN Vac air filtration system
LLETZ loop and ball electrodes
Electrosurgical accessories

Cook Ob/Gyn
Cook (UK) Ltd, 6 Such Close, Letchworth, Herts SG6 1JF, UK, Tel: +44 (0)462 481 290, Fax: +44 (0)462 480 944;
Cook Urological (Schweiz) AG, Tobelacklerstrasse 4, CH 8212 Neuhausen, Switzerland, Tel: +41 53 225 121, Fax: +41 53 227 549;
Cook Urological Inc, 1100 West Morgan Street, Spencer, IN 47460, USA, Tel: +1 (812) 829 4891, Fax: +1 (812) 829 2022

Accessories for laparoscopy and hysteroscopy

CooperSurgical
CooperSurgical, Chaussée de Louvain 484, 5004 Namur (Bouge), Belgium, Tel: +32 81 214 812, Fax: +32 81 215 900;
CooperSurgical, 770 River Road, PO Box 855, Shelton, CT 06484, USA, Tel: +1 (203) 929 6321, Fax: +1 (203) 926 9435

Hysteroscopy diagnostic system 3000
Resectoscope
Surgical laparoscopy instrument – EuroMed

Cory Bros (Hospital Contracts) Co Ltd
See Circon and Cabot Medical

Dexide Inc
Distributor: Rimmer Bros, 18 Aylesbury Street, Clerkenwell, London EC1R 0DD, UK, Tel: +44 (0)71 251 6494, Fax: +44 (0)71 253 7585;
7509 Flagstone Drive, Fort Worth, TX 76118, USA, Fax: +1 (817) 595 3300

Disposable equipment for minimally invasive surgery, including:
Disposable trocars
Endobag – specimen gathering equipment
FRED – anti-fogging solution
Cannula
Electro-surgical probe

Diagnostic Sonar Ltd
Kirkton Campus, Livingstone, West Lothian, EH54 7BX, UK, Tel: +44 (506) 411 877, Fax: +44 (0)506 412 410

Ultrasound scanners with vaginal transducers ("Imager 3")

Dornier Medizintechnik (formerly MBB)
Distributor: Keymed, Keymed House, Stock Road, Southend on Sea, Essex SS2 5QH, UK, Tel: +44 (0)702 616 333, Fax: +44 (0)702 465 677;
Dornier Medizintechnik GmbH, Laser Surgery Division, Industriestrasse 15, D-8034 Germering, Munchen, Germany, Tel: +49 89 8410 80506, Fax: +49 89 8410 8555;

Dornier Medical Systems, 1155 Roberts Boulevard, Kennesaw, GA, 30144, USA, Tel: +1 (404) 426 1315, Fax: +1 (404) 426 6115

Nd-YAG laser systems

DP Medical Systems Ltd
Sutton Business Centre, Restmore Way, off Hackbridge Road, Wallington, Surrey SM6 7AH, UK, Tel: +44 (0)81 669 0011, Fax: +44 (0)81 773 0406

Sterilizable micro video camera and lenses
Automatic video light source
Fibre optic cables
Custom video cabinets
Suppliers of monitors, recorders, printers etc

Electroscope Inc
4890 Sterling Drive, Boulder, CO 80301, USA, Tel: +1 (303) 444 2600, Fax: +1 (303) 444 2693

Electroshield monitoring system
Laparoscopic accessories: hooks, spatulas, irrigation suction, graspers, dissectors, scissors

Elmed
60 West Fay Avenue, Addison, IL 60101–5106, USA, Tel: +1 (708) 543 2792, Fax: +1 (708) 543 2102

Laparoscopes – single and double puncture
Hysteroscopes and accessories
Light sources including video
Instruments for pelvic surgery single and double puncture
Insufflators – conventional and digital
Electrosurgical generators for unipolar and bipolar pelvis surgery with accessories
Microsurgical instruments

Endoscopic Manufacturing and Services Ltd
Mercury House, 859 Coronation Road, Park Royal, London NW10 7QE, UK, Tel: +44 (0)81 965 0600, Fax: +44 (0)81 961 1234

Rod lens telescopes
Hysteroscope sheaths
Telescope bridge
Catheterizing slide
Resectoscopes for endometrium resection
Continuous flow irrigation sheath
Flexible forceps

Eschmann Equipment
Peter Road, Lancing, West Sussex BN15 8TJ, UK, Tel: +44 (0)903 753 322, Fax: +44 (0)903 766 793

Operating tables
Sterilizers
Electrosurgical unit
Pumps and accessories

Ethicon Endo-Surgery (subsidiary of Johnson and Johnson)
Ethicon Ltd, PO Box 408, Bankhead Avenue, Edinburgh EH11 4HE, UK, Tel: +44 (0)31 453 5555, Fax: +44 (0)31 453 6011;
Ethicon Endo-Surgery, 4545 Creek Road, Cincinnati, OH 45242, USA, Tel: +1 (513) 786 7000, Fax: +1 (513) 786 7080

Endotrainers (endoscopic simulation)
ENDOPATH – surgical trocars, adjustable stability, threads, scissors, graspers, dissectors, extractors
LIGACLIP and ABSOLOK – endoscopic clip appliers
Electrosurgery devices – probes and active cords
Ligatures
Endoscopic staplers
Veress needles

Euro-Med
Distributor: CooperSurgical, Chaussée de Louvain 484, 5004 Namur (Bouge), Belgium, Tel: +32 81 214 812, Fax: +32 81 215 900;
8561 154th Avenue, NE, Redmond, WA 98052 3557, USA, Tel: +1 (206) 861 9008, Fax: +1 (206) 861 9438

Lateral vaginal retractor

Euron Ltd
72 New Bond Street, London W1 9DD, UK, Tel: +44 (0)81 959 3611, Fax: +44 (0)81 455 9535

Laparoscopes
Surgical tools
Insufflator
Light source
Micro-video camera

European Information Technology (UK) Ltd
240 Brox Road, Ottershaw, Surrey KT16 0RA, UK, Tel: +44 (0)932 874 642, Fax: +44 (0)932 873 655

Euroking system – software

Eurosurgical Ltd
The Common, Cranleigh, Surrey GU6 8LU, UK, Tel: +44 (0)483 267 363, Fax: +44 (0)483 267 281

Filshie clip system for female sterilization
Fallopian ring system for female sterilization
Vacuum pumps
Tubing
Curettes
Pipelle sampling device for endometrial tissue

Femcare Ltd
67 St Peter's Street, Nottingham NG7 3EN, UK, Tel: +44 (0)602 786 322, Fax: +44 (0)602 420 234

Female sterilization clip and associated applicators for minilaparotomy
Single and double puncture laparoscopy

Fry Surgical International
Unit 17, Goldsworth Park Trading Estate, Woking, Surrey GU21 3BA, UK, Tel: +44 (0)483 721 404 Fax: +44 (0)483 755 282;
Manufacturer: AB Stille Werner, PO Box 90115, Ostmästargränd 10, S-120 21 Stockholm, Sweden. Tel: +46 8602 2000, Fax: +46 8913 187

Stille endoscopic surgical instruments

Fujinon Inc
Heerdter Lohweg 89, 4000 Dusseldorf 11, Germany. Tel: +49 2115 2050, Fax: +49 2115 20519;
10 High Point Drive, Wayne NJ 07470, USA, Tel: +1 (201) 633 5600, Fax: +44 (201) 633 8818

Diagnostic hysteroscope – HYS-R
Therapeutic hysteroscope – HYS-RT
Electronic flexible video laparoscope
Electronic rigid video laparoscope

GU Manufacturing
841 Coronation Road, Park Royal, London NW10 7QJ, UK, Tel: +44 (0)81 961 9000, Fax: +44 (0)31 963 1728

Fragenheim laparoscope
Instruments and equipment for hysteroscopy
Integrated hysteroscope

Heraeus Equipment Limited
9 Wates Way, Brentwood, Essex CM15 9TB, UK, Tel +44 (0)277 231 511, Fax: +44 (0)277 261 856;
Heraeus Instruments GmbH, Heraeusstrasse 12–14, W-6450 Hanau 1, Germany, Tel: +49 (0) 6181 350, Fax: +49 (0) 6181 35711;
Heraeus Lasersonics Inc, 575 Cottonwood Drive, Milpitas, CA, 95035–7434, USA, Tel: +1 (408) 954 4000, Fax: +1 (408) 954 4040

CO$_2$ laser equipment

Johnson & Johnson Medical Limited
Coronation Road, Ascot, Berks SL5 9EY, UK, Tel: +44 (0)344 872 626, Fax: +44 (0)344 212 47;
Ethicon Inc, US Route 22, Sommerville, NJ 08876, USA, Tel: +1 (908)218 0707

INTERCEED (TC7) absorbable adhesion barrier

Karl Storz GmbH and Co
UK Agents: Rimmer Brothers, 18 Aylesbury Street, Clerkenwell, London EC1R 0DD, UK, Tel: +44 (0)71 251 6494, Fax: +44 (0)71 253 7585;
Karl Storz GmbH & Co, Mittelstrasse 8, Postfach 230, D-7200 Tuttlingen, Germany, Tel: +49 7461 7080, Fax: +49 7461 708105;
Karl Storz Endoscopy-America Inc, 10111 W Jefferson Blvd, Culver City, CA 90232–3578, USA, Tel: +1 (213) 558 1500, Fax: +1 (213) 280 2504

Conventional and fibre optically illuminated surgical, scientific instruments and miniature lamps

Keymed
(See Olympus)

Kirwan Surgical
83 East Water Street, PO Box 35, Rockland, MA, USA, Tel: +1 (617) 871 1876, Fax: +1 (617) 871 2816

Endoscopic cables – disposable and reusable

Lasermatic Oy
UK Distributor: Lambda Photometrics Ltd, Lambda House, Batford Mill, Harpenden, Herts AL5 5BZ, UK, Tel: +44 (0)582 764334, Fax: +44 (0)582 72084;
Lasermatic Oy, Koivumäentie 14, SF-00680 Helsinki, Finland, Tel: +358 752 1433, Fax: +358 752 2878;
Photon Science Instruments, 1 Avenue Louis Delage, Z A de l'Autodrome, Linas, F- 91310 Mortlhery, France, Tel: +33 644 93487, Fax: +33 644 93489;
Lasermatic Inc, 10575 Newkirk St, Suite 740, Dallas TX 75220, USA, Tel: +1 (214) 556 2555, Fax: +1 (214) 556 1417

Surgical lasers
Combined CO$_2$ and YAG lasers
Combined CO$_2$/Nd YAG
Single Nd:YAG
Fibres and laser accessories

Laserscope
Laserscope (UK) Ltd, Raglan House, Llantarnam Park, Cwmbran, Gwent NP44 3AX, UK, Tel: +44 (0)633 838081, Fax: +44 (0)633 838161;
Laserscope, 3052 Orchard Drive, San Jose, CA 95134, USA, Tel: +1 (408) 943 0636 (or 800 356 7600 USA only), Fax: +1 (408) 943 1051

Surgical laser systems

Lederle Labs
(See Acufex)

Linvatec
Zimmer UK Ltd, Dunbeath Road, Elgin Drive, Swindon, Wilts SN2 6EA, UK, Tel: +44 (0)793 481 441, Fax: +44 (0)793 513 478;
Linvatec Europe, Zimmer International Ltd, Harrington House, Milton Road, Ickenham, Uxbridge UB10 8PU, UK, Tel: +44 (0)895 677 322, Fax: +44 (0)895 622 529;
Linvatec Corporation, 11311 Concept Blvd, Largo, FL 34643, USA, Tel: +1 (813) 392 6464/ +1 (800) 237 0169, Fax: +1 (813) 399 5256

Baggish hysteroscope, including instrumentation: sheath, scissors, forceps
Resectoscope
CDIS (Control dimension irrigation system)

Litechnica Ltd
Adamson House, Shambles Square, Manchester M3 1RE, UK, Tel: +44 (0)61 834 8432, Fax: +44 (0)61 832 1868

Surgical lasers: CO$_2$ and YAG lasers and accessories
Video systems

Luxar
Sigmacon, Heriots Wood, The Common, Stanmore, Middlesex HA7 3HT, UK, Tel: +44 (0)81 950 9501, Fax: +44 (0)81 950 9199;
Carl Zeiss, POB 1380, 7082 Oberkochon, Germany, Tel: +49 7 364 20 3514, Fax: +49 7 364 20 4346;
Luxar Corporation, 19204 North Creek Parkway. Bothell, WA 98011-8205, USA; Tel: +1 (206) 483 4142, Fax: +1 (206) 483 6844

CO$_2$ delivery system including both rigid and flexible waveguides

Marlow Surgical Technologies Inc
1810 Joseph Lloyd Parkway, Willoughby, OH 44094, USA, Tel: 800 992 5581, Fax: +1 (216) 946 1997

Martin
See Albert Waeschle Co, distributors in UK

Medical Advance Ltd
PO Box 4, Banbury, Oxon OX17 1TQ, UK, Tel: +44 (0)295 738 244/(0)978 755 840, Fax: +44 (0)295 269 188

SONOCO – ultrasonic dissector/aspirator
ASCO – inert gas coagulator and cutter (monopolar/bipolar)
ILCO – infrared light coagulator

Medical Dynamics
UK Distributor: Video South Medical Ltd, 5 Kingsmead Square, Bath, Avon BA1 2AB, UK, Tel: +44 (0)225 461 985, Fax: +44 (0)225 444 425;
99 Inverness Drive East, Englewood, Colorado 80112, USA, Tel: +1 (303) 790 2390, Fax: +1 (303) 799 1378

5990 Optical catheter system
5940 SVHS solid state surgical video camera

Micro-France
3 rue du Chateau, 03160 Bourbon L'Archambault, France, Tel: +33 70 670451, Fax: +33 70 671562

MISCOMedical
19 Station Road, Thorpe Bay, Southend on Sea, Essex SS1 3JY, UK, Tel: +44 (0)702 582764, Fax: +44 (0)702 586031;
Ranfac Corp, 30 Doherty Avenue, PO Box 635, Avon, MA, 02322–0635, USA, Tel: +1 (508) 588 4400, Fax: +1 (508) 584 8588

Laparoscopic surgical instrumentation and equipment for minimally invasive surgery

Northgate Technologies Inc
GU Manufacturing, 841 Coronation Road, Park Royal, London NW10 7QJ, UK, Tel: +44 (0)81 961 9000, Fax: +44 (0)81 963 1728;
Seda SPA, Via Tolstoi 7/B, Trezzano, Milano, Italy 20101, Tel: +39 2 445 6441, Fax: +39 2 445 6322;
Northgate Technologies Inc, 3930 Ventura Drive, Arlington Heights, Il 60004, USA, Tel: +1 (707) 506 0242, Fax: +1 (708) 506 9891

OMNIFLATOR automatic insufflator for gynaecological laparoscopy

Olympus
Olympus-Keymed, Keymed House, Stock Road, Southend on Sea, Essex SS2 5QH, UK, Tel: +44 (0)702 616333, Fax: +44 (0)702 465677;
Olympus Optical Co (Europa) GmbH, Postfach 104908, Wendenstrasse 14–16, W-2000, Hamburg 1, Germany, Tel: +49 40 237 730, Fax: +49 40 233 765;
Olympus Corporation, 4 Nevada Drive, Lake Success, NY 11042–1179, USA, Tel:1 (516) 488 3880, Fax: +1 (516) 326 9085

Full range of hysteroscopes, hystero-resectoscopes, laparoscopes, hand instrumentation and imaging systems

Pennco Medical Ltd
Heathgate, Agincourt Road, London NW3 2NT, UK, Tel: +44 (0)71 284 2824, Fax: +44 (0)71 284 2675

Colposcopes
Cryofreezers
Irrigation systems for endometrial ablation

Philips Medical Systems
Kelvin House, 63–75 Glenthorne Road, Hammersmith, London W6 0LJ, UK, Tel: +44 (0)81 741 1666, Fax: +44 (0)81 741 8716;
Philips Medical Systems, PO Box 10,000, Best DA 5680, The Netherlands, Tel: +31 430 762 734, Fax: +31 4076 2555;
Philips Medical Systems North America, 710 Bridgeport Avenue, Shelton, CT 06484, USA, Tel: +1 (203) 926 7475, Fax: +1 (203) 926 1272

Mobile X-ray imaging systems

Reznik Instruments Inc
7337 N Lawndale, Skokie, IL 60076, USA, Tel: +1 (708) 673 3444, Fax: +1 (708) 673 3447

Laparoscopes
Hysteroscopes
Related machinery and accessories

Richard Wolf (UK) Ltd
PO Box 47, Mitcham, Surrey CR4 4TT, UK, Tel: +44 (0)81 640 3054, Fax: +44 (0)81 640 9709;
Richard Wolf GmbH, Postfach 40, Knittlingen, Germany D7134, Tel: +49 (0) 7043 350, Fax: +49 (0) 7043 35300;
Richard Wolf Medical Instruments Corp, 353 Corporate Woods Parkway, Vernon Hills, IL, USA, Tel: +1 (708) 913 1113, Fax: +1 (708) 913 1488

All endoscopes and accessories

Rimmer Brothers
(See Karl Storz)

Rocket of London Ltd
Imperial Way, Watford, Herts WD2 4XX, UK, Tel: +44 (0)923 239 791, Fax: +44 (0)923 230 212

Hand instruments
Disposable instruments
Laparoscopes
Insufflators

Sigmacon UK Ltd
Heriots Wood, The Common, Stanmore, Middx HA7 3HT, UK, Tel: +44 (0)81 950 9501, Fax: +44 (0)81 950 9199

Hand instruments
CO$_2$ lasers
Laparoscopes
Videos
Light sources
Insufflators

Simpson/Basye
Henleys Medical, Headquarters Road, West Wilts Trading Estate, Westbury, Wilts BA13 4JR, UK, Tel: +44 (0)373 858 008, Fax: +44 (0)373 858 833;
Simpson Basye Inc, 430 Ayre Street, Wilmington DE 19804, USA, Tel: +1 (302) 995 7191, Fax: +1 (302) 995 1195

Hand instruments

Shanning Laser Systems
Sales office: Ashlyns Hall, Berkhamsted, Herts HP4 2ST, UK, Tel: +44 (0)442 863 301, Fax: +44 (0)442 873 743;
Units 1–2, Heol Rhoysn, Dafen Industrial Estate, Llanelli, Dyfed SA14 8LX, UK, Tel: +44 (0)554 755 444, Fax: +44 (0)554 755 333

CO$_2$ surgical lasers

Smith and Nephew Dyonics Inc
Smith and Nephew Richards Ltd, 6 The Techno Park, Newmarket Road, Cambridge CB5 8PB, UK, Tel: +44 (0)223 853 321, Fax: +44 (0)220 536 03;
160 Dascomb Road, Andover, MA 01810, USA, Tel: +1 (508) 470 2800, Fax: +1 (508) 470 2227

DYOCAM video camera system: single chip cameras, 3 chip cameras
Video laparoscope: 10 mm, 0°
                       5 mm, 0°
Laparoscope: 10 mm, 0°
                       5 mm, 0°

Solos Endoscopy Inc
4775 River Green Pkwy, Duluth, GA 30136, USA, Tel: +1 (404) 623 1000, Fax: +1 (404) 623 8944

ENDOTYER – suturing for advanced laparoscopic techniques

SPA Medical
119 Barden Road, Tonbridge, Kent TN9 1UU, UK, Tel: +44 (0)732 362 848, Fax: +44 (0)892 530 538

Hand instruments
Laparoscopes
Cameras

Stryker UK
2 Eros House, Calleva Industrial Park, Aldermaston, Reading, Berks RG7 4OW, UK, Tel: +44 (0)734 819 991, Fax: +44 (0)734 813 318;
Stryker SA, 19 Av de Belmont, 1820 Montreaux, Switzerland, Tel: +41 21 963 8701, Fax: +41 21 963 8700;
Stryker Corporation, 2725 Fairfield Road, PO Box 4085, Kalamazoo, MI 49003, USA, Tel: +1 (616) 385 2600, Fax: +1 (616) 385 1062

Complete video systems for gynaecological endoscopy

Sun Medical Inc
1179 Corporate Drive West, Suite 100, Arlington. TX 76006, USA, Tel: +1 (817) 633 1373, Fax: +1 (817) 640 1840

Sun Medical SFE-200 smoke and fluid evacuation system (a closed circuit smoke evacuator system designed specifically for laparoscopic surgery with no loss of pneumoperitoneum)

Surgilase Inc
33 Plan Way, Warwick, RI 02886, USA, Tel: +1 (401) 732 6440, Fax: +1 (401) 732 6445

CO$_2$ surgical laser with a high powered super pulse for infertility surgery

United States Surgical Corporation
(See Auto Suture Company UK)

Valleylab
Valleylab UK, Pfizer Hospital Products Group, Unit 5, Royal London Estate, 29–35 North Acton Road, London NW10 6FE, UK, Tel: +44 (0)81 961 9955, Fax: +44 (0)81 963 1310;
Valleylab Europe, Pfizer Hospital Products Group, Hoge Wei 8, B-1930 Zaventem, Belgium, Tel: +32 2 722 0375, Fax: +32 2 725 1085;
Valleylab Inc Pfizer Hospital Products Group, 5920 Longbow Drive, Boulder, CO 80301, USA, Tel: +1 (303) 530 2300, Fax: +1 (303) 530 6285

Electrosurgical generators and accessories (Diathermy)

Video South Medical Ltd
5 Kingsmead Square, Bath, Avon BA1 2AB, UK, Tel: +44 (0)225 461 985, Fax: +44 (0)225 444 425

Videos
Monitoring equipment

Walker Filtration Ltd
Spire Road, Glover East, Washington, Tyne and Wear NE37 3ES, UK, Tel: +44 (0)91 417 7816, Fax: +44 (0)91 415 3743

Laservac smoke evacuation equipment
High efficiency filtration units for removal of smoke plume and odour from laser surgery

WISAP Gesellschaft für Wissenschaftuchen Apparatebau
Rocket of London Ltd (UK Agent), Imperial Way, Watford, Herts WD2 4XX, UK, Tel: +44 (0)923 239 791, Fax: +44 (0)923 230 212;
Rudolf-Diesel Riv 20, 8209 Saverlach 6, München, Germany, +49 (8104) 1067, Fax: +49(8104) 9694;
WISAP USA, 14227 Sandy Lane, Tomball, TX 77375, USA, Tel: +1 (713) 351 2629; Fax: +1 (713) 255 6213

Laparoscopes

Zeppelin GmbH
UK Distributor: DPHMC, 7 Godstow Road, Upper Wolvercote, Oxford, OX2 8AJ, UK, Tel: +44 (0)865 510 111, Fax: +44 (0)865 514 751;
Zeppelin GmbH, Gistlstrasse 99, D-8023 Pulluch, Munich. Germany, Tel: +49 89 793 0619, Fax: +49 89 793 8545

Zeppelin surgical instruments

Zimmer
Zimmer Ltd, Dunbeath Road, Elgin Drive, Swindon, Wilts SN2 6EA, UK, Tel: +44 (0)793 481 441, Fax: +44 (0)793 486 092;
Zimmer International Ltd, Harrington House, Milton Road, Ickenham, Uxbridge UB10 8PU, UK, Tel: +44 (0)895 677 322, Fax: +44 (0)895 677 656;
Zimmer Patient Care Division, 200 West Ohio Avenue, Dover, OH 44622, USA, Tel: +1 (216) 343 8801, Fax: +1 (216) 343 0995

Zimmer CDIS (control distension irrigation system)
Dual spike disposable irrigation set
Cannula sets, 6mm, 7mm, 10mm
T adaptor

Zinnanti Surgical Instruments Inc
UK Agent: Cory Brothers Co Ltd, 4 Dollis Park, London N3 1HG, UK, Tel: +44 (0)81 349 1081, Fax: +44 (0)81 349 1962;
Zinnanti GmbH, Kuferweg 4, D-7208 Spaichingen, Germany, Tel: +49 7424 501 482, Fax: +49 7424 501 481;
Zinnanti Surgical Instruments Inc, 21540 B Prairie St, Chatsworth, CA 91311, Tel: +1 (818) 700 0090, Fax: +1 (818) 770 0575

Stainless steel instruments
ZUMI (Zinnanti uterine manipulator/injector)
ZUI-4.0 & 2.0 (Zinnanti uterine injector – 4.0 mm and 2.0 mm)
Z-sampler (endometrial suction curette)

Index

ABC *see* argon beam coagulator
abdomen
    cavity 23
    distension 22
    entry 240–1
ablation
    laser 305, 317–25
    thermal 305
    see also endometrial ablation
abscess, tubo-ovarian 154–7
absorption 288
adenocarcinoma 265
adhesiolysis 182
adhesions 342
    bowel *see* enterolysis
    cul-de-sac 226
    endometriosis 202, 203
    fatty 96
    fertility-promoting procedures 100
    formation *de novo* 245–5
    ovarian endometriomas 142
    pelvic 103, 125
    periadnexal 96–7, 101, 102, 103,
        216–17
    peritoneal endometriosis 212
    postoperative 140, 242
    prevention 38
    reformation prevention 245–9
        adjuvants 247–9
        laparoscopy versus laparotomy
            246
        laser surgery 246–7
        microsurgery 246
        second-look laparoscopy 247
        versus *de novo* adhesion
            formation 245–6
    subovarian 203
    see also intrauterine adhesions
adjuvants 247–9
adnexa 182
    cyst 128
    pain 230
    pathology, suspected 180
Allen–Master defects or windows 219
amenorrhoea 315
Amenorrhoea traumatica (aretica) 338

anaesthesia
    diagnostic laparoscopy 22
    endometrial electroablation 311
    endometrial transcervical resection
        295–6
    general 360
    local 359–60
    mass sterilization 117
    recommended doses 359
angiolysis 224–5
animal investigations 72
anovulation treatment and ovarian
        drilling 147–52
appendicectomy 187–9
aquadissection 31–2
    enterolysis 242
    tubo-ovarian abscess 156, 157
    uterine and pelvic surgery 189
argon
    beam coagulator 6, 32–3, 45–6, 63,
        65–8, 71–6
        adhesion reformation prevention
            247
        clinical use, early 73–4
        cutting modalities 97
        early animal investigation 72
        endometriosis 74, 215
        enterolysis 75, 239
        future 75–6
        hysteroscopic metroplasty 291
        laparoscopic presacral neurectomy
            74
        method of action 71–2
        modifications 72–3
        myomectomy 75
        ovarian drilling 148, 150
        ovarian endometriomas 145, 146
        techniques 73
        tissue effects 64
        uterine nerve ablation 162
    contact and non-contact 66
    fluoride (ArF) 383
    pumped dye laser 391
artery, umbilical 25
Asherman's syndrome *see* intrauterine
        adhesions

aspirating cannula 257, 258
atrophy 151

back focal length (BFL) 40–1, 44
backstops 42
beam misalignment and back focal
        length, long 41
BFL *see* back focal length
bilateral ovarian wedge resection
        (BOWR) 147, 148, 152
biopsy forceps 257
bipolar versus monopolar high
        frequency surgery 62–3
bladder 233
    lesions 217
    peritoneum 183, 203
bleeding
    post-surgical 308
    profuse 26
    uterine 263–5, 310–11, 360, 365
    vaginal 315
blend (1,2 and 3) 53–4
bowel 225–7
    adhesions *see* enterolysis
    injury 38–9, 347
    preparation 221
BOWR *see* bilateral ovarian wedge
        resection
bulldog clamps 30–1
Burch colposuspension 189–90

CA 125 135, 136
caesarean section, previous 180
camera
    guided surgery 47–8
    see also photography; video
cancer 125–6, 264
    see also adenocarcinoma; neoplasm;
        tumours
capacitive coupling 58
carbon dioxide
    distension 4, 269–70, 282–4
    endometrial ablation 323
    hysteroscopy 79
    insufflation 16, 81, 250–1
        diagnostic hysteroscopy 270

carbon dioxide (*cont.*)
  insufflation (*cont.*)
    diagnostic laparoscopy 23
    fertility-promoting procedures 99
    high flow 29
    laser 15, 18, 40–5, 63–5, 77, 84
      adhesion reformation prevention 247
      advanced endometriosis 231, 232, 233
      back focal length 40–1
      cutting modalities 97
      ectopic pregnancy 106, 107
      endometriosis 86, 215, 216, 219
      enterolysis 239, 243
      fibres, flexible hollow wave guides and rigid probes 43–5
      incision 65
      mechanical and optical backstops 42
      myomectomy 331
      neosalpingostomy and fimbrioplasty 92–3
      ovarian drilling 148, 149, 150, 152
      ovarian endometriomas 145
      power density 41–2, 43
      pregnancy rates, cumulative 87
      reflection 44
      salpingostomy 103
      smoke evacuation 42–3
      suction-irrigation probes 45
      tissue effects 64
      uterine nerve ablation 161, 163, 165, 166
    operative hysteroscopy 356
    pneumoperitoneum 187
cardiorespiratory disease 360
care, postoperative
  diagnostic laparoscopy 26–7
  laparoscopic assisted vaginal hysterectomy (LAVH) 184
  tubo-ovarian abscess 156–7
cart, biomedical 17, 19
catheter, coaxial 351
cautery
  bipolar 16
  ovarian 149–50
  videolaparoscopic ovarian 151
  see also electrocautery
cell fusion 384–5
cellular laser microsurgery 379–80
cellulo lymphatic flap 173–4
cervix
  dilation 311–12, 355–6
  see also transcervix
channel sheath, isolated 256
char build-up 312
chimney system 78
Chlamydia spp 247, 349
Chlamydia trachomatis 91, 154, 155
chocolate cyst *see* endometrial cyst
choledochoduodenoscope 278
circulating nurse 12–13
circumferential Nd:YAG endometrial destruction 372–7
  experimental work 374–6
  hyperthermia 373
  interstitial laser hyperthermia 373–4
clamps, bulldog 30–1
Clarke Knot-Pusher 33, 34
CO_2 *see* carbon dioxide
coagulation 62
  bipolar 232
  current 32
  effects 313
  mode 63, 97

versus vaporization 67, 68
  see also electrocoagulation; endocoagulation; photocoagulation
colon 218–19, 231
colourflow 129–30
colposuspension 189–90
colpotomy
  anterior and posterior 184
  incision 36
combo laser units 49
complications
  diagnostic laparoscopy 21
  endometrial electroablation 308, 309–11
  endometrial laser ablation 321, 322–4
  endometrial transcervical resection 300–5
  endometriosis, advanced 236
  enterolysis 242
  intraoperative 175–6
  laparoscopic ovarian surgery and ovarian torsion 140
  laparoscopy 21
  local anaesthesia 359–60
  mass sterilization 119
  non-laser resection endometriosis 227
  operative hysteroscopy 355–6
  pelvic lymphadenectomy 174–5, 176–7
  postoperative 176
  radiofrequency endometrial ablation (RaFEA) 370–1
  transcervical resection 300–5
  uterine nerve ablation 163
computed tomography (CT) 28, 130
  laparoscopic assisted vaginal hysterectomy 179
  pelvic lymphadenectomy 174
  tubo-ovarian abscess 154, 155
conception, assisted 198
consent *see* patient
contact
  argon 66
  hysteroscopy 268
  laser surgery 46
  Nd:YAG 66–9
  quality monitors 56
continence 189
continuous
  flow (CF) 264, 269, 286
  variable defocus (CVD) 41
  wave (CW) 43, 53, 380
contraception 197
  see also intrauterine contraceptive device
contraindications
  diagnostic laparoscopy 21–2
  ectopic pregnancy 107–8
  general anaesthesia 360
Corson needle 150, 151
counselling *see* patient
crescent shape spot 42
cul-de-sac 234
  adhesions 226
  disease 218
  method 118
culdotomy 36
curettage 312
  see also dilatation and curettage
current 32
  electrical 313, 331–2
  monopolar 16
cutting

current 32
electrodes 61
electrosurgery 52, 53
modalities 97
speed 61
cyclical pain 304, 370
cystectomy, ovarian 138–9
cystic lesion 127
cystoscopy 137
  ovarian 143–4
cysts
  adnexal 128
  benign 131, 136
  blood-filled 124, 127, 131
  dermoid 128–9
  echo free 124
  endometrial 143
  functional 136
  haemorrhagic corpus luteum 144
  lining 137, 139
  malignant 131
  ovarian 126, 127–9, 136, 139
  peripheral 126
  simple 128, 130–1, 135
  trilocular 128
  unilocular 127–8, 136
  wall 138

D and C *see* dilatation and curettage
danazol 297
de novo adhesion formation 245–6
delivery systems *see* laser laparoscopy delivery systems
dermoid cyst 128–9
desiccation 52, 54–5
  bipolar 32, 55
devascularization 368
development 3–6
dextran 70 283, 284, 356
dextran-induced anaphylactic reaction (DIAR) 357
dextrose 283, 339
diagnosis
  endometriosis 200–5
  intrauterine adhesions 339
  laparoscopy 201
  tubo-ovarian abscess (laparoscopic treatment) 154
diagnostic
  hysteroscopy 3–4, 263–76
    documentation 270–7
    indications 263–7
    instrumentation 267–9
    intrauterine procedures, minor 270
    method 270
    techniques 269
  laparoscopy 5, 21–7
    anaesthesia considerations 22
    carbon dioxide insufflation 23
    closure 26
    complications and consenting the patient 21
    contraindications 21–2
    initial inspection 24–5
    patient preparation and positioning 22–3
    postoperative care 26–7
    second operative trocar insertion 25–6
    suprapubic probe insertion 25
    trocar introduction and profuse bleeding 26
    umbilical trocar insertion and laparoscope 24
  ovarian 224

sheath 256
diathermy 149–50
see also electrodiathermy
dilatation and curettage (D & C) 235, 263, 264, 265, 320
dilation
  cervix 311–12, 355–6
  rectal 235
dissection see aquadissection; hydrodissection
distension media 79, 269–70, 356–7
  and fluid systems 282–9
    carbon dioxide 4, 269–70, 282–4
    dextrose in water (5%) 283
    fluid absorption 286–9
    fluid instillation 285–6
    glycine (1.5%) 283–4
    high-viscosity fluids 283
    Hyskon 269–70
    hysteroscopes 284–6
    low-viscosity fluids 283
    sodium chloride (0.9%) 284
    sorbitol 284
  hazards 356
  hysteroscopy 279
  uterine 318
Donnez backstop 42, 43
Doppler machine 129–30, 131
Doyle's procedure 160–1, 164
dynamic phase 312, 313
dysfunctional uterine bleeding (DUB) 365
dysmenorrhoea, endometrial electroablation 159–67, 267, 308

ectopic pregnancy 105–11
  fertility 108–10
  isthmic 108
  operative results, indications and contraindications 107–8
  techniques 105–7
  treatment 106–7, 109, 110
  tubal occlusion 347
EEA see end-to-end anastomotic dilator
electricity
  current 331–2
    endometrial electroablation 313
  energy and tissue temperature 51–2
  energy transmission 332
  loops 257
  needles 257
electroablation, endometrial 307–16
electrocautery 196
  hazards 358–9
  ovarian 149
electrocoagulation
  endometriosis 221
  mass sterilization 114
  pregnancy rates 87
  roller-ball 305, 315
electrodes 61, 312
electrodiathermy 60–3, 162–3
electrogenerator 82
electroresection, fibroids 327–30
electrosurgery 32, 51–9
  accidents 310
  blend (1,2 and 3) 53–4
  cut 52, 53
  desiccation 52, 54–5
  electrical energy and tissue temperature 51–2
  fulgurate 52, 54
  generator 14–15, 18, 75
  inherent risks 55–6
  instruments 97

laparoscopic issues 56–9
  and laser 84–8
  outputs, isolated 56
  temperature and tissue 51
  tower 52
embolism 303–4
en bloc resection 226
end-to-end anastomotic (EEA) dilator 235
endo-irrigation unit 78
endo-ovarian laser surgery 144–6
endocoagulation 84, 162–3
endometrial
  ablation 81, 280
    carbon dioxide 323
    clinical results 322
    complications 323
    fluid absorption 286
    infusion systems 284
    operative details 322, 324
    published results 323
    radiofrequency 365–71
    techniques 305
    tissue effects 319
    see also radiofrequency endometrial ablation
  adenocarcinoma 265
  cancer 264
  cyst 143
  destruction 390–1
    circumferential Nd:YAG 372–7
  electroablation 307–16
    complications 308
    electrical current 313
    operative technique 311–15
    patient counselling 308–11
    patient selection 307–8
    results 315–16
    suppression 311
  Nd:YAG laser ablation 317–25
  photodynamic therapy 391
  polyp 264
  resected 295, 297
  transcervical resection 294–305
    ablation techniques comparison 305
    anaesthesia 295–6
    complications 300–5
    fluid balance 297
    long-term outcome 300
    menstruation 298–9
    operating time 297
    operative procedures, concurrent 297
    preoperative recovery 297–8
    resected endometrium examination 297
    resectoscopic surgery in uterus 294–5
    surgery 296–7
    technique 295
    treatment criteria 296
    uterine cavity 299–300
endometrioma 142, 143
  see also ovarian endometriomas
endometriosis 144, 192–8, 201
  adhesions 202, 203
  advanced 229–37
    bladder and ureteral involvement 233
    complications 236
    deep infiltration 231–3
    equipment 229
    laparotomy 236
    ovarian endometriomas 229–31
    rectosigmoid infiltration 233–6

atypical 24
diagnosis 200–5
  anatomical distribution 201–2
  laparoscopic appearance 202–5
disease identification 222
excision 216, 217
fibrotic 203, 205
instrumentation 221–2
invasive 204
laparoscopic
  assisted vaginal hysterectomy (LAVH) 180–1
  pathology 194–5
  treatment 74
in laparoscopy scar, previous 26
large bowel 225–7
laser and electrosurgery 86–7
laser vaporization 215–19
lesions 194, 195, 202, 204, 211–12
microscopic 194–5
no treatment 87
non-laser resection 220–8
  advantages 220–1
  bowel preparation 221
  complications 227
  patient outcome 227–8
  techniques 222–7
non-pigmented and microscopic 194–5
ovarian surgery 125
pathogenesis and predisposition 192–4
patient positioning 221
peritoneal 207–13, 223
powderburn 204
residual vaporization 217
severity classification 196
staging 195
treatment 195–8
  endometriotic tissue 196–7
  ovarian support withdrawal 197
  photodynamic therapy 389–90
  symptomatic approaches 197–8
endometrium: transcervical resection, symptoms recurrence 304
endoscopic surgery instrumentation 13–17, 278–9
endosurgery, intrauterine 267
endovaginal scanner 123
enterolysis 75, 238–43
  abdominal entry 240–1
  aquadissection 242
  armamentarium available 238–9
  complications 242
  future 243
  history 238
  laparoscopic 75, 238–43
  method 241–2
  operating room preparation 240
  patient evaluation and selection 239–40
  postsurgical adhesions 242
  preoperative preparation 240
  results 243
environmental influences and endometriosis 192–3
enzyme wash 260
epigastric vessels, inferior 25
equipment
  endometriosis, advanced 229
  hysteroscopic tubal occlusion 346
  laparoscopic ovarian surgery 123–5, 138
  laparoscopic techniques, new 29–30
  mass sterilization 116
  operative hysteroscopy 19

equipment (*cont.*)
  radiofrequency endometrial ablation
    (RaFEA) 366–7
  summary 16–17
  tubo-ovarian abscess 156
  see also video equipment
ESU 54, 55, 56, 58
excision 197, 216, 217
excrescences 212

fallopian tube 90–1
fertility 108–10, 335
  promoting procedures *see* non-laser
fertilization
  polyspermic 384
  see also in vitro fertilization
fibre
  bare 66, 68
  flexible 48
  guides 46
  laser 43–5, 66, 162
  quartz 318, 319
  tip, modified 374
fibreoptics
  hysteroscope, flexible 268
  laser 261
  light cable 254–5
fibroids 36, 280
  electroresection 327–30
  intramural 333
  submucosal 264, 266, 333–5
  subserous 127
  uterine 75
fibrosis 204
fimbrioplasty 92, 94, 101, 103
  see also laser neosalpingostomy and
    fimbrioplasty
finger laparoscopy 241
fluid
  absorption 286–9, 297
  balance 297
  delivery methods 339
  flow actuator system 350
  high-viscosity 283, 356–7
  instillation 285–6
  low-viscosity 283, 357
  overload 302, 309–10
focus depth 40, 41
focus length *see* back focal length
forceps 16, 150, 257, 258
fulgurate 52, 54

gas embolism 303–4
generator 14–15, 18, 75, 255
glycine 309
  1.5% 283–4, 303, 329, 332, 357
  tagged 302
GnRH *see* gonadotrophin releasing
  hormone
gonadotrophin-releasing hormone
  (GnRH)
    4, 210–11, 332
  endometrial ablation 320
  endometriosis 197, 216
  fibroid electroresection 328
  myomectomy 171, 332, 334, 335, 336
  ovarian drilling 148

haematometra 304
haematoporphyrin derivative (HPD)
  387, 388, 390, 391
haemorrhage 144, 302–3, 373
haemostasis 105, 232
Hamou Hysteromat 285, 318, 329
hCG 107, 108

helium-neon (He-Ne) laser 63, 319
HF *see* high frequency
hiatus hernia 22
high-frequency
  interference 275
  surgery 61, 62–3
high-viscosity fluids 283, 356–7
history of endoscopy 3–6
hollow wave guides, flexible 43–5
Hopkins' laparoscope 201
hormones
  independence 210
  therapy evaluation 332
HSG *see* hysterosalpingography
hydrodissection 216, 217, 232
hydrosalpinx 91, 127
hydrostatic pressure 285
hyperthermia 373–4
hypomenorrhoea 315
hyponatraemia 373
Hyskon 258–9, 269–70, 309, 356
hysterectomy 198, 301, 324
  vaginal 179–86
hysterographic-hysteroscopic
  classification 342–3
hysterosalpingography (HSG) 91, 98,
  262, 265, 266, 319, 342
  intrauterine adhesions 340, 341
hysteroscopes
  continuous flow (CF) 269
  distension media and fluid systems
    284–6
  flexible 268, 277–81
  operative 279–80
  rigid 268–9, 277–81
  set 270
  single flow (SF) 268–9
  uterus 278
  Weck-Baggish 285, 287, 318
hysteroscopy 3–5
  contact 268
  diagnostic 263–76
  distension media 279
  dual image video 20
  endometrial ablation 198
  instrumentation 254–60, 332
    fibreoptic light cable 254–5
    Hyskon pump 258–9
    light generator 255
    medium instillation 258
    nipples and plugs for operating
      channel 258
    operating accessories 257–8
    pumps 259, 260
    sheaths 255–7
    telescopes 254
    video equipment 259–60
  insufflation and smoke evacuation
    79–80
  laparoscopic techniques, new 30–1
  laser types 77
  Luer-lock plugs 259
  lysis 343
  metroplasty 291–3
  myomectomy 331–6
  needles 257, 258
  operator position 278
  panoramic 268–9
  programme 253–62
    data documentation 261–2
    instrumentation 254–60
    office hysteroscopy 260–1
    special instruments 261
  rigid and flexible optical systems
    277–81
  surgery 253–360

tubal occlusion 345–54
  equipment 346
  Ovabloc system 349–54
  techniques 346–8
  uterine tubal ostia 345–6
two-step operative 334
see also hysteroscope; operative
  hysteroscopy

iliac vein, external 173
imaging 47–8
  chain 271, 272
in vitro fertilization 48, 103, 198, 383,
  384
incision 31
  carbon dioxide laser 65
  colpotomy 36
  endometriosis 224
  high frequency current 61
  instruments 60
  peritoneal 173, 223
incontinence 189
infection 304, 360
infertility 265–7, 280–1
infiltration, deep 231–3
infundibulopelvic ligament 232
infusion systems 284
initiation phase 312, 313
injection tube 258
instillates 247, 248, 258
instrumentation 13–17, 257–8
  basic 16
  diagnostic hysteroscopy 267–9
  electrosurgery 97
  endometriosis 221–2
  endoscopic surgery 12–13
  hysteroscopy 254–60, 261
  incision 60
  individual operating 16
  injuries 357–9
  laser neosalpingostomy and
    fimbrioplasty 92–3
  non-laser fertility-promoting
    procedures 97–8
  table 17, 18
insufflation 77–9
  and smoke evacuation 77–82
    hysteroscopy 79–80
    laparoscopy 77–9
    new developments 81–2
  see also carbon dioxide
intercostal space 31
interstitial
  laser hyperthermia 373–4
  pregnancy 107
intratubal devices 348
intrauterine
  adhesions 265, 266, 267, 338–44
    classification 342–3
    diagnosis 339
    ESH classification 266, 267
    hysteroscopic lysis 343
    pathophysiology 338
    symptomatology 338
    treatment 339–42
  contraceptive device, missing 267
  device 292, 321
  endosurgery 267
  manipulations, complicated 267
  pregnancy (IUP) 108, 110
  procedures, minor 270
intravasation 309–10
irrigation 16
  probes *see* suction-irrigation
  see also endo-irrigation
IUA *see* intrauterine adhesions

IUCD *see* intrauterine contraceptive device

knot
  placement 37
  pushing 33, 34
  tying 190
Krukenberg tumours 129
KTP laser 6, 15, 19, 45–6, 65–6
  adhesion reformation prevention 247
  cutting modalities 97
  endometriosis 215
  enterolysis 239, 241, 242
  hysteroscopic metroplasty 291
  microsurgery 379
  myomectomy 331
  operative hysteroscopy 358
  ovarian drilling 148, 150, 151, 152
  ovarian endometriomas 145, 146
  photodynamic therapy 390
  uterine nerve ablation 162, 163, 165

laparoscopy 5–6, 24, 201
  appearance 202–5
  appendicectomy 187–9
  argon beam coagulator 74
  assisted vaginal hysterectomy (LAVH) 179–86
  cart 17, 18
  delivery systems 40–9
  diagnosis 201
  dual image video 20
  enterolysis 75, 238–43
  fimbrioplasty 94
  finger 241
  insufflation and smoke evacuation 77–9
  issues 56–9
  laser types 77
  myomectomy 75, 169–71
  operating room 14, 17–19, 49
  operative 5–6, 14
  ovarian surgery 123–31, 134–41
    colourflow and duplex Doppler 129–30
    complications 140
    computerized tomography 130
    cyst lining destruction 139
    cystectomy 138–9
    equipment 123–5, 138
    general principles 137–8
    magnetic resonance imaging 130
    mass 126–9
    neoplasm assessment 136–7
    oncological considerations 134–5
    oophorectomy 139–40
    ovary, normal 126
    pelvic mass management 130–1
    pre-laparoscopic assessment 135–6
    technique 123–5
    ultrasound 125–6
  pathology 194–5
  pelvic lymphadenectomy 172–8
  portals position 187, 188
  presacral neurectomy 74
  salpingectomy 106
  salpingo-ovariolysis 85
  sterilization 116, 119
  surgery 11–249
    dual image video 20
    instrumentation 13–17
    operating room design 14, 17–19, 49
    operative hysteroscopy 19–20

overall concept 11–12
setting up a service 11–20
techniques 12–13, 28–39
  equipment 29–30
  hysteroscopy 30–1
  incisions 31
  operative techniques 31–9
  patient positioning 30
  preoperative preparation 28–9
  scrubbing 30
  video equipment positioning 30
treatment
  conservative 105–6
  ectopic pregnancy 106–7, 109, 110
  endometriosis, advanced 229–37
  with methotrexate 106
  ovarian torsion 140
  polycystic ovarian syndrome 87–8
  tubo-ovarian abscess 154–7
uterine nerve ablation (LUNA) 87, 159–67
uterine and pelvic surgery 187–91
versus laparotomy 246
see also diagnostic laparoscopy; laser laparoscopy; second-look laparoscopy
laparotomy
  ectopic pregnancy 109
  endometriosis, advanced 236
  versus laparoscopy 246
laser 15, 33, 63–9
  ablation 305, 317–25
  beam intracellular application 382
  channel 42
  and electrosurgery 84–8
  fibreoptic 261
  flexible fibre 162
  hazards 358–9
  hyperthermia, interstitial 373–4
  and laparoscopic treatment of ectopic pregnancy 106–7
  laparoscopy delivery systems 40–9
  microsurgery 379–85
    beam intracellular application 382
    cell fusion 384–5
    optical trap 380–2
    pelvic organ laser surgery to cellular laser microsurgery 379–80
    polyspermic fertilization 384
    zona drilling (LZD) 382–4
  neosalpingostomy and fimbrioplasty 90–4
  non-laser fertility-promoting procedures 97
  ovarian drilling 150–1
  pregnancy rates 87
  surgery
    adhesion reformation prevention 246–7
    contact and non-contact 46
    endo-ovarian 144–6
    pelvic organ 379–80
  systems 64
  techniques 66–9
  units 49
  uterine nerve ablation (LUNA) 161–4
  vaporization 196, 215–19, 221
  zona drilling (LZD) 382–4
  see also argon beam coagulator; carbon-dioxide laser; endo-ovarian laser surgery; KTP; Nd:YAG
LAVH *see* laparoscopic assisted vaginal hysterectomy

lens 255
lesions
  advanced endometriosis 233, 234
  bladder 217
  cystic 127
  endometriosis 194, 195, 202, 204
  overlapping 375–6
  peritoneal endometriosis 208, 211, 212
  red flame-like 208, 212
  single 374–5
  subtle 209, 211–12
  typical 207
LHRH agonists 297
ligament 197, 230, 231, 232
  uterosacral 184, 222–3, 325
light
  cable 254–5
  generator 255
  mass sterilization 117
  scalpel 42
  source 14, 19–20, 271–2
liquid
  distension media 79, 356–7
  pumps 259
loops 257
low-viscosity
  fluids 283, 339, 357
  liquid pumps 259
LUNA *see* laparoscopy, uterine nerve ablation; laser uterine nerve ablation
lymph nodes, missing 176
lymphadenectomy, pelvic 172–8
lysis, hysteroscopic 343
LZD *see* laser zona drilling

magnetic resonance imaging (MRI) 28, 130, 154
malignancy
  cyst 131
  occult cervical 360
  uterine 304–5
manipulators, uterine 29
mannitol sorbitol 357
MAP *see* mean arterial blood pressure
mass sterilization 113–21
  adverse factors 121
  anaesthesia 117
  camp 114–17
  complications 119
  economic considerations 121
  failure 120–1
  follow-up 120
  method, choice of 113–14
  mortality 119–20
  pneumoperitoneum 117–18
  postoperative 118, 119
  procedure 118
  reversal 121
  tubal occlusion 114
MBL *see* menstrual blood loss
mean arterial blood pressure (MAP) 287–8
medical
  team 115
  therapy and endometriosis 220
Menostat radiofrequency endometrial ablation unit 367
menstruation 298–9
  endometrial electroablation 308
  endometriosis 192, 193
  menstrual blood loss (MBL) 301, 370
  retrograde 193
  transcervical resection 298–9, 300, 301

methotrexate 106, 107
metroplasty 291–3
microbeam facility 385
microsurgery 246, 379
    see also laser microsurgery
mini-laparotomy 113
minilight 117
monopolar
    current 16
    scissors 224
    versus bipolar high frequency
        surgery 62–3
morbidity, potential 175–7
mortality 119–20
multi-channel operating sheath 257
muscularis 236
myoma 328
    intramural 82
    screw 257
    submucous 82
    surgical procedures 336
    uterine 180
myomectomy
    hysteroscopic 331–6
    laparoscopic 75, 169–71
myometrial reticulated structures 328

Nd:YAG laser 6, 15, 19, 45–6, 63, 65
    adhesion reformation prevention
        247
    contact 66–9
    cutting modalities 97
    diagnostic hysteroscopy 268
    distension media 283
    ectopic pregnancy 106, 107
    endometrial ablation 317–25
        clinical experience
            United Kingdom 321–4
            USA 319–21
        photocoagulation 317–19
    endometrial destruction,
        circumferential 372–7
    endometriosis 86
    enterolysis 239
    fibroid electroresection 328
    hysteroscopy 279, 280, 281
        metroplasty 291, 292
        myomectomy 331–6
            electrical current 331–2
            hysteroscopic equipment 332
            preoperative therapy 332
            techniques 333–5
            tissue effects 331
        programme 261
    infusion systems 284, 285
    insufflation and smoke evacuation
        90
    microsurgery 379, 380, 383, 384
    non-contact 66–9
    operative hysteroscopy 358
    ovarian drilling 148
    ovarian endometriomas 145
    photodynamic therapy 390
    tissue effects 64
    tubal occlusion 347
    uterine nerve ablation 162, 163
needle
    Corson 150, 151
    electrical 257
    hysteroscopic 257, 258
    needle-holder 35
    Veress 21, 23, 24
Neisseria gonorrhoea 91, 154, 155
neodymium yttrium-aluminium-
    garnet see Nd:YAG
neoplasm, ovarian 134, 136–7

neosalpingostomy 92–3
    see also laser neosalpingostomy
nerve injury 176
neurectomy, presacral 74
nipples for operating channel 257–8
non-laser fertility-promoting
        procedures 96–103
    instruments 97–8
    investigation 98
    periadnexal adhesive disease 96–7
    results 102–3
    surgical technique 98–102
        fimbrioplasty 101
        general principles 98–9
        salpingo-ovariolysis 99–101
        salpingostomy
            (neosalpingostomy) 101–2
non-laser resection 220–8
non-thermal effects on tissue 45

obturator
    muscle 173
    tip 352
occlusion 103
    tubal 113, 114, 116, 345–54
occult cervical malignancy 360
office hysteroscopy 260–1
oophorectomy 139–40
operating
    instruments 16, 257–8
    room 11, 12
        endometrial electroablation 311
        enterolysis 240
        laparoscopy 14, 17–19, 49
        table 29
        team 13, 19
        technique 92–3
operation
    advanced endometriosis 230
    endometrial electroablation 314–15
operative
    hysteroscopy 4–5, 19–20, 279–80,
        329, 355–60
        anaesthesia 359–60
        carbon dioxide complications 356
        classification 355
        complications 355–9
        equipment 19
        light source 19–20
        liquid distension media
            complications 356–7
        operating room team 19
    laparoscopy 5–6, 14
    procedure
        endometrium: transcervical
            resection 297
        uterine nerve ablation for
            intractable dysmenorrhoea
            161–4
    results 107–8
    techniques
        adhesion prevention 38
        aquadissection 31–2
        argon beam coagulation 32–3
        bowel injury 38–9
        Burch colposuspension 189–90
        culdotomy 36
        electrosurgery 32
        hysteroscopic metroplasty 291–3
        laparoscopic appendicectomy
            187–9
        laparoscopic techniques, new 31–9
        laser 33
        scissors that cut 32
        staples 34–5
        suturing 33–4

tissue removal 36–7
    underwater surgery at close of
        surgery 37
optical systems 277–81
    backstops 42
    endometrial ablation 280
    fibroids 280
    flexible endoscopes 278–9
    infertility 280–1
    operative hysteroscope 279–80
    results 279
    trap 380–2
OR see operating room
orogastric tube 30
ostium, tubal 318
    outflow channel 288
Ovabloc system 349–54
ovarian drilling see ovary
ovary 85, 99–101, 102, 126, 232
    atrophy 151
    cancer 125–6
    cautery 149–50, 151
    cyst 126, 127–9, 136, 139
    cystectomy 138–9
    cystoscopy 143–4
    drilling and anovulation treatment
        87–8, 147–52
        dangers 151–2
        hormonal changes 148–9
        mechanism of action 148
        methodology 149–51
    electrocautery and unipolar
        diathermy 149
    endometriomas 142–4, 151, 152, 225,
        229–31
    endometriosis 224
    malignancy 135
    mass 126–9, 135–6
    neoplasm 136–7
    polycystic 87–8, 151, 152
    support withdrawal 197
    surgery see laparoscopy, ovarian
    suture 138, 139
    syndrome 87–8
    torsion 140
    tumour 129, 130, 134
    wedge resection 147, 148, 152
    see also endo-ovarian

PAA see plasminogen activator
        activity
pain
    adnexal 230
    cyclical 304, 370
    pelvis 74, 125, 180, 204, 308–9
paramedical staff 115
paravesical space 173
pathology, macroscopic 194
patient
    consent 21, 160–1
    counselling, endometrial
        electroablation 160, 308–11
    evaluation 239–40
    management, perioperative 227
    outcome 227–8
    positioning
        diagnostic laparoscopy 22–3
        endometrial electroablation 311
        endometriosis 221
        laparoscopic techniques, new 30
        preparation 22–3
    selection
        endometrial electroablation 307–8
        enterolysis 239–40
        radiofrequency endometrial
            ablation (RaFEA) 367

pelvis
  adhesions 103, 125
  imaging 134
  inflammatory disease (PID) 96, 181
  lymphadenectomy 172–8
    complications 174–7
    indications 177
    morbidity, potential 175–7
    results 174
    surgical technique 172–4
  mass 125, 130–1, 181
  organ laser surgery 379–80
  pain 180, 204
    endometrial electroablation 308–9
    midline 74
    ultrasound 125
  postoperative 185
  preoperative 182
  surgery 49, 180, 187–91, 380
  uterine nerve ablation 160–1
perforation
  operative hysteroscopy 357
  uterine 301–2, 310, 373
peritoneum 216–17
  bladder 183, 203
  defects 204
  endometriosis 207–13, 223
    different appearances 208
    histological study 209–10
    hormonal independence 210
    hypothesis 212–13
    lesions 207, 209, 211–12
    subtle appearance 207–9
    three-dimensional (3–D)
      architecture 212–13
    two-dimensional (2–D) evaluation
      210–11
    typical 209
    unsuspected 209–10
  incision 173, 223
  resection 222
  toilet 106
  see also pneumoperitoneum
phimosis 101
photocoagulation 317–19
photodynamic therapy 387–91
  endometriosis treatment 389–90
  endometrium destruction 390–1
  principles 387–9
photography 271, 272–3
plasma sodium concentration 303
plasminogen activator activity (PAA)
  245, 246, 247
plugs 257–8, 259, 353
pneumoperitoneum 117–18, 187
pneumothorax, spontaneous 315
polyp, endometrial 264
postsurgical see postoperative
potassium-titanyl-phosphate see KTP
powderburn endometriosis 204
power
  attenuation during laparoscopic
    laser surgery 43
  density 41–2, 52
  formula 52
  settings 312–14
pre-laparoscopic assessment 135–6
pregnancy
  endometrial electroablation 311
  endometrium: transcervical
    resection 304
  interstitial 107
  intrauterine 108, 110, 267
  operative hysteroscopy 360
  rates, cumulative 87
  salpingostomy 103

see also pseudopregnancy; ectopic
  pregnancy
premenstrual syndrome 309
preoperative
  evaluation
    laparoscopic techniques, new 28
    laser neosalpingostomy and
      fimbrioplasty 91–2
    tubo-ovarian abscess 155
    pelvis 182
  preparation
    enterolysis 240
    laparoscopic techniques, new
      28–9
    operative hysteroscopy 358
  recovery 297–8
  therapy with GnRH agonist 332
pressure cuff 285
probe
  argon beam coagulator 72
  blunt 224, 232
  rectal 29, 218, 235
  rigid 43–5
  suction-irrigation 45, 241, 242
  suprapubic 25
  thermal 366, 368
  vaginal 29, 218
progestogens 197
pronucleus 384
pseudopregnancy 197
pubic bone 173
pulsatility index (PI) 129, 130
pump 258–9, 260, 285

quality monitors 56

radiofrequency endometrial ablation
  (RaFEA) 365–71
  complications 370–1
  equipment 366–7
  experimental studies 367
  future development 371
  patient selection 367
  physical principle 365–6
  results 369–70
  treatment technique 368–9
radiofrequency generating apparatus
  366
radiofrequency-induced thermal
  ablation (RITEA) 305
RaFEA see radiofrequency
  endometrial ablation
rectosigmoid infiltration 233–6
rectum
  dilator 235
  probe 29, 218, 235
reproduction output 85, 86
resection
  endometrium 295, 297
  non-laser 220–8
  peritoneum 222
  transcervical 294–305
resectoscope 261
  fibroid electroresection 328
  operative hysteroscopy 358
  surgery see underwater
  uterine 284
resistance index (RI) 129, 130
roller-ball electrocoagulation (RBE)
  305, 315

salpingectomy 106
salpingitis 96
salpingo-oophorectomy 139
salpingo-ovariolysis 85, 99–101, 102

salpingostomy 85–6, 94, 101–2, 103,
  105
sapphire tips 47, 66, 68, 323
scalpel 42
scanner 123, 124
scissors 16, 32, 232
  hysteroscopy 257
  monopolar 224
  non-laser fertility-promoting
    procedures 97
  semi-rigid 258, 341
scoring system
  therapeutic 110, 111
  tubal 92
scrub nurse 12, 13
scrubbing 30
second look laparoscopy (SLL) 245,
  246, 247
Semm's forceps 150
septae 280–1
service, setting up of 11–20
sheaths 255–7
single
  cell manipulation 379–85
  flow (SF) hysteroscopes 268–9
SLL see second look laparoscopy
smoke evacuation 15, 42–3, 78–9
  see also insufflation
sodium 303
  chloride (0.9%) 284
  hyaluronate 242
sonography see pelvic imaging
sorbitol 284, 309, 357
sperm micromanipulation 380–2
spotting 315
Staphylococcus aureus 23
staples 34–6
star burst effect 215
sterilization see mass sterilization
stripping technique 230
suction 16
suction-irrigation probe 45, 241, 242
superpulse 233
surgery 296–7
  assistant 13
  high frequency 61, 62–3
  hysteroscopic 253–360
  laparoscopic 11–249
  modalities 84–5
  pelvis 49, 180, 187–91, 380
  procedure
    myomas 336
    Nd:YAG laser ablation of
      endometrium 317–19
    non-laser fertility-promoting
      98–102
  surgeon 13
  see also laser surgery; microsurgery;
    electrosurgery
suturing 33–4, 36, 190
  intracorporeal 236
  ovary 138, 139
synechiae 280–1, 320
syringes 285, 350

table see operating table
TCRE see transcervix, resection of
  endometrium
technician, biomedical 12, 13
techniques
  argon beam coagulator 73
  bladder lesions 217
  colon 218–19
  cul-de-sac disease 218
  diagnostic hysteroscopy 269
  ectopic pregnancy 105–7

techniques (*cont.*)
  endometrium: transcervical resection 295
  fibroids electroresection 328–9
  hysteroscopic tubal occlusion 346–8
  laparoscopic assisted vaginal hysterectomy (LAVH) 181–4
  laparoscopic ovarian surgery 123–5
  laparoscopic surgery 12–13, 28–39
  large bowel endometriosis 225–7
  laser 66–9
  myomectomy by laparoscopy 169
  Nd:YAG laser hysteroscopic myomectomy 333–5
  non-laser resection 227
  ovarian endometriosis 224
  peritoneal resection 222
  peritoneum and soft tissue 216–17
  tubo-ovarian abscess 156–7
  ureter and uterine vessels 217–18
  ureterolysis and angiolysis 224–5
  uterosacral ligament resection 222–3
  see also operative techniques
telangiectases 166
telescope 15–16, 19, 254, 272
temperature 51, 60, 368
thecomas 129
therapeutic scoring system 110, 111
three-dimensional (3–D) architecture 212–13
tips 352, 353
tissue
  effects 60
    endometrial ablation 319
    high frequency surgery 62, 63
    lasers 64
    Nd:YAG laser 65, 331
  electrosurgery 51
  removal 36–7
  soft 216–17
  temperature and electrical energy 51–2
  thermal and non-thermal effects 45
torsion, ovarian 140
transabdominal scanner 123, 124
transcervix
  resection of endometrium 294–305
  tubal occlusion 346–8
transducer 123, 125, 126
transurethral resection (TUR) syndrome 302
transvaginal ultrasound 123–4, 125, 126, 127, 129, 131
treatment
  endometriosis 87, 195–8
  endometrium: transcervical resection 296, 304
  intrauterine adhesions 339–42
  radiofrequency endometrial ablation (RaFEA) 368–9
  tubo-ovarian abscess 155–7

see also laparoscopic treatment
trocar 25–6
  sleeve 29–30, 35
  umbilical 24
trophoblast extraction 106
tubal wall 333, 334
tuboscope 278
tumours 130
  borderline ovarian 134
  with characteristic features 128–9
  Krukenberg 129
  microscopic 135
TUR *see* transurethral resection syndrome
two-dimensional (2–D) evaluation 210–11

ultrapulse 65
ultrasound 125–6
ultrastop 15
underwater resectoscope surgery 31, 37–8, 294–5
unipolar
  Corson needle 150, 151
  current 32
  diathermy 149
  Semm's forceps 150
United Kingdom 321–4
United States 113, 114, 319–24
ureter 217–18, 232, 233
  injury 176
ureterolysis 224–5
uterine
  artery 183
  bleeding
    abnormal 263–5
    dysfunctional 365
    excessive 310–11
    operative hysteroscopy 360
  cavity 287
    endometrium: transcervical resection 299–300
    fundus 319
    intrauterine adhesions 340, 341
    myomectomy 333, 334
    radiofrequency endometrial ablation 369
    submucosal fibroid 333–4
  distension system 318
  fibroids 75
  haemorrhage 302–3
  horn 374, 375, 376
  malignancy 304–5
  manipulators 29
  mobility, minimal 181
  mobilizer 235
  myoma 180
  nerve ablation 87, 159–67, 197
    Doyle's procedure 160–1
    nerve supply anatomy 159–60
    operative procedure 161–4
  perforation 301–2, 310, 373
  pressure 287

resectoscope 284
surgery 187–91
  Burch colposuspension 189–90
  laparoscopic appendicectomy 187–9
tubal ostia 345–6
vessels 217–18
wall 334–5
see also intrauterine
uterus
  fibromatous 335
  hysteroscope 278
  photodynamic therapy 391
  resectoscopic surgery 294–5
  retroverted 349
  see also uterine

vagina
  bleeding 315
  cuff 184
  guard 366, 368
  hysterectomy 179–86
  probe 29, 218
  transducer 126
  see also endovaginal; transvaginal
vaporization 161, 217
  versus coagulation 67, 68
vascular injury 175–6
vascularization 210–11
vasoconstrictive agents 311
Veress needle 21, 23, 24
vesicovaginal fistula 370
video 13
  camera 274–5
  documentation 273–5
  dual image 20
  equipment 30, 259–60
  hysteroscopy 261, 271, 272
  monitor 18, 275
  printing 275
  recorder 275
  standards 273
  systems 274
  videolaparoscopic ovarian cautery 151
voltage modulations 61

water tower 52
wave guides 43–5
waveform selection 312–14
Weck–Baggish hysteroscope 285, 287, 318

xenon chloride (XeCl) 383, 384

YAG laser ovarian drilling 151

Z-puncture technique 22, 24
zona pellucida 383, 384